04 Bn 0

Handbook of Experimental Pharmacology

Volume 167

Inhibitors of Protein Kinases and Protein Phosphates

Contributors
D.R. Alexander, H.S. Andersen, N.R. Banner, R. Battistutta, A.M. Berghuis, S.M. Blake, D. Bossemeyer, C. Breitenlechner, D. L. Burk, A. Cheng, P. Cohen, S.W. Cowan-Jakob, B.J. Druker, R. Engh, D. Fabbro, G. Fendrich, D.H. Fong, P. Furet, M. Gaßel, J.D. Griffin, V. Guez, S. Herrero, H. Hidaka, R.E. Honkanen, L.F. Iversen, C.B. Jeppesen, S. Kumar, C. Kunick, C. Lampron, D.S. Lawrence, M. Leost, O. Lozach, H. Lyster, P.W. Manley, L. Meijer, J. Mestan, T. Meyer, N.P.H. Møller, S. Sarno, Y. Sasaki, S. Schmitt, M. Shibuya, Y. Suzuki, M.L. Tremblay, N. Uetani, A. Wakeling, M.H. Yacoub, G. Zanotti

Editors
Lorenzo A. Pinna and Patricia T.W. Cohen

Springer

Professor
Lorenzo A. Pinna
Università di Padova
Dipartimento di Chimica Biologica
Via Trieste 75
Padova 35121
Italy
e-mail: lorenzo.pinna@unipd.it

Patricia T.W. Cohen, Ph.D.
Professor of Molecular Biology,
MRC Protein Phosphorylation Unit,
School of Life Sciences
University of Dundee
MSI/WTB Complex, Dow St.
Dundee, DD1 5EH
Scotland, U.K.
e-mail: p.t.w.cohen@dundee.ac.uk

With 95 Figures and 17 Tables

Library of Congress Control Number: 2004103428

ISSN 0171-2004

ISBN 3-540-21242-6 Springer Berlin Heidelberg New York

Springer-Verlag is a part of Springer Science+Business Media
springeronline.com

Printed in Germany

Editor: Dr. R. Lange, Heidelberg, Germany
Desk Editor: S. Dathe, Heidelberg, Germany
Production Editor: H. Schwaninger, Heidelberg, Germany
Cover design: design & production GmbH, Heidelberg, Germany
Typesetting: Stürtz GmbH, Würzburg, Germany

Printed on acid-free paper 27/3150 hs – 5 4 3 2 1 0

Preface

Nearly all aspects of cell life (and death) are controlled by the phosphorylation of proteins, which is catalysed by protein kinases (PKs) and reversed by protein phosphatases (PPs). The role of PKs can be likened to that of interpreters, who translate stimuli and signals into biochemical events. For this reason, PKs and PPs are themselves interlinked and highly regulated, forming complex communicative networks. Not surprisingly, therefore, the deregulation of PKs results in cell malfunction, eventually resulting in neoplastic growth and other diseases. This makes PKs attractive targets for drugs not only to combat cancer, but also for other global diseases, notably diabetes, inflammatory and infectious diseases, stroke, hypertension and Alzheimer's. Actually about half of all proto-oncogenes so far identified encode PKs, and oncogenesis frequently results from the activation and/or overexpression of PKs. For example, overexpression of the epidermal growth factor receptor tyrosine kinase is the cause of many cancers of epithelial cell origin. In other instances, however, the link of PKs with neoplasia is not so straightforward, and depends on defective interactions with cellular partners of PKs, susceptibility to particular metabolic conditions, abnormal levels of other regulatory components or the combination of several of these factors.

The attractiveness of PKs as targets is enhanced by the fact that they are enzymes, which are targetable molecules par excellence. Thus their biological activity can be turned off very easily and precisely by drugs that block the catalytic site. Virtually all PKs belong to the largest single family of enzymes, numbering over 500 and accounting for almost 2% of the proteins encoded by the human genome. They share similar catalytic domains that catalyse the transfer of phosphate from ATP to serine, threonine or tyrosine residues in key regulatory proteins. Nevertheless, the structures of the catalytic domains of PKs are sufficiently distinctive that it is possible to develop compounds that are highly selective for a particular PK. Even the highly conserved binding site for the substrate ATP is surrounded by structural elements with variable features that can be exploited for the design of specific inhibitors, and most of the PK inhibitors currently undergoing human clinical trials are of this type. Two PK inhibitors are already in clinical use for the treatment of cancers (Gleevec and Iressa), while another is the immunosuppressant of choice to prevent tissue rejection after organ transplantation (rapamycin). At least 30 other PK inhibitors are undergoing human clinical trials to treat cancers and other diseases. These have the potential to provide a significant impact on the management of epithelial cancers, such as breast and lung cancer. The approval of Gleevec for the treatment of a form of leukaemia by the FDA in May 2001 and more recently for the treatment of stomach cancers was a landmark because it is the first drug to be developed by targeting specific PKs. Moreover, its spectacular clinical effects, with minimal side effects, have had an enormous impact on the pharmaceutical and biotechnology industry. As a result, PKs have become the second most important family of drug targets, 20%–30% of all drug development programmes now being concentrated in this area. Although most PK inhibitors currently under investigation as potential drugs are ATP site-directed ligands, the field is still in its infancy, and there is tremendous potential to develop different types of drugs that target the binding sites for the protein substrates or which prevent the activation of PKs, since many of these enzymes are arranged in 'cascades' in which one PK activates or inhibits another one. Longer-term strategies would involve approaches based on gene therapy in which the mutant PK would be replaced by the wild-type enzyme.

PPs have received less attention to date as potential drug targets than PKs. The empirical discovery of an immunosuppressant drug that revolutionised organ transplantation (ciclosporin) and the subsequent recognition that it is a specific inhibitor of one PP indicates that PPs can be effective drug targets. An anticancer agent also discovered empirically (fostriecin) is now recognised to be a PP inhibitor. Other PPs, such as PTP1B, are currently under active investigations as drug targets for the treatment of diabetes and other diseases. As with PKs, known PP inhibitors at present target the active site but since many PPs are complexes with regulatory subunits, there is a potential for developing drugs that target the binding site of these regulatory subunits or their interaction with regulators. Thus the expansion of PPs as suitable drug targets may eventually follow that of PKs.

This volume of HEP highlights the tremendous pharmacological potential of PK and PP inhibitors, by providing a thorough overview of the most remarkable achievements in the field and illustrating how beneficial these studies can be for the advancement of both basic knowledge on biological regulation and deregulation and for the clinical treatment of a wide spectrum of diseases.

List of Contributors

(Addresses stated at the beginning of respective chapters)

Alexander, D.R. 263
Andersen, H.S. 215

Banner, N.R. 321
Battistutta, R. 125
Berghuis, A.M. 157
Blake, S.M. 65
Bossemeyer, D. 85
Breitenlechner, C. 85
Burk, D.L. 157

Cheng, A. 191
Cohen, P. 1
Cowan-Jacob, S.W. 361

Druker, B.J. 391

Engh, R. 85

Fabbro, D. 361
Fendrich, G. 361
Fong, D.H. 157
Furet, P. 361

Gaßel, M. 85
Griffin, J.D. 361
Guez, V. 361

Herrero, S. 85
Hidaka, H. 411
Honkanen, R.E. 295

Iversen, L.F. 215

Jeppesen, C.B. 215

Kumar, S. 65
Kunick, C. 47

Lampron, C. 191
Lawrence, D.S. 11
Leost, M. 47
Lozach, O. 47
Lyster, H. 321

Manley, P.W. 361
Meijer, L. 47
Mestan, J. 361
Meyer, T. 361
Møller, N.P.H. 215

Sarno, S. 125
Sasaki, Y. 411
Schmitt, S. 47
Shibuya, M. 411
Suzuki, Y. 411

Tremblay, M.L. 191

Uetani, N. 191

Wakeling, A.E. 433

Yacoub, M.H. 321

Zanotti, G. 125

List of Contents

HEP (2005) 167:1–7

Protein Kinase Inhibitors for the Treatment of Disease: The Promise and the Problems

P. Cohen

Medical Research Council Protein Phosphorylation Unit,
University of Dundee, MSI/WTB Complex, Dundee, Scotland, DD1 5EH, UK
p.cohen@dundee.ac.uk

1 The Promise

The reversible phosphorylation of proteins, catalysed by protein kinases and phosphatases, was first identified as a regulatory device in the 1950s, and it has been established for many years that this control mechanism regulates most aspects of cell life. However, it was only in the 1990s that interest in developing inhibitors of protein kinases and phosphatases started to enter centre stage (see Cohen 2002a,b for historical reviews). The first two drugs shown to target these classes of enzyme were cyclosporin, an inhibitor of protein phosphatase 2B (PP2B, also called calcineurin) (Liu et al. 1991) and rapamycin, an inhibitor of the protein kinase mTOR (mammalian target of rapamycin) (Heitman et al. 1991), which are the immunosuppressants that have permitted the widespread use of organ transplantation. However, these drugs were developed and approved for clinical use before their mechanism of action was identified. Fasudil, an isoquinoline sulphonamide that inhibits several protein kinases with relatively low potency, such as the Rho-dependent protein kinases (ROCK) (Davies et al. 2000), was developed by Hiroyoshi Hidaka in the 1980s and approved in Japan in 1995 for the treatment of cerebral vasospasm. ROCK can constrict blood vessels by inhibiting smooth muscle myosin phosphatase, but whether the clinical efficacy of fasudil results from its inhibition of ROCK, another protein kinase(s) or a completely different target, is unclear. Current information about this drug is discussed by Hidaka et al. (in Part 4).

Glivec (also called imatinib and STI-571), developed by Nick Lydon and his colleagues at Novartis, was the first drug to be developed by targeting a specific protein kinase and was approved for clinical use in the USA in 2001. It targets the protein tyrosine kinase c-Abl, which is mutated to the constitutively active BCR-Abl fusion protein in nearly all cases of chronic myelogenous leukaemia (CML). The spectacular efficacy and minimal side effects of Glivec, first highlighted by Brian Druker, resulted in the most rapid approval of a drug in FDA history and was a landmark event in this area. The development of Glivec and its implications for the future of drug discovery in this area are discussed by Fabbro et al. (in Part 4). Interestingly, Abl is not the only protein tyrosine kinase targeted by Glivec. It also inhibits the c-Kit receptor tyrosine kinase and the platelet-derived growth factor (PDGF) receptor. The c-Kit receptor is mutated to an abnormally active form in many gastrointestinal stromal tumours (GISTs) and the efficacy of Glivec for the treatment GISTs is equally impressive, resulting in its approval for this therapeutic use in 2002. The potential of Glivec to treat several types of cancer is discussed by Druker (in Part 4).

Following on from the successful launch of Glivec, Iressa a potent inhibitor of the epidermal growth factor (EGF) receptor tyrosine kinase was approved in Japan in 2002 and in the USA in 2003 for the treatment of some types of lung cancer. Developed by AstraZeneca, this drug is discussed by Wakeling (in Part 4). Drugs that inhibit the vascular endothelial-growth factor (VEGF) or fibroblast growth factor (FGF) receptor tyrosine kinases are undergoing phase III clinical trials and may be among the next protein kinase inhibitors to be approved for clinical use. VEGF and FGF play key roles in angiogenesis, and inhibitors of their receptors destroy the tumour's vascular supply. For this reason these compounds may be useful for the treatment of several types of cancer.

Compounds that inhibit protein serine/threonine kinases are also undergoing human clinical trials in a number of therapeutic areas. For example, at least four companies have inhibitors of p38 mitogen-activated protein (MAP) kinase in the clinic. These compounds suppress the production of tumour necrosis factor (TNF) and some other proinflammatory cytokines and show efficacy for the treatment of rheumatoid arthritis and other chronic inflammatory diseases. These programmes are discussed by Kumar and Blake (in Part 2). In the same section, Meijer (in Part 2) discusses inhibitors of cyclin-dependent protein kinases (CDKs), which are undergoing clinical trials as anti-cancer agents, and inhibitors of GSK3 which, although at the preclinical stage, have shown potential for the treatment of several diseases including type II diabetes (Cline et al. 2002; Ring et al. 2003) and stroke (Cross et al. 2001). Inhibitors of MAP kinase kinase 1 (MKK1, also called MEK) and RAF (product of the proto-oncogene *Raf*) are undergoing clinical trials as anti-cancer agents, and inhibitors of mixed lineage kinase 3 (MLK3) to prevent neurodegeneration (reviewed in Cohen 2002b). However, this is only the 'tip of the iceberg'. Over the past few years protein kinases have become the second most studied group of drug targets after G protein-coupled receptors, accounting for a quarter or more of drug discovery programmes worldwide. The number of protein kinase inhibitors undergoing human clinical trials at the present time almost certainly exceeds 100.

The discovery that PP2B, a serine/threonine-specific protein phosphatase, was inhibited specifically by cyclosporin highlighted the potential of protein phosphatases as drug targets, and programmes to develop specific inhibitors of several of these enzymes are underway. Protein tyrosine phosphatase IB (PTP1B) appears to be one of the enzymes that dephosphorylates and inactivates the insulin receptor, because mice that do not express it are hypersensitive to insulin and maintain normal blood glucose levels at half the normal circulating of insulin (Elchebly et al. 1999). In addition, these mice do not become obese when fed a high-fat, high-carbohydrate diet. For these reasons, PTPIB is potentially an attractive target for the development of a drug to treat diabetes and/or obesity, as discussed by Cheng et al. (in Part 3). However, although interesting compounds have been developed that are relatively specific inhibitors of PTP1B, as discussed by Møller (in Part 3), no inhibitors of this enzyme appear to have entered clinical trials. CD45 is another protein tyrosine phosphatase that is potentially an attractive drug target, because it is only expressed in cells of the immune system and is essential for T cell activation. Inhibitors of CD45 therefore have the potential to be effective immunosuppressants, but may lack the side effects associated with cyclosporin and rapamycin whose targets (PP2B and TOR) are expressed in nearly all cells and tissues. This topic is discussed by Alexander (in Part 3).

A number of toxins and tumour promoters are potent inhibitors of several members of one of the major classes of protein serine/threonine phosphatases, termed the PPP subfamily. They include the marine toxins responsible for diarrhetic seafood poisoning (okadaic acid and related compounds) and the algal toxins that are a threat to water supplies (microcystins) (reviewed in MacKintosh and MacKintosh 1994). Indeed, microcystins are the most potent liver carcinogens known to man. One might therefore predict that compounds which inhibit the catalytic subunits of these protein phosphatases would frequently be oncogenic and of little use as therapeutic agents. However, as discussed by Honkanen (Part 3), both fostriecin and cantharidin, which inhibit the same protein phosphatases, are cytotoxic for tumour cells and have been tested in phase I human clinical trials as anti-cancer agents. Not surprisingly, there are a number of side effects associated with the use of these compounds, and it seems more likely that drugs will eventually be developed that disrupt the functions of protein serine/threonine phosphatases in more subtle and specific ways. For example, the ability of the serine/threonine-specific protein phosphatase 1 (PP1) to dephosphorylate many proteins is controlled by its interaction with a great variety of 'targeting' subunits that direct it to specific subcellular locations and confer unique regulatory properties upon it. The form of PP1 associated with liver glycogen, which dephosphorylates and activates glycogen synthase, comprises the catalytic subunit of PP1 complexed to a glycogen-targeting subunit G_L. The ability of the PP1–G_L complex to dephosphorylate glycogen synthase is prevented when the active form of glycogen phosphorylase (termed phosphorylase a) binds to the extreme C-terminus of G_L, providing a mechanism for inhibiting glycogen synthesis when glycogenolysis is activated and vice versa (Armstrong et al. 1998). A drug that prevented the interaction of phosphorylase a with G_L would have the potential to lower the concentration of glucose in the blood by activating glycogen synthase and so stimulating the conversion of glucose into liver glycogen.

1.1 The Problems

There are over 500 protein kinases encoded by the human genome, most of which are members of the same superfamily. This has created a plethora of potential targets that can be studied in a unified way, but has highlighted the difficulty in developing compounds that are capable of inhibiting one of these enzymes specifically. The development of Glivec has shown that inhibition of more than one protein kinase can sometimes be beneficial, allowing the same drug to have more than one therapeutic use. However, more frequently one would expect such a lack of specificity to give rise to unwanted or unacceptable side effects. The recent availability of large panels of protein kinases (e.g. Davies et al. 2000; Bain et al. 2003) has been of considerable help in assessing the specificities of protein kinase inhibitors, and it is to be expected that such panels will continue to expand and eventually include the entire repertoire of protein kinases.

Lack of specificity may also mean that the therapeutic effect of a drug is actually mediated by inhibition of another protein kinase and not by inhibition of the kinase for which it was originally developed. For example, inhibitors of the cell cycle regulator CDK2 have been developed that suppress the proliferation of tumour cells, but these compounds may actually exert their therapeutic effects by inhibiting other protein kinases, such as CDK7 and/or CDK9, which are regulators of RNA polymerase II. It is therefore unclear whether the effects of these compounds are really mediated via CDK2. In order establish that the therapeutic effect of a drug is mediated by inhibition of a particular protein kinase one needs to show that the effects of the drug disappear in cells that express a drug-resistant mutant of the protein kinase (Eyers et al. 1999). It is possible to convert protein kinases to drug-resistant forms by single amino acid replacements (Brown et al. 1995; Eyers et al. 1998) so that, as for other types of drug, the development of drug resistance is a potential hazard. Mutations in Abl that make it resistant to Glivec are the cause of relapse in patients with chronic myelogenous leukaemia (Gorre et al. 2001). However, resistance to Glivec is mainly seen in patients with the most advanced stage of this disease, where extensive genomic instability has already taken place.

Most of the protein kinase inhibitors developed thus far target the ATP-binding site and must therefore be of sufficient potency to compete with the millimolar concentrations of ATP that are present in the intracellular milieu. Clearly, it is possible to develop compounds with the requisite in vivo potency, as shown by the number of compounds undergoing human clinical trials. However, this remains a challenging problem, especially for protein kinases that bind ATP particularly tightly. Some of the most interesting protein kinase inhibitors developed thus far, including Glivec (Schindler et al. 2000) and the p38 MAP kinase inhibitor BIRB 796 (Pargellis et al. 2002), not only target the ATP-binding site, but also trigger structural changes that induce the inactive conformations of these protein kinases. Two other compounds, PD 98059 and U0126, do not target the ATP-binding site at all, but bind to the inactive conformation of MKK1, preventing it from being activated by the protein kinase Raf (Alessi et al. 1995; Davies et al. 2000). The development of more compounds that prevent one protein kinase from activating another may be a promising strategy for novel drug development in this area, since many of these enzymes are components of protein kinase 'cascades'. Another way of generating compounds that are not ATP-competitive would be to target the binding sites for protein substrates, a topic discussed by Lawrence (in Part 1).

There are about 150 protein phosphatase catalytic subunits encoded by the human genome, and they fall into three main superfamilies. The generation of compounds that discriminate between different protein phosphatases is therefore also a challenging one. However, in contrast to protein kinases, the option of targeting an ATP binding pocket does not exist. Moreover, the protein substrate-binding cleft can be very polar, as in the case of PTP1B (Kellie 2003). This has made it difficult to develop compounds that combine high potency with cell permeability. The only protein phosphatase inhibitor that has advanced to human clinical trials, cyclosporin, inhibits PP2B in an unusual way; it binds to the protein cyclophilin, and the cyclosporin–cyclophilin complex then inhibits the protein phosphatase (Liu et al. 1991). As discussed earlier, it seems more likely that the future of drug discovery in this area may lie in targeting the regulatory subunits of serine/threonine-specific protein phosphatases.

Finally, it is important to mention that inhibitors of protein kinases are not only becoming important for the treatment of disease, but also as reagents for the study of cell signalling. The huge number of citations garnered by the publications that have introduced these compounds to the scientific community are a reflection of the widespread need for these compounds by the scientific community. For example, I was surprised to learn from the Institute for Scientific Information that the paper we published in 1995 with David Dudley and Alan Saltiel at Parke Davis on the mechanism of action of PD 98059 (Alessi et al. 1995) was the UK's most frequently cited original research paper over the past 10 years in the fields of biology and biochemistry, while our publication with Peter Young and John Lee at SmithKline Beecham on the specificity of SB 203580 (Cuenda et al. 1995), a prototypic p38 MAP kinase inhibitor, was the UK's sixth most cited original research paper over this period. Although many compounds are advertised for sale as 'specific protein kinase inhibitors', in practice many have turned out to inhibit so many protein kinases that conclusions drawn from their use are likely to be erroneous (Davies et al. 2000; Bain et al. 2003). The number of really useful protein kinase inhibitors that are available commercially is still rather limited, but the number will increase considerably over the next few years. I believe that pharmaceutical companies have much to gain from the discoveries that will be made by exploiting these compounds, and it is to be hoped that many more will be released for general use in the future.

References

Alessi DR, Cuenda A, Cohen P, Dudley DT, Saltiel AR (1995) PD98059 is a specific inhibitor of the activation of mitogen-activated protein kinase kinase in vitro and in vivo. J Biol Chem 270:27489–27494

Armstrong CG, Doherty MJ, Cohen PTW (1998) Identification of the separate domains in the hepatic glycogen-targeting subunit of protein phosphatase 1 that interact with phosphorylase a, glycogen and protein phosphatase 1. Biochem J 336:699–704

Bain J, McLauchlan H, Elliott M, Cohen P (2003) The specificities of protein kinase inhibitors: an update. Biochem J 371:199–204

Brown EJ, Beal PA, Keith CT, Chen J, Shin TB, Schreiber SL (1995) Control of p70S6 kinase by kinase activity of FRAP in vivo. Nature 377:441–446

Cline GW, Johnson K, Regittnig W, Perret P, Tozzo E, Xiao L, Damico C, Schulman GI (2002) Effects of a novel glycogen synthase kinase-3 inhibitor on insulin-stimulated glucose metabolism in Zucker diabetic fatty (fa/fa) rats. Diabetes 51:2903–2910

Cohen P (2002a) The origins of protein phosphorylation. Nat Cell Biol 4:E127–E130

Cohen P (2002b) Protein kinases—the major drug targets of the twenty-first century? Nat Rev Drug Discov 1:309–315

Cross DA, Culbert AA, Chalmers KA, Facci L, Skaper SD, Reith AD (2001) Selective small molecule inhibitors of glycogen synthase kinase-3 activity protect primary neurons from death. J Neurochem 77:94–102

Cuenda A, Rouse J, Doza YN, Meier R, Cohen P, Gallagher TF, Young PR, Lee JC (1995) SB 203580 is a specific inhibitor of a MAP kinase homologue which is stimulated by cellular stress and interleukin-1. FEBS Lett 364:229–233

Davies SP, Reddy H, Caivano M, Cohen P (2000) Specificity and mechanism of action of some commonly used protein kinase inhibitors. Biochem J 351:95–105

Elchebly M, Payette P, Michaliszyn E, Cromlish W, Collins S, Loy AL, Normandin D, Cheng A, Himms-Hagen J, Chan CC, Ramachandran C, Gresser MJ, Tremblay ML, Kennedy BP (1999) Increased insulin sensitivity and obesity resistance in mice lacking the protein tyrosine phosphatase 1B gene. Science 282:1544–1548

Eyers PA, Craxton M, Morrice N, Cohen P, Goedert M (1998) Conversion of SB-203580-insensitive MAP kinase family members to drug-sensitive forms by a single amino acid substitution. Chem Biol 5:321–328

Eyers PA, Van den Ijssel P, Quinlan R, Goedert M, Cohen P (1999) Use of a drug resistant mutant of stress activated protein kinase 2a/p38 to validate the in vivo specificity of SB203580. FEBS Lett 451: 191–196

Gorre ME, Mohammed M, Ellwood K, Hsu N, Pacquette R, Rao PN, Sawyers CL (2001) Clinical resistance of STI 571 cancer therapy caused by BCR-ABL gene mutation or amplification. Science 293:876–880

Heitman J, Mowa NR, Hall MN (1991) Targets for cell cycle arrest by the immunosuppressant rapamycin in yeast. Science 253:905–909

Kellie S (2003) Protein tyrosine phosphatases: potential roles in disease. In: Watling KJ (ed) Celltransmissions. Sigma-Aldrich, St Louis, pp 3–8

Liu J, Farmer JD, Lane WS, Friedman J, Weissman I, Schreiber SL (1991) Calcineurin is a common target of cyclophilin-cyclosporin A and FKBP-FK506 complexes. Cell 66:807–815

MacKintosh C, MacKintosh RW (1994) Inhibitors of protein kinases and phosphatases. Trends Biochem Sci 19:444–447

Pargellis C, Tong L, Churchill L, Cirillo PF, Gilmore T, Graham AG, Grob PM, Hickey ER, Moss N, Pav S, Regan J (2002) Inhibition of p38 MAP kinase by utilising a novel allosteric binding site. Nat Struct Biol 9:268–272

Ring DB, Johnson KW, Henriksen EJ, Nuss JM, Goff D, Kinnick TR, Ma ST, Reeder JW, Samuels I, Slabiak T, Wagman AS, Hammond M-EW, Harrison SD (2003) Selective glycogen synthase kinase 3 inhibitors potentiate insulin activation of glucose transport and utilisation in vitro and in vivo. Diabetes 52:588–595

Schindler T, Bornmann W, Pellicena P, Miller WT, Clarkson B, Kuriyan J (2000) Structural mechanism for STI 571 inhibition of Abelson tyrosine kinase. Science 289:1938–1942

Part I
General Aspects of PKs Inhibition

HEP (2005) 167:11–44

New Design Strategies for Ligands That Target Protein Kinase-Mediated Protein–Protein Interactions

D. S. Lawrence

Department of Biochemistry, The Albert Einstein College of Medicine,
1300 Morris Park Ave, Bronx, NY 10461, USA
lawrence@medusa.bioc.aecom.yu.edu

Abstract Protein–protein interactions serve as the molecular engine that drives the formation and disassembly of intracellular signaling pathways. Antagonists of these interactions could play key roles as both biological reagents and therapeutic compounds. However, much of the early work in this area with peptides revealed that these species, in general, bind with modest affinity to their protein targets. In addition, when these studies first commenced nearly 20 years ago, the technology for the intracellular delivery of peptides and modified analogs thereof was rudimentary. In the intervening years, not only has this technology dramatically improved, but the global role that protein–protein interactions play in transducing intracellular signals has become simply too obvious to ignore. With the introduction of combinatorial library methods, it is now a simple matter to identify consensus sequences recognized by protein interaction domains. An array of strategies has now been developed to transform these otherwise modest binding consensus sequences into high-affinity ligands. These strategies include the design of high-affinity replacements for key amino acid residues in consensus peptides, the construction of multidomain-binding peptides, and the structural modification of consensus sequence peptides. In several of these instances, unprecedented affinity (<nM) and selectivity (>1,000-fold versus closely related protein targets) have been achieved.

Keywords Signal transduction · Antagonists of protein–protein interactions · Peptide-based inhibitors · Protein kinases and phosphatases · Combinatorial libraries · Amino acid analogs · Bivalent inhibitors · Structurally modified peptides

1 Introduction

Protein–protein interactions serve as the adhesive that drives the assembly of signaling pathways. However, this adhesive is transient in nature. Once the cell has acknowledged the environmental stimulus, signaling pathways must rapidly disassemble to restore the cell to its resting state. At first glance, agents that selectively target key protein–protein interactions would appear to serve as ideal inhibitors of cell signaling as well as potential therapeutics. First, protein–protein interactions are typically exemplified by well-defined consensus sequences, which can often be reasonably selective for a given protein–protein pair. Consequently, the preparation of inhibitors of protein–protein interactions appears, at least on paper, to be reasonably straightforward since, the acquisition of preferred consensus sequences employs simple and well-defined methods. Second, the intracellular levels of protein–protein-binding partners rarely surpass low micromolar amounts, thereby rendering competition with endogenous substrates relatively unimportant. In spite of these apparent advantages, the overwhelming majority of reported protein kinase inhibitors target the ATP-binding site, a region common to all protein kinases, non-protein kinases, and many other ATP-binding proteins. Furthermore, the intracellular concentration of ATP (~1–10 mM) is much larger than its K_m (serine/threonine kinases ~1–10 μM; tyrosine kinases ~20–50 μM), which all but assures that the ATP-binding site will be saturated with ATP. The consequence of the latter is that inhibitors that target the ATP-binding site must be present at intracellular concentrations that significantly exceed their in vitro-determined K_i values. Finally, the acquisition of ATP analogs that specifically target individual protein kinases requires the initial screening of a large starting library of potential inhibitor candidates. This is then followed by a substantial synthetic effort that involves the preparation of secondary and tertiary libraries based on initially identified leads. The notion of disrupting signaling pathways via antagonists of protein–protein interactions has been unpopular for a number of reasons, including issues related to potency, intracellular stability and uptake, and general bioavailability (i.e., with respect to therapeutics). However, recent advances in various delivery technologies coupled with our increasing understanding of the widespread participation of protein-binding domains in signaling, has led to a renewed interest in the development of anti-signaling agents that disrupt intracellular protein–protein interactions.

Given the long-dormant state of this field, which is characterized by a recent reawakening, a broad overview of the general area of protein kinase-mediated protein–protein interactions and their corresponding antagonists is provided. This includes a summary of the methods employed to obtain consensus sequence information, a general synopsis of protein-binding domains, and finally a description of antagonists of protein–protein interactions as well as emerging strategies to acquire ever more potent and selective inhibitory agents.

2 Identification of Consensus Sequences

2.1 Degradation of Protein Ligands

Amino acid recognition sequences that drive protein–protein interactions were initially identified via partial digestion of one of the protein-binding partners. Fragments that were determined to retain binding potency were then sequenced. Further refinement of the amino acid recognition sequence could then be explored via the preparation of synthetic peptides. This strategy is best exemplified by the work described in the 1980s on the potent "heat-stable" inhibitor of the cyclic adenosine monophosphate (cAMP)-dependent protein kinase (PKA) known as PKI (protein kinase inhibitor). Krebs, Walsh, and their colleagues (Scott et al. 1985a,b; Cheng et al. 1986; Scott et al. 1986; Van Patten et al. 1986; Glass et al. 1989) identified a series of peptides that serve as extraordinarily potent inhibitors (K_i<50 nM) of PKA. Protease digestion of the isolated protein furnished a 20-mer peptide that acts as a competitive inhibitor versus peptide substrate with a K_i in the subnanomolar range. These investigators demonstrated that the sequence Gly-Arg-Thr-Gly-Arg-Arg-Asn-<u>Ala</u>-Ile is the active site-directed component of PKI, where the <u>Ala</u> residue is positioned at the site normally reserved for the phosphorylatable serine. Indeed, subsequent studies demonstrated that insertion of serine in active site-directed sequences derived from PKI generates powerful peptide substrates (Mitchell et al. 1995). However, the new library-based methods introduced in the 1990s have largely supplanted the biochemical approaches for identifying amino acid sequences recognized by protein interaction domains. The new methodologies are not only significantly less labor intensive than their classical counterparts, but are also able to bypass the need for large quantities of both binding partners (for digestion and sequencing purposes).

2.2 Synthetic Peptide Libraries

A large number of different library strategies using synthetic peptides have been described. These approaches include one-bead/one-peptide libraries (Wu et al. 1994), solution mixtures of peptides (Songyang et al. 1994), one-well/one-peptide strategies (Lee and Lawrence 1999), peptides on chips (Houseman et al. 2002), and even proteins on chips (Zhu et al. 2000). A detailed description of the vast array of peptide library strategies now available is well beyond the scope of this review. However, all of these methods offer a rapid means to quickly identify preferred amino acid sequences in what is typically a single experiment. Peptide-based libraries also permit the use of amino acid derivatives beyond the standard genetically encoded residues (e.g., post-translationally modified residues such as phosphoTyr, hydroxyPro, etc.). In addition, many of the methods not only identify a preferred consensus sequence, but also often furnish an assessment of the range of residues permitted at a given position on the peptide ligand.

Each of the peptide library strategies enjoys certain advantages while enduring specific disadvantages:

1. One-bead/one-peptide libraries are extremely easy to prepare via split-and-pool synthesis (Lam et al. 2003). However, these libraries are commonly composed of a mixture of millions of beads, with each bead possessing a unique peptide sequence. Consequently, a screening method must be devised so that the bead containing the tightest binding ligand can be readily identified. Possibilities include the use of a target protein that contains an appended fluorophore or is conjugated to an enzymatic reporter. Beads can also be identified via the introduction of radioactivity (i.e., the use of [γ-^{32}P]ATP). Once leads have been identified, the beads are isolated and the bound peptides identified by microsequencing. Given the heavy reliance upon the latter, the use of uncommon hypermodified residues is severely restricted.
2. Soluble peptide library mixtures have also been utilized to identify consensus sequences (Songyang and Cantley 1998). These libraries are prepared by treating the growing peptide chain with a mixture of the standard amino acid derivatives. The actual ratio of the amino acids introduced during the coupling reaction is based upon the relative coupling efficiencies of the individual residues. Consequently, a particular residue that couples sluggishly (e.g., Arg) is present at a greater relative ratio than one that couples readily (e.g., Gly). Following completion of the synthesis, the peptide mixture is cleaved from the resin and subsequently employed for consensus sequence identification. The latter is achieved by selective enrichment of the binding sequence, often using an affinity column. For example, protein kinase-catalyzed phosphorylation of the mixture is allowed to proceed until a small fraction (<1%) of the total peptide is phosphorylated. The phosphopeptide

mixture is subsequently isolated and sequenced as a mixture. Each position on the peptide is not identified as a single residue, but rather as the relative abundance of all the amino acid residues at a particular site. The residue present in the largest amount at a given position is taken as the one most favored at that site. However, since a peptide mixture, as opposed to a single peptide, is sequenced, this strategy does not yield sequences of unique peptides but merely determines the preferences for particular residues at specific positions. An inherent assumption of this method is that selection at each position is independent of the adjacent amino acids. Consequently, this technique ignores the possibility that two or more residues can act in a synergistic fashion to promote target protein affinity.

3. The one-well/one-peptide approach ("parallel synthesis") (Granier 2002) employs pure peptides that are spatially segregated from one another (Lee and Lawrence 1999). This technique has the advantage that the sequence of each peptide in each well is verified in advance. Furthermore, a wide assortment of hypermodified amino acid residues can be employed, since the synthesis history of each peptide in each well in known. An obvious disadvantage is that the size of these libraries, by necessity, is much smaller than those described in points *1* and *2* above. Variations that employ spatially segregated mixtures ("positional scanning") have been reported that address this concern (Houghten et al. 1996).
4. Peptide chips represent the solid phase version of the method described in *3* (Houseman et al. 2002). The added advantage of this system is the higher spatial density, and therefore smaller chip size [membranes have been employed in this technique as well (Frank 2002)]. However, the increased spatial density of the individual peptide "colonies" can come at a cost. Although methods that employ fluorescence detection of target protein binding will work well in this system, other common methods, such as those that utilize radioactivity, cannot be applied to ultra high-density chips.

2.3 Phage Display

Phage display is a genetically encoded peptide library strategy (Scott and Smith 1990; Smith and Scott 1993). In brief, peptides are displayed on the capsid protein of filamentous phage. Each virion particle displays a unique peptide sequence on its surface. Millions of phage clones are exposed to the protein target of interest and the affinity purified particles then amplified in *Escherichia coli*. Subsequent rounds of selection furnish a few "lead" clones, from which the displayed sequences can be determined via sequencing of the viral DNA coding region. Phage display has been used to acquire peptide ligand sequences for a wide variety of protein interaction domains (Smothers et al. 2002). The obvious limitation here is that the genetic basis for this method restricts the range of amino acids to the 20 standard residues.

3
The Protein-Binding Domains of Protein Kinases

Protein kinases are, first and foremost, catalysts that promote the transfer of a phosphoryl group from ATP to the acceptor hydroxyl moiety of serine, threonine, and/or tyrosine. The serine, threonine, and tyrosine residues must be embedded within the proper amino acid sequence in order to be recognized by a given protein kinase, a fact exemplified by the large number of synthetic peptide-based substrates that have been devised for scores of protein kinases. Of all the protein-binding domains contained within protein kinases, the active site region displays the greatest diversity in terms of sequence recognition. However, since all members of the protein kinase family utilize the same phosphoryl donor (ATP) and acceptors (serine, threonine, tyrosine), it is perhaps not too surprising that the conformation of the active site region is remarkably well-conserved (Johnson et al. 1998; Huse and Kuriyan 2002). The "protein kinase fold" is composed of two separate lobes, commonly designated as the N- and C-terminal lobes. The former is the smaller of the two and is composed of five antiparallel β-strands and a single α-helix. The larger C-terminal lobe is primarily α-helical in structure. ATP resides in a cleft that lies at the interface between the N- and C-terminal lobes. By contrast, the peptide/protein phosphoryl acceptor is primarily associated with the C-terminal lobe. The catalytic domain of protein kinases can assume active and inactive conformational states. The lobes in the former migrate toward one another, thereby closing the active site and promoting catalysis.

Protein kinases are commonly differentiated on the basis of their preferred phosphoryl acceptor group on the protein substrate: either the aliphatic hydroxyl moieties of serine and threonine ("serine/threonine protein kinases") or the aromatic phenol of the tyrosine residue ("tyrosine protein kinases"). A few protein kinases display the property of "dual specificity" in terms of their ability to recognize and phosphorylate both aliphatic and aromatic alcohols on peptides or proteins in vitro (fewer still display this property in living cells) (Dhanasekaran and Premkumar Reddy 1998; Marin et al. 1999). However, in a very strict sense, the segregation of protein kinases into these separate camps most likely has less to do with the protein kinases themselves and more to do with the fact that the genetic code is limited to only 20 different amino acids. For example, PKA, a well-known serine/threonine-specific protein kinase, phosphorylates appropriately designed aromatic alcohols (e.g., **1**–**3**) (Lee et al. 1994).

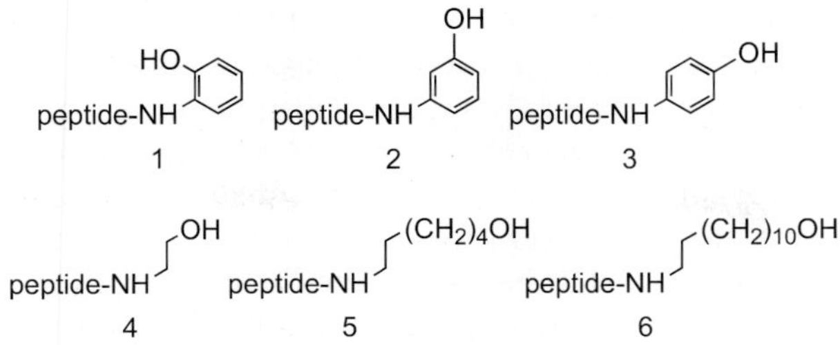

Furthermore, Src, an equally well-established tyrosine-specific protein kinase, phosphorylates aliphatic alcohols (e.g., **4–6**) (Lee et al. 1995a,b). Obviously, from the biological point of view, compounds **1–6** are mere curiosities. However, in terms of designing sensors, substrates, and antagonists of protein kinase-mediated protein–protein interactions, derivatives **1–6** are an important reminder that, unlike cells, chemists are not limited to the standard 20 amino acids fixed by the genetic code. Indeed, early work with consensus sequence peptides *containing conventional amino acids* is, in large part, responsible for the prevailing notion that inhibiting signaling pathways via disruption of protein–protein interactions is a strategy doomed to failure.

In addition to the "active site specificity" (i.e., serine/threonine versus tyrosine) of protein kinases, these enzymes display a preference for the amino acid sequence that encompasses the phosphorylatable residue (the "sequence specificity"). Compilations of sequences phosphorylated by protein kinases are available and these will not be recapitulated here (Pinna and Ruzzene 1996). However, certain trends are apparent:

1. The overwhelming majority of protein kinases will also phosphorylate simple peptides, thereby rendering the in vitro assay of these enzymes fairly straightforward. In addition, this demonstrates that the protein-binding region of these enzymes is sufficiently structurally well established to recognize substrates on its own (i.e., large intact protein substrates are not required for the protein kinase to assume an active state). However, the notion that the protein-binding region is the only site on the protein kinase that is responsible for substrate specificity is decidedly untrue.
2. Absolute protein kinase specificity is not encoded within the substrate-binding site. In other words, the consensus sequence surrounding the phosphorylatable residue, although an important parameter of protein kinase recognition, is not the sole determinant of specificity. For example, the cyclic guanosine monophosphate (cGMP)-dependent protein kinase (PKG) and PKA, members of the same protein kinase subfamily, display largely overlapping specificities with respect to simple peptide substrates (Mitchell et al. 1995; Wood et al. 1996). Certain protein kinase C (PKC) isoforms likewise phosphorylate the same peptides as PKA and PKG; however, the sequence preference of PKC is broad enough that PKC peptide substrates have

been devised that are recognized by neither PKA nor PKG (Yan et al. 2000). In short, it is unlikely that a peptide composed of only conventional amino acids will serve as an absolutely specific substrate for any given protein kinase. Indeed, Cohen and his colleagues have used this notion to generate a small set of peptides that serve as general substrates for more than three dozen different protein kinases (Ross et al. 2002).

3. Consensus sequence-containing active site-directed peptides are generally poor inhibitors. This fact is responsible for much of the common belief that targeting the substrate recognition site in particular, and protein–protein interactions in general, is an untenable strategy. Perhaps the best-known example is kemptide, Leu-Arg-Arg-Ala-Ser-Leu-Gly, which serves as an excellent substrate for PKA. The K_m for this peptide is less than 20 μM, a value that was (incorrectly) taken as a reflection of the binding constant of the peptide. However, the corresponding nonphosphorylatable peptide, Leu-Arg-Arg-Ala-Ala-Leu-Gly, is an exceedingly poor PKA inhibitor (K_i=320 μM) (Whitehouse et al. 1983). Much of the early discussion concerning the ineffectiveness of the Ala-substituted peptide centered on the possibility that the serine hydroxyl group (missing in the inhibitor) promotes binding affinity by two orders of magnitude. However, subsequent detailed enzymological studies revealed that the K_m value is a complex parameter that is dependent upon more than just the microscopic rate constants that control the active site association and dissociation of peptide substrate (Adams and Taylor 1992). In an analogous vein, poor inhibitors of tyrosine kinases (in which the phosphorylatable tyrosine residue was replaced with a phenylalanine) have been noted. Nevertheless, a few exceptions to the "rule" that active site-directed peptides serve as poor inhibitors are known. A naturally occurring "heat stable" protein-based inhibitor (PKI) of PKA is a powerful inhibitor (K_i<1 nM) (Whitehouse and Walsh 1983). A peptide fragment of PKI, most notably Gly-Arg-Thr-Gly-Arg-Arg-Asn-Ala-Leu-Gly-amide (where the Ala represents the site that would be reserved for serine) was reported to have a K_i of 36 nM (Glass et al. 1989). As an aside, the K_i for this peptide was originally determined under conditions of low salt; when the inhibitory potency of this peptide was subsequently reexamined several years later under more physiologically conditions, the K_i was found to be 500 nM (Wood et al. 1998). Nevertheless, the latter value does suggest that it is feasible to devise reasonably potent inhibitors based on standard amino acid residues alone. Indeed, perhaps the most outstanding example of this is the extraordinarily potent 24 amino acid-containing PKG selective inhibitor Arg-Gln-Ile-Lys-Ile-Trp-Phe-Gln-Asn-Arg-Arg-Met-Lys-Typ-Lys-Lys-Leu-Arg-Lys-Lys-Lys-Lys-Lys-His (Dostmann et al. 2000). This peptide is likely engaged in interactions beyond the immediate vicinity of the active site. Indeed, there appears to be a general consensus of opinion that, unlike targeting the ATP-binding site, effective inhibitors of protein–protein interactions must coordinate to a relatively large surface area.

In addition to the active site, there are several other protein interaction domains that are commonly affixed to protein kinases. These include the SH2 and SH3 domains, which are prevalent among the tyrosine protein kinases. PDZ, LIM, WW, PTB, and others are found in many protein kinases and/or in the adaptor proteins that help to transduce the activity of these enzymes. In addition, protein kinases themselves serve as ligands for protein interaction domains present on anchoring proteins. Indeed, peptide-derived inhibitors that bind to these anchoring proteins and thereby block protein kinase docking, have been described (Csukai and Mochly-Rosen 1999). The primary focus of this chapter is on the acquisition of active site-directed peptide-based inhibitors and the emerging strategies to acquire ever more potent and selective agents.

4 Strategies for the Acquisition of Potent and Selective Peptide-Based Inhibitors of Protein Kinases

Although a few exceptions are known, in general, conventional peptides display modest affinities and poor selectivities for the protein interaction domains contained within protein kinases. Biological systems appear to have little need for high-affinity ligands for active sites, SH2, SH3, LIM, PDZ, and other protein-interaction domains due to the transient nature of signaling pathways. However, it is abundantly clear that biological systems have mastered the issue of selectivity. Selective expression of only certain protein kinases in specific cell types, or at precise intervals during the lifetime of the cell, offers one means to navigate the tricky waters of intracellular selectivity. Spatial segregation of protein kinases to specific intracellular sites represents another means by which selectivity can be achieved. Finally, given the comparatively large size of these proteins, and their correspondingly well-defined structures, selectivity may simply be attained via a highly precise three-dimensional choreography of interactions between binding partners. Consequently, the design of potent and selective artificial antagonists of protein–protein interactions represents a significant challenge, albeit an exciting one. The primary advantage enjoyed by the chemist is that he or she is not restricted to the 20 standard amino acids designated by the genetic code.

The acquisition of agents that target protein–protein interaction sites has the potential to be relatively straightforward. Consensus sequences are easy to identify. However, it is necessary to develop the tools and/or strategies that can convert peptides containing these sequences into agents that recapitulate the high selectivities observed in biochemical pathways while significantly surpassing the affinities that intracellular binding partners display for one another. The tools and strategies to achieve the twin goals of potency and selectivity, within the framework of relatively small ligands (cf., proteins), are outlined below in three separate, but interrelated sections.

4.1 Mimetics of Key Residues in Consensus Sequence Peptides

4.1.1 Serine Analogs

As noted above, one of the first indications that the acquisition of effective peptide-based inhibitors for protein kinases might be problematic was the replacement of the phosphorylatable serine residue in the PKA substrate kemptide with an alanine to create a dead-end inhibitor. The latter proved to be an unexpectedly weak inhibitory agent (K_i>300 μM versus the K_m for kemptide <20 μM). One of the explanations offered for the low affinity, namely loss of the hydroxyl serine side chain as a potential hydrogen bond donor, was subsequently shown to be incorrect. However, this notion does suggest that there may be ways to improve upon the use of alanine as a non-phosphorylatable replacement for serine.

Coward and his colleagues were the first to suggest that the phosphorylatable residue in an active site-directed peptide could be substituted with an analog that is able to also engage the ATP-binding site (i.e., a bisubstrate inhibitor) (Lashmet et al. 1983).

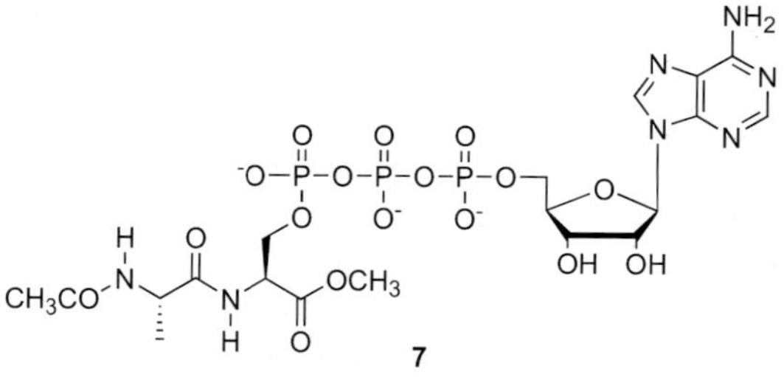

7

Although the ATP-γ-Ala-Ser ester 7 does not possess the requisite peptide framework for it to serve as a protein kinase inhibitor, it is a model of the type of compounds that were eventually prepared more than a decade later.

Gibson and his colleagues were the first to report the synthesis of adenosine phosphopeptides in a solid phase format (Medzihradszky et al. 1994).

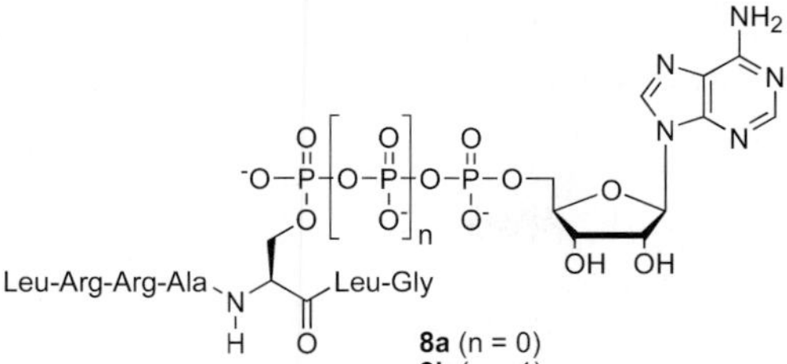

8a (n = 0)
8b (n = 1)
8c (n = 2)

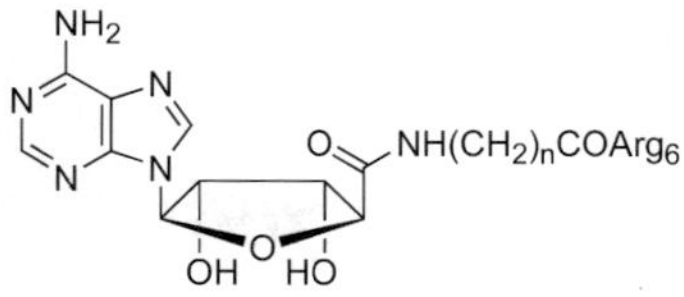

9

These investigators described the preparation and characterization of several analogs (**8**) of kemptide. Although the IC_{50} values of **8a**, **8b**, and **8c** (935 μM, 226 μM, and 68 μM, respectively) are modest, these inhibitors are significantly more effective than the simple Ala-containing analog Leu-Arg-Arg-Ala-Ala-Leu-Glu. The authors found that **8** displays a competitive inhibition pattern versus variable ATP, but such a pattern was not observed with respect to variable peptide substrate. One might expect that a bisubstrate analog would exhibit competitive patterns versus both ATP and phosphorylatable peptide. However, the absence of double competitive behavior does not necessarily rule out the two-site binding model. Strictly speaking, competitive behavior is observed for an inhibitor only if that inhibitor and the corresponding substrate bind in a mutually exclusive fashion to the *same enzyme form*. PKA is known to exhibit a primarily ordered mechanism with ATP binding first (Whitehouse et al. 1983). Consequently, one would expect compound **8** and ATP to associate with the same enzyme form, namely the free enzyme, and thereby exhibit competitive behavior. By contrast, given the nature of the ordered mechanism, peptide substrate preferentially coordinates to the enzyme–ATP complex, which would thereby rule out a competitive pattern with **8**.

Recently Uri and his colleagues have described a series of bisubstrate analogs that dispenses with the phosphoric anhydride portion of the ATP moiety (Loog et al. 1999). These investigators employed an adenosine-5′-carboxylic acid derivative as the ATP mimic which, using a variety of linkers, was appended to the N-terminus of an arginine rich peptide (**9**). The most effective analogs displayed IC_{50} values of between 100 and 300 nM for PKA and PKC. These bisubstrate analogs have been used to affinity-purify protein kinases (Loog et al. 2000). In addition, membrane-permeable fluorophore-labeled bisubstrate derivatives have been prepared (Uri et al. 2002; Viht et al. 2003).

In a departure from the ATP-based bisubstrate strategy, Sergheraert and colleagues designed (ATP mimics)-linker-substrate analogs (Ricouart et al. 1991). Isoquinoline and naphthalene sulfonic acid derivatives served as ATP replacements. The most potent of the several derivatives prepared was compound **10**.

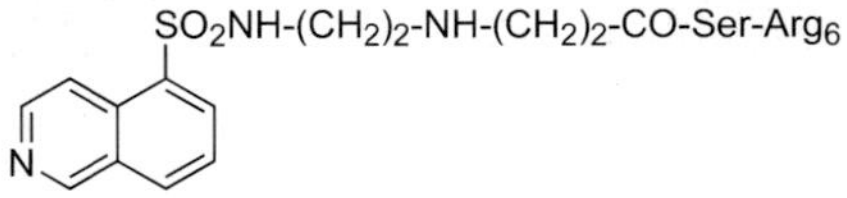

10

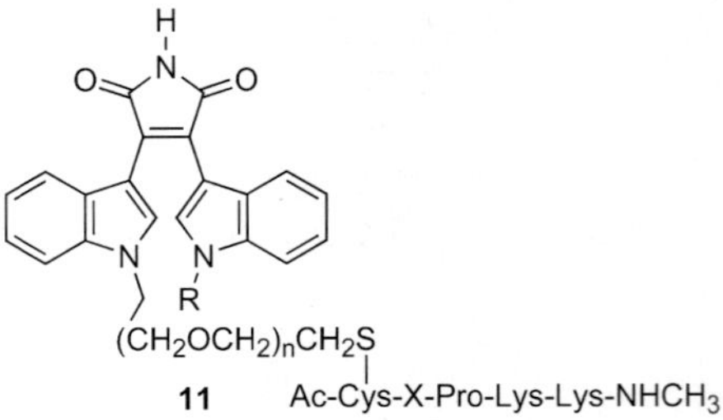

11

The latter exhibits a 25-fold selectivity in favor of PKA (K_i=4 nM) versus PKC (K_i=100 nM). The inhibitory potency of this derivative is impressive when one considers the fact that the ATP mimic alone is a nearly three orders of magnitude poorer inhibitor than **10**. However, since the ATP analog is appended off the N-terminus of the peptide, an unanswered question is the nature of the requisite structural requirements to replace a serine moiety that is contained within the interior of a consensus sequence. Finally, **10** acts as a competitive inhibitor versus variable ATP, but is not competitive with respect to variable peptide substrate. Sasaki, Maeda, and their coworkers likewise utilized an ATP analog (a bisindolylmaleimide) to prepare a series of bisubstrate inhibitors **11** that are designed to target the cyclin-dependent protein kinase, cdc2 (Sasaki et al. 1998). The best inhibitors display IC_{50} values in the low micromolar range (where X=no amino acid). However, when X=Ser, the inhibitory potency is reduced by two orders of magnitude.

4.1.2
Tyrosine Analogs

In an analogous vein to serine/threonine protein kinases, peptide-based inhibitors of tyrosine kinases were initially prepared by substituting the phosphorylatable tyrosine with the nonphosphorylatable phenylalanine. In general, the phenylalanine-for-tyrosine replacement generates exceedingly poor inhibitory agents (K_i>1 mM).

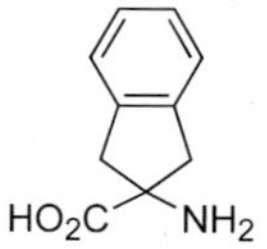

12

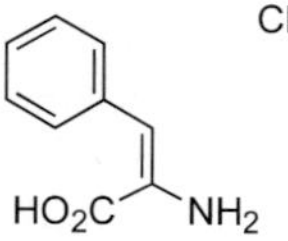

13

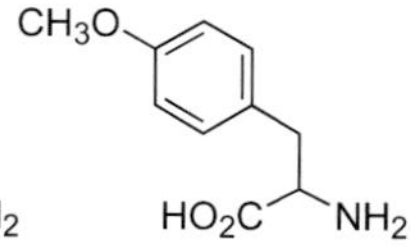

14

Several peptides containing tyrosine analogs (**12**–**14**) were reported in the 1980s, but these derivatives proved to be ineffective as inhibitors (Wong and Goldberg 1984; Shoelson et al. 1989).

Graves and his colleagues described the first example of an effective peptide-based tyrosine kinase inhibitor (Yuan et al. 1990).

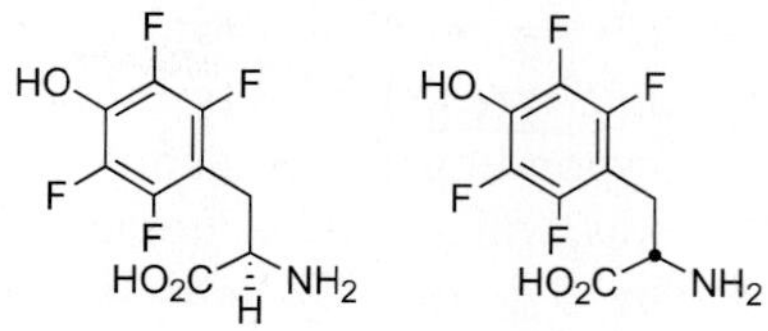

15 **16**

The inhibitory agent, which contains the tetrafluorotyrosine moiety **15**, targets the insulin receptor with a K_i of 4 μM. The rationale for the use of the fluorinated tyrosine analog was based on the presumed mechanism of catalysis. These investigators reasoned that an active site base partially removes the aromatic hydroxyl proton during the transition state of the enzyme-catalyzed phosphoryl transfer reaction from ATP to the acceptor phenol. Presumably, the enzyme stabilizes this partial-negative charge on the phenol/phenoxide during the transition state, which suggests that a tyrosine analog that is negatively charged might be well accommodated within the active site. The four fluorine substituents not only lower the pK_a of the phenol, thereby promoting ionization to the phenoxide at physiological pH, but in addition they render the phenoxide less nucleophilic than its natural counterpart. These investigators also prepared the corresponding d-analog **16**, which also displays promising inhibitory activity (K_i=20 μM). Interestingly, although both **15** and **16** serve as competitive inhibitors versus variable peptide substrate, the l-analog directly competes with ATP as well, whereas the d-derivative does not.

Subsequent work by Fry and his colleagues at Parke-Davis confirmed the usefulness of the tetrafluorotyrosine moiety as a nonphosphorylatable analog, in this case for peptides that target the epidermal growth factor receptor (EGFR) (Fry et al. 1994). The phenylalanine-containing "parent" peptide acetyl-Leu-Ala-Glu-Glu-Ser-Ala-Phe-Glu-Glu displays a K_i of 150 μM, whereas the corresponding l- and d-tetrafluorotyrosine-containing derivatives exhibit relative inhibitory enhancements of threefold and eightfold, respectively. The Parke-Davis group also prepared peptides that contained other l-tyrosine analogs, including 3-fluorotyrosine, 3-iodotyrosine, and d-tyrosine, but all of these derivatives were ineffective EGFR inhibitors. Curiously, 3-iodotyrosine was subsequently found to serve as an excellent tyrosine replacement in a cyclic peptide targeting Src (Alfaro-Lopez et al. 1998).

Walsh, Cole, and their colleagues also examined the use of tetrafluorotyrosine as a tyrosine replacement in a C-terminal Src kinase (CSK)-targeted peptide (Cole et al. 1995; Kim and Cole 1998). However, in this case, the peptide serves as a substrate, rather than as an inhibitor, for CSK. These results suggest that the applicability of tetrafluorotyrosine as a nonphosphorylatable tyrosine replacement is kinase-dependent.

Lam and his collaborators have prepared a series of active site-directed peptides that target the Src tyrosine protein kinase (Lou et al. 1997). These investigators employed both d- and l-napthylalanine (Nal) derivatives in place of the phosphorylatable tyrosine moiety in the sequence Gly-Ile-Tyr-Trp-His-His-Tyr. The corresponding phenylalanine derivative was not prepared; however, the d-Tyr was, which gives a measure of the inherent affinity of the peptide for Src. The IC_{50} for Gly-Ile-d-Tyr-Trp-His-His is 50 μM, which indicates that the peptide framework is, comparatively speaking, a remarkably effective peptide-based inhibitor. The corresponding Gly-Ile-Nal-Trp-His-His derivative exhibits only a twofold improvement in IC_{50} relative the d-Tyr analog. However, the doubly substituted Gly-Ile-Nal-Trp-His-His-Nal exhibits an IC_{50} of 4 μM, suggesting that the C-terminal Nal is able to access sites outside of the immediate active site region. Interestingly, one of the less effective inhibitors Gly-Ile-Nal-Trp-His-His-Tyr (IC_{50}=27 μM) proved to be remarkably selective for Src versus other closely related members of the Src kinase family (Lyn and Lck; IC_{50}>1 mM).

One of the difficulties associated with the acquisition of nonphosphorylatable tyrosine surrogates is their synthesis, which typically resorts to the use of achiral starting material. Following a resolution step, the analogs must then be appropriately protected for use in solid phase peptide synthesis. Some of these difficulties have been circumvented by Kim and Cole, who employed the enzyme tyrosine phenol lyase to prepare gram quantities of an assortment of fluorinated tyrosine analogs (Kim and Cole 1998). The Lawrence group has developed a library-driven strategy, which allows one to prepare and subsequently screen a wide assortment of commercially available aryl-containing amines as peptide-based nonphosphorylatable tyrosine analogs (Niu and Lawrence 1997a,b). In spite of the fact that these are peptide derivatives, issues related to synthesis, resolution, and protection of these tyrosine substitutes are all bypassed.

Although the most common protein kinase peptide substrates possess a phosphorylatable residue embedded within the interior of the peptide, protein kinases will also phosphorylate peptides containing tyrosine, serine, and threonine moieties appended off the N- or C-terminus of these substrates. For example, Src catalyzes the phosphorylation of Arg-Arg-Arg-Arg-Arg-Leu-Glu-Glu-Leu-Leu-Tyr-amide (the arginine residues are present for assay purposes, not enzyme recognition). C- and N-terminal residues can be readily appended onto the active site-directed peptide after solid phase peptide synthesis. This allows one to employ potential tyrosine analogs that are not protected, possess functionality that might not survive the harsh conditions of peptide synthesis, and even lack the standard α-stereocenter. The synthetic strategy utilizes a solid phase peptide synthesis support (Kaiser's oxime resin) that allows the tyrosine analog to be attached to the synthesized peptide in a fashion that simultaneously promotes cleavage from the resin (Kaiser et al. 1989). For example, a wide assortment of phenylethylamine derivatives was attached to the C-terminus of a Src active site-directed peptide (Niu and Lawrence 1997a,b).

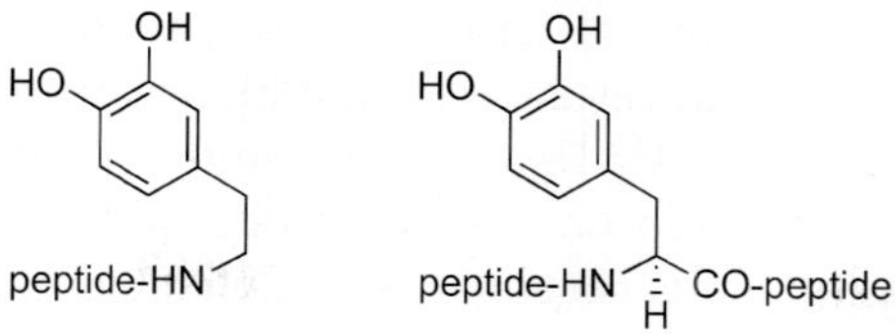

17 18

These were screened for inhibitory potency, and the lead analog was identified as the dopamine derivative **17** (which, in spite of a *p*-substituted aromatic alcohol, does not serve as a substrate). A peptide containing the amino acid analog of dopamine, l-dopa (**18**), was subsequently synthesized and shown to display an inhibitory potency (K=16 μM) that exceeds the parent phenylalanine-containing peptide by 60-fold.

Cole and his colleagues have reported a high-affinity bisubstrate analog for the insulin receptor protein kinase (IRK) (Parang et al. 2001).

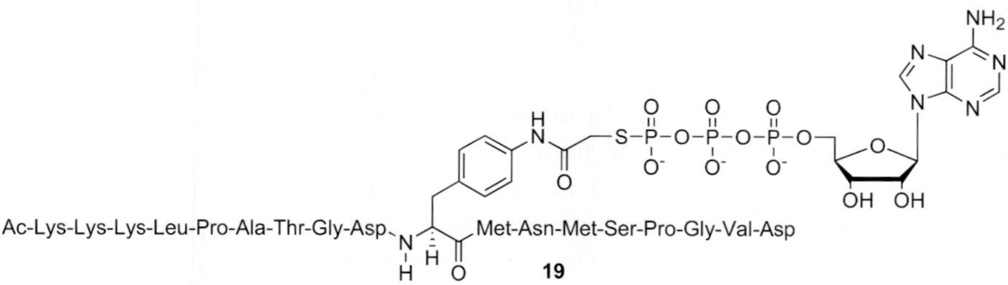

19

Compound **19** was designed based upon a dissociative mechanism for phosphoryl transfer in the IRK active site. The authors reasoned that the approximately 5 Å that separates the aromatic amine nitrogen from the γ-thiophosphate phosphorous roughly recapitulates the distance between acceptor and donor in a metaphosphate-like dissociative mechanism. Unlike the bisubstrate analogs reported to date for the serine/threonine-protein kinases, compound **19** serves as a competitive inhibitor versus both variable ATP and peptide substrate. The K_i of **19** is 370 nM, which corresponds to a binding energy that is roughly equal to the sum of the ATP- and protein-binding site portions of the inhibitor. As one might expect for an inhibitor that contains a peptide sequence targeting IRK, compound **19** is ineffective versus CSK (K_i~40 μM). These investigators also obtained the crystal structure of the inhibitor bound to the tyrosine kinase domain of IRK. The latter confirmed that the inhibitor is bound in a bisubstrate-like mode with the expected distance between the anilino nitrogen and the γ-phosphorous. In addition, the anilino nitrogen is engaged in a hydrogen bond to a key active site Asp residue.

Budde, McMurray, and their collaborators reported an N-myristoylated peptide, myr-Glu-Phe-Leu-Tyr-Gly-Val-Phe-Asp-amide, that serves as an apparent bisubstrate analog for Src (Ramdas et al. 1999). Surprisingly, the corresponding peptide with a free N-terminus is a Src substrate. However, upon acylation the substrate is converted into an inhibitor with the caveat that the acyl group must be lauryl ($C_{11}H_{23}CO$-) or longer. Clearly, the unexpected structure/activity relationship of this inhibitory species places it in an unusual category in that there is no obvious consolidated nonphosphorylatable tyrosine mimetic present in the peptide framework. Nonetheless, the fatty acyl-peptide serves as a competitive inhibitor with respect to both variable ATP and peptide substrate (poly Glu_4Tyr), thereby rendering it, like compound **19**, a bisubstrate analog. The nonacylated peptide itself blocks phosphorylation of poly Glu_4Tyr with a K_i of 260 μM via a competitive pattern. Myristic acid also serves as an inhibitor of the Src-catalyzed phosphorylation of poly Glu_4Tyr, but in this instance the fatty acid competes with ATP (K_i=35 μM).

The conjoined myr-Glu-Phe-Leu-Tyr-Gly-Val-Phe-Asp-amide exhibits bisubstrate inhibition with K_i values of 3 μM (variable Glu_4Tyr) and 6 μM (variable ATP). Consequently, the fatty acyl-peptide is unable to serve as a Src substrate because ATP is unable to bind to the active site in the presence of the myristyl group. Unfortunately, this inhibitory species does not display selectivity against other protein kinases (CSK, PKA, and the FGF receptor). However, it may ultimately be possible to enhance either selectivity or potency by placing the fatty acid moiety at different sites along the peptide chain to minimize the distance between the site of phosphorylation (i.e., the Tyr residue) and the ATP-binding site. These results stand in interesting contrast to earlier work described by Ward and O'Brian (O'Brian et al. 1990; O'Brian et al. 1991; Ward and O'Brian 1993). PKC peptide substrates, upon *N*-myristoylation, are converted into inhibitors with IC_{50} values of between 3–10 μM, depending upon the amino acid sequence. However, unlike the myristoylated peptides that inhibit Src, Ward and O'Brian's PKC inhibitors do not display a competitive pattern versus variable ATP, nor do they serve as competitive inhibitors versus peptide substrate. The authors conclude that their myristoylated peptides bind to a different enzyme form (i.e., the free enzyme) than the peptide substrate (i.e., the enzyme-ATP complex). This accounts for the noncompetitive inhibition pattern versus peptide substrate. In addition, Ward, O'Brian, and their colleagues have suggested that the inhibitory effect conferred by the myristoyl appendage is due, at least in part, to its interaction with the phosphatidylserine cofactor of PKC (O'Brian et al. 1990). However, more recent studies suggest that a myristyl-binding region is located in close proximity to the peptide-binding region of the active site (Zaliani et al. 1998). Consequently, it appears likely that the inhibitory behavior of myristoylated peptides toward PKC is at least partly due to the presence of a near active site hydrophobic region that is able to accommodate the lipophilic fatty acid moiety.

4.1.3
Phosphotyrosine Analogs

SH2 and PTB domains, as well as protein tyrosine phosphatases, recognize sequences that encompass phosphotyrosine. However, since the latter is hydrolyzable, peptides that contain this residue serve only as transient antagonists of protein–protein interactions. A number of nonhydrolyzable phosphotyrosine mimetics have been described, in large part due to the effort of Burke and his collaborators at the NIH. Since phosphotyrosine analogs have been the topic of recent reviews, only a cursory discussion of their current status will be presented (Burke et al. 2001; Burke and Lee 2003).

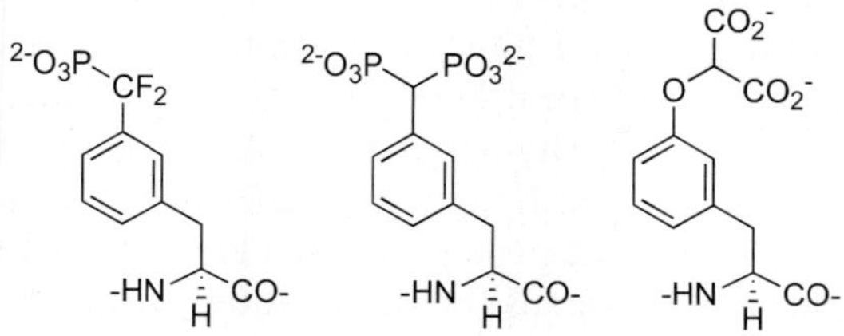

20 **21** **22**

Perhaps the most extensively employed of all phosphotyrosine analogs is the difluorophosphonate derivative **20**. The synthesis of this analog was first described by Burke and his colleagues (Smyth et al. 1992; Burke et al. 1993) and was subsequently introduced into peptides and evaluated as SH2 ligands in 1994 (Burke et al. 1994; Gilmer et al. 1994). The phosphonate moiety is not only resistant to hydrolysis by adventitious intracellular phosphatases, but the electron-withdrawing effect of the difluoro substituents ensures that the phosphonate is doubly ionized at physiological pH. In addition to the difluoromethylene moiety, a variety of other groups have been used to link the phosphoryl moiety to the aromatic nucleus, including methylene, hydroxymethylene, and fluoromethylene (Burke et al. 1994). The -OPO_3H group on phosphotyrosine has also been replaced with -CH_2COOH (Gilmer et al. 1994; Tong et al. 1998), -OCH_2COOH (Burke et al. 1999), -CHOHCOOH (Beaulieu et al. 1999), -CF_2COOH (Burke et al. 1999), -CH_2SO_3H (Gilmer et al. 1994), -$CH_2CH_2COCOCH_3$ (Gilmer et al. 1994), and NO_2 (Gilmer et al. 1994). In addition, the phosphoryl group has been directly attached to the aromatic ring (i.e., no bridging group) (Stankovic et al. 1997). A number of geminal analogs [e.g., **21** (Bohacek et al. 2001) and **22** (Kole et al. 1995; Ye et al. 1995)] have been prepared and examined as well. Although the general statement that peptides containing **20** in place of phosphotyrosine possess the greatest affinity for their intended targets may be true, there is sufficient variability among the protein-binding domains that any generalization concerning binding preferences is dangerous. For example, the monocarboxylic acid analogs of phosphotyrosine appear to have reasonable affinity for certain SH2 domains, but are poor inhibitors for the protein tyrosine phosphatase family member PTP1B (Gao et al. 2000).

4.1.4
Proline Analogs

Proline is commonly thought of as a turn-promoting residue. Indeed, a large number of turn-inducing proline mimetics have been described, some of which have been synthetically incorporated into peptides. Sarcosine, also known as *N*-methyl glycine (CH_3NHCH_2COOH), is a commonly employed proline replacement. Indeed, the latter has been used in substrates for cyclin-dependent protein kinases, enzymes that require a proline residue on its intended substrate to direct phosphorylation to an adjacent serine moiety. For example, Ando and coworkers showed that peptides containing the sequence from vimentin, Leu-Gly-Ser-Ala-Leu-Arg-Arg-Arg-amide, in which the alanine moiety is replaced by either proline or sarcosine, serve as enhanced substrates for the cdc2 protein kinase (V/K 600-fold for Pro-peptide and 90-fold for Sar-peptide versus the Ala-peptide) (Ando et al. 1993). These investigators subsequently examined the specificity of the cdc2 and cdk5 proline-directed protein kinases with respect to a variety of N-substituted proline replacements including, *N*-methyl alanine, *N*-methyl leucine, *N*-methyl valine, and the four (azetidine carboxylic acid) and six ring (piperidine carboxylic acid) analogs of proline (Ando et al. 1997). Perhaps not too surprisingly, the peptides containing the ring analogs of proline were among the best substrates for these protein kinases, with the proline-containing parent serving as the most efficient substrate. Nevertheless, the sarcosine derivative serves as a substrate as well, albeit somewhat more efficiently for the cdc2 versus cdk5 enzyme. The latter observation is significant since sarcosine is the parent of N-substituted glycine derivatives. Peptides containing the latter ("peptoids") are readily prepared using standard solid-phase peptide synthesis conditions (Figliozzi et al. 1996; Burkoth et al. 2003). Indeed, recent improvements have reduced the coupling time to a few minutes (Olivos et al. 2002). Consequently, it is now possible to prepare large libraries of peptoid-based derivatives in an essentially automated fashion.

Lim and his colleagues have reported that N-substituted amino acids serve as proline replacements in peptide-based ligands targeting both SH3 and WW domains (Nguyen et al. 1998; Nguyen et al. 2000). These investigators demonstrated that the proline selectivity for these domains is due to a preference for N-substituted residues and not simply a function of the rigid cyclic structure that is unique to proline. The SH3 domain from Sem5 recognizes the motif PPPVPPR, whereas the WW domain from Yap prefers GTPPPPYTVG (where the "essential" prolines are underlined). The initial strategy employed a scanning approach in which both essential and nonessential prolines were replaced by either the C^{α}-substituted alanine or the N-substituted sarcosine. Replacement of the essential prolines with sarcosine is well tolerated, whereas introduction of alanine at these sites is not. The three-dimensional structures of these protein recognition domains are known. The ligand binds as a polyproline type II left-handed helix, which contains three residues per turn. The binding grooves on these protein domains can accommodate substituents from the type II helix, but only in a closely packed fashion. The latter can be achieved by a motif in which a C^{α}-substituent is adjacent to an N-substituted residue. A small library was prepared that consisted of peptides containing 11 different N-substituted glycines at the two essential proline sites in an SH3-targeted ligand. These were screened against the SH3 domains from Src, Grb2, Crk, and Sem5.

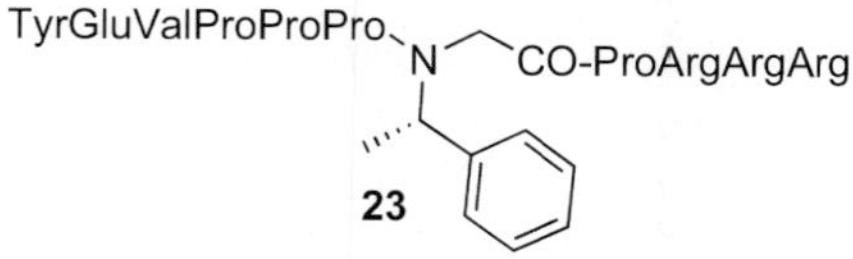

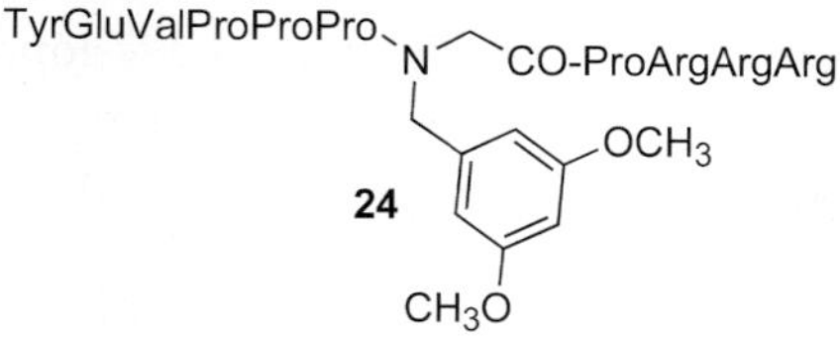

The lead peptide for Grb2, **23**, exhibits a K_D of 40 nM, more than 100-fold better than that of the corresponding proline-containing derivative. A subsequently prepared library, containing N-substituted glycine residues with oxygen- and nitrogen-containing substituents, was also evaluated (Nguyen et al. 2000). The latter functionality was chosen for their ability to interact with polar residues that reside near the ligand-binding grooves of the SH3 domain. Compound **24** exhibits a 30 nM K_D for the Grb2 SH3 domain and high selectivity versus Crk (300-fold) and Src (1,500-fold). A high-affinity ligand with impressive selectivity was also identified for the Crk SH3 domain. Double proline-substituted derivatives were also prepared, but these ligands failed to show an additive improvement in affinity for their protein targets. The latter is likely because the N-substituted glycines at the two different "essential" proline sites were identified independently of one another. Introduction of an N-derivatized glycine at one position likely induces a conformational change between ligand and protein that influences the interaction at the second proline site. Nevertheless, these results demonstrate that "essential" residues cannot only be replaced with unnatural analogs, but that the latter can furnish dramatically enhanced potency and selectivity.

4.2
Multidomain-Targeting Peptides

Many protein kinases contain two or more independent protein-binding domains. This includes the best-known example, Src, which contains SH1 (active site), SH2, and SH3 domains. Others, such as the LIM-kinase (LIM, PDZ, and active site regions) likewise contain multiple domains (Stanyon and Bernard 1999). The twin issues of potency and specificity can potentially be addressed by simultaneously targeting two protein interaction domains on the same enzyme. First, a single bivalent peptide that concomitantly interacts with two binding domains should display an enhanced affinity for the protein kinase target relative to either monovalent peptide alone. Second, although the sequence homology within closely related domains can be very high, the relative three-dimensional disposition of two protein interaction domains in the intact protein may differ substantially from one protein kinase to the next. Consequently, the linker that connects the two monovalent consensus sequences could play an important role in conveying enzyme selectivity. At this point in time, however, the potential of bivalent (or multivalent) peptides that can interact with two or more protein interaction domains is at an early stage in development and has not yet been fully realized.

One of the first papers to describe the preparation of bivalent ligands for signaling proteins dealt with the SH-PTP2 protein tyrosine phosphatase (Pluskey et al. 1995). The latter contains two SH2 domains. Occupancy of these domains is known to stimulate phosphatase activity. Previous studies had identified peptides SLNpYIDLDLVK and LSTpYASINFQK that specifically target the N-terminal and C-terminal SH2 domains, respectively (Case et al. 1994; Sugimoto et al. 1994). These monovalent species were linked with one another via an aminocaproic acid bridge to create a consolidated derivative, LNpYIDLDLVK-(6-aminocaproic acid)$_4$-LSTpYASINFQK, that can simultaneously interact with both SH2 domains. The latter does not act as an inhibitor, since it was designed to promote phosphatase activity. Nevertheless, it stimulates the phosphatase by 37-fold, compared with the 9- to 16-fold displayed by the monovalent consensus peptides. In addition, the heterodimeric peptide displays a 60- to 90-fold higher affinity for SH-PTP2 than either monomer peptide alone.

Cowburn, Barany, and their colleagues have described peptides that simultaneously target the SH2 and SH3 domains of Abl (Cowburn et al. 1995). The SH2-targeting sequence (PVpYENV-amide; K_D=2.0±0.2 μM) was attached to the SH3-targeting sequence (PPAYPPPPVP; K_D=10.5±0.2 μM) via a lysine side chain as illustrated in **25**. The latter exhibits a K_D of 249±5 nM for the SH2–SH3 domain construct, which is approximately 10- to 80-fold greater than that of individual monovalent consensus peptides. These investigators subsequently prepared a series of bivalent ligands containing the individual monomers in the four possible orientations illustrated in Scheme 1 25*A–D* (Xu et al. 1999). The highest affinity ligand, **25***C*, exhibits a K_D of 190 nM for the Abl SH2-SH3 (where LINKER=Gly$_7$K).

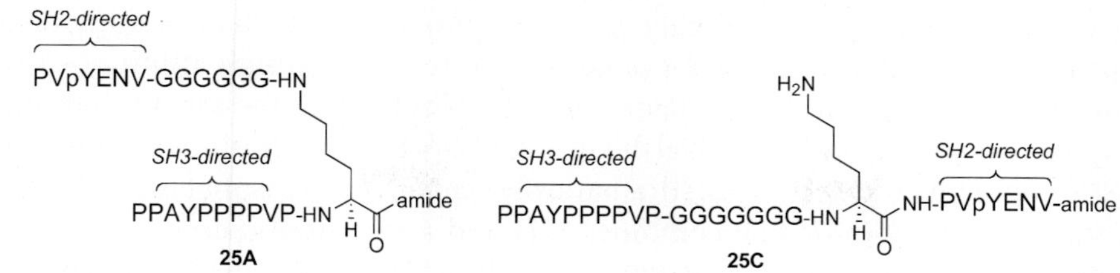

25A **25C**

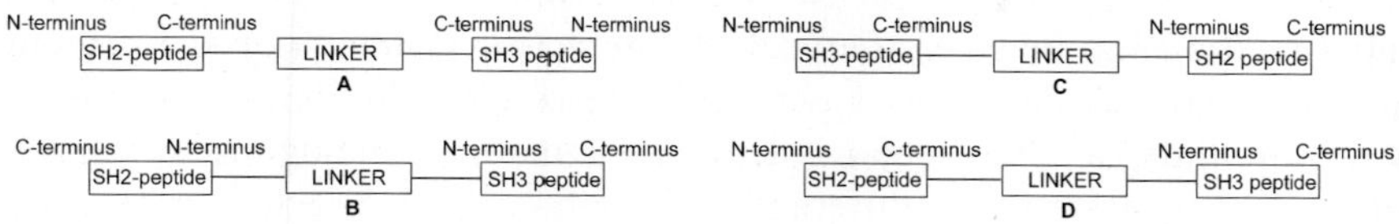

Roques, Garbay, and coworkers prepared peptides that interact with the two SH3 domains of Grb2 (Cussac et al. 1999). As with the bivalent analogs described in this section, the strategy employed coupling two monomer units via a linker. Two SH3-binding monomer units, Val-Pro-Pro-Val-Pro-Pro-Arg-Arg-Arg, were attached to each other via their C-termini using the lysine-based strategy described by Cowburn and Barany. The bivalent species exhibits an affinity (K_D=40 nM) that is two to three orders of magnitude greater than that exhibited by the corresponding monomer (N-terminal SH3 domain: K_D=2.6 μM; C-terminal SH3 domain: K_D=40 μM). These investigators demonstrated that the peptide dimer blocks Grb2-Sos complex formation in cell lysates, can selectively pull down Grb2 from lysate versus other double SH3 domain-containing proteins, and interferes with neurite formation in nerve growth factor-treated PC12 cells.

Miller and his coworkers prepared a series of SH2 domain-assisted *substrates* for the Abl tyrosine kinase (Pellicena et al. 1998). These investigators found that the presence of an SH2 domain binding sequence appended to the active site-directed sequence enhances substrate efficacy, specifically via a tenfold reduction in K_m. For example, a peptide of the general structure (active site-directed peptide)–(SH2-directed peptide) displays a K_m of 69±11 μM and a V_{max} of 3.0±0.1 μmol/min-mg. The key residue in the SH2-directed component is phosphoTyr, which is essential for SH2 recognition. When a Phe replaces this critical residue, the peptide displays a significantly larger K_m of 680±90 μM, yet a V_{max} (3.0±0.1 μmol/min-mg) that is essentially unaltered. A peptide containing an inversed orientation, namely (SH2-directed peptide)–(active site-directed peptide), likewise displays a relatively low K_m value (72±5 μM), which is presumably a reflection of enhanced affinity via coordination to the SH2 domain.

Lawrence and his collaborators employed the multidomain targeting approach to create combined active site/SH2 domain-directed inhibitors of Src (Profit et al. 1999; Profit et al. 2001). Peptide-based inhibitors of tyrosine kinases must confront at least two challenges. First, peptides that target the active site tend to be exceedingly poor inhibitory agents. Second, although peptides that bind to the SH2 domain are of reasonably high affinity (~low μM) they have the unintended consequence of activating the kinase. Indeed, by analogy, Shoelson's and Walsh's bivalent ligand, which binds to the two SH2 domains of SH-PTP2, dramatically enhances phosphatase activity. However, an inhibitor that combines SH2 and active site-binding properties should simultaneously display enhanced affinity and inhibitory potency. In addition, bivalent analogs can furnish an assessment of the distance and spatial relationship between the protein interaction domains on the protein under evaluation. Indeed, the Lawrence team referred to their small library (16 compounds) as "molecular rulers." In a manner analogous to Barany and Cowburn, a series of differentially oriented SH2-directed and active site-directed bivalent ligands were prepared. γ-Aminobutyric acid (GABA) residues were employed in the linker region to connect the monovalent ligands. The active site-directed fragment, -Glu-Glu-Leu-Leu-(F_5Phe)-, contains pentafluorophenylalanine, which had been previously identified as a nonphosphorylatable tyrosine surrogate (*vide supra*) (Niu and Lawrence 1997a). The SH2 sequence, -pTyr-Glu-Glu-Ile-, was based on the well-known preference of the SH2 domain from Src for a sequence motif containing pTyr followed by at hydrophobic amino acid at the P+3 position (Songyang et al. 1993).

SH2-directed (acetyl-pTyr-Glu-Glu-Ile-) *A.S.-directed* (Glu-Glu-Leu-Leu-F5Phe)

acetyl-**pTyr**-Glu-Glu-Ile-Glu-(GABA)$_n$-Glu-Glu-Leu-Leu-**F_5Phe**-amide

26A

A.S.-directed (Glu-Glu-Leu-Leu-F5Phe) *SH2-directed* (pTyr-Glu-Glu-Ile)

acetyl-Glu-Glu-Leu-Leu-**F_5Phe**-(GABA)$_n$-**pTyr**-Glu-Glu-Ile-Glu-amide

26B

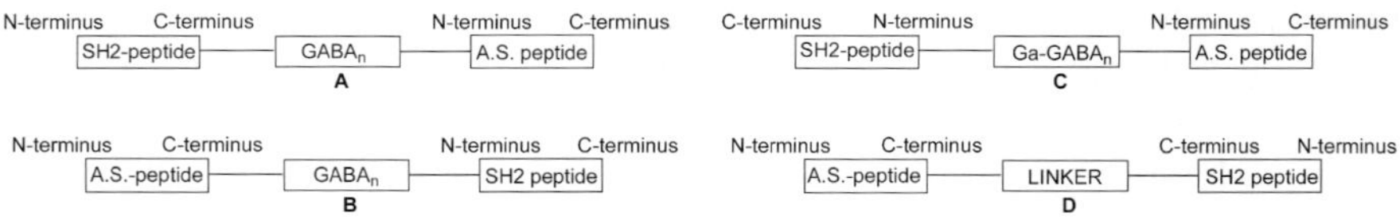

Of the four possible relative orientations between the SH2- and active site-directed fragments (Scheme 2), only three were prepared (*A–C*) since the fourth (*D*) was subsequently ruled out as suboptimal (*vide infra*). The orientation illustrated in *C* requires that the peptide chains in the two monovalent units run anti-parallel to one another. This reversal of chain polarity was achieved via insertion of a glutaric anhydride (Ga) residue between the SH2-directed sequence and the GABA linker. Orientation *B* furnished the most effective inhibitors possessing the shortest linkers (optimal: $GABA_n$= $GABA_3$). In this particular case, the tyrosine surrogate F_5Phe (occupying the active site) lies only three residues from the pTyr moiety which resides in the SH2 domain (see **26***B*).

This suggests that the active site region and the SH2 domain are situated close to one another in the active form of the enzyme. The series **26***D* was not prepared since, even in the absence of a GABA linker, the key F_5Phe and pTyr moieties are positioned at least five residues apart. The latter is suboptimal relative to the relationship in **26***B*. The lead bivalent analog **26***B* (where $GABA_n$=$GABA_3$) displays an enhanced 120-fold inhibitory potency relative to the simple active site-directed monomer (IC_{50}=13±1 μM versus IC_{50}= 1590±170 μM, respectively).

4.3
Structural Modification of Consensus Sequence Peptides

4.3.1
Conformationally Biased Peptides

Cyclization of peptides improves stability against proteases while affording conformational constraints that may enhance inhibitory potency. Research teams at M.D. Anderson and the University of Arizona have explored the efficacy of this structurally distinct class of active site-directed protein kinase inhibitors.

Lam and his colleagues have shown that the Tyr-Ile-Tyr-Gly-Ser-Phe-Lys-amide motif serves as an effective Src substrate (Lam et al. 1995) and that the peptide might bind to the active site in the form of a *β*-turn (Lou et al. 1997). In order to assess the reasonableness of this notion, Lam, Hruby, and their coworkers prepared a series of disulfide bridge-cyclized inhibitory peptides that target Src (Alfaro-Lopez et al. 1998). In addition, these investigators took advantage of the observation that 2-naphthylalanine (Sect. 11) serves as a nonphosphorylatable tyrosine mimetic (Wu et al. 1996).

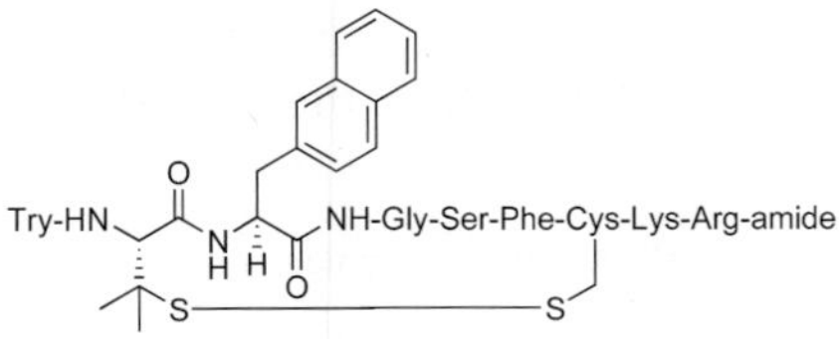

27

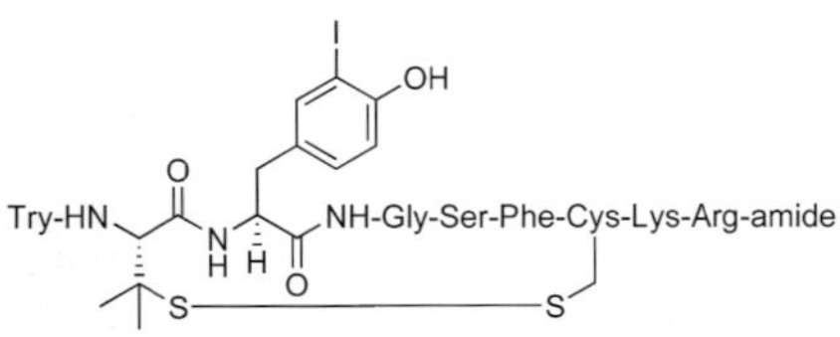

28

Compound **27** exhibits an IC_{50} of 1.6 μM. Interestingly, and somewhat surprisingly, potency was further improved by tenfold when the naphthylalanine was replaced with 3-iodotyrosine (**28**). This observation stands in marked contrast to the ineffectiveness of 3-iodotyrosine as a tyrosine mimetic in an EGFR-targeted inhibitory peptide (Fry et al. 1994). Peptide **28** is not only an effective Src kinase inhibitor but also exhibits impressive selectivity in favor of Src versus other Src kinase family members (20-fold versus

Lck and >1,300-fold versus Lyn). In addition, these investigators found that several of their less potent Src kinase inhibitors (IC_{50} values 1–3 μM range) exhibit even better selectivity profiles than **28.**

McMurray, Budde, and coworkers likewise examined the effectiveness of cyclic peptide inhibitors on the Src kinase. These investigators first examined the affinity of a series of cyclic peptide substrates for Src (i.e., the ability of these substrates to block the phosphorylation of poly Glu_4Tyr) (McMurray et al. 1998). One of the lead compounds, cyclo[Asp-Asn-Glu-Tyr-Ala-Phe-Phe^7-Gln-D-Phe-Pro) displays a K_i of 150 μM, which is nearly identical to its Michaelis constant as a substrate (140 μM). Insertion of an arginine residue at position 7 resulted in a dramatic loss in enzyme affinity, whereas a glutamic acid residue at this site is well tolerated. On the basis of this observation, these investigators concluded that residues at this site are positioned within a positively charged region of the enzyme. Indeed, when Phe^7 was subsequently replaced with a series of 14 different analogs, the lead inhibitors contained a negatively charged residue at this position [4-carboxyphenylalanine (K_i=0.85 μM) and phosphotyrosine (K_i=1.1 μM)] (Wang et al. 2000). The carboxylphenylalanine-containing cyclic peptide displays an impressive selectivity profile in favor of Src (>100-fold against Yes; >300-fold versus Lck; >1,000-fold versus PKA; 1,200-fold versus FGF receptor; 1,800-fold versus Abl; >2,000-fold versus CSK).

Watterson and his group described a different strategy for topologically biasing an active site-directed peptide (Lukas et al. 1999). Myosin light chain kinase (MLCK) was the target in this particular case. These investigators first identified a nonapeptide sequence, Arg-Lys-Lys-Tyr-Lys-Tyr-Arg-Arg-Lys-amide that exhibits both a remarkable affinity (IC_{50}=50 nM) and selectivity (~4,000-fold versus CaM kinase II) for MLCK. Based on the screening results of closely related peptides, in combination with molecular modeling, it was proposed that the peptide might bind to the active site region in an extended conformation. The structural constraints inherent within 4-aminocyclohexanecarboxylic acid were used to promote this desired conformation by inserting the residue at specific sites within the peptide sequence.

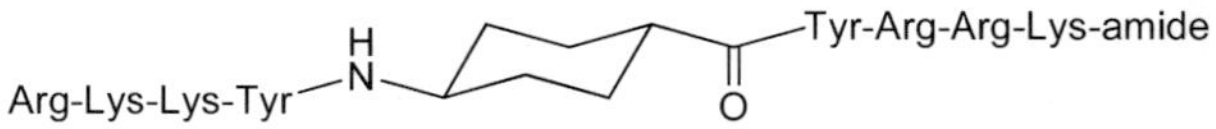

29

The most potent of these derivatives (**29**) exhibits an IC_{50} (40 nM) similar to that of the parent nonapeptide. Although improved potency and selectivity were not observed versus the already formidable peptide parent, the results in this study suggest that conformational constraints could serve as scaffolds upon which an array of functionality can be appended.

4.3.2
Terminally Modified Peptides

The fatty acid-modified peptides described in Sect. 4.1.2 are examples of terminally modified consensus sequences. Addition of the long alkyl chain furnishes enhanced active site affinity via coordination to ancillary binding pockets. However, it should be possible to access potential sites of interaction that are extensions of the protein-binding pocket with non-natural substituents. Schreiber's group explored this concept utilizing N-terminally modified peptides that target the SH3 domain of Src (Combs et al. 1996). The three-dimensional structure of the protein was employed as a guide to focus structural diversity into a potential binding region adjacent to the site at which a peptide ligand of the SH3 domain is known to reside. Structural diversity was created using a split-and-pool approach. Pro-Leu-Pro-Pro-Leu-Pro-resin was split into 33 equal amounts and each fraction subsequently modified at the peptide N-terminus with one of 32 different non-natural amino acids (plus no residue at all). The fractions were recombined and the process repeated two additional times. The one-bead/one-compound library was then exposed to a phosphatase-modified SH3 domain. Beads possessing high-affinity ligands were visually identified under the microscope using the phosphatase as a colorimetric reporter.

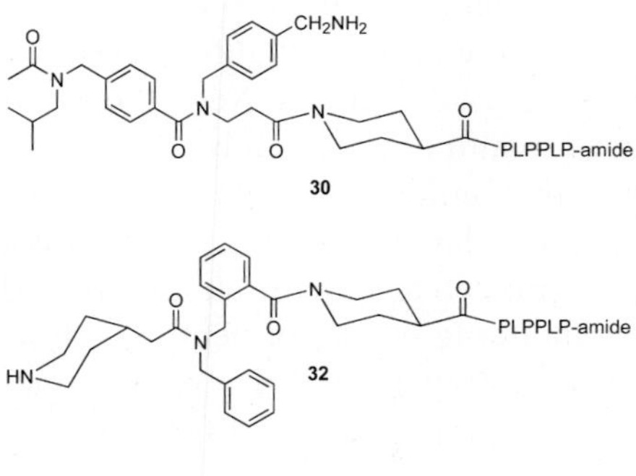

30

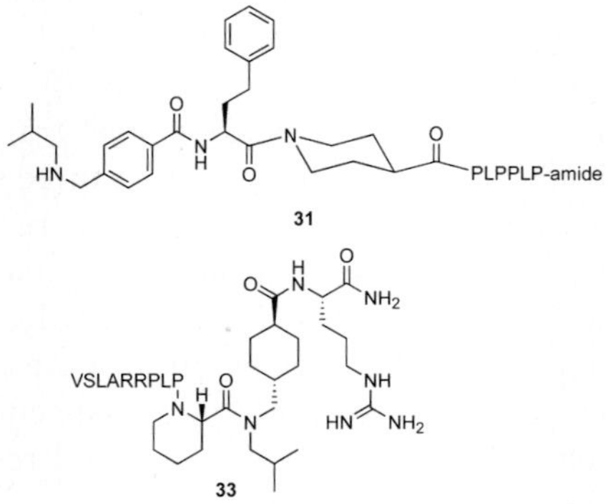

31

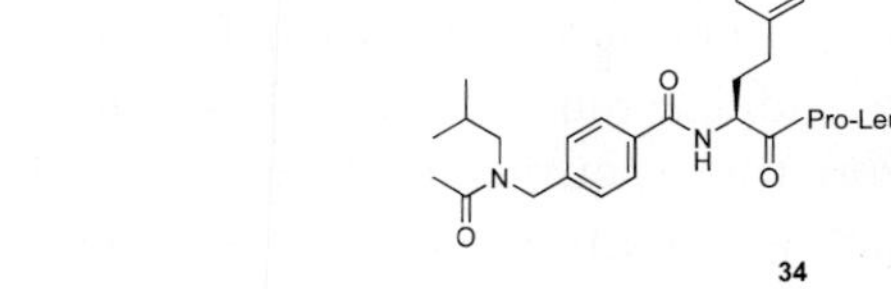

32

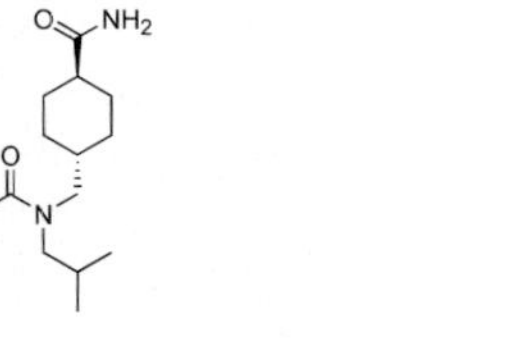

33

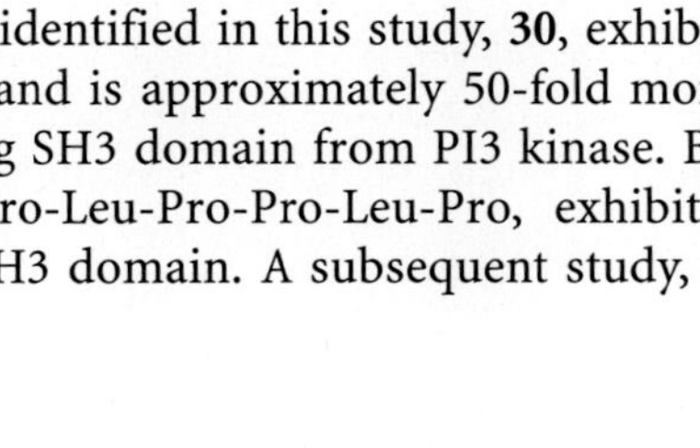

34

The lead peptide identified in this study, **30**, exhibits a K_D of 3.4 μM for the Src SH3 domain and is approximately 50-fold more selective for Src versus the corresponding SH3 domain from PI3 kinase. By comparison, the parent peptide, acetyl-Pro-Leu-Pro-Pro-Leu-Pro, exhibits a K_D of greater than 1 mM for Src's SH3 domain. A subsequent study, using a slightly larger set of non-natural monomers and greater structural diversity at each position, identified additional ligands for the Src SH3 domain (**31**; K_D=0.9 μM) as well as leads for the closely related SH3 domain of Hck (**32**; K_D=1.0 μM) (Kapoor et al. 1998). Some of these ligands proved to be moderately selective (e.g., **32** is 46-fold more selective for Hck than Src).

The Schreiber group extended the concept of structural diversity to the C-terminus of the SH3-directed ligand as well (Morken et al. 1998). In this instance, the library took the form of Val-Ser-Leu-Ala-Arg-Arg-Pro-Leu-Pro-M3-M2-M1-resin, where M3, M2, and M1 represent 50 different residues, which included 49 monomers plus an omitted residue. The goal of this work was to identify a replacement for the C-terminal Leu-Pro dyad in the parent peptide -Pro-Leu-Pro-Pro-Leu-Pro-. The lead **33** displays a K_D of 2.6 μM for the SH3 domain from Src. A portion of the C-terminal non-natural component from **33** was then appended, along with the N-terminal non-natural component in **31**, to the Pro-Leu-Pro core (**34**). The latter compound displays a K_D of 1.1 μM for Src's SH3 domain.

4.3.3
Globally Modified Peptides

Protein interaction domains have evolved to accommodate specific sequences of preferred amino residues on their protein-binding partner. However, each amino acid site on the bound sequence is limited to a genetically encoded molecular diversity of 20. In reality, the latter is slightly larger due to a small array of possible post-translational modifications. Nevertheless, it is not difficult to imagine that there exist a wealth of potential binding interactions that lie just outside of the reach of this limited set of naturally occurring residues. One strategy to enhance molecular diversity is to prepare a wide assortment of Fmoc and side chain-protected, unnatural, amino acid derivatives and then synthesize the corresponding library of peptides. However, a reasonable 50-fold enhancement in molecular diversity vis-à-vis genetically encoded residues would require the preparation of 1,000 different monomers, a nontrivial task.

Lawrence and his colleagues outlined an approach that creates high diversity at any desired site along a peptide chain using readily available carboxylic acid-containing compounds (Lee and Lawrence 1999). The strategy, as outlined in Scheme 3, employs a consensus sequence peptide containing 2,3-diaminopropionic acid ("Dap"), appropriately inserted at key sites along the peptide chain.

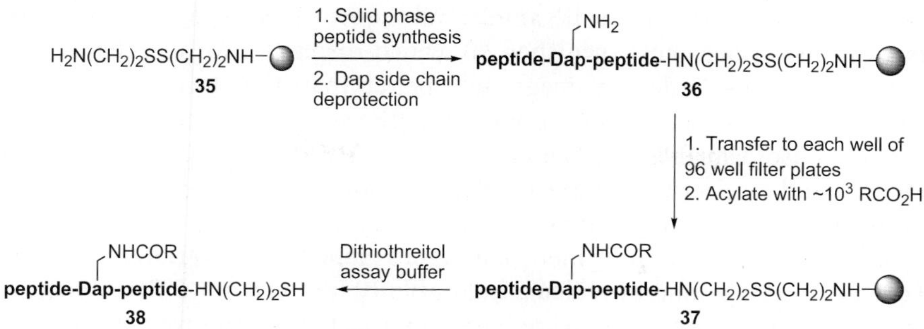

The peptide is synthesized on a disulfide-substituted Tentagel resin. Once prepared, the peptide-resin is distributed in equal amounts to the individual wells of a 96-multiwell plate designed for organic synthesis (i.e., the bottom of each well contains a frit that allows multiple washings without loss of the peptide-resin). Each well is then exposed to one of approximately 1,000 different carboxylic acid compounds. In short, the library is prepared in parallel, thereby obviating the necessity of molecular deconvolution. Once the modification in the Dap residue is complete, any side chain protecting groups on the peptide are removed with trifluoroacetic acid. After multiple washings to remove residual acid, the individual peptides are cleaved from the resin with assay buffer, which contains dithiothreitol. The peptides can then be directly assessed for potency.

Lawrence and his team employed a structure-based strategy, in combination with the synthetic approach outlined in Scheme 3, to identify high-affinity ligands for the SH2 domain from Lck (Lee and Lawrence 1999, 2000; Yeh et al. 2001). The three-dimensional structure of the Lck SH2 ligand, acetyl-pTyr-Glu-Glu-Ile-amide, bound to its protein target, had been previously reported (Tong et al. 1996). Three sites on the ligand, the N-terminal acetyl moiety and the two Glu side chains, are oriented into regions of the SH2 surface that could potentially accommodate modified analogs of the acetyl and glutamic acid moieties.

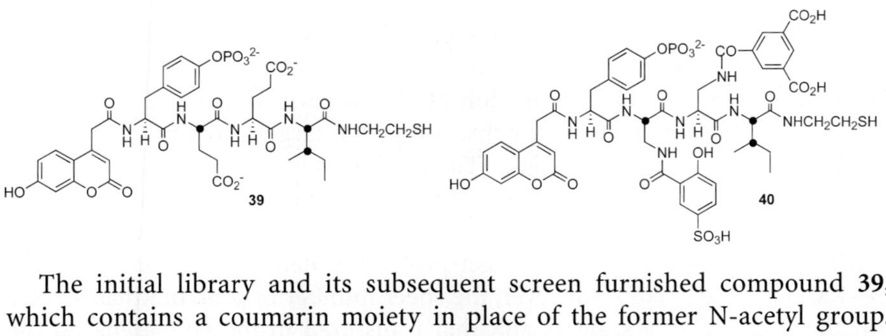

The initial library and its subsequent screen furnished compound **39**, which contains a coumarin moiety in place of the former N-acetyl group. The coumarin-derivatized peptide exhibits a K_D of 35 nM for the Lck SH2 domain, approximately two orders of magnitude greater than the parent peptide aceyl-pTyr-Glu-Glu-Ile-amide. Subsequent identification of the glutamic acid replacements furnished **40**, which displays a K_D of 200 pM, approximately four orders of magnitude better than the starting consensus peptide. An analogous approach was recently used to construct an inhibitor for the α isoform of PKC (Lee et al. 2004). The inhibitor displays a K_i of 800 pM and a selectivity of greater than 400-fold versus other conventional, novel, and atypical PKC isoforms.

Lawrence, Zhang, and their colleagues reported a variation on the Scheme 3 strategy that provided a high-affinity inhibitor for PTP1B (Shen et al. 2001). Once again, a structure-based approach was employed that directed molecular diversity toward potential binding sites on the target protein surface. In this particular case, PTP1B had been previously shown to bind phosphotyrosine at two distinct sites, one at the active site and the other at a position adjacent to the active site (Puius et al. 1997).

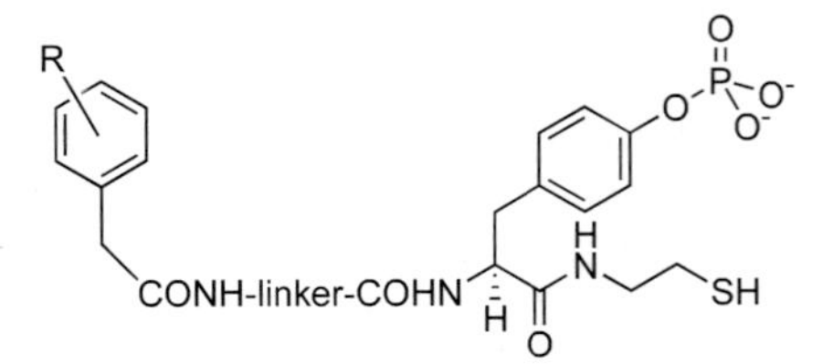

peripheral site-targeted **41** active site-targeted

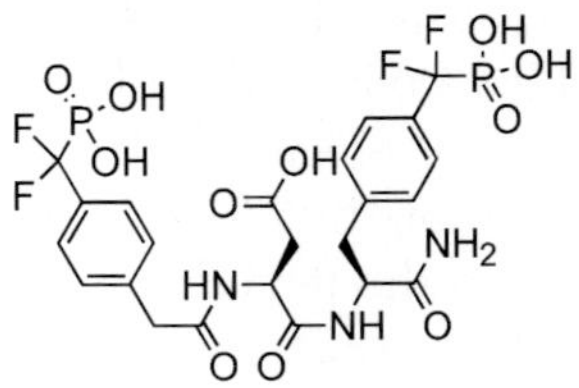

42

A library of the general form **41** was prepared using the disulfide Tentagel resin **35**. Molecular diversity was inserted at the N-terminal and linker positions. The lead compound **42** exhibits a K_i of 2.6 nM for PTP1B and a selectivity of between 1,000- and 10,000-fold versus a panel of fifteen other protein phosphatases.

5
Summary

An exceedingly important, but time-consuming area of drug design is the conversion of consensus recognition sequences into small molecules with drug-like properties. The acquisition of peptidomimetics requires a combination of detailed structural information of the target protein, an intensive synthetic effort, and gifted insight. The rapid development of human immunodeficiency virus (HIV) protease inhibitors stands as a testimony to the fact that, given enough resources, it is possible to successfully create potent small molecule inhibitors that target protein–protein interaction sites (Abdel-Rahman et al. 2002). However, the sheer number of protein kinases rules out the kind of large-scale assault that transpired in the HIV arena on the protein kinase family as a whole. Nevertheless, at a minimum, a worthwhile goal is the acquisition of high-affinity reagents for as many signaling proteins as possible. Although consensus sequences represent an obvious starting point, their transmogrification into high-affinity ligands remains an ongoing struggle. Given the large number of possible targets, simple rules or strategies for the conversion of modest-binding peptides into high-affinity reagents are a much sought after commodity. Amino acid analogs, which serve as high-affinity replacements for their natural counterparts, represent one such approach (Sect. 4.1). Alternatively, the notion of targeting two or more protein–protein interaction domains on a single protein kinase, represents a decidedly different tactic (Sect. 4.2). Finally, structurally modified consensus sequences that are either topologically biased or are able to access sites simply unavailable to standard amino acid residues represents a third strategy (Sect. 4.3). Inherent within all of these approaches is the possibility of general applicability to the family of protein kinases. Unfortunately, the route from peptide to a high-affinity species with equally high selectivity is often anything but straightforward. The disadvantage with protein kinases is their large number. However, this disadvantage is also an advantage in that they are all closely related. Consequently, inhibitor design rules that emerge from the study of a few representative members of this large enzyme family may ultimately prove applicable to the family as a whole.

References

Abdel-Rahman HM, Al-karamany GS, et al (2002) HIV protease inhibitors: peptidomimetic drugs and future perspectives. Curr Med Chem 9:1905–22

Adams JA, Taylor SS (1992) Energetic limits of phosphotransfer in the catalytic subunit of cAMP-dependent protein kinase as measured by viscosity experiments. Biochemistry 31:8516–22

Alfaro-Lopez J, Yuan W, et al (1998) Discovery of a novel series of potent and selective substrate-based inhibitors of p60c-src protein tyrosine kinase: conformational and topographical constraints in peptide design. J Med Chem 41:2252–60

Ando S, Tsujimura K, et al (1993) Phosphorylation of synthetic vimentin peptides by cdc2 kinase. Biochem Biophys Res Commun 195:837–43

Ando S, Ikuhara T, et al (1997) Role of the pyrrolidine ring of proline in determining the substrate specificity of cdc2 kinase or cdk5. J Biochem [Tokyo] 122:409–14

Beaulieu PL, Cameron DR, et al (1999) Ligands for the tyrosine kinase p56lck SH2 domain: discovery of potent dipeptide derivatives with monocharged, nonhydrolyzable phosphate replacements. J Med Chem 42:1757–66

Bohacek RS, Dalgarno DC, et al (2001) X-Ray structure of citrate bound to Src SH2 leads to a high-affinity, bone-targeted Src SH2 inhibitor. J Med Chem 44:660–3

Burke TR Jr, Smyth MS, et al (1993) Preparation of fluoro-4-(phosphonomethyl)-D,L-phenylalanine and hydroxy-4-(phosphonomethyl)-D,L-phenylalanine suitably protected for solid phase synthesis of peptides containing hydrolytically stable analogues of O-phosphotyrosine. J Org Chem 58:1336–40

Burke TR Jr, Smyth MS, et al (1994) Nonhydrolyzable phosphotyrosyl mimetics for the preparation of phosphatase-resistant SH2 domain inhibitors. Biochemistry 33:6490–4
Burke TR Jr, Luo J, et al (1999) Monocarboxylic-based phosphotyrosyl mimetics in the design of GRB2 SH2 domain inhibitors. Bioorg Med Chem Lett 9:347–52
Burke TR Jr, Yao ZJ, et al (2001) Phosphoryltyrosyl mimetics in the design of peptide-based signal transduction inhibitors. Biopolymers 60:32–44
Burke TR Jr, Lee K (2003) Phosphotyrosyl mimetics in the development of signal transduction inhibitors. Acc Chem Res 36:426–33
Burkoth TS, Fafarman AT, et al (2003) Incorporation of unprotected heterocyclic side chains into peptoid oligomers via solid-phase submonomer synthesis. J Am Chem Soc 125:8841–5
Case RD, Piccione E, et al (1994) SH-PTP2/Syp SH2 domain binding specificity is defined by direct interactions with platelet-derived growth factor beta-receptor, epidermal growth factor receptor, and insulin receptor substrate-1-derived phosphopeptides. J Biol Chem 269:10467–74
Cheng HC, Kemp BE, et al (1986) A potent synthetic peptide inhibitor of the cAMP-dependent protein kinase. J Biol Chem 261:989–92
Cole PA, Grace MR, et al (1995) The role of the catalytic base in the protein tyrosine kinase Csk. J Biol Chem 270:22105–8
Combs AP, Kapoor TM, et al (1996) Protein structure-based combinatorial chemistry: discovery of non-peptide binding elements to Src SH3 domain. J Am Chem Soc 118:287–8
Cowburn D, Zheng J, et al (1995) Enhanced affinities and specificities of consolidated ligands for the Src homology (SH) 3 and SH2 domains of Abelson protein-tyrosine kinase. J Biol Chem 270:26738–41
Csukai M, Mochly-Rosen D (1999) Pharmacologic modulation of protein kinase C isozymes: the role of RACKs and subcellular localisation. Pharmacol Res 39:253–9
Cussac D, Vidal M, et al (1999) A Sos-derived peptidimer blocks the Ras signaling pathway by binding both Grb2 SH3 domains and displays antiproliferative activity. FASEB J 13:31–8
Dhanasekaran N, Premkumar Reddy E (1998) Signaling by dual specificity kinases. Oncogene 17:1447–55
Dostmann WR, Taylor MS, et al (2000) Highly specific, membrane-permeant peptide blockers of cGMP-dependent protein kinase Ialpha inhibit NO-induced cerebral dilation. Proc Natl Acad Sci U S A 97:14772–7
Figliozzi GM, Goldsmith R, et al (1996) Synthesis of N-substituted glycine peptoid libraries. Methods Enzymol 267:437–47
Frank R (2002) The SPOT-synthesis technique. Synthetic peptide arrays on membrane supports—principles and applications. J Immunol Methods 267:13–26
Fry DW, McMichael A, et al (1994) Design of a potent peptide inhibitor of the epidermal growth factor receptor tyrosine kinase utilizing sequences based on the natural phosphorylation sites of phospholipase C-gamma 1. Peptides 15:951–7
Gao Y, Wu L, et al (2000) Examination of novel non-phosphorus-containing phosphotyrosyl mimetics against protein-tyrosine phosphatase-1B and demonstration of differential affinities toward Grb2 SH2 domains. Bioorg Med Chem Lett 10:923–7
Gilmer T, Rodriguez M, et al (1994) Peptide inhibitors of src SH3-SH2-phosphoprotein interactions. J Biol Chem 269:31711–9
Glass DB, Cheng HC, et al (1989) Primary structural determinants essential for potent inhibition of cAMP-dependent protein kinase by inhibitory peptides corresponding to the active portion of the heat-stable inhibitor protein. J Biol Chem 264:8802–10

Glass DB, Lundquist LJ, et al (1989) Protein kinase inhibitor-(6–22)-amide peptide analogs with standard and nonstandard amino acid substitutions for phenylalanine 10. Inhibition of cAMP-dependent protein kinase. J Biol Chem 264:14579–84

Granier C (2002) Special issue on methods of parallel peptide synthesis and their contributions to deciphering molecular interactions in the immune system. J Immunol Methods 267:1–2

Houghten RA, Blondelle SE, et al (1996) Libraries from libraries: generation and comparison of screening profiles. Mol Divers 2:41–5

Houseman BT, Huh JH, et al (2002) Peptide chips for the quantitative evaluation of protein kinase activity. Nat Biotechnol 20:270–4

Huse M, Kuriyan J (2002) The conformational plasticity of protein kinases. Cell 109:275–82

Johnson LN, Lowe ED, et al (1998) The Eleventh Datta Lecture. The structural basis for substrate recognition and control by protein kinases. FEBS Lett 430:1–11

Kaiser ET, Mihara H, et al (1989) Peptide and protein synthesis by segment synthesis-condensation. Science 243:187–92

Kapoor TM, Andreotti AH, et al (1998) Exploring the specificity pockets of two homologous SH3 domains using structure-based, split-pool synthesis and affinity-based selection. J Am Chem Soc 120:23–9

Kim K, Cole PA (1998) Kinetic analysis of a protein tyrosine kinase reaction transition state in the forward and the reverse directions. J Am Chem Soc 120:6851–8

Kole HK, Akamatsu M, et al (1995) Protein-tyrosine phosphatase inhibition by a peptide containing the phosphotyrosyl mimetic, L-O-malonyltyrosine. Biochem Biophys Res Commun 209:817–22

Lam KS, Wu J, et al (1995) Identification and characterization of a novel synthetic peptide substrate specific for Src-family protein tyrosine kinases. Int J Pept Protein Res 45:587–92

Lam KS, Liu R, et al (2003) Applications of one-bead one-compound combinatorial libraries and chemical microarrays in signal transduction research. Acc Chem Res 36:370–7

Lashmet PR, Tang K-C, et al (1983) The synthesis of an ATP-gamma-peptidyl ester as a potential probe of c-AMP-dependent protein kinase. Tetrahedron Lett 24:1121–4

Lee TR, Lawrence DS (1999) Acquisition of high-affinity, SH2-targeted ligands via a spatially focused library. J Med Chem 42:784–7

Lee TR, Lawrence DS (2000) SH2-directed ligands of the Lck tyrosine kinase. J Med Chem 43:1173–9

Lee TR, Niu J, et al (1994) Phenol kinase activity of the serine/threonine-specific cAMP-dependent protein kinase: steric and electronic effects. Biochemistry 33:4245–4250

Lee TR, Niu J, et al (1995a) The extraordinary active site substrate specificity of pp60c-src. A multiple specificity protein kinase. J Biol Chem 270:5375–80

Lee TR, Till JH, et al (1995b) Precision substrate targeting of protein kinases v-Abl and c-Src. J Biol Chem 270:27022–6

Lee JH, Nandy SK, et al (2004) A highly potent and selective PKCalpha inhibitor generated via combinatorial modification of a peptide scaffold. J Am Chem Soc 126:3394–5

Loog M, Uri A, et al (1999) Adenosine-5'-carboxylic acid peptidyl derivatives as inhibitors of protein kinases. Bioorg Med Chem Lett 9:1447–52

Loog M, Uri A, et al (2000) Bi-substrate analogue ligands for affinity chromatography of protein kinases. FEBS Lett 480:244–8

Lou Q, Leftwich ME, et al (1997) Potent pseudosubstrate-based peptide inhibitors for p60(c-src) protein tyrosine kinase. Cancer Res 57:1877–81

Lukas TJ, Mirzoeva S, et al (1999) Identification of novel classes of protein kinase inhibitors using combinatorial peptide chemistry based on functional genomics knowledge. J Med Chem 42:910–9

Marin O, Meggio F, et al (1999) Tyrosine versus serine/threonine phosphorylation by protein kinase casein kinase-2. A study with peptide substrates derived from immunophilin Fpr3. J Biol Chem 274:29260–5

McMurray JS, Budde RJ, et al (1998) Cyclic peptides as probes of the substrate binding site of the cytosolic tyrosine kinase, pp60c-src. Arch Biochem Biophys 355:124–30

Medzihradszky D, Chen SL, et al (1994) Solid-phase synthesis of adenosine phosphopeptides as potential bisubstrate inhibitors of protein kinases. J Am Chem Soc 116:9413–9

Mitchell RD, Glass DB, et al (1995) Heat-stable inhibitor protein derived peptide substrate analogs: phosphorylation by cAMP-dependent and cGMP-dependent protein kinases. Biochemistry 34:528–34

Morken JP, Kapoor TM, et al (1998) Exploring the leucine-proline binding pocket of the Src SH3 domain using structure-based, split-pool synthesis and affinity selection. J Am Chem Soc 120:30–6

Nguyen JT, Turck CW, et al (1998) Exploiting the basis of proline recognition by SH3 and WW domains: design of N-substituted inhibitors. Science 282:2088–92

Nguyen JT, Porter M, et al (2000) Improving SH3 domain ligand selectivity using a non-natural scaffold. Chem Biol 7:463–73

Niu J, Lawrence DS (1997a) L-dopa: a potent nonphosphorylatable tyrosine mimetic for pp60c-src. J Am Chem Soc 119:3844–5

Niu J, Lawrence DS (1997b) Nonphosphorylatable tyrosine surrogates. Implications for protein kinase inhibitor design. J Biol Chem 272:1493–9

O'Brian CA, Ward NE, et al (1990) N-myristyl-Lys-Arg-Thr-Leu-Arg: a novel protein kinase C inhibitor. Biochem Pharmacol 39:49–57

O'Brian CA, Ward NE, et al (1991) A novel N-myristylated synthetic octapeptide inhibits protein kinase C activity and partially reverses murine fibrosarcoma cell resistance to adriamycin. Invest New Drugs 9:169–79

Olivos HJ, Alluri PG, et al (2002) Microwave-assisted solid-phase synthesis of peptoids. Org Lett 4:4057–9

Parang K, Till JH, et al (2001) Mechanism-based design of a protein kinase inhibitor. Nat Struct Biol 8:37–41

Pellicena P, Stowell KR, et al (1998) Enhanced phosphorylation of Src family kinase substrates containing SH2 domain binding sites. J Biol Chem 273:15325–8

Pinna LA, Ruzzene M (1996) How do protein kinases recognize their substrates? Biochim Biophys Acta 1314:191–225

Pluskey S, Wandless TJ, et al (1995) Potent stimulation of SH-PTP2 phosphatase activity by simultaneous occupancy of both SH2 domains. J Biol Chem 270:2897–900

Profit AA, Lee TR, et al (1999) Bivalent inhibitors of protein tyrosine kinases. J Am Chem Soc 121:280–3

Profit AA, Lee TR, et al (2001) Molecular rulers: an assessment of distance and spatial relationships of Src tyrosine kinase Sh2 and active site regions. J Biol Chem 276:9446–51

Puius YA, Zhao Y, et al (1997) Identification of a second aryl phosphate-binding site in protein-tyrosine phosphatase 1B: a paradigm for inhibitor design. Proc Natl Acad Sci U S A 94:13420–5

Ramdas L, Obeyesekere NU, et al (1999) N-myristoylation of a peptide substrate for Src converts it into an apparent slow-binding bisubstrate-type inhibitor. J Pept Res 53:569–77

Ricouart A, Gesquiere JC, et al (1991) Design of potent protein kinase inhibitors using the bisubstrate approach. J Med Chem 34:73–8

Ross H, Armstrong CG, et al (2002) A non-radioactive method for the assay of many serine/threonine-specific protein kinases. Biochem J 366:977–81

Sasaki S, Hashimoto T, et al (1998) Design of new inhibitors for cdc2 kinase based on a multiple pseudosubstrate structure. Bioorg Med Chem Lett 8:1019–22

Scott JD, Fischer EH, et al (1985a) Identification of an inhibitory region of the heat-stable protein inhibitor of the cAMP-dependent protein kinase. Proc Natl Acad Sci U S A 82:4379-83

Scott JD, Fischer EH, et al (1985b) Amino acid sequence of the heat-stable inhibitor of the cAMP-dependent protein kinase from rabbit skeletal muscle. Proc Natl Acad Sci U S A 82:5732–6

Scott JD, Glaccum MB, et al (1986) Primary-structure requirements for inhibition by the heat-stable inhibitor of the cAMP-dependent protein kinase. Proc Natl Acad Sci U S A 83:1613–6

Scott JK, Smith GP (1990) Searching for peptide ligands with an epitope library. Science 249:386–90

Shen K, Keng YF, et al (2001) Acquisition of a specific and potent PTP1B inhibitor from a novel combinatorial library and screening procedure. J Biol Chem 276:47311–47319

Shoelson SE, White MF, et al (1989) Nonphosphorylatable substrate analogs selectively block autophosphorylation and activation of the insulin receptor, epidermal growth factor receptor, and pp60v-src kinases. J Biol Chem 264:7831–6

Smith GP, Scott JK (1993) Libraries of peptides and proteins displayed on filamentous phage. Methods Enzymol 217:228–57

Smothers JF, Henikoff S, et al (2002) Tech.Sight. Phage display. Affinity selection from biological libraries. Science 298:621–2

Smyth MS, Ford H, et al (1992) A general method for the preparation of benzylic alpha, alpha-difluorophosphonic acids; non-hydrolyzable mimetics of phosphotyrosine. Tetrahedron Lett 33:4137–40

Songyang Z, Shoelson SE, et al (1993) SH2 domains recognize specific phosphopeptide sequences. Cell 72:767–78

Songyang Z, Blechner S, et al (1994) Use of an oriented peptide library to determine the optimal substrates of protein kinases. Curr Biol 4:973–82

Songyang Z, Cantley LC (1998) The use of peptide library for the determination of kinase peptide substrates. Methods Mol Biol 87:87–98

Stankovic CJ, Surendranc N, et al (1997) The role of 4-phosphonodifluoromethyl- and 4-phosphonon-phenylalanine in the selectivity and cellular uptake of SH2 domain ligands. Bioorg Med Chem Lett 7:1909–14

Stanyon CA, Bernard O (1999) LIM-kinase1. Int J Biochem Cell Biol 31:389–94

Sugimoto S, Wandless TJ, et al (1994) Activation of the SH2-containing protein tyrosine phosphatase, SH-PTP2, by phosphotyrosine-containing peptides derived from insulin receptor substrate-1. J Biol Chem 269:13614–22

Tong L, Warren TC, et al (1996) Crystal structures of the human p56lck SH2 domain in complex with two short phosphotyrosyl peptides at 1.0 A and 1.8 A resolution. J Mol Biol 256:601–10

Tong L, Warren TC, et al (1998) Carboxymethyl-phenylalanine as a replacement for phosphotyrosine in SH2 domain binding. J Biol Chem 273:20238–42

Uri A, Raidaru G, et al (2002) Identification of the ability of highly charged nanomolar inhibitors of protein kinases to cross plasma membranes and carry a protein into cells. Bioorg Med Chem Lett 12:2117–20

Van Patten SM, Fletcher WH, et al (1986) The inhibitor protein of the cAMP-dependent protein kinase-catalytic subunit interaction. Parameters of complex formation. J Biol Chem 261:5514–23

Viht K, Padari K, et al (2003) Liquid-phase synthesis of a pegylated adenosine-oligoarginine conjugate, cell-permeable inhibitor of cAMP-dependent protein kinase. Bioorg Med Chem Lett 13:3035–9

Wang W, Ramdas L, et al (2000) Cyclic peptides incorporating 4-carboxyphenylalanine and phosphotyrosine are potent inhibitors of pp60(c-)(src). Biochemistry 39:5221–8

Ward NE, O'Brian AA (1993) Inhibition of protein kinase C by N-myristoylated peptide substrate analogs. Biochemistry 32:11903–9

Whitehouse S, Walsh DA (1983) Mg X ATP2-dependent interaction of the inhibitor protein of the cAMP-dependent protein kinase with the catalytic subunit. J Biol Chem 258:3682–92

Whitehouse S, Feramisco JR, et al (1983) Studies on the kinetic mechanism of the catalytic subunit of the cAMP-dependent protein kinase. J Biol Chem 258:3693–701

Wong TW, Goldberg AR (1984) Kinetics and mechanism of angiotensin phosphorylation by the transforming gene product of Rous sarcoma virus. J Biol Chem 259:3127–31

Wood J, Koszelak M, et al (1998) A caged protein kinase inhibitor. J Am Chem Soc 120:7145–7146

Wood JS, Yan X, et al (1996) Precision substrate targeting of protein kinases. The cGMP- and cAMP-dependent protein kinases. J Biol Chem 271:174–9

Wu J, Ma QN, et al (1994) Identifying substrate motifs of protein kinases by a random library approach. Biochemistry 33:14825–33

Wu J, Phan H, et al (1996) Development of a selective pseudosubstrate-based peptide inhibitor of $p60^{c\text{-}src}$. Lett Pept Sci 3:309–16

Xu Q, Zheng J, et al (1999) Flexibility of interdomain contacts revealed by topological isomers of bivalent consolidated ligands to the dual Src homology domain SH(32) of abelson. Biochemistry 38:3491–7

Yan X, Curley K, et al (2000) The specificity of the protein kinase C alpha, betaII and gamma isoforms as assessed by an unnatural alcohol-appended peptide library. Biochem J 349 Pt 3:709–15

Ye B, Akamatsu M, et al (1995) L-O-(2-malonyl)tyrosine: a new phosphotyrosyl mimetic for the preparation of Src homology 2 domain inhibitory peptides. J Med Chem 38:4270–5

Yeh RH, Lee TR, et al (2001) From consensus sequence peptide to high affinity ligand, a library scan strategy. J Biol Chem 276:12235–40

Yuan CJ, Jakes S, et al (1990) A rationale for the design of an inhibitor of tyrosyl kinase. J Biol Chem 265:16205–9

Zaliani A, Pinori M, et al (1998) The interaction of myristylated peptides with the catalytic domain of protein kinase C revealed by their sequence palindromy and the identification of a myristyl binding site. Protein Eng 11:803–10

Zhu H, Klemic JF, et al (2000) Analysis of yeast protein kinases using protein chips. Nat Genet 26:283–9

Part II

Pharmacological Potential and Inhibitors of Individual Classes of Protein Kinases

HEP (2005) 167:47–64

The Paullones: A Family of Pharmacological Inhibitors of Cyclin-Dependent Kinases and Glycogen Synthase Kinase 3

L. Meijer[1] (✉) · M. Leost[1] · O. Lozach[1] · S. Schmitt[1] · C. Kunick[2]

[1] C.N.R.S., Cell Cycle Group and UPS-2682, Station Biologique, B.P. 74, 29682 Roscoff cedex, Bretagne, France
meijer@sb-roscoff.fr
[2] Institut für Pharmazie, Universität Hamburg, Bundesstraße 45, 20146 Hamburg, Germany

Abstract Cyclin-dependent kinases (CDKs) regulate multiple pathways such as the cell division cycle, apoptosis, transcription, and neuronal functions. Glycogen synthase kinase 3 (GSK-3) plays a key role in Wnt signaling, cellular response to insulin, cell death, cell proliferation, maintenance of "stemness." Both families of kinases are clearly involved in the onset and development of major human diseases like cancer, neurodegenerative disorders (Alzheimer's and Parkinson's disease, stroke), diabetes, restenosis, viral infections, etc. Homologues of these kinases also regulate the proliferation of unicellular parasites. For these reasons an intensive search for pharmacological inhibitors of these protein kinases has been carried out during the last decade. Numerous small molecular weight compounds have been described that directly compete with ATP for binding to the catalytic site of the kinases. We here illustrate the development of this research area by reviewing the paullones, a family of potent and rather selective inhibitors of CDKs and GSK-3, from their discovery and optimisation to their molecular and cellular characterisation. The potential medical applications of CDK/GSK-3 inhibitors are presented.

Keywords Cyclin-dependent kinase · Glycogen synthase kinase · Cancer · Neurodegenerative disorders · Paullone · Malaria

Abbreviations

CDK	Cyclin-dependent kinase
CoMSIA	Comparative molecular similarity indices analysis
GSK-3	Glycogen synthase kinase 3
QSAR	Quantitative structure/activity relationship
MDH	Malate dehydrogenase
SAR	Structure/activity relationship

1 Introduction

1.1 Protein Kinases and Phosphatases

About 30% of human proteins contain covalently bound phosphate. Protein phosphorylation is considered one of the main post-translational mechanisms used by cells to finely tune their metabolic and regulatory pathways. Protein kinases catalyse the phosphorylation of serine, threonine and tyrosine residues of proteins, using ATP or guanosine triphosphate (GTP) as the phosphate donor, while protein phosphatases are responsible for dephosphorylation, the opposite reaction (Fig. 1). With the completion of the sequencing of several important genomes, we are starting to have a better view of the total range of kinases and phosphatases required in an organism. There are about 518+ kinases in man (Adams 2001; Krupa and Srinivasan 2002; Manning et al. 2002; Hanks 2003). Protein kinases are classified according to their primary sequence, the amino acids they target (tyrosine vs

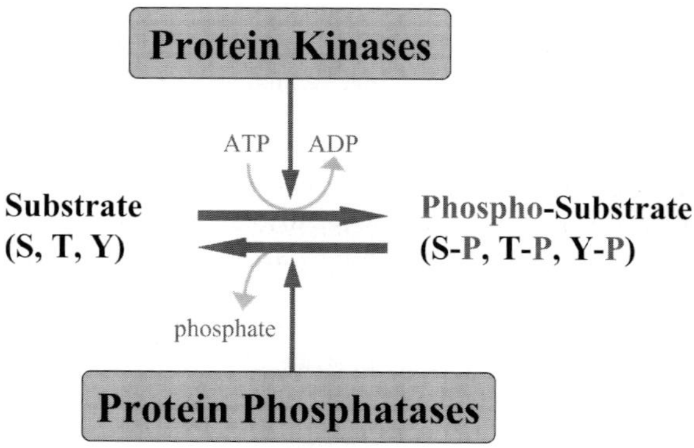

Fig. 1 Phosphorylation and dephosphorylation reactions are catalysed, respectively, by protein kinases and protein phosphatases

serine/threonine) and the nature of their activator. There are approximately 180 phosphatases in the human genome. Protein phosphatases are classified according to the amino acid they dephosphorylate (tyrosine or serine/threonine or dual-specificity phosphatases), and their sensitivity to various inhibitors and ions (PP1, PP2A, PP2B, PP2C) (Jackson and Denu 2001; Kennelly 2001; Sim and Ludowyke 2002; Lyon et al. 2002).

1.2
Protein Phosphorylation and Disease

In view of the importance of phosphorylation in essentially all physiological and cellular events, it is not surprising that abnormal phosphorylation turns out to be a cause or consequence of human disease. A number of diseases actually result from mutations in specific protein kinases and phosphatases (Cohen 2001; Cohen 2002). Of the kinase genes, 244 map to disease loci or cancer amplicons (Manning et al. 2002). In addition, many naturally occurring toxins also exert their effects by altering the phosphorylation state of proteins. Abnormal phosphorylation of proteins is now known to be closely associated with or even a cause of major diseases such as cancers, diabetes, rheumatoid arthritis, Alzheimer's disease, and Parkinson's disease.

These are the reasons why screening for and optimising potent and selective inhibitors of protein kinases and phosphatases has intensified over the last 10 years (review in Adams and Lee 1999; Garcia-Echeverria et al. 2000; Sridhar et al. 2000; Dumas 2001; Bridges 2001; Cohen 2002). However the idea that one could actually target kinases and phosphatases to develop drugs to treat disease was slow to develop. The discovery of the mechanism of action of cyclosporin, the immunosuppressive drug that made transplantation of organs possible, was a strong contributor to this development. Cyclosporin binds to a protein called cyclophilin. The cyclophilin/cyclosporin complex turned out to be a potent and specific inhibitor of PP2B, a calcium/calmodulin-dependent protein phosphatase. As one of the latest examples, the Novartis compound STI-571, or Gleevec, a potent inhibitor of the Abelson tyrosine kinase, has shown remarkable efficacy in human clinical trials against chronic myelocytic leukaemia (Capdeville et al. 2002a,b). At present, three kinase inhibitors have been approved for clinical use and more than 25 are undergoing clinical trials. The potential of pharmacological inhibitors of kinases and the current status of the inhibitors that are in clinical development have been recently reviewed (Cohen 2002).

1.3
Screening for Protein Kinase Inhibitors

Currently, all major pharmaceutical companies and many biotechnology start-ups run kinase screening assays. Briefly, the screening process involves six different steps (summarised in Doerig et al. 2002): (1) selecting a kinase as an appropriate and disease-relevant target, (2) expressing and purifying the kinase (either a recombinant, tagged enzyme or a native enzyme), (3) configuring the kinase assay using a convenient substrate, (4) assembling a library of compounds (synthetic or natural) or extracts of natural sources (plants, animals, microorganisms), (5) running the screen by assaying the kinase in the presence of the library compounds, (6) characterising the selectivity of the hits by secondary screens on additional targets (and perhaps also on the target cell/organism) and their mechanism of action (enzymology and crystallography approaches). This process is reiterated by synthesis of analogues and testing, leading to the optimisation of the chemical family [structure–activity relationship (SAR) studies], and ultimately allowing the synthesis of a lead compound which can be evaluated on cellular and animal models before clinical trials can be initiated.

In this chapter we would like to present an overview of the strategy developed to identify, optimise and characterise pharmacological inhibitors of two classes of disease-relevant kinases, namely the cyclin-dependent kinases (CDKs) and glycogen synthase kinase-3 (GSK-3). To avoid duplication with numerous reviews published elsewhere, we will here illustrate this field by reviewing a class of well-characterised inhibitors, the paullones.

2
CDKs and GSK-3 as Kinase Screening Targets

We have focused our screening efforts on two families of kinases, the CDKs and GSK-3, as well as *Pf*GSK-3, the GSK-3 homologue kinase in *Plasmodium falciparum* (the agent responsible for the lethal form of malaria) (Droucheau et al. 2004). CDKs are involved in controlling the cell cycle (CDK1, CDK2, CDK3, CDK4, CDK6, CDK7), apoptosis (CDK1, CDK2, CDK5), neuronal functions and neurodegeneration (CDK5, CDK11), transcription (CDK7, CDK8, CDK9) and exocytosis (review in Morgan 1997; Pavletich 1999; Malumbres et al. 2000; Dhavan and Tsai 2001; Harper and Adams 2001; Maccioni et al. 2001; Malumbres and Barbacid 2001; Knockaert et al. 2002a). GSK-3, an essential element of the Wnt signalling pathway, is involved in multiple physiological processes including cell cycle regulation by controlling the levels of cyclin D1 and β-catenin, dorso-ventral patterning during development, insulin action on glycogen synthesis, axonal outgrowth, HIV-1 Tat-mediated neurotoxicity, apoptosis, Alzheimer's disease characteristic phosphorylation of tau and amyloid-β production, and maintenance of "stemness" (review in Cohen and Frame 2001; Grimes and Jope 2001; Eldar-Finkelman 2002; Kaytor and Orr 2002; Doble and Woodgett 2003).

Potential applications of CDK/GSK-3 inhibitors are being evaluated for the treatment of cancers, neurodegenerative disorders such as Alzheimer's disease, Parkinson's disease and stroke, diabetes, restenosis, proliferation of protozoan parasites, and viral infections.

2.1 Kinase Purification and Assay

As a general rule, whenever possible, we are working with native enzymes purified from natural sources rather than with recombinant enzymes. Indeed, recombinant enzyme preparations are sometimes not very active and contain a significant proportion of misfolded, inactive, yet inhibitor-binding, enzyme. For this purpose we have developed several affinity purification methods that allow the easy purification of CDKs and GSK-3. CDK1/cyclin B is purified from starfish oocytes by affinity chromatography on immobilised $p9^{CKShs1}$ (Borgne and Meijer 1996). GSK-3α/β is purified from pork brain by affinity chromatography on an immobilised axin fragment (Primot et al. 2000) (Fig. 2).

Our kinase assays are based on the radioactive labelling of a substrate with ^{33}P from [γ-^{33}P]-ATP (Fig. 2). We are currently running our assays in a robotic system allowing the automated handling of liquid samples, in a 96-well format (Fig. 3). The use of a robotised set-up allows for the running of high numbers of compounds in duplicates and to cope with the generation of large quantities of data. Our 96-well plates are organised in a fairly standard way: 80 samples/plate, the first and last columns being occupied by positive and negative controls (non-inhibited enzyme, background and control in the presence of a potent and previously characterised inhibitor).

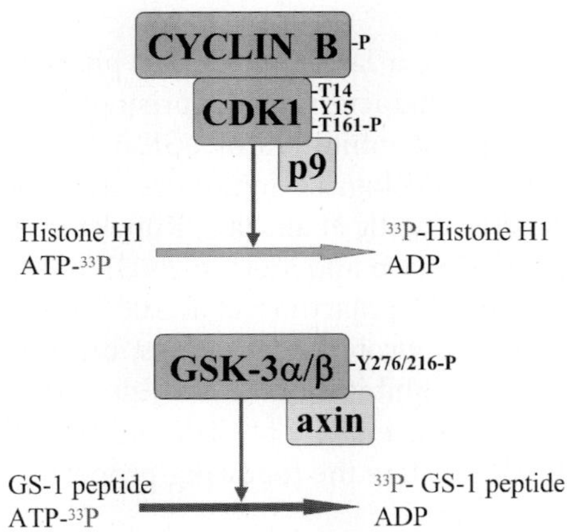

Fig. 2 Principle of the kinase assays. *Top*: active CDK1/cyclin B kinase is purified by affinity chromatography on $p9^{CKShs1}$-sepharose. It is assayed by measuring the incorporation of radioactive phosphate from radiolabelled ATP into the histone H1 substrate. *Bottom*: active GSK-3α/β is purified by affinity chromatography on axin-agarose. Its activity is measured using the GS-1 peptide as a substrate

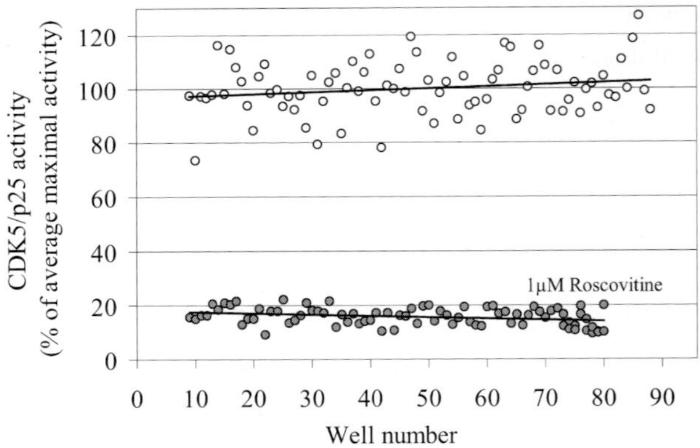

Fig. 3 Validation of the CDK5/p25 assay in a 96-well plate format. All wells, except those from the first and last columns, are filled with kinase assay mix. The kinase assays are run in the absence or presence of 1 μM roscovitine. The assay allows the unambiguous detection of an inhibitor

As a general rule we first screen the compounds in duplicates at a single concentration (10 μM for identified compounds; 10 μg/ml for extracts). Compounds are considered inactive when less than 50% inhibition is observed at this concentration. When a compound displays over 50% inhibition, a second run of assays is carried out to determine the IC_{50} value from dose–response curves.

2.2 Pharmacological Inhibitors of CDKs and GSK-3

Using these simple methods, a large number of pharmacological inhibitors have been discovered and characterised. Surprisingly many CDK inhibitors, but not all, are also excellent inhibitors of GSK-3 (Leclerc et al. 2001). The properties of these pharmacological inhibitors have been extensively reviewed both for CDKs (Hardcastle et al. 2002; Knockaert et al. 2002a; Sausville 2002; Fischer et al. 2003; Monaco and Vallano 2003) and for GSK-3 (Leclerc et al. 2001; Dorronsoro et al. 2002; Martinez et al. 2002; L. Meijer et al., in preparation). We will thus not duplicate these reviews, but instead summarise the properties shared by these inhibitors in a few lines and provide a more detailed review on the paullones, a family of CDK and GSK-3 dual inhibitors.

Essentially all inhibitors share the following properties:

- They are small molecular weight compounds (<600 Da).
- They are flat, rather hydrophobic, heterocycles.
- They act by competing with ATP for binding to the catalytic site of the kinase.

- They bind in the ATP-binding pocket, located between the small and large lobe of the kinase.
- The interactions with the kinase are predominantly hydrophobic and Van der Waals type.
- The inhibitors also bind through two or three hydrogen bonds with backbone atoms of leucine-83 and glutamic acid 81 (in CDK2) and the corresponding valine-135 and aspartic acid 133 in GSK-3 (Meijer et al. 2003).

3
Paullones as CDK and GSK-3 Inhibitors

3.1
Discovery of Paullones

The National Cancer Institute (NCI) Human Tumor Cell Line Anti-Cancer Drug Screen was established in the late 1980s with the purpose of identifying new anti-cancer drugs (review in Monks et al. 1997). To date the antiproliferative activity of over 70,000 compounds has been measured on the 60 human tumour cell lines panel. Dr. Kenneth Paull conceived a computerised pattern-recognition algorithm, named COMPARE, to allow the identification of new chemotypes that can act through a cellular target similar to that of a reference or "seed" compound (Paull 1992, 1995). In 1997 we used COM-

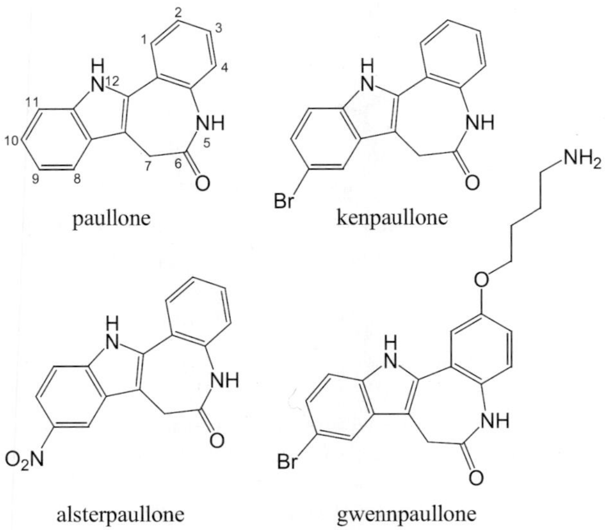

Fig. 4 Chemical structure of the most frequently used paullones. The description of their synthesis has been described in detail: paullone (Kunick 1992), kenpaullone (Kunick 1992; Schultz et al. 1999), alsterpaullone (Schultz et al. 1999), gwennpaullone (Wieking et al. 2002)

PARE with the CDK inhibitor flavopiridol (NSC-649890) as a reference to identify compounds in the NCI collection that might act through CDK inhibition (Zaharevitz 1999). The highest COMPARE correlation coeffi-cient (0.67) was found to be with another CDK inhibitor, olomoucine (NSC-666096) (Vesely et al. 1994). Among five other compounds displaying a correlation coefficient with flavopiridol superior to 0.60, one compound (NSC-664704) was by far the most active against CDK1/cyclin B (IC_{50}: 0.4 μM). This benzazepinone, 9-bromo-7,12-dihydro-indolo[3,2-*d*]benzazepin-6(5H)-one (Fig. 4), had been synthesised earlier by one of us (Kunick 1992). We renamed it kenpaullone to honour the memory of Dr. Kenneth Paull. Paullone was the name given to the unsubstituted ring structure.

3.2 Molecular Mechanism of Interaction of Paullones with Kinases—Structure/Activity Relationship Studies

Kinetic studies revealed that paullones inhibit kinases by competition with ATP for binding to the catalytic site (Zaharevitz et al. 1999). Since the initial

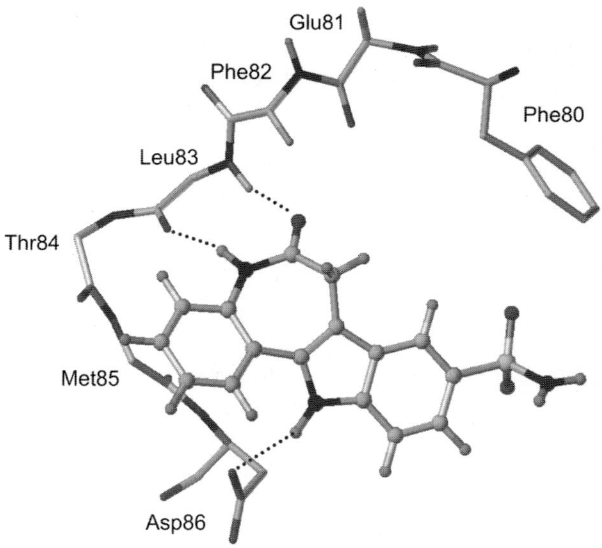

Fig. 5 Hydrogen bonds between CDK1/cyclin B and a 9-sulphamoyl-substituted paullone docked to the ATP-binding pocket. This illustration was created using SYBYL (Version 6.7, Tripos Inc. St. Louis, Missouri 63144, USA), employing the CDK1/cyclin B homology model developed by R. Gussio (Gussio et al. 2000). The manual docking and the subsequent minimisation process, performed using the MAB force field implemented in the program MOLOC (Gerber 1998), were carried out by T. Lemcke, University of Hamburg. To improve clarity of the illustration, the side chains of the amino acids glutamic acid-81 through methionine-85 are not depicted. The *dotted lines* represent the hydrogen bonds formed between the paullone molecule and the amino acids leucine-83 and aspartic acid-86. (This figure comes from the dissertation thesis of T. Pies)

discovery of paullones, more than 60 analogues have been synthesised, leading to compounds active in the nanomolar range (Schultz et al. 1999; Kunick et al. 2000; Leost et al. 2000). In addition, this SAR study has provided some information on the mechanism of interaction of paullones with their kinase targets. Recently, 3D-QSAR CoMSIA models were developed for the inhibition of CDK1/cyclin B, CDK5/p25 and GSK-3β by the paullones family (Kunick et al. 2004). The models were based on the kinase inhibition data of 52 paullones, docked into the ATP-binding site of a CDK1 homology model (Gussio et al. 2000) (Fig. 5). Recently, alsterpaullone has also been crystallised with GSK-3β (Bertrand et al. 2003). The co-crystal structure confirms that alsterpaullone is binding in the ATP-binding pocket. The interactions include hydrogen bonds with aspartic acid 133 and valine 135, as observed for other inhibitors recently crystallised with GSK-3β, 6-bromo-indirubin-3′-oxime (Meijer et al. 2003), indirubin-3′-oxime, I-5 and staurosporine (Bertrand et al. 2003) and the thiazole AR-A014418 (Bhat et al. 2003) (see review in Fischer 2003).

3.3 Selectivity of Paullones

Running the initial hits on a small panel of 25 enzymes provided a first view on the selectivity of paullones as shown in Table 1. Clearly paullones appear to be rather specific inhibitors (when compared with staurosporine or flavopiridol, for example) which display exquisite selectivity for CDKs (Schultz et al. 1999; Zaharevitz et al. 1999) and GSK-3 (Leost et al. 2000). Using a set of 28 kinases, Bain et al. (2003) confirmed the CDK/GSK-3 selectivity of paullones and showed that the src-family tyrosine kinase LCK was somewhat sensitive to paullones, and, surprisingly, that kenpaullone was more selective than alsterpaullone. It was suggested that the use of roscovitine (Meijer et al. 1997) and kenpaullone may be useful for identifying substrates and functions of CDKs, while the combined use of kenpaullone and lithium may be useful for identifying substrates and functions of GSK-3 (Bain et al. 2003).

However, this time- and money-consuming kinase panel approach has also strong limitations, since most existing kinases (518+) have not been tested. Other potential, non-kinase, targets are not even considered. This is why we recently developed an affinity chromatography method using immobilised compound to "fish out" the real targets of a defined compound (Fig. 6) (Knockaert et al. 2002b; Knockaert and Meijer 2002). This method has also been illustrated recently with the p38 kinase inhibitor SB 203580 (Godl et al. 2003).

Gwennpaullone was thus covalently bound to agarose beads, and extracts of various cell types and tissues were run on this matrix. Bound proteins were analysed by sodium dodecyl sulphate polyacrylamide gel electrophoresis (SDS-PAGE) followed by Western blotting and microsequencing of inter-

Table 1 Investigation of the selectivity of paullones by the classical "enzyme panel" method. Kenpaullone and alsterpaullone are tested for their effects on a series of purified kinases and their IC_{50} values (expressed in μM) are determined from the dose–response curves. A ranking, in accordance with IC_{50} values, highlights the inhibition potency of the paullones on various kinases

Protein kinases	Ken paullone Inhibition potency	Alster paullone Inhibition potency
GSK-3β	0.023	0.004
CDK1/cyclin B	0.40	0.035
CDK2/cyclin A	0.68	0.015
CDK4/cyclin D1	>100	>10.0
CDK5/p25	0.85	0.040
erk1	20.0	22.0
erk2	9.0	4.5
c-raf	38.0	10–100
MAPKK	>100	>100
c-Jun N-terminal kinase	>100	10–100
Protein kinase C α	>100	>100
Protein kinase C β1	>100	>100
Protein kinase C β2	>100	>100
Protein kinase C γ	>100	>100
Protein kinase C δ	>100	>100
Protein kinase C ϵ	>100	>100
Protein kinase C η	>100	>100
Protein kinase C ζ	>100	>100
cAMP-dependent PK	>100	7
cGMP-dependent PK	>100	>100
Casein kinase 1	>100	>100
Casein kinase 2	20.0	>100
Insulin receptor Tyr kinase	>100	>100
c-src	15.0	n.t.
v-abl	>100	n.t.

n.t., Not tested.

nal peptides. This analysis confirmed that GSK-3α and GSK-3β are prominent targets of paullones. Quite unexpectedly, mitochondrial malate dehydrogenase (MDH) was found to bind to the paullone matrix. This was observed with various biological sources ranging from sea urchin eggs, *Xenopus* oocytes, mammalian brain and various cell lines, to unicellular parasites (*Leishmania*).

MDH catalyses the conversion of malate into oxaloacetate. It plays a role in a variety of essential metabolic pathways such as the citric acid (Krebs) cycle, the tricarboxylic acid cycle, gluconeogenesis and amino acid synthesis. Paullones inhibit purified MDH by competing with NAD (Knockaert et al. 2002b). The interaction of paullones with MDH may contribute to the anti-mitotic properties of these compounds, although this needs to be investigated. In this respect, one of the targets of E7070, a sulphonamide com-

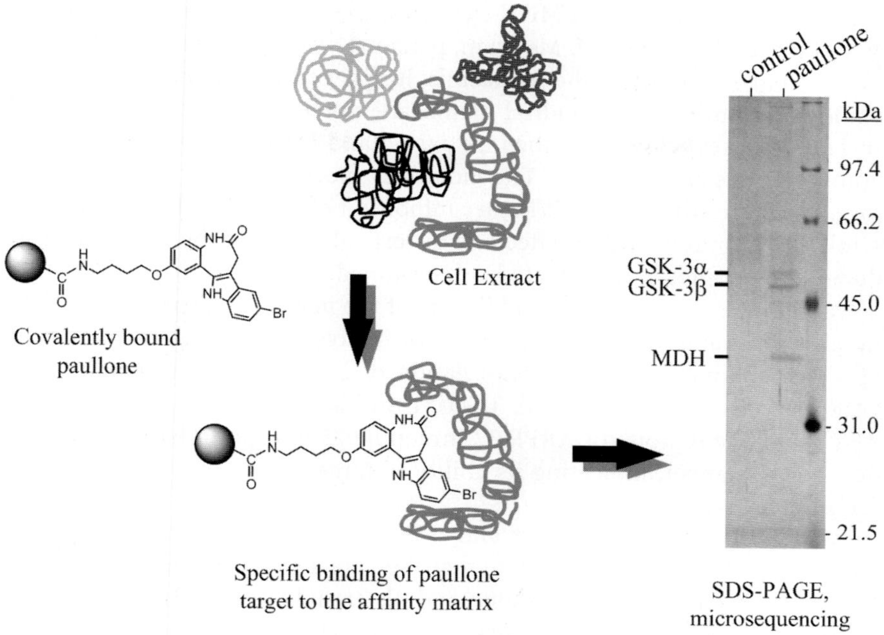

Fig. 6 Affinity chromatography purification of paullone targets. Gwennpaullone is immobilised to agarose beads. Cell extracts are incubated with this matrix as well as a control matrix. After extensive washing, the matrix-bound proteins are resolved by sodium dodecyl sulphate polyacrylamide gel electrophoresis (SDS-PAGE) and silver-stained. The proteins are then excised from the gel and identified by microsequencing of internal peptides. (Aadapted from Knockaert and Meijer 2002)

pound currently undergoing phase II clinical trials against cancer, was recently identified as cytosolic MDH (Oda et al. 2003). E7070 is suggested to act by competing with NADH binding. Cytosolic and mitochondrial MDH may thus constitute new targets for drugs with anti-tumour properties.

3.4 Cellular Effects of Paullones

Paullones have been tested as potential anti-tumour agents. They indeed inhibit mammalian cell proliferation in culture (Schultz et al. 1999; Zaharevitz et al. 1999; Gussio et al. 2000) with an accumulation of cells both in G1 and G2, as would be expected from an inhibition of both CDK1 and CDK2. However, the fact that paullones inhibit CDKs in vivo still remains to be demonstrated. Paullones also inhibit the proliferation of *Leishmania mexicana* (Knockaert et al. 2002). Two potential targets were purified from this unicellular parasite using gwennpaullone agarose beads, and one of them was identified as mitochondrial MDH (Knockaert et al. 2002), the other as a new MAP kinase-like protein (J. Mottram, personal communication).

A recent study using the leukaemia Jurkat cell line showed that alsterpaullone perturbs mitochondrial membrane potential, induces activation of several caspases (caspase-9, then caspase-8 and caspase-3) and triggers apoptosis (Lahusen et al. 2003). The molecular mechanisms beyond this apoptosis effect are still unclear. Whether inhibition of mitochondrial MDH plays a role in the mitochondrial effects of alsterpaullone, and the subsequent induction of apoptosis, remains to be determined.

Paullones are rather potent inhibitors of the nervous system kinase CDK5 in vitro. To evaluate whether this was true in vivo, we investigated the effects of alsterpaullone on the phosphorylation of DARPP-32 on threonine 75, a CDK5-selective site (Bibb et al. 1999), using isolated brain striatum slices. Alsterpaullone inhibited DARPP-32 threonine 75 phosphorylation in a dose-dependent manner, indicating its ability to target CDK5 in a cellular setting (Leost et al. 2000).

As described above, GSK-3α and GSK-3β are also two major targets of paullones in vitro. To demonstrate that they are also in vivo targets, we have analysed the effects of kenpaullone and alsterpaullone on SH-SY5Y cells in culture (Fig. 7). As expected, kenpaullone and alsterpaullone, even more potently, induce an accumulation of β-catenin, a direct consequence of its stabilisation by dephosphorylation. Increased dephospho-β-catenin (detected with an antibody that cross-reacts with β-catenin only when it is not phosphory-

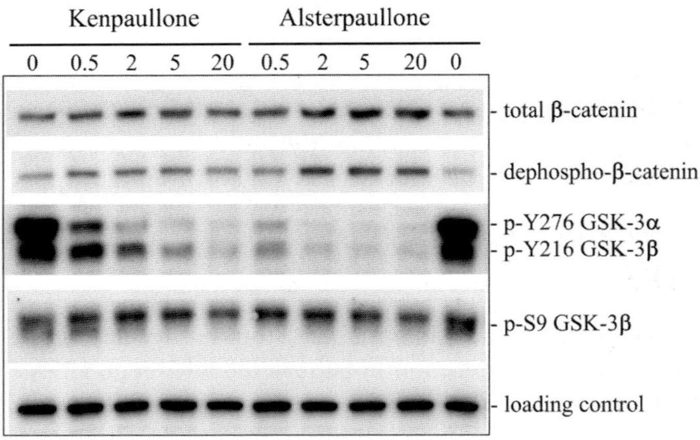

Fig. 7 Paullones are selective GSK-3 inhibitors in cell cultures. SH-SY5Y cells were untreated (*0*) or exposed to 0.5–20 μM kenpaullone or alsterpaullone for 24 h. Proteins were then separated by SDS-PAGE followed by Western blotting with antibodies directed (*top to bottom*) against β-catenin, dephospho-β-catenin, phospho-tyrosine 276 (GSK-3α)/-tyrosine 216 (GSK-3β), phospho-serine 9 GSK-3 and a loading control (non-specific band detected with the dephospho-β-catenin). (Courtesy of Dr. Xiaozhou P. Ryan)

lated on GSK-3 specific sites) is also seen with both paullones. Finally, both paullones inhibit the phosphorylation of GSK-3α and GSK-3β on tyrosine 276 and tyrosine 216, respectively. Phosphorylation of these sites is directly involved in GSK-3 activation, and their inhibition by paullones (through a yet-unknown mechanism) further contributes to GSK-3 inhibition.

Recently, the GSK-3 inhibitory property of kenpaullone has been used to support data demonstrating that GSK-3α regulates the production of amyloid-β peptides (Phiel et al. 2003). Amyloid-β peptides derive from the amyloid precursor protein through the proteolytic action of β- and γ-secretases. Amyloid-β peptides accumulate and aggregate in Alzheimer's disease, and the formation of amyloid plaques is thought to play a major role in the development of the disease (De Strooper and Woodgett 2003). Very interestingly, both lithium (millimolar concentrations), a classical inhibitor of GSK-3, and kenpaullone (micromolar concentrations), but not roscovitine (inactive on GSK-3), inhibit the production of amyloid-β peptides in cell lines (Phiel et al. 2003). Depletion of GSK-3α by RNAi together with overexpression studies confirm that GSK-3α is required for the generation of amyloid-β peptides.

Hyperphosphorylation of the microtubule-binding protein tau, and its subsequent aggregation in paired helical filaments (neurofibrillary tangles) is also a landmark of Alzheimer's disease (De Strooper and Woodgett 2003). GSK-3 and CDK5 are two major kinases implicated in abnormal tau hyperphosphorylation. Using Sf9 cells overexpressing human tau, we found that alsterpaullone is able to inhibit tau phosphorylation on epitopes which represent major GSK-3 phosphorylation sites detected in Alzheimer's disease (cross-reacting with PHF-1 and AT100 antibodies) (Leost 2000).

3.5 Future Development of Paullones

Although numerous analogues of paullones have been synthesised, there is probably space for improvement in both efficacy and selectivity. This would be greatly guided by the co-crystallisation of paullones with a CDK or GSK-3. Hopefully paullones can be designed that are mono-specific for CDKs, GSK-3 or MDH inhibition. This will then allow us to relate the observed cellular effects of paullones to inhibition of a specific molecular target.

Paullones also need to be improved with respect to their solubility. Indeed, like most kinase inhibitors, paullones bind by hydrophobic interactions within the ATP-binding pocket of kinases. They are thus quite hydrophobic and therefore poorly soluble in aqueous media. As this problem could seriously preclude their clinical development, ways to improve the solubility of paullones must be identified. There are several possible solutions, such as the development of water-soluble analogues, nano-encapsulation, insertion into liposomes, and the formation of water-soluble pro-drugs.

4 Conclusion

The identification of paullones as a family of CDK inhibitors has been followed by several unexpected findings, specifically their stronger affinity for GSK-3, and their interactions with mitochondrial MDH. This, in fact, has opened the way to alternative applications beyond the initial anti-cancer application (Zaharevitz et al. 1999), which had not been initially predicted, namely the use against neurodegenerative disorders. As CDK/GSK-3 dual specificity inhibitors, paullones could be highly advantageous, since both CDK5/p25 (Cruz et al. 2003; Noble et al. 2003) and GSK-3 (Caricasole 2003; De Strooper and Woodgett 2003; Phiel et al. 2003) have been shown to play essential roles in the development of Alzheimer's disease. CDK5 has also been shown to mediate dopaminergic neuron loss in Parkinson's disease (Smith et al. 2003). Recently modulation of *N*-methyl-d-aspartate receptors by CDK5 has been shown to represent a primary event underlying the ischaemic injury of CA1 pyramidal neurons as observed in stroke (Wang et al. 2003). Therefore CDK inhibitors like paullones may have an input in the treatment of Parkinson's disease and stroke as well. Finally, as GSK-3-selective drugs, paullones may find applications in the treatment of diabetes type 2 and as a tool to maintain undifferentiated embryonic stem cells (Sato et al. 2004).

Acknowledgements This research was supported by the "Association pour la Recherche sur le Cancer" (L.M.) and the Ministère de la Recherche/INSERM/CNRS "Molécules et Cibles Thérapeutiques" Programme. This review was written during a sabbatical leave at Rockefeller University, in the laboratory of Paul Greengard, who is warmly acknowledged. Supported by CNRS, Rockefeller University and NATO.

References

Adams JA (2001) Kinetic and catalytic mechanisms of protein kinases. Chem Rev 101:2271–2290

Adams JL, Lee D (1999) Recent progress towards the identification of selective inhibitors of serine/threonine protein kinases. Curr Opin Drug Discov Devel 2:96–109

Bain J, McLauchlan H, Elliott M, et al (2003) The specificities of protein kinase inhibitors: an update. Biochem J 371:199–204

Bertrand JA, Thieffine S, Vulpetti A, et al (2003) Structural characterization of the GSK-3β active site using selective and non-selective ATP-mimetic inhibitors. J Mol Biol 333:393–407

Bhat R, Xue Y, Berg S, et al (2003) Structural insights and biological effects of glycogen synthase kinase 3-specific inhibitor AR-A014418. J Biol Chem 278:45937–45945

Bibb JA, Snyder GL, Nishi A, Yan Z, Meijer L, Fienberg AA, Tsai LH, Kwon YT, Girault JA, Czernik AJ, Huganir RL, Hemmings HC Jr, Nairn AC, Greengard P (1999) Phosphorylation of DARPP-32 by Cdk5 modulates dopamine signalling in neurons. Nature 402:669–671

Borgne A, Meijer L (1996) Sequential dephosphorylation of p34(cdc2) on Thr-14 and Tyr-15 at the prophase/metaphase transition. J Biol Chem 271:27847–27854

Bridges AJ (2001) Chemical inhibitors of protein kinases. Chem Rev 101:2541–2571

Capdeville R, Silberman S, Dimitrijevic S (2002a) Imatinib: the first 3 years. Eur J Cancer 38(Suppl 5):77–82

Capdeville R, Buchdunger E, Zimmermann J, et al (2002b) Glivec (STI571, imatinib), a rationally developed, targeted anticancer drug. Nat Rev Drug Discov 1:493–502

Caricasole A (2003) The Wnt pathway, cell-cycle activation and beta-amyloid: novel therapeutic strategies in Alzheimer's disease? Trends Pharmacol Sci 24:233–238

Cohen P (2001) The role of protein phosphorylation in human health and disease. The Sir Hans Krebs Medal Lecture. Eur J Biochem 268:5001–5010

Cohen P (2002) Protein kinases—the major drug targets of the twenty-first century? Nat Rev Drug Discov 1:309–315

Cohen P, Frame S (2001) The renaissance of GSK3. Nat Rev Mol Cell Biol 2:769–776

Cruz JC, Tseng HC, Goldman JA, et al (2003) Aberrant Cdk5 activation by p25 triggers pathological events leading to neurodegeneration and neurofibrillary tangles. Neuron 40:471–483

De Strooper B, Woodgett J (2003) Alzheimer's disease: mental plaque removal. Nature 423:392–393

Dhavan R, Tsai L-H (2001) A decade of CDK5. Nat Rev Mol Cell Biol 2:749–759

Doble BW, Woodgett JR (2003) GSK-3: tricks of the trade for a multi-tasking kinase. J Cell Sci 116:1175–1186

Doerig C, Meijer L, Mottram J (2002) Protein kinases as drug targets in parasitic protozoa. Trends Parasitol 18:366–371

Dorronsoro I, Castro A, Martinez A (2002) Inhibitors of glycogen synthase kinase-3: future therapy for unmet medical needs? Expert Opin Ther Patents 12:1527–1536

Droucheau E, Primot A, Thomas V, Mattei D, Knockaert M, Richardson C, Sallicandro P, Alano P, Jafarshad A, Baratte B, Kunick C, Parzy D, Pearl L, Doerig C, Meijer L (2004) Plasmodium falciparum glycogen synthase kinase-3: molecular model, expression, intracellular localisation and selective inhibitors. Biochim Biophys Acta 1697:181–96

Dumas J (2001) Protein kinase inhibitors: emerging pharmacophores 1997–2000. Expert Opin Ther Patents 11:405–429

Eldar-Finkelman H (2002) Glycogen synthase kinase 3: an emerging therapeutic target. Trends Mol Med 8:126–132

Fischer PM (2003) CDK versus GSK-3 inhibition: a purple haze no longer? Chem Biol 10:1144–1146

Fischer PM, Endicott J, Meijer L (2003) Cyclin-dependent kinase inhibitors. Prog Cell Cycle Res 5:235–248

Garcia-Echeverria C, Traxler P, Evans DB (2000) ATP site-directed competitive and irreversible inhibitors of protein kinases. Med Res Rev 20:28–57

Gerber PR (1998) Charge distribution from a simple molecular orbital type calculation and non-bonding interaction terms in the force field MAB. J Comput Aided Mol Des 12:37–51

Godl K, Wissing J, Kurtenbach A, et al (2003) An efficient proteomics method to identify the cellular targets of protein kinase inhibitors. Proc Natl Acad Sci USA 100:15434–15439

Grimes CA, Jope RS (2001) The multifaceted roles of glycogen synthase kinase 3beta in cellular signaling. Prog Neurobiol 65:391–426

Gussio R, Zaharevitz D, McGrath CF, et al (2000) Structure-based design modifications of the paullone molecular scaffold for cyclin-dependent kinase inhibition. Anticancer Drug Des 15: 53–66

Hanks SK (2003) Genomic analysis of the eukaryotic protein kinase superfamily: a perspective. Genome Biol 4:111:1–7

Hardcastle IR, Golding BT, Griffin RJ (2002) Designing inhibitors of cyclin-dependent kinases. Annu Rev Pharmacol Toxicol 42:325–348

Harper JW, Adams PD (2001) Cyclin-dependent kinases. Chem Rev 101:2511–2526

Jackson MD, Denu JM (2001) Molecular reactions of protein phosphatases–insights from structure and chemistry. Chem Rev 101:2313–2340

Kaytor MD, Orr HT (2002) The GSK3 beta signaling cascade and neurodegenerative disease. Curr Opin Neurobiol 12:275–278

Kennelly PJ (2001) Protein phosphatases–a phylogenetic perspective. Chem Rev 101:2291–2312

Knockaert M, Meijer L (2002) Identifying in vivo targets of cyclin-dependent kinase inhibitors by affinity chromatography. Biochem Pharmacol 64:819–825

Knockaert M, Greengard P, Meijer L (2002a) Pharmacological inhibitors of cyclin-dependent kinases. Trends Pharmacol Sci 23:417–425

Knockaert M, Viking K, Schmitt S (2002b) Intracellular targets of paullones. Identification following affinity purification on immobilized inhibitor. J Biol Chem 277:25493–25501

Krupa A, Srinivasan N (2002) The repertoire of protein kinases encoded in the draft version of the human genome: atypical variations and uncommon domain combinations. Genome Biol 3:Research0066.1–006614

Kunick C (1992) Synthese von 7,12-Dihydro-indolo[3,2-*d*][1]benzazepin-6-(5 *H*)-onen und 6,11-Dihydro-thieno-[3',2':2,3]azepino[4,5-*b*]indol-5(4 *H*)-on. Arch Pharm (Weinheim) 325:297–299

Kunick C, Schultz C, Lemcke T (2000) 2-Substituted paullones: CDK1/cyclin B-inhibiting property and in vitro antiproliferative activity. Bioorg Med Chem Lett 10:567–569

Kunick C, Lauenroth K, Wieking K, et al (2004) Evaluation and comparison of 3D-QSAR-models for CDK1, CDK5 and GSK-3 inhibition by paullones. J Med Chem 47:22–36

Lahusen T, De Siervi A, Kunick C (2003) Alsterpaullone, a novel cyclin-dependent kinase inhibitor, induces apoptosis by activation of caspase-9 due to perturbation in mitochondrial membrane potential. Mol Carcinog 36:183–194

Leclerc S, Garnier M, Hoessel R (2001) Indirubins inhibit glycogen synthase kinase-3 beta and CDK5/p25, two protein kinases involved in abnormal tau phosphorylation in Alzheimer's disease. A property common to most cyclin-dependent kinase inhibitors? J Biol Chem 276:251–260

Leost M, Schultz C, Link A (2000) Paullones are potent inhibitors of glycogen synthase kinase-3beta and cyclin-dependent kinase 5/p25. Eur J Biochem 267:5983–5994

Lyon MA, Ducruet AP, Wipf P, et al (2002) Dual-specificity phosphatases as targets for antineoplastic agents. Nat Rev Drug Discov 1:961–976

Maccioni RB, Otth C, Concha II, et al (2001) The protein kinase Cdk5. Structural aspects, roles in neurogenesis and involvement in Alzheimer's pathology. Eur J Biochem 268:1518–1527

Malumbres M, Barbacid M (2001) To cycle or not to cycle: a critical decision in cancer. Nat Rev Cancer 1:222–231

Malumbres M, Ortega S, Barbacid M (2000) Genetic analysis of mammalian cyclin-dependent kinases and their inhibitors. Biol Chem 381:827–838

Manning G, Whyte DB, Martinez R, et al (2002) The protein kinase complement of the human genome. Science 298:1912–1934

Martinez A, Castro A, Dorronsoro I, et al (2002) Glycogen synthase kinase 3 (GSK-3) inhibitors as new promising drugs for diabetes, neurodegeneration, cancer, and inflammation. Med Res Rev 22:373–384

Meijer L, Borgne A, Mulner O, et al (1997) Biochemical and cellular effects of roscovitine, a potent and selective inhibitor of the cyclin-dependent kinases cdc2, cdk2 and cdk5. Eur J Biochem 243: 527–536

Meijer L, Skaltsounis AL, Magiatis P, et al (2003) GSK-3 selective inhibitors derived from Tyrian purple indirubins. Chem Biol 10: 1–12

Monaco EA 3rd, Vallano ML (2003) Cyclin-dependent kinase inhibitors: cancer killers to neuronal guardians. Curr Med Chem 10:367–379

Monks A, Scudiero DA, Johnson GS, et al (1997) The NCI anti-cancer drug screen: a smart screen to identify effectors of novel targets. Anti-Cancer Drug Des 12:533–541

Morgan D (1997) Cyclin-dependent kinases: engines, clocks, and microprocessors. Annu Rev Cell Dev Biol 13:261–291

Noble W, Olm V, Takata K, et al (2003) Cdk5 is a key factor in tau aggregation and tangle formation in vivo. Neuron 38:555–565

Oda Y, Owa T, Sato T, et al (2003) Quantitative chemical proteomics for identifying candidate drug targets. Anal Chem 75:2159–2165

Paull KD (1992) Identification of novel antimitotic agents acting at the tubulin level by computer-assisted evaluation of differential cytotoxicity data. Cancer Res 52:3892–3900

Paull KD (1995) Prediction of biochemical mechanism of action from the in vitro antitumor screen of the National Cancer Institute. In: Foye WO (ed) Cancer Chemotherapeutic Agents. American Chemical Society Books, Washington, pp 8–45

Pavletich NP (1999) Mechanisms of cyclin-dependent kinase regulation: structures of Cdks, their cyclin activators, and Cip and INK4 inhibitors. J Mol Biol 287:821–828

Phiel CJ, Wilson CA, Lee VM, et al (2003) GSK-3alpha regulates production of Alzheimer's disease amyloid-beta peptides. Nature 423:435–439

Primot A, Baratte B, Gompel M, et al (2000) Purification of GSK-3 by affinity chromatography on immobilized axin. Protein Expr Purif 20:394–404

Sausville EA (2002) Complexities in the development of cyclin-dependent kinase inhibitor drugs. Trends Mol Med 8:S32–S37

Schultz C, Link A, Leost M, et al (1999) Paullones, a series of cyclin-dependent kinase inhibitors: synthesis, evaluation of CDK1/cyclin B inhibition, and in vitro antitumor activity. J Med Chem 42:2909–2919

Sim AT, Ludowyke RI (2002) The complex nature of protein phosphatases. IUBMB Life 53:283–286

Smith PD, Crocker SJ, Jackson-Lewis V, et al (2003) Cyclin-dependent kinase 5 is a mediator of dopaminergic neuron loss in a mouse model of Parkinson's disease. Proc Natl Acad Sci USA 100:13650–13655

Sridhar R, Hanson-Painton O, Cooper DR (2000) Protein kinases as therapeutic targets. Pharm Res 17:1345–1353

Vesely J, Havlicek L, Strnad M, et al (1994) Inhibition of cyclin-dependent kinases by purine analogues. Eur J Biochem 224:771–786

Wang J, Liu SH, Fu YP, et al (2003) Cdk5 activation induces hippocampal CA1 cell death by directly phosphorylating NMDA receptors. Nat Neurosci 6:1039–1047

Wieking K, Knockaert M, Leost M, et al (2002) Synthesis of paullones with aminoalkyl side chains. Arch Pharm (Weinheim) 335:311–317

Zaharevitz D, Gussio R, Leost M, et al (1999) Discovery and initial characterization of the paullones, a novel class of small-molecule inhibitors of cyclin-dependent kinases. Cancer Res 59:2566–2569

HEP (2005) 167:65–83

Pharmacological Potential of p38 MAPK Inhibitors

S. Kumar (✉) · S. M. Blake

GlaxoSmithKline, UP1340, 1250 South Collegeville Rd., P.O. Box 5089, Collegeville, PA 19426-0989, USA
sanjay.2.kumar@gsk.com

Abstract A key component of the intracellular signaling pathways involved in cellular response to environmental stress and inflammatory cytokines is the p38 family of mitogen-activated protein kinases (MAPKs). Of the four isoforms of the p38 family of MAPKs identified thus far, p38α is the most characterized enzyme. Since the discovery of p38α MAPK as a target of a series of compounds that inhibited the production of inflammatory cytokines, an intense effort has been applied to further identify, develop, and refine highly potent and selective inhibitors of this enzyme. In addition, availability of p38α MAPK inhibitors has allowed the investigators to dissect this signaling pathway and to examine its role in various pathologies. A large body of biochemical as well as genetic evidence indicates a critical role of p38α MAPK in both the production of inflammatory cytokines such as interleukin (IL)-1 and tumor necrosis factor (TNF) and subsequent signaling initiated in response to these cytokines. This suggests that inhibition of p38α MAPK pathway will have utility in pathological settings where tissue inflammation and pro-inflammatory cytokines have been implicated. Indeed, several p38α MAPK inhibitors have been shown to be efficacious in preclinical animal models of a variety of diseases, including rheumatoid arthritis, pulmonary diseases, neuronal protection, and cancer. In the past few years, several groups have advanced inhibitors into early clinical studies for rheumatoid arthritis, but none thus far has reached the critical phase III efficacy stage. In this chapter, we review the p38 MAPK pathway and pharmacological potential of p38α MAPK inhibitors in various pathologies with particular emphasis on inflammatory diseases.

Keywords p38 MAPK · Inhibitors · Inflammation · Interleukin 1 · Tumor necrosis factor · Cytokines · Rheumatoid arthritis · Respiratory · Neuronal

1 Introduction

The ability of living cells to respond to the multitude of signals emanating from its environment rests with a variety of signaling pathways inside the cell. The components involved and their assembly in a pathway are dependent upon the type, duration, and magnitude of the signal and ensure the appropriate integrating and processing of the signal resulting in a stimulus-specific response. One of the major intracellular signaling pathways is the mitogen-activated protein kinase (MAPK) pathway. A central component of this pathway is the MAPKs. The MAPK signaling cascade consists of three protein kinases (Pearson et al. 2001), MAPK and two upstream components, MAPK kinase (MAPKK or MKK) and MAPKK kinase (MAPKKK) (Fig. 1). Three MAPK pathways have so far been described in mammalian cells. The first to be discovered was the extracellular signal-related kinases, ERK1 and ERK2. Subsequently, c-jun amino terminal kinase (JNK) and p38 MAPK

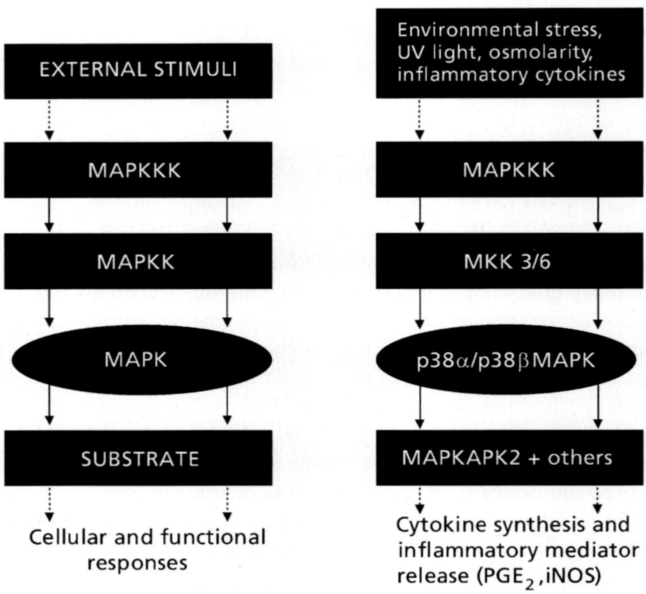

Fig. 1 p38 MAPK pathways with activators and substrates

were described. These kinases exhibit between 60% and 70% amino acid identity to one another. Differences have been demonstrated in the sequence and size of their activation loop as well as their responsiveness to different stimuli. Each of the MAPK sub-families has been shown to consist of multiple isoforms and sub-family members. Activation of the kinases occurs through the dual phosphorylation of Thr and Tyr residues in a "TXY" motif (X being Glu, Pro or Gly in ERKs, JNKs and p38 respectively) by a dual specificity MAPKK (Pearson et al. 2001). A serine threonine kinase, MAPKKK, is responsible for the phosphorylation of MAPKK. As previously stated, the MAPK can be differentiated by their responsiveness to stimuli. In general, the ERKs have been shown to respond to mitogenic and proliferative stimuli, whereas the JNKs and p38 MAPKs respond to environmental stresses such as UV light, heat, osmotic shock and exposure to inflammatory cytokines (Pearson et al. 2001).

The elucidation of the p38 MAPK pathway began almost a decade ago, when the murine p38 was identified as a major phosphoprotein activated as a result of bacterial lipopolysaccharide (LPS) challenge (Han et al. 1994). Shortly following this discovery, human p38 was identified as the molecular target for members of the pyridinylimidazole class of compounds which were known to inhibit the biosynthesis of inflammatory cytokines in LPS-stimulated human monocytes (Lee et al. 1994). The extensive use of bioinformatics has led to the identification p38β2, p38γ, and p38δ. Of the four isoforms of human p38 so far described, p38α is both the best characterized and potentially the most relevant in its involvement in the inflammatory response. Tissue distribution data for p38α and β2 demonstrate them to be widely expressed across a variety of tissues. Functionally, however, they appear to be distinct. For example, while both p38α and p38β2 were shown to be elevated in a mouse model of ventricular hypertrophy, increased p38α activity was associated with cardiomyocyte apoptosis, whereas elevated p38β2 led to an induction of cardiomyocyte hypertrophy (Braz et al. 2003). Much less is known about the functional role of the other two kinases, p38γ and δ. A wide tissue distribution in both adult and developing tissues has been shown for p38δ, whereas p38γ showed a more restricted distribution in skeletal muscle. A possible role for p38γ in cardiac pathophysiology has recently been postulated with the discovery of its expression in normal and diseased human heart tissue and in normal and hypertrophic rat myocytes (Court et al. 2002).

Activation of p38α and β2 MAPK occurs through the dual phosphorylation of Thr180 and Tyr182 by the upstream MAPKK, MKK6. Another MAPKK, MKK3 has also been shown to activate p38α MAPK. MKK3/6 are, in turn, activated by several MAPKKK in response to a variety of stimuli (Adams et al. 2001a; Kyriakis and Avruch 2001) (Fig. 1). These multiple activation pathways serve to illustrate the complexity of this cascade. Recently, a MAPKK-independent pathway of p38α MAPK activation has been described. This involves the transforming growth factor-β-activated protein kinase-1

(TAK-1) binding protein 1, TAB1 (Ge et al. 2002). Using a yeast two-hybrid system, TAB1 was shown to associate with p38α and induce its intramolecular autophosphorylation. The substrates of the p38 MAPK include other kinases, transcription factors, and cytosolic proteins. Various protein phosphatases including protein phosphatase 2A have been shown to dephosphorylate p38 MAPK, resulting in its downregulation. p38α MAPK is also downregulated through the dephosphorylation activity of MAPK phosphatase (MKP)-7 and MKP-5 (Theodosiou et al. 1999; Masuda et al. 2001; Tanoue et al. 2001).

2 Discovery of p38 Inhibitors

Lee et al. first reported a series of bicyclic imidazoles that inhibited both 5-lipoxygenase/cyclooxygenase (LO/COX) and inflammatory cytokines production (Lee et al. 1988, 1993, 1994, 1999). SKF 86002 was one of the first compounds that exhibited potent anti-inflammatory activity and suppression of inflammatory cytokines. In 1995, Gallagher et al. described SB 203580 and other 2,4,5-triaryl imidazoles that were used as pharmacological tools to identify p38 MAPK as the molecular target of these compounds. SB 203580 has since been widely used as a pharmacological tool to elucidate and understand p38 MAPK pathways and p38 MAPK's physiological role (Lee et al. 1994; Gallagher et al. 1995, 1997). These early compounds, however, were not very selective, and further modification of the imidazole template led to improved selectivity and developability characteristics. For example, imidazoles with substitution of two-substituted pyridine in place of pyridine resulted in reduced cytochrome P450 inhibition (Adams et al. 1998). Further improvement of kinase selectivity and potency was accomplished by several groups (Boehm et al. 1996; Liverton et al. 1999; Adams et al. 2001b). The central imidazole core has been replaced by other heteroaryl (Jackson and Bullington 2002) as well as novel non-aryl-pyridinyl scaffolding (Cirillo et al. 2002). The key interaction with a majority of these inhibitors and p38 MAPK is between a carbonyl group acting as a hydrogen bond acceptor to Met 109 in p38α MAPK and a fluorinated phenyl group fitting in the aryl selectivity pocket of the compound. As is the case with imidazoles, these diverse sets of new compounds also potently inhibit p38α in an ATP-competitive manner. However, recently scientists at Boehringer Ingelheim have identified *N-N'*-diaryl ureas exemplified by BIRB-796 that binds to the ATP binding site and kinase specificity pocket but not in an ATP-competitive manner, forcing a conformational change in p38α MAPK. However, unlike imidazoles, BIRB-796 binds in a time-dependent manner and has slow association kinetics of binding (Pargellis et al. 2002; Regan et al. 2002). Some recent examples of indoles (Scios, WO0071535), tetrasubstituted imidazoles (Merck, WO9712876), and heteroaryl fused pyrimidinones (GlaxoSmithKline, WO02059083 and Merck, WO02058695) from patent literature are given in Fig. 2. A detailed descrip-

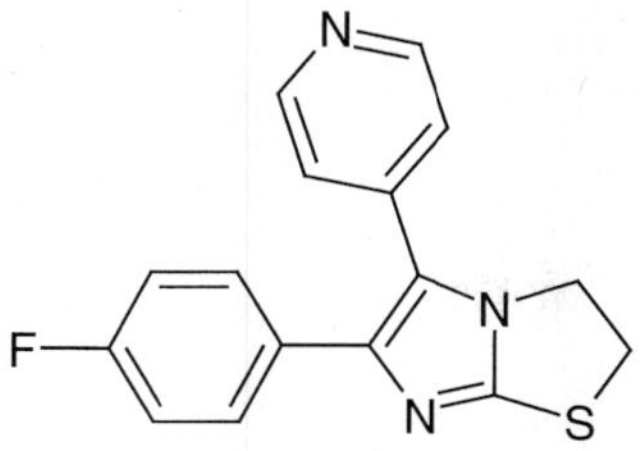

SKF-86002

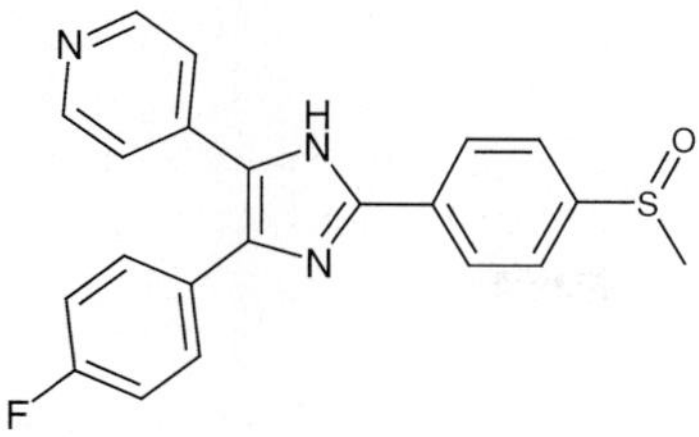

SB-203580

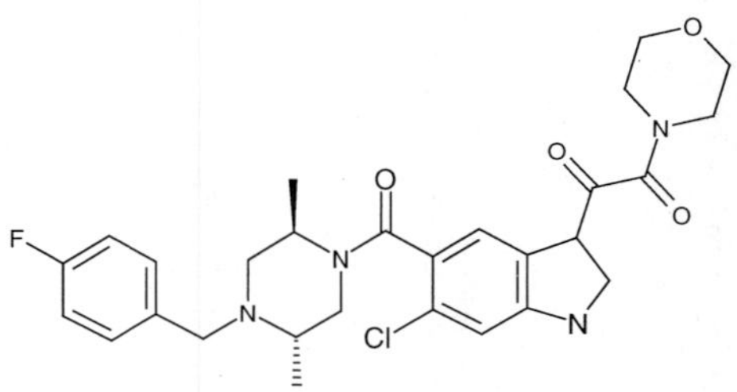

1 Scios
(WO0071535)

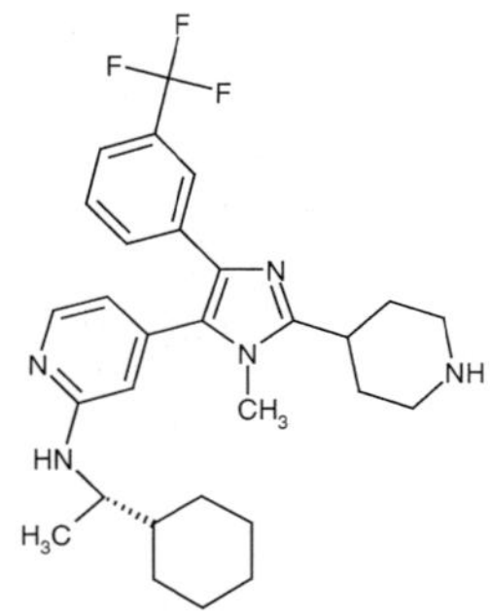

2 Merck
(WO9712876)

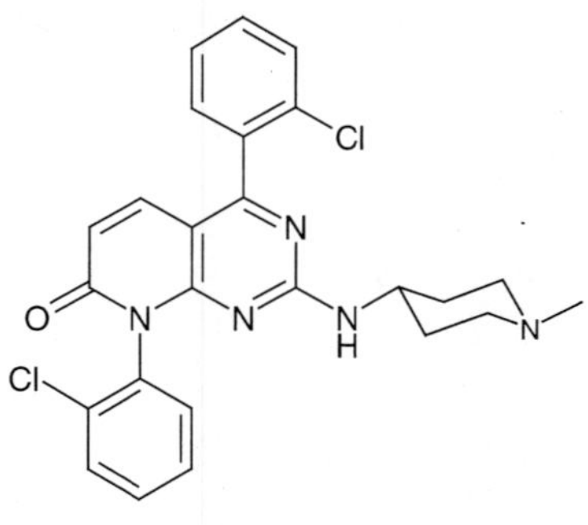

3 GSK
(WO02059083)

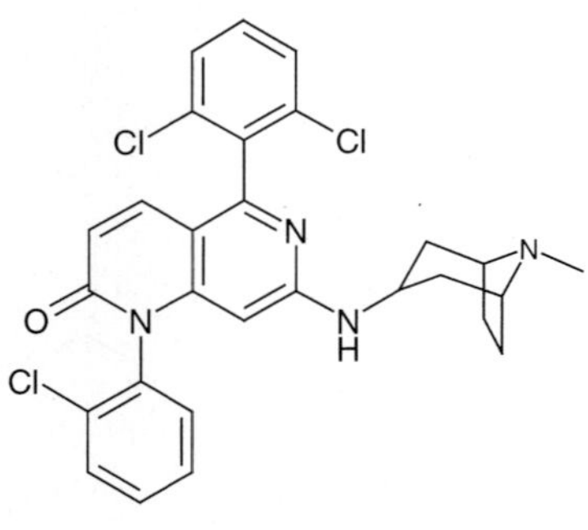

4 Merck
(WO02058695)

Fig. 2 Structures of representative classes of p38 MAPK inhibitors

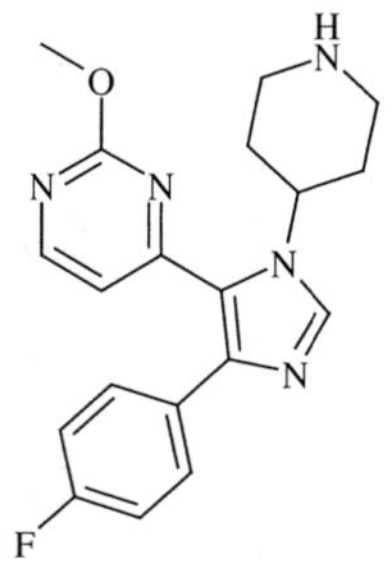

SB-242235

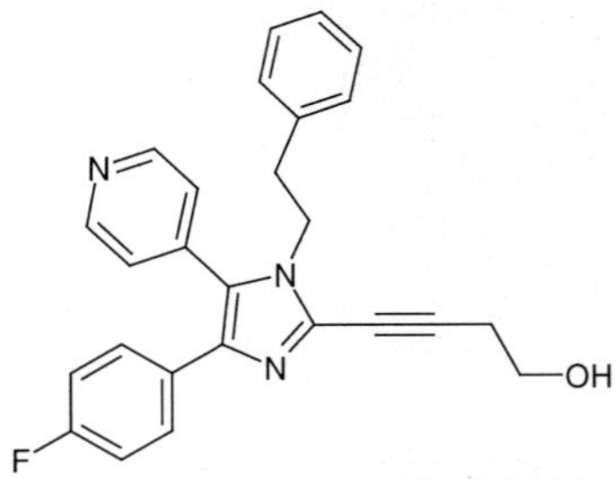

RWJ-67657

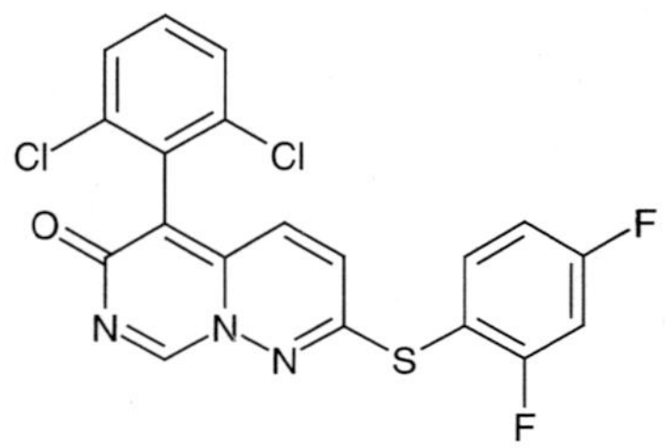

VX-745

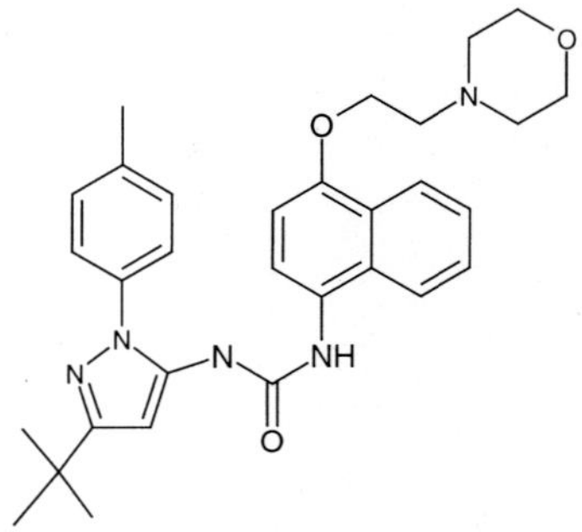

BIRB-796

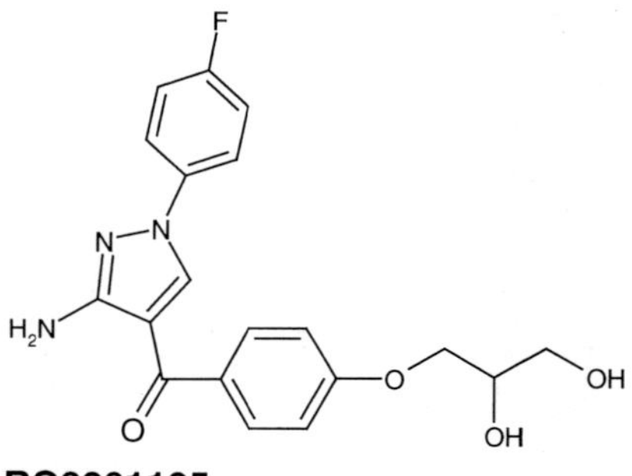

RO3201195

Fig. 2 (continued)

tion of the discovery of p38 inhibitors and their structure activity relationships can be found in Kumar et al. (2003).

Several p38 MAPK inhibitors have reached early clinical studies. SB 242235 was tested in healthy human volunteers. A dose-dependent inhibition of tumor necrosis factor (TNF)-α, interleukin (IL)-1β, IL-6, and IL-8 production was observed in an ex vivo study with isolated PBMNCs from drug treated individuals (Fullerton et al. 2000). Similarly, the effect of RWJ65657 was evaluated on clinical symptoms and cytokine production in response to LPS in healthy human volunteers. Both flu-like clinical symptoms and an increase in serum levels of TNFα, IL-6, and IL-8 were dose-dependently inhibited (Fijen et al. 2001). VX745 from vertex has been evaluated in patients with active rheumatoid arthritis. Although a significant effect of drug was observed on the clinical arthritis score, it was associated with elevated liver enzymes (Weisman et al. 2002). Other compounds reported to be in clinical studies are BIRB796, RO-320-1195 and Scio-469 (Polmar and al. 2002). The structures of several p38 MAPK inhibitors undergoing clinical studies are presented in Fig. 2.

3 Regulation of Cytokine Expression

Evidence for the pivotal role of the p38α/MAPK-activated protein kinase 2 (MAPKAP K2) pathway in cytokine production and signaling has been obtained from mouse genetic studies. Embryonic stem cells from p38α knockout mice demonstrated both a reduced capacity to produce IL-6 in response to IL-1 and a reduction in MAPKAP K2 activation in response to chemical stress (Allen et al. 2000). Additionally, MAPKAP K2-null mice exhibited a diminished ability to produce both IL-1 and IL-6 (Kotlyarov et al. 1999). The mechanisms involved in this inhibition appear to involve activity at both the levels of transcription and translation. The 3′ UTR (untranslated) regions of the mRNA for inducible cytokines such as IL-1, IL-8, and TNF contain an AU-rich element that has been shown to be responsible for their short half-life (Caput et al. 1986; Shaw and Kamen 1986). Under normal physiological conditions it is believed that these AU-rich regions are occupied by AU-binding proteins, rendering them non-translatable. It is hypothesized that these AU-binding proteins become phosphorylated in a p38α MAPK-dependent manner in response to appropriate inflammatory stimuli, such as LPS, resulting in the stabilization and translation of these mRNAs. Since MAPKAP K2 deficiency is also able to block the production of these short-lived mRNAs, it appears that p38α MAPK is indirectly responsible for stability of these short-lived cytokine mRNAs (Winzen et al. 1999; Ming et al. 2001). Therefore, the current working hypothesis is that the p38α/

Table 1 Summary table of pre-clinical pharmacology studies with various p38 MAPK inhibitors

Compound	Company	Study/model	Reference(s)
SB-203580	GlaxoSmithKline	AA rat and CIA mice, ischemia/reperfusion in rat heart, follicular lymphoma, rat spinal injury	Badger et al. 1996; Ma et al. 1999; Elenitoba-Johnson et al. 2003; Horiuchi et al. 2003
SB-242235	GlaxoSmithKline	AA rats	Badger et al. 2000
Selective imidazole (L-167307)	Merck	AA rats	Liverton et al. 1999
RWJ 67657	RW Johnson Pharmaceutical	AA rats	Wadsworth et al. 1999
Pyridinyloxazole inhibitor	Novartis	CIA in rats	Revesz et al. 2000
RPR-200765A	Aventis	Streptococcal cell wall-induced arthritis in rats	McLay et al. 2001
RPR-238677	Aventis	Streptococcal cell wall-induced arthritis in rats	McKenna et al. 2002
BIRB 796	Boehringer Ingelheim Pharmaceuticals	LPS challenge in mice	Regan et al. 2002
FR167653	Fujisawa Pharmaceuticals	Ischemia/reperfusion of lung and liver in rats	Kawashima et al. 2001; Kobayashi et al. 2002; Nishikawa et al. 2003
SB-239063	GlaxoSmithKline	Cardiac hypertrophy and dysfunction in rats, cerebral focal ischemia in rats, balloon injury in rabbit	Barone et al. 2001; Behr et al. 2001; Ju et al. 2002

AA, adjuvant arthritic (rat model); CIA, collagen-induced arthritis (mouse and rat models).

MAPKAP K2 pathway is involved in the phosphorylation of these AU-binding proteins (Neininger et al. 2002; Frevel et al. 2003).

4 Data with p38 Inhibitors

The discovery that members of the pyridinylimidazole class of compounds could inhibit the biosynthesis of inflammatory cytokines in LPS-stimulated human monocytes has led to an abundance of preclinical studies which point to a critical role for p38α MAPK in the inflammatory process. Studies have investigated the potential clinical value of inhibiting this pathway in therapeutic areas including rheumatoid arthritis, pulmonary disease, and neuroprotection. The diversity of these studies is exemplified by the listing in Table 1.

4.1 Rheumatoid Arthritis

In addition to its role in inflammatory cytokine synthesis, the p38α MAPK pathway is also involved in the induction of other genes encoding inflammatory mediators including COX-2 and inducible nitric oxide synthase (iNOS) (Guan et al. 1998; Badger et al. 2000). These findings have resulted in much of the preclinical and clinical research being focused upon its role in the chronic inflammatory joint disease rheumatoid arthritis (RA). RA is characterized by the infiltration of immunocompetent cells into the synovial tissue and fluid, proliferation of synovial fibroblasts, and the formation of pannus tissue, which invades and degrades the articular cartilage and subchondral bone. The etiology of this disease is unknown. However, many of the cellular and molecular mechanisms underlying the inflammation and associated degradation of the extracellular matrix of the articular cartilage and subchondral bone are becoming more clearly understood (Lee and Weinblatt 2001). A large body of evidence has emerged over the last two decades to implicate the inflammatory cytokines TNF and IL-1 as playing a pivotal role in the pathogenesis of this disease. As illustrated by Fig. 3, these pleiotropic inflammatory cytokines have been shown to promote cartilage degradation and bone resorption in vitro (Arend and Dayer 1995), stimulate the release of prostaglandin E_2 and collagenase from synovial fibroblasts (Dayer et al. 1985), and induce the expression of adhesion molecules on vascular endothelium and inflammatory cells leading to diapedesis (Cavender et al. 1987). Biological agents that effectively neutralize the activity of these cytokines have been shown to be highly effective in the clinic (Lee and Kavanaugh 2003). The chimeric anti-TNF antibody Remicade and the TNF-R-Fc fusion protein Enbrel both bind to TNF and prevent it from binding to its receptor

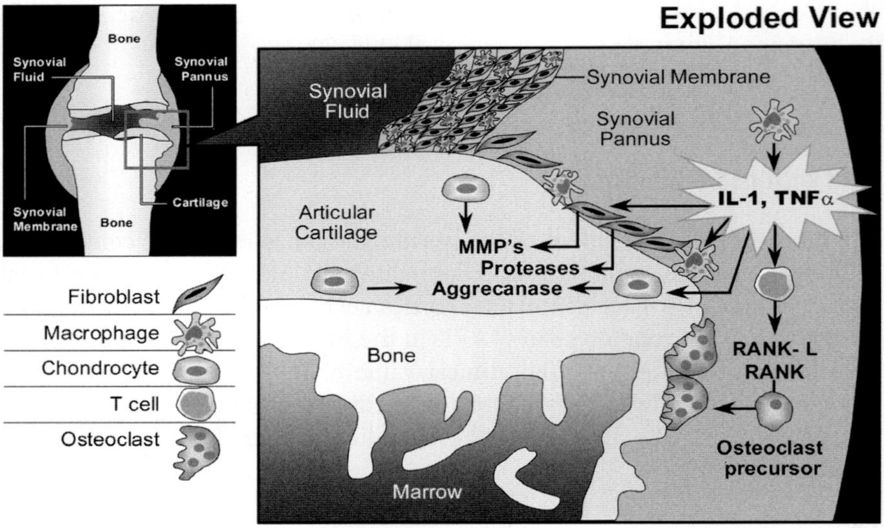

Fig. 3 A simplified diagrammatic representation of the rheumatoid joint (*upper left*). An exploded view of the major cellular and molecular events occurring within the synovial pannus is shown in the *large panel*. The central role of pro-inflammatory cytokines IL-1 and TNF in the expression of downstream mediators of inflammation and joint damage is highlighted. (Reprinted from Kumar et al. 2001a, with permission from Elsevier)

and exerting its biological effects. Anakinra, the IL-1 receptor antagonist (IL-1RA), binds to the IL-1 receptor but does not signal, thereby inhibiting the biological activity of IL-1. However, these therapies are relatively expensive and need to be parenterally administered. It is also clear from the clinical studies that not all patients respond to these therapies (Lee and Kavanaugh 2003). Preclinical data strongly suggest that dual antagonism of both of these mediators would offer a more synergistic benefit than antagonism of either cytokine alone (Bendele et al. 2000). Therefore, an orally active agent that can inhibit either the production or activity of these inflammatory mediators may offer superior therapeutic benefit in the treatment of RA.

4.1.1
In Vitro Data Supporting a Role for p38α MAPK in RA

Inflammatory cytokine production from many of the cell types present in the rheumatoid joint has been shown to be dependent on the p38α MAPK pathway. The ability of monocytes, synovial fibroblasts, chondrocytes, and osteoblasts to generate IL-6 and IL-8 was shown to be attenuated by p38α MAPK inhibition (Suzuki et al. 2000; Adams et al. 2001a). It is of note that p38α MAPK inhibition does not result in the prevention of proteoglycan loss from IL-1-stimulated articular cartilage (Badger et al. 2000). However, a significant inhibitory effect on iNOS production was demonstrated. Both IL-1 and TNF can stimulate osteoclast-mediated bone resorption through their ability to act directly or indirectly on the osteoclast or their precursors. This indirect activation results from an upregulation of the receptor activator of nuclear factor (NF)-κB ligand (RANK-L), an important osteoclast differentiation, activation, and survival factor present on osteoblasts and stromal cells. Osteoclast-mediated bone resorption stimulated either by IL-1, TNF, or RANK-L have all been shown to be attenuated by p38α MAPK inhibition (Matsumoto et al. 2000; Kumar et al. 2001b). These data offer support to the hypothesis that inhibition of p38α MAPK may not only provide effective anti-inflammatory therapy through their attenuation of cytokine release but may also offer joint protection.

4.1.2
In Vivo Data Supporting a Role for p38 MAPK in RA

The p38 MAPK inhibitor SB 203580 has been used extensively to study the therapeutic potential of this approach in RA preclinical models. Badger and co-workers (1996) demonstrated the anti-inflammatory effects of this molecule in the adjuvant arthritic (AA) rat model of inflammatory joint disease. They reported that it was effective at reducing paw inflammation in the AA rat with an optimum dose of 60 mg/kg administered in a prophylactic dosing regimen. Evidence of a joint-protective effect was also noted using measurements of bone mineral density and histology. A further extension of these studies using the more selective p38 MAPK inhibitor SB 242235 demonstrated that this effect was not only apparent when the compound was administered in a prophylactic dosing regimen, prior to the establishment of lesion, but also using a more clinically relevant therapeutic treatment regimen once the lesion had become established (Badger et al. 2000). This study further highlighted the effect of such treatment in preventing the loss of joint integrity using measurements of bone mineral density, histology, and magnetic resonance imaging. The effectiveness of p38 MAPK inhibition is not limited to the AA rat model. Studies by Aventis Pharmaceuticals have shown the p38 MAPK inhibitors RPR200765A and RPR238677 to also be effective anti-inflammatory and joint protective agents in the streptococcal cell wall-induced arthritis in the rat (McLay et al. 2001; McKenna et al. 2002). Studies using the rat model of collagen-induced arthritis (CIA) have also demonstrated a significant anti-inflammatory effect of p38 MAPK inhibitors (Revesz et al. 2000). Most recently, FR167653, a p38 MAPK inhibitor from Fujisawa Pharmaceuticals, was shown to prevent the onset and progression of CIA in the rat. This molecule also inhibited osteoclastogenesis induced by RANK-L and TNF (Nishikawa et al. 2003).

4.2 Pulmonary Disease

As in RA, inflammatory cytokines play a crucial role in the pathogenesis of airways inflammation. Cytokines such as TNF, interferon (IFN)-γ, IL-4, IL-5, and chemokines such as IL-8, regulated upon activation normal T cells expressed and secreted (RANTES) and eotaxin have all been demonstrated to be capable of generating or supporting airways inflammation (Barnes et al. 1998). The generation and signaling of many of these mediators has also been shown to be dependent on the MAPK cascade. It is therefore postulated that inhibition of p38α MAPK may have a beneficial effect in the treatment of pulmonary diseases including asthma, chronic obstructive pulmonary disease (COPD), and idiopathic pulmonary fibrosis (IPF).

4.2.1 In Vitro Data Supporting p38 MAPK Activation in Pulmonary Disease

The infiltration of the lungs by eosinophils is a prominent feature of asthma. These bone marrow-derived granulocytes can promote airway remodeling and tissue damage through the release of cytotoxic proteins and oxygen radicals (Giembycz and Lindsay 1999). The differentiation, recruitment, and activation of these cells result from the activity of an array of cytokines and chemokines including IL-3, IL-5, and eotaxin. Data generated using the p38 MAPK inhibitor SB 202190 demonstrated an inhibitory effect upon eosinophil differentiation, degranulation, and cytokine release, suggesting a role for this pathway in eosinophil effector functions (Adachi et al. 2000). Changes in airway osmolarity have been hypothesized to contribute to exercise-induced bronchoconstriction and the late-phase airway response. Exposure of bronchial epithelial cells to hyperosmolar medium has been shown to induce expression of the neutrophil chemoattractant chemokine IL-8, which is inhibited by SB 203580 (Shapiro and Dinarello 1995; Matsumoto et al. 1998; Hashimoto et al. 1999).

4.2.2 In Vivo Data Supporting p38 MAPK Activation in Pulmonary Disease

Consistent with the findings outlined above from in vitro studies with eosinophils, the second generation p38 MAPK inhibitor SB 239063 induced eosinophil apoptosis and significantly reduced antigen-induced lung eosinophilia in both mice and guinea pigs in vivo (Underwood et al. 2000). In contrast to these findings, studies using L-790070, another p38 MAPK inhibitor, revealed no effect on eosinophil numbers or cytokine levels in bronchoalveolar lavage (BAL) from antigen-sensitized and challenged mice. These studies, though, did demonstrate a reduction in neutrophilia and a reversal in the antigen-induced increase in mucus-secreting cell numbers (Nick et al. 2002).

IPF, a member of the heterogeneous group of pulmonary fibroses whose etiology is unknown, is a chronic, progressive, and often fatal disorder. In a murine model of this disease, induced by bleomycin, administration of the p38 MAPK inhibitor FR-167653 prior to induction of fibrosis resulted in an amelioration of the fibrosis and pulmonary cachexia (Matsuoka et al. 2002).

4.3 Neurodegeneration

There is a substantial amount of evidence linking the MAPK pathways JNK and p38 with neuronal cell death and Alzheimer's disease. Although much of this evidence supports JNK as being the primary pathway, studies also point to a role for p38 MAPK in these processes (Harper and LoGrasso 2001). Both p38α and p38β2 MAPK are expressed in the hippocampus and cortex of brain by immunoblotting techniques (Mielke et al. 1999; Mielke and Herdegen 2000). Using an antibody to the phosphorylated form of p38α MAPK, studies demonstrated its association with neuritic plaques, neuropil threads, and neurofibrillary tangles, all of which are characteristic features of Alzheimer's disease (Hensley et al. 1999).

4.3.1 In Vitro Data Supporting a Role for p38 MAPK in Neurodegeneration

Much of the in vitro evidence for a role for p38 MAPK in neuronal cell death comes from studies with PC12 cells, a rat pheochromocytoma cell line which responds to nerve growth factor (NGF). Withdrawal of NGF from these cells results in apoptosis and a concomitant induction of p38α and JNK MAPK activity. Furthermore, these studies also demonstrated that this cell death could be inhibited by the p38α MAPK inhibitor PD169316 (Kummer et al. 1997). It is becoming clear from a number of studies that activation of p38α MAPK and its relative role in neuronal cell death is stimulus dependent. The induction of apoptosis by calyculin in cortical cultures could partially be reversed by PD169316, whereas the induction of excitotoxic cell death by *N*-methyl-d-aspartate (NMDA) was not (Ko et al. 2000). Furthermore, SB 203580 could not rescue apoptotic rat ganglion neurons deprived of neurotrophins (Maas et al. 1998), whereas in a separate study it did extend the survival of retinal ganglion neurons exposed to NMDA (Kikuchi et al. 2000). Most recently, Legos and colleagues demonstrated that the selective p38 MAPK inhibitor SB 239063 could confer neuroprotection to cultured primary neurons exposed to NMDA for 5 min, but not for 60 min (Legos et al. 2002).

4.3.2
In Vivo Data Supporting p38 MAPK Activation in Neurodegeneration

Only a limited number of studies involving p38 MAPK inhibition in vivo have been described. Despite this, much of the data generated in vivo supports the assertion above that various stresses result in the activation of different pathways with subsequent cell death. For example, the p38 MAPK inhibitors SB 203580 and SB 239063 have been shown to reduce both brain injury and neurological deficits in models of ischemic brain injury (Barone et al. 2001; Piao et al. 2003), whereas SB 203580 demonstrated no protective effects in a murine model of traumatic brain injury (Mori et al. 2002). Most recently, a study in a rat spinal injury model demonstrated that inhibition of p38α MAPK activity could prevent the delayed progressive degeneration of oligodendrocytes in the injured area, and a recovery in motor function if the cord damage was not complete (Horiuchi et al. 2003).

4.4
Other Indications

The therapeutic potential of p38α MAPK inhibitors is not confined to the therapeutic indications outlined above. Preclinical in vivo data also point to a potential effect of p38α inhibition in indications as diverse as ischemia-reperfusion injury (Barancik et al. 2000; Kawashima et al. 2001; Kobayashi et al. 2002), polymicrobial sepsis (Song et al. 2001), lymphoma (Elenitoba-Johnson et al. 2003), and inflammatory bowel disease (Waetzig et al. 2002).

5
Conclusion

Over the past decade, the p38 MAPKs have been the subject of intense multidisciplinary research. The discovery of potent selective inhibitors of this pathway has led to a greater understanding of their role in signal transduction and response pathways. The role of these enzymes, particularly p38α MAPK in the generation of pro-inflammatory mediators, including cytokines, PGE_2, and iNOS, has led to an intensive effort among the pharmaceutical industry to identify clinical candidates for the treatment of a variety of inflammatory diseases. Several of these inhibitors have now entered human clinical trials and demonstrated good pharmacokinetic and pharmacodynamic effects. To date no compound has entered phase III trials; however, several have reached the phase II stage. In all studies, reported administration of drug has resulted in an inhibition of either in vivo or ex vivo endotoxin-induced inflammatory cytokine release. Concern over safety issues has stopped many of these studies. A possible reason for these adverse events may be a cross-reactivity of these compounds with other kinases or enzymes. A majority of the p38 MAPK inhibitors described within this article are ATP competitive. One exception is BIRB-796 that binds to the ATP site but not in an ATP-competitive manner. The BIRB-796 series of inhibitors, which are non-competitive for ATP, may offer better selectivity. The interaction of p38 MAPK with TAB1 (Ge et al. 2002) offers the intriguing possibility that disruption of such an association may also have benefits over the ATP-competitive inhibitors. Further research on the role of the other p38 homologs may also offer an alternative approach for intervention in the future. For example, all four isoforms have shown to be activated as a result of myeloid cell exposure to inflammatory stimuli. There is no doubt that the plethora of preclinical data so far amassed for this molecular target certainly warrants further investigations, not only to identify a clinical candidate but also the appropriate therapeutic indication.

Acknowledgements The authors wish to thank Drs. John Lee and Jeffrey Boehm for their invaluable assistance in the preparation of this manuscript. In addition, they would like to acknowledge the assistance of Marti-Jean Daly in the preparation of artwork.

References

Adachi T, Choudhury BK, et al (2000) The differential role of extracellular signal-regulated kinases and p38 mitogen-activated protein kinase in eosinophil functions. J Immunol 165:2198–2204

Adams JL, Boehm JC, et al (1998) Pyrimidinylimidazole inhibitors of CSBP/p38 kinase demonstrating decreased inhibition of hepatic cytochrome P450 enzymes. Bioorg Med Chem Lett 8:3111–3116

Adams JL, Badger AM, et al (2001a) p38 MAP Kinase: molecular target for the inhibition of pro-inflammatory cytokines. Prog Med Chem 38:1–60

Adams JL, Boehm JC, et al (2001b) Pyrimidinylimidazole inhibitors of p38: Cyclic N-1 imidazole substituents enhance p38 kinase inhibition and oral activity. Bioorg Med Chem Lett 11:2867–2870

Allen M, Svensson L, et al (2000) Deficiency of the stress kinase p38a results in embryonic lethality: characterization of the kinase dependence of stress response of enzyme-deficient embryonic stem cells. J Exp Med 191:859–869

Arend WP, Dayer JM (1995) Inhibition of the production and effects of interleukin-1 and tumor necrosis factor alpha in rheumatoid arthritis. Arthritis Rheumatism 38:151–60

Badger AM, Bradbeer JN, et al (1996) Pharmacological Profile of SB 203580, a Selective Inhibitor of Cytokine Suppressive Binding Protein/p38 Kinase, in Animal Models of Arthritis, Bone Resorption, Endotoxin Shock and Immune Function. J Pharmacol Exp Therap 279:1453–1461

Badger AM, Griswold DE, et al (2000) Disease-modifying activity of SB 242235, a selective inhibitor of p38 mitogen-activated protein kinase, in rat adjuvant-induced arthritis. Arthritis Rheumatism 43:175–183

Badger AM, Roshak AK, et al (2000) Differential effects of SB 242235, a selective p38 mitogen-activated protein kinase inhibitor, on IL-1 treated bovine and human cartilage/chondrocyte cultures. Osteoarthritis Cartilage 8:434–443

Barancik M, Htun P, et al (2000) Inhibition of the cardiac p38-MAPK pathway by SB203580 delays ischemic cell death. J Cardiovasc Pharmacol 35:474–483

Barnes PJ, Chung KF, et al (1998) Inflammatory mediators of asthma: An update. Pharmacol Rev 50:515–596

Barone FC, Irving EA, et al (2001) SB 239063, a second-generation p38 mitogen-activated protein kinase inhibitor, reduces brain injury and neurological deficits in cerebral focal ischemia. J Pharmacol Exp Ther 296:312–321

Behr TM, Nerurkar SS, et al (2001) Hypertensive end-organ damage and premature mortality are p38 mitogen-activated protein kinase-dependent in a rat model of cardiac hypertrophy and dysfunction. Circulation 104:1292–1298

Bendele AM, Chlipala ES, et al (2000) Combination benefit of treatment with the cytokine inhibitors interleukin-1 receptor antagonist and PEGylated soluble tumor necrosis factor receptor type I in animal models of rheumatoid arthritis. Arthritis Rheum 43:2648–2659

Boehm JC, Smietana JM, et al (1996) 1-substituted 4-aryl-5-pyridinylimidazoles: a new class of cytokine suppressive drugs with low 5-lipoxygenase and cyclooxygenase inhibitory potency. J Med Chem 39:3929–3937

Braz JC, Bueno OF, et al (2003) Targeted inhibition of p38 MAPK promotes hypertrophic cardiomyopathy through upregulation of calcineurin-NEAT signaling. J Clin Invest 111:1475–1486

Caput D, Beutler B, et al (1986) Identification of a common nucleotide sequence in the 3'-untranslated region of mRNA molecules specifying inflammatory mediators. Proc Natl Acad Sci U S A 83:1670–1674

Cavender D, Haskard D, et al (1987) Pathways to chronic inflammation in rheumatoid synovitis. Fed Proc 46:113–7

Cirillo PF, Pargellis C, et al (2002) The non-diaryl heterocycle classes of p38 MAP kinase inhibitors. Curr Top Med Chem 2:1021–1035

Court NW, dos Remedios CG, et al (2002) Cardiac expression and subcellular localization of the p38 mitogen-activated protein kinase member, stress-activated protein kinase-3 (SAPK3). J Mol Cell Cardiol 34:413–426

Dayer JM, Beutler B, et al (1985) Cachectin/tumor necrosis factor stimulates collagenase and prostaglandin E2 production by human synovial cells and dermal fibroblasts. J Exp Med 162:2163–8

Elenitoba-Johnson KS J, Jenson SD, et al (2003) Involvement of multiple signaling pathways in follicular lymphoma transformation: p38-mitogenactivated protein kinase as a target for therapy. Proc Natl Acad Sci U S A 100:7259–7264

Fijen JW, Zijlstra JG, et al (2001) Suppression of the clinical and cytokine response to endotoxin by RWJ-67657, a p38 mitogen-activated protein-kinase inhibitor, in healthy human volunteers. Clin Exp Immunol 124:16–20

Frevel MA E, Bakheet T, et al (2003) p38 mitogen-activated protein kinase-dependent and -independent signaling of mRNA stability of AU-rich element-containing transcripts. Mol Cell Biol 23:425–436

Fullerton T, Sharma A, et al (2000) Suppression of ex vivo cytokine production by SB-242235, a selective inhibitor of p38 MAP kinase. Clin Pharmacol Ther 101st Ann Meeting Am Soc Clin Pharmacol 67:Abstract O1-B-4

Gallagher T, Seibel GL, et al (1997) Regulation of stress-induced cytokine production by pyridinylimidazoles; inhibition of CSBP kinase. Bioorg Med Chem 5:49–64

Gallagher TF, Fierthompson SM, et al (1995) 2,4,5-Triarylimidazole Inhibitors of IL-1 Biosynthesis. Bioorg Med Chem Lett 5:1171–1176

Ge BX, Gram H, et al (2002) MAPKK-independent activation of p38 alpha mediated by TAB1-dependent autophosphorylation of p38 alpha. Science 295:1291–1294

Giembycz MA, Lindsay MA (1999) Pharmacology of the eosinophil. Pharmacol Rev 51:213–339

Guan ZH, Buckman SY, et al (1998) Induction of Cyclooxygenase-2 by the Activated Mekk1-]Sek1/Mkk4-]P38 Mitogen-Activated Protein Kinase Pathway. J Biol Chem 273:12901–12908

Han J, Lee JD, et al (1994) A MAP kinase targeted by endotoxin and hyperosmolarity in mammalian cells. Science 265:808–811

Harper SJ, LoGrasso P (2001) Signalling for survival and death in neurones—the role of stress-activated kinases, JNK and p38. Cell Signal 13:299–310

Hashimoto S, Matsumoto K, et al (1999) Hyperosmolarity-induced interleukin-8 expression in human bronchial epithelial cells through p38 mitogen-activated protein kinase. Am J Respir Critic Care Med 159:634–40

Hensley K, Floyd RA, et al (1999) p38 kinase is activated in the Alzheimer's disease brain. J NeuroChem 72:2053–2058

Horiuchi D, Ogata T, et al (2003) Continuous intrathecal infusion of SB203580, a selective inhibitor of p38 mitogen-activated protein kinase, reduces the damage of hindlimb function after thoracic spinal cord injury in rat. Neurosci Res 47:209–217

Jackson PF, Bullington JL (2002) Pyridinylimidazole based p38 MAP kinase inhibitors. Curr Top Med Chem 2:1011–1020

Ju HS, Nerurkar S, et al (2002) Sustained activation of p38 mitogen-activated protein kinase contributes to the vascular response to injury. J Pharmacol Exp Ther 301:15–20

Kawashima Y, Takeyoshi I, et al (2001) FR167653 attenuates ischemia and reperfusion injury of the rat lung with suppressing p38 mitogen-activated protein kinase. J Heart Lung Transplant 20:568–574

Kikuchi M, Tenneti L, et al (2000) Role of p38 mitogen-activated protein kinase in axotomy-induced apoptosis of rat retinal ganglion cells. J Neurosci 20:5037–5044

Ko HW, Han KS, et al (2000) Synergetic activation of p38 mitogen-activated protein kinase and caspase-3-like proteases for execution of calyculin A-induced apoptosis but not N-methyl-D-aspartate-induced necrosis in mouse cortical neurons. J NeuroChem 74:2455–2461

Kobayashi M, Takeyoshi I, et al (2002) P38 mitogen-activated protein kinase inhibition attenuates ischemia-reperfusion injury of the rat liver. Surgery 131:344–349

Kotlyarov A, Neininger A, et al (1999) MAPKAP Kinase 2 is essential for LPS-induced TNF-a biosynthesis. Nat Cell Biol 1:94–97

Kumar S, Blake SM, et al (2001a) Intracellular signaling pathways as a target for the treatment of rheumatoid arthritis. Curr Opin Pharmacol 1:307–13

Kumar S, Votta BJ, et al (2001b) IL-1 and TNF-induced bone resorption is mediated by p38 mitogen activated protein kinase. J Cell Physiol 187:294–303

Kumar S, Boehm J, et al (2003) p38 map kinases: key signalling molecules as therapeutic targets for inflammatory diseases. Nat Rev Drug Discov 2:717–726

Kummer JL, Rao PK, et al (1997) Apoptosis induced by withdrawal of trophic factors is mediated by P38 mitogen-activated protein kinase. J Biol Chem 272:20490–20494

Kyriakis JM, Avruch J (2001) Mammalian mitogen-activated protein kinase signal transduction pathways activated by stress and inflammation. Physiol Rev 81:807–869

Lee DM, Weinblatt ME (2001) Rheumatoid arthritis. Lancet 358:903–911

Lee JC, Griswold DE, et al (1988) Inhibition of monocyte IL-1 production by the anti-inflammatory compound, SK&F 86002. Int J Immunopharmacol 10:835–843
Lee JC, Badger AM, et al (1993) Bicyclic imidazoles as a novel class of cytokine biosynthesis inhibitors. Ann N Y Acad Sci 696:149–170
Lee JC, Laydon JT, et al (1994) A protein kinase involved in the regulation of inflammatory cytokine biosynthesis. Nature 372:739–746
Lee JC, Kassis S, et al (1999) p38 mitogen-activated protein kinase inhibitors-Mechanism and therapeutic potentials. Pharmacol Ther 82:389–397
Lee SJ, Kavanaugh A (2003) Pharmacological treatment of established rheumatoid arthritis. Best Pract Res Clin Rheumatol 17:811-29
Legos JJ, McLaughlin B, et al (2002) The selective p38 inhibitor SB-239063 protects primary neurons from mild to moderate excitotoxic injury. Eur J Pharmacol 447:37–42
Liverton NJ, Butcher JW, et al (1999) Design and synthesis of potent, selective, and orally bioavailable tetrasubstituted imidazole inhibitors of p38 mitogen-activated protein kinase. J Med Chem 42:2180–2190
Ma XL, Kumar S, et al (1999) Inhibition of p38 mitogen-activated protein kinase decreases cardiomyocyte apoptosis and improves cardiac function after myocardial ischemia and reperfusion. Circulation 99:1685–1691
Maas JW, Horstmann S, et al (1998) Apoptosis of central and peripheral neurons can be prevented with cyclin-dependent kinase mitogen-activated protein kinase inhibitors. J NeuroChem 70:1401–1410
Masuda K, Shima H, et al (2001) MKP-7, a novel mitogen-activated protein kinase phosphatase, functions as a shuttle protein. J Biol Chem 276:39002–39011
Matsumoto K, Hashimoto S, et al (1998) Proinflammatory cytokine-induced and chemical mediator-induced IL-8 expression in human bronchial epithelial cells through p38 mitogen-activated protein kinase-dependent pathway. J Allergy Clin Immunol 101:825–31
Matsumoto M, Sudo T, et al (2000) Involvement of p38 mitogen-activated protein kinase signaling pathway in osteoclastogenesis mediated by receptor activator of NF-kappa B ligand (RANKL). J Biol Chem 275:31155–31161
Matsuoka H, Arai T, et al (2002) A p38 MAPK inhibitor, FR-167653, ameliorates murine bleomycin-induced pulmonary fibrosis. Am J Physiol Lung Cell Mol Physiol 283:L103-L112
McKenna JM, Halley F, et al (2002) An algorithm-directed two-component library synthesized via solid-phase methodology yielding potent and orally bioavailable p38 MAP kinase inhibitors. J Med Chem 45:2173–2184
McLay IM, Halley F, et al (2001) The discovery of RPR 200765A, a p38 MAP kinase inhibitor displaying a good oral anti-arthritic efficacy. Bioorg Med Chem 9:537–554
Mielke K, Herdegen T (2000) JNK and p38 stresskinases—degenerative effectors of signal-transduction-cascades in the nervous system. Prog NeuroBiol 61:45–60
Mielke K, Brecht S, et al (1999) Activity and expression of JNK1, p38 and ERK kinases, c-Jun N-terminal phosphorylation, and c-jun promoter binding in the adult rat brain following kainate-induced seizures. Neuroscience 91:471–483
Ming XF, Stoecklin G, et al (2001) Parallel and independent regulation of interleukin-3 mRNA turnover by phosphatidylinositol 3-kinase and p38 mitogen-activated protein kinase. Mol Cell Biol 21:5778–5789
Mori T, Wang XY, et al (2002) Mitogen-activated protein kinase inhibition in traumatic brain injury: In vitro and in vivo effects. J Cereb Blood Flow Metabolism 22:444–452
Neininger A, Kontoyiannis D, et al (2002) MK2 targets AU-rich elements and regulates biosynthesis of tumor necrosis factor and interleukin-6 independently at different post-transcriptional levels. J Biol Chem 277:3065–3068

Nick JA, Young SK, et al (2002) Selective suppression of neutrophil accumulation in ongoing pulmonary inflammation by systemic inhibition of p38 mitogen-activated protein kinase. J Immunol 169:5260–5269

Nishikawa M, Myoui A, et al (2003) Prevention of the onset and progression of collagen-induced arthritis in rats by the potent p38 mitogen-activated protein kinase inhibitor FR167653. Arthritis Rheum 48:2670–2681

Pargellis C, Tong L, et al (2002) Inhibition of p38 MAP kinase by utilizing a novel allosteric binding site. Nat Struct Biol 9:268–272

Pearson G, Robinson F, et al (2001) Mitogen-activated protein (MAP) kinase pathways: regulation and physiological functions. Endocr Rev 22:153–183

Piao CS, Kim JB, et al (2003) Administration of the p38 MAPK inhibitor SB203580 affords brain protection with a wide therapeutic window against focal ischemic insult. J Neurosci Res 73:537–544

Polmar SH (2002) Safety and pharmacokinetics of an oral p38 MAP kinase inhibitor (BIRB 796 BS), administered twice daily for 14 days to healthy volunteers. J Allergy Clin Immunol 58th Ann Meeting Am Acad Allergy Asthma Immunol 109:S66:Abstract 167

Regan J, Breitfelder S, et al (2002) Pyrazole urea-based inhibitors of p38 MAP kinase: from lead compound to clinical candidate. J Med Chem 45:2994–3008

Revesz L, Di Padova FE, et al (2000) SAR of 4-hydroxypiperidine and hydroxyalkyl substituted heterocycles as novel p38 map kinase inhibitors. Bioorg Med Chem Lett 10:1261–1264

Shapiro L, Dinarello CA (1995) Osmotic regulation of cytokine synthesis in vitro. Proc Natl Acad Sci U S A 92:12230–12234

Shaw G, Kamen R (1986) A conserved AU sequence from the 3' untranslated region of GM-CSF mRNA mediates selective mRNA degradation. Cell 46:659–667

Song GY, Chung CS, et al (2001) MAPK p38 antagonism as a novel method of inhibiting lymphoid immune suppression in polymicrobial sepsis. Am J Physiol Cell Physiol 281:C662–C669

Suzuki M, Tetsuka T, et al (2000) The role of p38 mitogen-activated protein kinase in IL-6 and IL-8 production from the TNF-alpha- or IL-1 beta-stimulated rheumatoid synovial fibroblasts. FEBS Lett 465:23–27

Tanoue T, Yamamoto T, et al (2001) A novel MAPK phosphatase MKP-7 acts preferentially on JNK/SAPK and p38 alpha and beta MAPKs. J Biol Chem 276:26629–26639

Theodosiou A, Smith A, et al (1999) MKP5, a new member of the MAP kinase phosphatase family, which selectively dephosphorylates stress-activated kinases. Oncogene 18:6981–6988

Underwood DC, Osborn RR, et al (2000) SB 239063, a p38 MAPK inhibitor, reduces neutrophilia, inflammatory cytokines, MMP-9, and fibrosis in lung. Am J Physiol Lung Cell Mol Physiol 279:L895-L902

Wadsworth SA, Cavender DE, et al (1999) RWJ 67657, a potent, orally active inhibitor of p38 mitogen-activated protein kinase. J Pharmacol Exp Ther 291:680–7

Waetzig GH, Seegert D, et al (2002) p38 mitogen-activated protein kinase is activated and linked to TNF-alpha signaling in inflammatory bowel disease. J Immunol 168:5342–5351

Weisman M (2002) Double-blind, placebo-controlled trial of VX-745, an oral p38 mitogen activated protein kinase inhibitor, in patients with rheumatoid arthritis (RA). Ann Eur Congress Rheumatol:Abstract FR 10018

Winzen R, Kracht M, et al (1999) The p38 MAP kinase pathway signals for cytokine-induced mRNA stabilization via MAP kinase-activated protein kinase 2 and an AU-rich region-targeted mechanism. EMBO J 18:4969–4980

HEP (2005) 167:85–124

Inhibitors of PKA and Related Protein Kinases

M. Gaßel[3, 4] · C. Breitenlechner[1] · S. Herrero[3] · R. Engh[1, 2] ·
D. Bossemeyer[3] (✉)

[1] Abteilung Strukturforschung, Max-Planck-Institut fuer Biochemie, 82152 Martinsried, Germany
[2] Department of Medicinal Chemistry, Roche Diagnostics GmbH, 82372 Penzberg, Germany
[3] Department for Pathochemistry, German Cancer Research Centre, 69120 Heidelberg, Germany
D.Bossemeyer@DKFZ.de
[4] Present address: Drug Discovery—Assay Development, Intervet Innovation GmbH, 55270 Schwabenheim, Germany

Abstract The AGC group of protein kinases comprises a number of pharmacologically important members—targets for small molecule inhibitors of therapeutic value. Crystal structure data assist in the design of new or improved inhibitory molecules. Protein kinase A (PKA), one of the longest and best-known members of the AGC kinase group, has been cocrystallized with many AGC group inhibitors from highly diverse chemical groups, including isoquinoline derivatives, staurosporine and bisindolylmaleimide cognates, and balanol and pyridine derivatives, thus providing structural information about binding modes, selectivity and cross selectivity. The creation of 'ersatz' kinases by mutating the inhibitor binding site of PKA to resemble other fellow kinases from the AGC group and the cocrystallization of these ersatz kinases with small molecules as well as cocrystal structures of other AGC kinases like 3-phosphoinositide-dependent kinase 1 (PDK1) with staurosporine and bisindolylmaleimide derivatives helps in the identification and exploration of factors governing selectivity.

Keywords PKA · PKC · PDK1 · Rho kinase · Isoquinoline · H7 · H8 · H89 · H-1152P · HA-1077 · Fasudil · Y-27632 · Balanol · Staurosporine · UCN01 · Bisindolylmaleimide 2 · LY333531

1 Introduction

The central role of protein kinases in cellular regulation and signalling control is reflected in the frequent connection between failures in kinase control and serious disease, as is the case in the majority of human cancers. Because most protein kinases are active only when signalling, diseases typically arise from excess rather than loss of kinase activity, caused by mutation, overexpression or disabled cellular inhibition. Several protein kinases, in addition, contribute to disease in the course of their normal cellular function in cell survival, tumour vascularization, cell migration or vascular functions. Pharmacological targets include kinases from the group of AGC kinases, both because of excessive activity and also because of 'normal' functions. While the first protein kinase inhibitors, several of them directed against the classical AGC kinases PKA, PKG, and PKC, were used mostly to elucidate the role of protein phosphorylation in signal transduction pathways and cellular regulation, protein kinase inhibitors now have long reached general acceptance as pharmacological tools of proven high therapeutic value (Traxler 2003). The first protein kinase inhibitor with clinical approval was the AGC kinase inhibitor fasudil or HA1077 (see chapter of Hidaka et al. on fasudil in this volume). Of the 518 protein kinases in man, 62 belong to the subgroup of AGC kinases. Pharmacologically important members of the AGC branch include Aurora, PKB/Akt, 3-phosphoinositide-dependent kinase 1 (PDK1), Rho kinase, and the various isoforms of PKC. PKA, PKC and PKG were amongst the first protein kinases to be identified and isolated, and the accumulated research on these enzymes represents a large proportion of our present knowledge about protein kinase function. Most of the biochemical work was performed with PKA, the so-called 'prototype' protein kinase. PKA was isolated in 1968 (Walsh et al. 1968) and has been studied with respect to protein kinase function ever since. PKA is the central effector of cyclic adenosine monophosphate (cAMP), the second messenger involved in a myriad of signalling pathways for metabolism, gene transcription, memory function, ion channel regulation, cell proliferation and cell differentiation (Montminy 1997). PKA also is a marker and a target in malignant disease; antisense inhibitors targeting the RI subunits are in early clinical trials against a variety of tumours (Chen et al. 2000). The activity of the catalytic subunit also appears to be associated with the development of Alzheimer's disease (Marambaud et al. 1999).

PKA is a prototype enzyme for the protein kinase family for three reasons. (1) PKA is quite abundant in tissue, and efficient highly specific purification methods were discovered early (Kinzel and Kubler 1976; Kubler et al. 1979; Nelson and Taylor 1981) to enable biochemical investigation and also to provide highly homogeneous enzyme for subsequent crystallographic studies (Bossemeyer et al. 1993). (2) The catalytic subunit forms an inactive holoenzyme in the absence of cAMP, consisting of catalytic and regulatory subunits, but is monomeric in the presence of high cAMP concentrations. It consists almost entirely of the conserved catalytic core of protein kinases, constituted by 245 out of 350 residues of PKA (Hanks and Quinn 1991). (3) The monomeric C-subunit is always found phosphorylated at its activation loop threonine residue and is thus in an active state. Together, these circumstances make PKA ideally suited for studies on substrate recognition, catalytic pathway, order of substrate and cofactor binding, the identification of catalytic site residues, the cofactor specificity and its interaction with pseudosubstrate inhibitors, such as the protein kinase inhibitor and the R-subunits. Consequently, the first crystal structure of a protein kinase was from the catalytic subunit of PKA (Knighton et al. 1991).

Most known protein kinase inhibitors act in competition to ATP, binding in the ATP binding pocket, and mimicking many of the ATP enzyme interactions. The crystal structures of PKA in complex with MgATP or MnAMP-PNP and a pseudosubstrate peptide (Zheng et al. 1993; Bossemeyer et al. 1993) showed in detail the binding of the ATP molecule to protein kinases. These structures showed the functions to most of the residues, which are invariantly conserved in the kinase family. Together with the vast amount of previous data from biochemical and genetic studies, the structures explained in detail most principles of the catalytic mechanism of protein kinases, recently further confirmed by the structure of the putative transition state of the phosphorylation reaction (Madhusudan et al. 2002). In addition to the unique structural properties of the kinase-conserved glycine-rich loop, the structural origins of the synergistic binding of cofactor and pseudosubstrate inhibitors became apparent (Bossemeyer 1994). In this way, these early structures provided the first insights into the binding site relevant to the majority of all protein kinase inhibitors.

1.1 Specificity Features of the ATP Binding Site

The ATP binding site of protein kinases consists of two subsites with very different properties: the triphosphoryl subsite contains most of the invariantly conserved residues and is thus entirely conserved. All residues with sidechain contacts to the ATP molecule are either charged or electrophilic. The contacts of the triphosphoryl group to the enzyme form an extensive electrophilic network that involves the conserved sidechains either directly or via metal ions, and also involves several backbone atoms from the glycine-rich loop. Both the interactions with conserved sidechains and the loop interactions, because of the high structural homology of the protein kinases, seem likely to be conserved. Structures from other protein kinases with ATP or ATP analogues, however, showed that these contacts are not always identical. This is especially true for the metal ions, and the contacts to the glycine-rich loop (Russo et al. 1996; Hubbard 1997; Aubol et al. 2003; Nolen et al. 2003). Apparently, although at least within each of the subfamilies of the Ser/Thr and the Tyr-specific kinases amino acid residues in contact with the triphosphoryl group are strictly conserved, structural or electrical differences appear to exist and thus might contribute to the selectivity of suitable kinase inhibitors. In contrast to this highly conserved triphosphoryl subsite, the adenosine binding site contains only one invariant residue, the homologue of Val57, located at the C-terminus of the glycine-rich motif in PKA, and one very conserved residue, the homologue of Ala70 from β-strand 3. All other residues with sidechain contacts to ATP are variable but conservatively exchanged in the kinase family. Charged residues exist only in the ribose–hydroxyl subsite, Glu (corresponding to Glu127 of PKA), and Asp residues are common here. Apart from that, few residues are hydrophilic, such as Thr183 (PKA) and most are hydrophobic. The conserved polar interactions of adenosine in the binding site are again with backbone atoms, in PKA from N1 of the adenosine moiety to the amide of Val123 and from N6 to the carbonyl of Glu121. A functional reason for the variability of residues in the ATP site is not obvious. As all kinases bind ATP, differences might affect ATP binding and adenosine diphosphate (ADP) release rates, and could conceivably affect catalytic rates as well. As kinase (down)regulation often is accompanied by significant structural changes (Engh and Bossemeyer 2001; Huse and Kuriyan 2002), a specific role of ATP-site residues in inactivated conformations might also exist. A correspondence between the rotamer conformation of a residue on the enzyme surface and the sidechain change of a residue in the adenosine binding site has been shown recently with mutants of PKA. Gln181, usually in sidechain contact with hydrophilic residues on the surface, changed its conformation and partly obstructed the adenosine binding site after exchange of Val123, a variable hinge region residue, to alanine (Gaßel et al. 2003). As will be discussed in more detail later, a corresponding conformational change of such a Gln residue has been observed in the structure of PDK1 with UCN01 (Komander et al. 2003). PDK1 has alanine in the Val123 (PKA) position too. Exchange of Gln181 in PKA to the much more conserved lysine in the position of Gln181 resulted in a fixed surface orientation (Gaßel et al. 2003). This clearly demonstrates secondary functional consequences of single residue exchanges that require compensation of some sort. Thus, the high variability of residues which line the adenosine subsite may represent functional differences or may simply reflect less stringent evolutionary constraints in this region; in either case, it offers interesting opportunities to selectively target protein kinases with small molecule inhibitors by making use of the small differences in the individual shape and electronic environment in each protein kinase ATP pocket.

The sequence similarity of kinases within the same branch of kinases, such as the AGC kinases, leads to cross selectivity of protein kinase inhibitors. Obviously, closely related kinases appear to have a higher conservation of the kinase fold. A good example is the structures of active PKB (Yang et al. 2002), showing an ATP binding site which is almost indistinguishable from that of PKA. Mutagenesis of PKA and exchange of residues in the ATP pocket to PKB-specific residues emphasizes these similarities even further (Gaßel et al. 2003). Correspondingly, commercially available protein kinase inhibitors have very similar activities against both kinases (Davies et al. 2000). This is true for several protein kinase inhibitors that target AGC kinases. Though certainly a predicament for the design and development of selective protein kinase inhibitors, it can be turned into an advantage to achieve structural information about inhibitor/target interactions even if the primary target is difficult to deal with. PKA has been used as an ersatz kinase to study the binding mode of various AGC kinase inhibitors, mostly in cases were the actual target was structurally not available. For a long time PKA was the only AGC kinase with a known crystal structure. In the last 2 years, the crystal structures of several other members of the AGC branch have been solved, such as PKB/Akt (Yang et al. 2002), PDK1 (Biondi et al. 2002), Aurora (Bayliss et al. 2003) and Grk2 (Lodowski et al. 2003).

2
Inhibitor Cocrystal Structures

2.1
Structures of PKA with Isoquinoline Sulphonamide Derivatives

PKA was among the first kinases cocrystallized with protein kinase inhibitors (Schulze Gahmen et al. 1995; De Azevedo et al. 1996; Engh et al. 1996; Xu et al. 1996). The isoquinoline sulphonamide derivatives H7 (1-(5-isoquinolinesulfonyl)-2-methylpiperazine), H8 (N-[2-(methylamino)-ethyl]-

5-isoquinolinesulphonamide), and H89 (*N*-[2-(p-Bromocinnamylamino)ethyl]-5-isoquinolinesulphonamide) were chosen, because these inhibitors were at that time in wide use, and all of them inhibit PKA (PDB-codes 1YDR, 1YDS, 1YDT). H7 has a broad specificity within the AGC kinases and inhibits PKC as well as PKA in the micromolar range. Its ability to inhibit PKC (at 6 μM) was the reason for the enormous popularity of H7, used by many laboratories to dissect the role of PKC in signal transduction. Rho kinase, actually, is a 20-fold better target for H7 (Uehata et al. 1997) (300 nM), but this enzyme was not described before 1995 (Leung et al. 1995). H8, a micromolar inhibitor of PKA and PKC, inhibits PKG also. Still, H89 (48 nM for PKA) is one of the more selective PKA inhibitors, although when tested against a wider panel of protein kinases, some other AGC kinases, such as Rho kinase and PKB/Akt from the AGC group and S6K1 and MSK1 from other branches of the kinase family, are found to be inhibited by H89 too at comparable concentrations.

The H-inhibitors are characterized by an isoquinoline sulphonamide group, and a sidechain, where a two-carbon spacer separates two amide groups.

The binding of H7 to PKA is representative for some typical aspects of PKA inhibitor binding. The conserved isoquinoline moiety of the inhibitor, a planar double ring with one nitrogen atom acting as proton acceptor, occupies the position of the adenine purine of ATP and mimics the ATP N1 H-bond to the hinge region Val123 amide (Fig. 1). The planar isoquinoline group is embedded between the residues Val57, Ala70 and Leu49 from the small lobe, and Leu173 from the large lobe; these interactions contribute significantly to the number of van der Waals (VDW) contacts to the enzyme. Usually protein kinase inhibitors bind alike, with a proton accepting interaction from a planar structure. Few structures are known where the inhibitor does not follow this pattern. TBB (tetrabromo-2-benzotriazole) (PDB-code 1J91) is such an example, which makes no hinge atom contact in CK2 (Battistutta et al. 2001); however, this appears to be a specific feature of CK2,

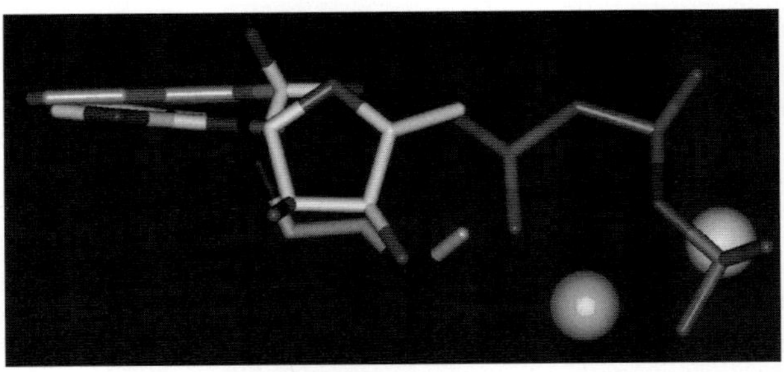

Fig. 1 Superimposition of H8 and MnAMP-PNP, showing spatial congruence with adenosine group and of function groups. (Engh et al. 1996)

because the same inhibitor binds in CDK2 according to the common pattern (De Moliner et al. 2003). Also the inhibitor BIRB 796 (PDB-code 1KV1) binds to a 'DFG-out' conformation of P38 in an atypical way without a hinge region contact (Pargellis et al. 2002). In many AGC kinases, such as PKA, or PKB, a residue from outside the catalytic core, Phe327, contributes to the completeness of the adenosine binding site. Phe327 or its homologue is positioned on a C-terminal polypeptide stretch that expands from the large lobe via the catalytic cleft to the N-terminal lobe and ends in the hydrophobic motif beside helix C. This aromatic residue is not conserved outside the group of AGC kinases, nor has a comparable contribution been observed in other kinases so far. The H-inhibitors mimic not only the purine of ATP, but also aspects of the ribose. The $2'$ and $3'$ OH groups of ATP in PKA make contacts to the backbone carbonyl of Glu170, and in addition to the sidechain of Glu127, the only charged residue in the adenosine pocket. The sulphonamide group together with the sidechain mimics a part of the ribose spatially, and the distal amine of the aminoethyl sidechain of most H-inhibitors forms a similar contact to the Glu170 carbonyl. Interestingly, one of the sulphonyl oxygens is in the same spatial position as the ring oxygen of the ribose. This is not only observed with H7, but is a general feature of H-inhibitor binding in PKA, and is observed also with the indolocarbazole staurosporine. In none of these cases is a typical H-bond contact formed from the oxygen, but the $C\alpha$-hydrogen of Gly50 is close enough for a weak CH–O interaction, as was postulated for staurosporine (Zhu et al. 1999). The triphosphoryl subsite, however, is not occupied by most of the PKA inhibitors, with the exception of balanol (see below), which makes electrophilic contacts to Lys72 (in its normal function involved in binding the phosphoryl groups) and the backbone amides of the glycine loop. The consequence is that, in the case of H7 and H8, the glycine-rich flap is not in contact with the inhibitors and has an increased mobility. This is different in the case of H89, which possesses a large bromocinnamyl sidechain, binding underneath and stabilizing the structure of the glycine flap (Fig. 2). The specificity of the H-inhibitors is defined by differences in their sulphonamide substituents, as all (with the exception of H-1152P) have identical isoquinoline sulphonamide head groups. Accordingly, the number of VDW contacts to the isoquinoline is almost identical for all three inhibitors, only H89 is packed slightly better. Differences are observed for the contacts of the amino group of the sidechains, although this group is present in all three inhibitors. Only H8 makes a contact from here to the sidechain of Asp184. Asp184 usually has a different rotamer and is in contact with the basic charge of Lys72, or, in the ATP-bound structure, with one of the metal ions. Apparently, the distal amine in the H8 sidechain attracts this residue more than the comparable nitrogens in H7 or H89, which even is structurally identical to H8 in this region. The bromocinnamoyl group and the piperazine ring weaken the partial-positive charge of the secondary amine, which

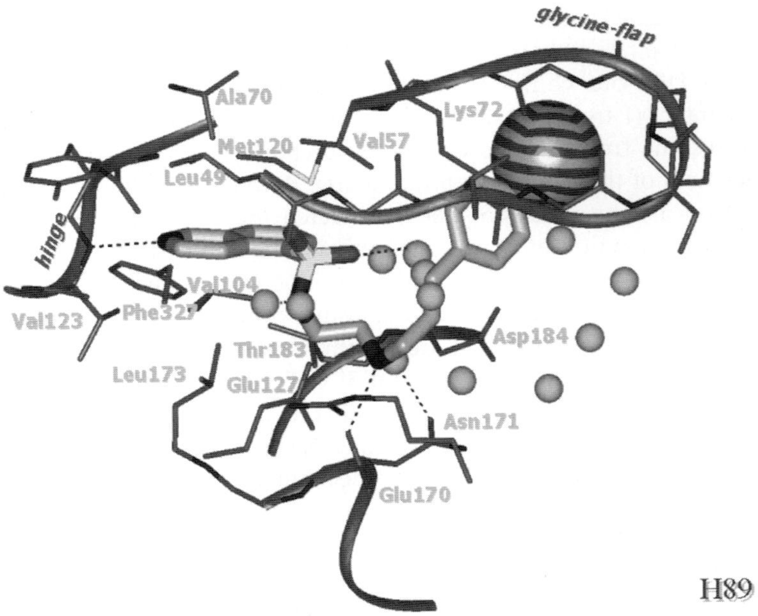

Fig. 2 H89 in the binding pocket of PKA. The bromocinnamoyl group interacts with the glycine-rich motif. (Engh et al. 1996)

then is less attractive for the Asp residue and does not induce a conformational change. The overall number of polar and VDW interactions of these inhibitors varies; H89 has three H-bond contacts to the enzyme and the highest number of VDW interactions. A correlation of structural features to the inhibitory activity was found in the total area of the buried surface of the inhibitor (Engh and Bossemeyer 2002). Inhibitor selectivity in closely related kinases is determined mostly by sidechain differences in the ATP pocket. One PKA related kinase, hardly inhibited by H89, is PDK1. Few residues differ in the ATP binding pocket between PDK1 and PKA: Val123 is Ala in PDK1, Met120 is Leu in PDK1; both residues, however, interact with the isoquinoline head group, and not with the H89-specific sidechain. A significant difference in a sidechain-critical region is Gly55, the first residue following the turn in the glycine-rich beta sheet. This residue is Ser in PDK1. Interestingly, Phkγ, although also quite similar to PKA in the binding pocket, is also much more weakly inhibited by H89 and also contains a serine residue in the Gly55 position. Another general difference between PKA and PDK1 is the absence of the C-terminal stretch with the phenylalanine residue which, as Phe327, makes contacts to the isoquinoline of all H-inhibitors. Perhaps the binding pocket for comparably small molecules such as H-inhibitors often requires some completeness, provided for most AGC kinases by this C-terminal phenylalanine residue. It cannot be excluded that this residue is one reason for the general preference of several H-inhibitors, such as H89, or HA1077 for AGC kinase, such as MSK1 or S6kinase (Davies et al. 2000). Several derivatives of the isoquinoline sulphonamides have been made which are active against protein kinases. A cognate of H7, HA-1077 or fasudil, was especially successful as an inhibitor of Rho kinase (see the chapter on fasudil by Hidaka et al., this volume). Fasudil and two other Rho kinase-selective inhibitors, H-1152P and Y-27632, were cocrystallized with PKA (Breitenlechner et al. 2003).

2.2 PKA as a Model for Rho Kinase: Structures of PKA with Rho Kinase Inhibitors Y-27632, Fasudil (HA-1077) and H-1152P

As a serine–threonine kinase of the AGC group, Rho kinase possesses a catalytic domain closely related to other AGC group kinases, among them PKA, PKB, PKC and PKG; although no crystal structure of Rho kinase has been reported yet. The close relationship between PKA and Rho kinase (37% identical) and the well-established crystallization conditions for PKA make PKA a suitable model system for studying Rho kinase inhibitors. Furthermore, cocrystallization of PKA with Rho kinase inhibitors helps identify factors governing cross selectivity of protein kinase inhibitors. The importance of sidechain differences in the ATP binding pocket for inhibitor selectivity has been shown previously with Erk2 (Fox et al. 1998).

To avoid confusion, we will use the term 'Rho kinase' for the two enzymes of this family: Rho-associated, coiled-coil-containing protein kinase p160ROCK (gene: *ROCK1*) and Rho kinase (gene: *ROCK2*). They are highly homologous in the kinase domain (96%), especially in ATP pocket and are identical in all residues in contact with the inhibitors.

2.2.1 Inhibitor Binding Site—ATP pocket

The inhibitors are ATP competitive and bind to the ATP pocket made up of residues from the glycine loop (Leu49, Gly50, Thr51, Val57), β-sheet 3 (Ala70), hinge region (Met120, Glu121, Tyr122, Val123, Glu127), catalytic loop (Glu170, Asn171, Leu173), beginning of the activation loop (Thr183, Asp184), and C-terminal stretch (Phe327) (Fig. 3).

The buried surface of the inhibitors in their pocket in PKA correlates with their affinity: H-1152P (1.1 μM) with the highest affinity also has the largest buried surface of the three inhibitors (215.7 Å^2); Y-27632 (25 μM) has the smallest buried surface of the three (188 Å^2). A correlation of buried inhibitor surface and binding affinity has previously been observed for PKA inhibitors (Engh and Bossemeyer 2002). Rho kinase and PKA differ, however, in eight positions in the ATP binding pocket. Four of their sidechains are

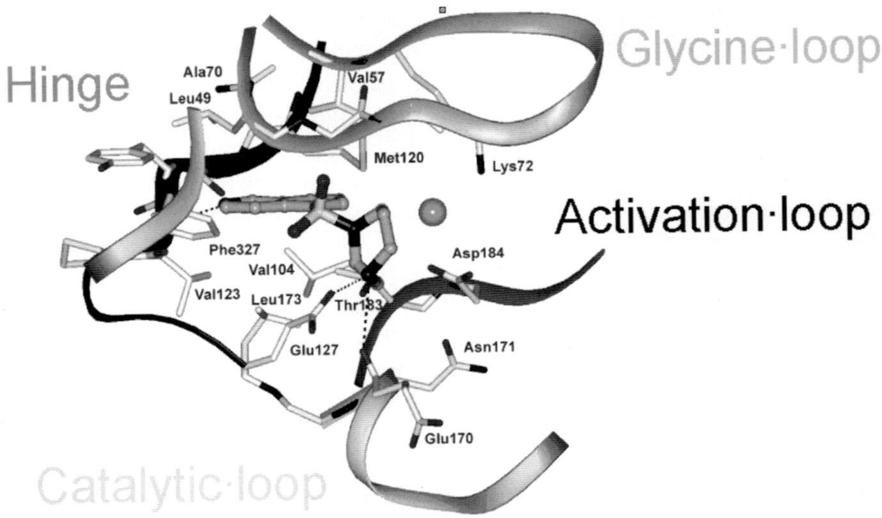

Fig. 3 Binding of HA-1077 (fasudil) in the ATP pocket (Breitenlechner et al. 2003). Hydrogen bonds between enzyme and inhibitor are depicted by *dotted lines*; conserved peptide strands of the kinase domain are shown as *ribbons*

in close (<4 Å) contact with the inhibitors, corresponding to the following PKA→Rho substitutions: Leu49Ile, Val123Met, Thr183Ala and Glu127Asp. Because the protein kinase fold is so highly conserved, variations of amino acid residues that line the ATP subsite belong to the most important factors in defining inhibitor selectivity.

2.2.2 Fasudil (HA-1077 or AT877)

Fasudil was the first protein kinase inhibitor approved for clinical use (1995). It is effective—with very little side effects—for cerebral vasospasm, the painful and sometimes deadly after-effect of subarachnoid haemorrhage. Fasudil has significant vasodilatory activity (Ono-Saito et al. 1999) and is now in clinical trials for the treatment of angina pectoris (Shimokawa et al. 2001). Fasudil's activity has been attributed to inhibition of Rho kinase (Matsui et al. 1996) and its role in signalling for myosin light chain phosphorylation and arterial smooth muscle contraction (Amano et al. 1996; Takemoto et al. 2002), although the in vitro activity of fasudil is not strictly limited to Rho kinase. Other Rho kinase-related protein kinases, such as PKA, PRK2, MSK1 and S6K1, are also inhibited by fasudil, although to a lesser extent (Davies et al. 2000). Rho kinase may be an important pharmacological target also for cancer because of its role in the invasion and migration of cancer cells (Amano et al. 2000; Fukata et al. 2001).

Table 1 Crystal structures of PKA–Rho kinase inhibitor complexes

PDB code	Inhibitor	Resolution (Å)	Chemical structure	K_i [μM] (PKA)[a]	K_i [μM] (Rho kinase)[a]
1Q8 W	HA-1077	2.2	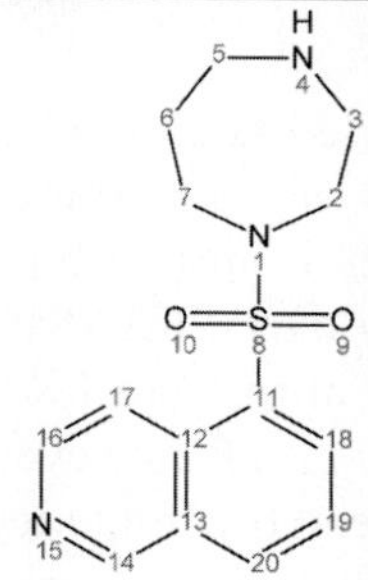	1	0.33
1Q8U	H-1152P	1.9	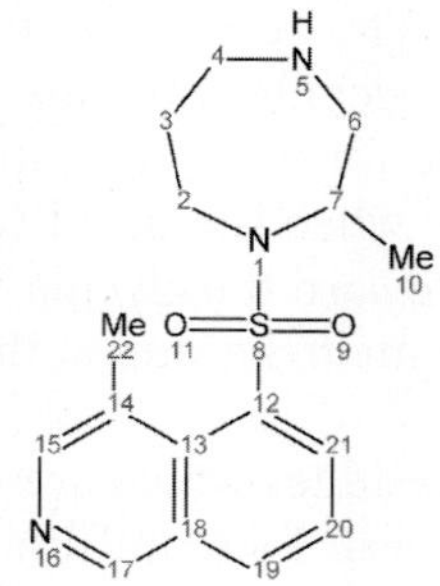	0.63	0.0016
1Q8T	Y-27632	2.0	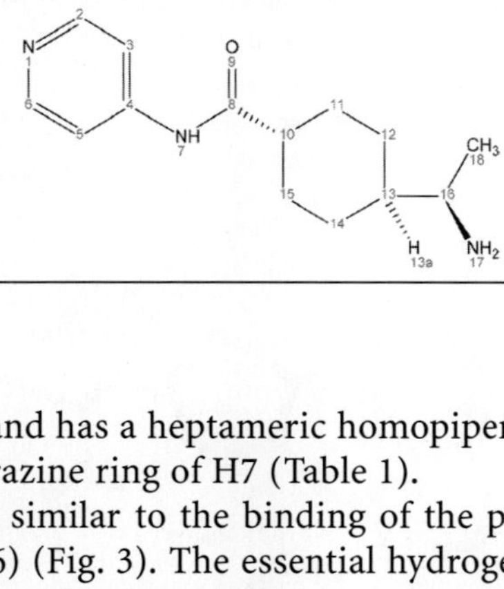	25	0.14

[a] Ikenoya et al. 2002.

Fasudil is related to H7, and has a heptameric homopiperazine ring at the position of the methyl-piperazine ring of H7 (Table 1).

The binding of fasudil is similar to the binding of the parental molecule H7 to PKA (Engh et al. 1996) (Fig. 3). The essential hydrogen bond between the peptide backbone amide of Val123 and the nitrogen atom of the isoquinoline ring is formed. As H7, the secondary amine of the homopiperazine ring makes a hydrogen contact to the peptide backbone carbonyl of Glu170. This contact, usually reserved for the 3′ OH of ATP, is present in the PKA/H7 structure too. Not provided by H7, fasudil can make, in addition, a contact of the homopiperazine nitrogen to the sidechain of Glu127. In the

ATP structure this contact is also present, to the 2′ and 3′ OH groups of the ribose.

2.2.3 H-1152P

Further derivatization of fasudil led to H-1152P, with two additional methyl groups, one at the isoquinoline ring and the other at the homopiperazine ring (Tanaka et al. 1998). H-1152P inhibits Rho kinase in the low nanomolar range, with a 400-fold selectivity over PKA (Sasaki et al. 2002). Fasudil and H-1152P bind both with similar affinity to PKA in the same orientation in the adenosine pocket (Fig. 4). H-1152P, however, has only one H-bond contact to the enzyme, the one between the hinge region amide group to the isoquinoline ring nitrogen. No H-bonds are formed with the nitrogen atom of the homopiperazine ring. The reason for this difference in binding of H-1152P and fasudil to PKA becomes obvious from an overlay of both inhibitor structures. In order to form the 'essential' H-bond to the hinge region, H-1152P can only bind, when the distal (as seen from the hinge) homopiperazine ring is shifted toward the glycine-rich loop in order to avoid a steric clash between the extra methyl group at the homopiperazine ring, and the sidechain of Thr183.

Thr183 is one of the four residues which are in sidechain contact to ATP-side inhibitors and differ between PKA and Rho kinase. An alanine residue in this position, as in Rho kinase, would provide enough space for a closer

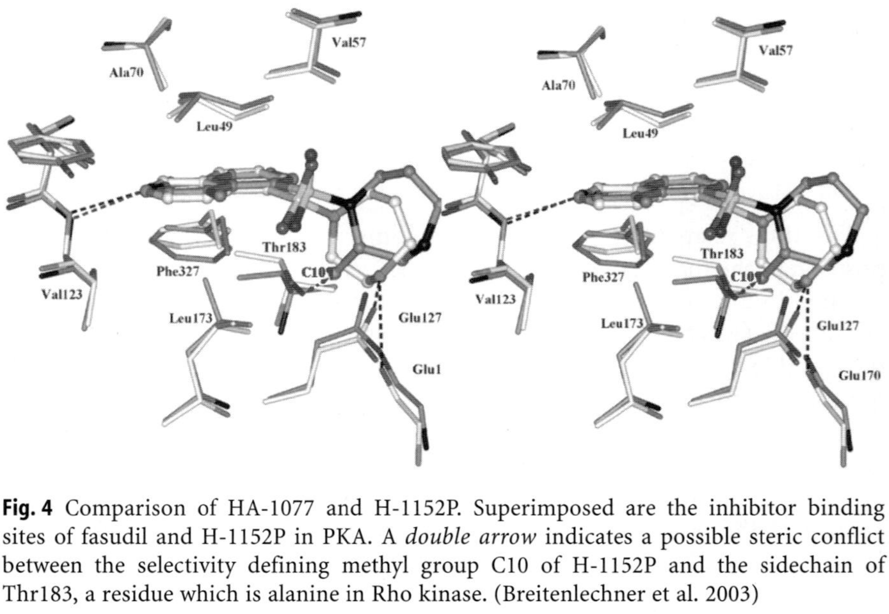

Fig. 4 Comparison of HA-1077 and H-1152P. Superimposed are the inhibitor binding sites of fasudil and H-1152P in PKA. A *double arrow* indicates a possible steric conflict between the selectivity defining methyl group C10 of H-1152P and the sidechain of Thr183, a residue which is alanine in Rho kinase. (Breitenlechner et al. 2003)

approach of the H-1152P homopiperazine ring towards the H-bond-forming groups of Glu170, and Gly127 (Fig. 4). Also, the exchange of the Leu49 residue to isoleucine could be an advantage for H-1152P, by increasing the number of VDW contacts and the hydrophobic interactions. The extra methyl group at the isoquinoline ring could benefit from the branching of the isoleucine sidechain at the Cβ atom. The two other differences, Val123Met and Glu127Asp, are difficult to interpret in terms of selectivity for Rho kinase. The valine residue makes the largest number of contacts with fasudil, and the second largest number of contacts with H-1152P. As seen in protein kinase crystal structures with a methionine residue in the homologous position, the sidechain points away from the ATP binding pocket such that only Cβ or Cγ atoms can interact with an ATP-site ligand. The methionine therefore does not likely contribute to Rho kinase selectivity for HA-1077 or H-1152P, since its effect, if any, would be to remove interactions and lower the binding affinity (S. Bonn, S. Herrero, M. Gaßel, C.B. Breitenlechner, R. Engh, D. Bossemeyer, in preparation). An exchange of Glu127 to Asp is also expected to change little, because the shorter sidechain can still make the H-bond contacts to the homopiperazine nitrogen atoms. Overall, the contacts from the residues which differ between PKA and Rho kinase in the ATP binding site contribute most significantly to the interactions between the inhibitors and PKA.

Because sidechain interactions form the major kinase selectivity determinant of active conformations to ATP-site inhibitors, the conservation of Thr183, Val123, Leu49 and Glu127 should be predictive of H-1152P selectivity. None of these four residues is rare or exceptional (Table 2). However, this combination occurs in only six other kinases, none of which belong to the AGC group of protein kinases. Consideration of a fifth residue renders Rho kinases unique. AGC kinases, including PKA and Rho kinase, possess a C-terminal strand that inserts a phenylalanine sidechain in to the ATP binding site. The phenylalanine interacts in known AGC kinase structures with the purine base of ATP and most ATP-site ligands, and also with fasudil and H-1152P. The ATP-site ligand contacts to Phe327 are typically edge–edge aromat aromat contacts that affix the ligand to the adenine site. Thus, the

Table 2 Differences in Rho kinase and PKA and occurrence (according to Hanks and Quinn 1991; Manning et al. 2002)

PKA	Residue number	Rho-kinase	Occurrence (%)
Thr	183	Ala	34/29
Val	123	Met	29/25
Leu	49	Ile	44/38
Glu	127	Asp	38/32

combination of Thr183, Val123, Leu49 and Glu127 together with Phe327 is unique to Rho kinase.

2.2.4
Second Binding Site for H-1152P

In addition, for H-1152P a second binding site exists in a surface region with contact to the phosphoryl group of Thr197 and to Lys189 (Fig. 5), both from the activation loop and to Glu86 from helix C, a region critical for kinase activity and protein–protein interaction with the regulatory R-subunit (Gibbs et al. 1992; Orellana et al. 1993). Although a functional relevance of H-1152P

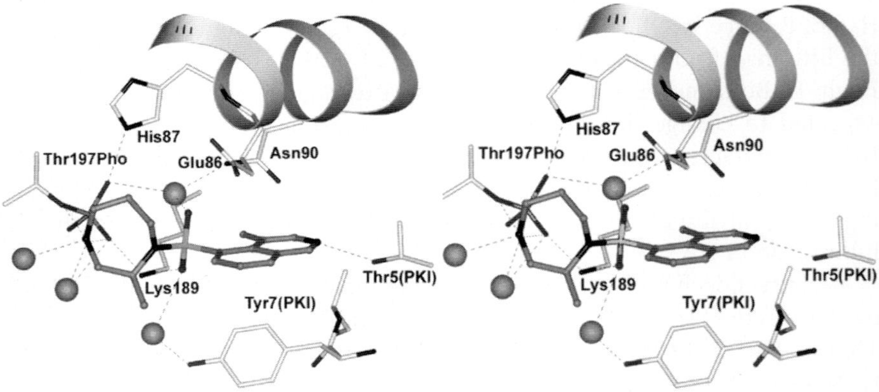

Fig. 5 H-1152P binds in a second position on the surface of the protein in contact with activation loop phospho-Thr197, and helix C

in this second position for PKA is not clear yet, this site might be attractive as a new target site for drugs that interfere with kinase regulatory elements or regulatory subunits.

2.2.5
Y-27632

Y-27632, a pyridine derivative, represents a chemical class distinct from the H inhibitors described above. It has a K_i of 140 nM for Rho kinase and 25 μM for PKA (Table 1) (Ishizaki et al. 2000) and is ATP competitive, like the H inhibitors (Ikenoya et al. 2002; Trauger et al. 2002). Y-27623 is a widely used Rho kinase inhibitor and several effects could be observed in vitro and in vivo (for review see Ishizaki et al. 2000; Narumiya et al. 2000). It prevents phosphorylation of focal adhesion kinase and paxillin (Sinnett-Smith et al. 2001), inhibits the migration of rat MM1 hepatoma cancer cells (Itoh et al.

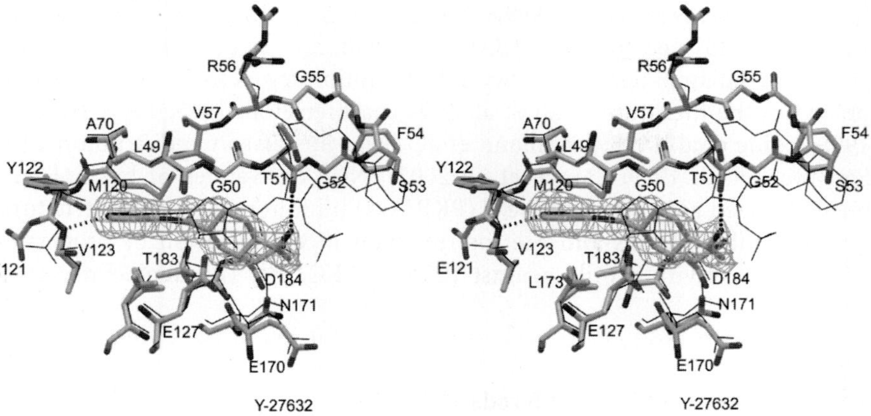

Fig. 6 Binding of Y-27632 to PKA to the ATP binding site. Electron density is displayed at 2 σ. (Breitenlechner et al. 2003)

1999), and leads to smooth muscle contraction and normalization of blood pressure in rats (Uehata et al. 1997). A pyridine ring is connected by an amide to a saturated para-aminoethyl cyclohexane ring. The pyridine similarly occupies the adenine subsite and with the canonical H-bond contacts to the hinge region the Val123 amide group (Fig. 6). The cyclohexane is situated in the ribose subsite. A hydrogen bond is formed from the terminal aminoethyl group to the carbonyl oxygen of Thr51. As the cyclohexane moiety can bind in two slightly different orientations, alternatively, hydrogen bonds from the terminal aminoethyl group to the sidechains of Asp171 and Asp184 are possible too.

The selectivity of Y-27632 for Rho kinase over PKA is 200-fold, a property not immediately rationalized by the structure. It seems, however, likely that the Leu49Ile exchange can enhance hydrophobic interactions. At the same time, the exchange Thr183Ala in Rho kinase offers a wider pocket and greater freedom for the inhibitor to optimize binding interactions.

2.3 Balanol and Derivatives

The balanols represent a class of potentially therapeutic PKC inhibitors. They are derived from the natural product (−)-balanol, which was first isolated as a metabolite of the fungus *Verticillium balanoides* at Sphinx Pharmaceuticals (Eli Lilly) (Kulanthaivel et al. 1993) and from a species of *Fusarium* at Nippon Roche (Ohshima et al. 1994). (−)-Balanol inhibits PKC and PKA in the low nanomolar range (K_i=6.4 nM for PKCα, K_i=1.8 nM for PKCβII and K_i=3.9 nM for PKA) and other serine/threonine kinases less potently (e.g. 74 nM for CaMKII and 742 for MAPK); tyrosine kinases are not inhibited (Setyawan et al. 1999). A cocrystal structure of (−)-balanol with PKA was published in 1999 (1BX6) (Hunenberger et al. 1999; Narayana et al. 1999). Balanol derivatives with PKC inhibitory activity have been reported in the literature (Hall et al. 1994; Barbier et al. 1995, 1997; Hu et al. 1995; Koide et al. 1995; Jagdmann et al. 1996; Gustafsson and Brunton 1999; Setyawan et al. 1999; Lampe et al. 2002). New derivatives of balanol have been reported as protein kinase B (PKB/Akt) inhibitors. Cocrystal structures reveal binding modes and are instrumental in optimization of properties, such as selectivity profile against PKA or PKC, etc. (Breitenlechner et al. 2004).

2.3.1
X-Ray Structure of Balanol (PDB-code 1BX6)

The complex of the natural (−)-balanol with PKA (PDB-code 1BX6) was solved in 1999 (Narayana et al. 1999). The molecule (Fig. 7) can be considered in terms of occupation of three regions of the ATP binding pocket: a phenol (Fig. 7, ring *A*) in the adenine subsite, an azepane (*B*) in the ribose subsite and the benzophenone (*C* and *D*) occupies the triphosphate subsite.

The phenol makes two H-bonds from the –OH group to the hinge region Val123(N) and Glu121(O); VDW contacts exist to Leu49, Ala70, Glu121, Tyr122, Val123, Thr183 and Phe327. The amide that links to the azepane ring makes one H-bond to a water molecule with its amide nitrogen and to Thr183 with its carbonyl oxygen. The azepane ring is in VDW contact with Gly50, Glu127 and Glu170, and additionally forms an H-bond with Gly170. The benzophenone part interacts with Thr51, Gly52, Ser53, Phe54, Gly55, Arg56, Lys72, Leu74, Gln84, Glu91, Asp184, Gly186, Phe187. Benzophenone substituents are involved in several H-bonds: to Gly52, Ser53, Phe54, and

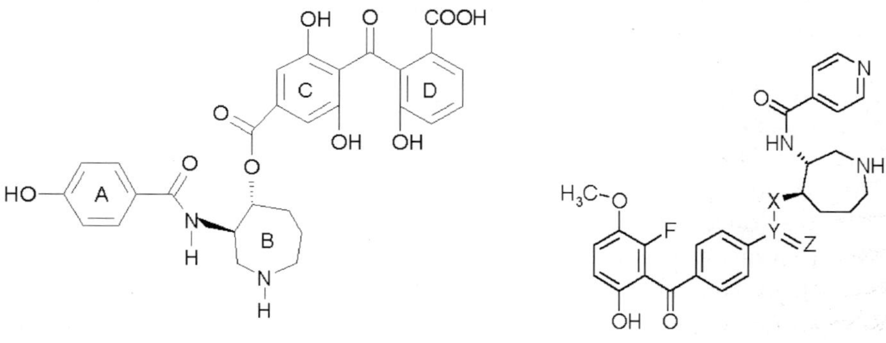

Fig. 7 Chemical structure of the natural (−)-balanol and the novel balanol derivatives. (Breitenlechner et al. 2004)

Gly55 from the glycine loop, to the conserved residues Lys72 and Glu91, and to Asp184 from the beginning of the activation loop.

In total, there are 21 H-bonds and 114 VDW interactions, whereas most occur with the triphosphate subsite (Narayana et al. 1999; Setyawan et al. 1999; Wong et al. 2001).

2.3.2
X-Ray Structures and Binding Mode of Balanol Derivatives

Novel azepane derivatives have been synthesized and the X-ray structures of the PKA-PKI-complexes solved (Breitenlechner et al. 2004). The chemical structures involve variations of different parts of the natural balanol: the phenol has been replaced by a pyridine ring, the substituents on the benzophenone have been modified and the ester linker between ring *B* and *C* has been extensively modified in order to optimize pharmacokinetic properties.

Three binding regions were defined in reference to the balanol-type interactions: the pyridine pocket, the azepane pocket and the benzophenone pocket (Fig. 8). These regions correspond closely to the adenine, ribose and phosphate binding sites (Breitenlechner et al. 2004).

The pyridine pocket contains the pyridine moiety and the amide connecting it to the azepane ring. This space is occupied by the adenine in the complex of AMP–PNP and PKA (Bossemeyer et al. 1993) (Fig. 8) and accepts in general aromatic groups. The glycine loop (Leu49, Val57), β-sheet 3 (Ala70), the hinge region (Met120, Tyr122, Val123, Glu127), the catalytic loop (Leu173), the beginning of the activation loop (Thr183), and Phe327 from the C-terminal stretch are involved in VDW contacts to the pyridine and amide portion of compound 1 (Fig. 9).

The hinge region residue Val123 makes an H-bond to the pyridine via its main chain amide. This H-bond to Val123 (or its homologue in other kinases) is nearly universal amongst protein kinase inhibitor complexes and is

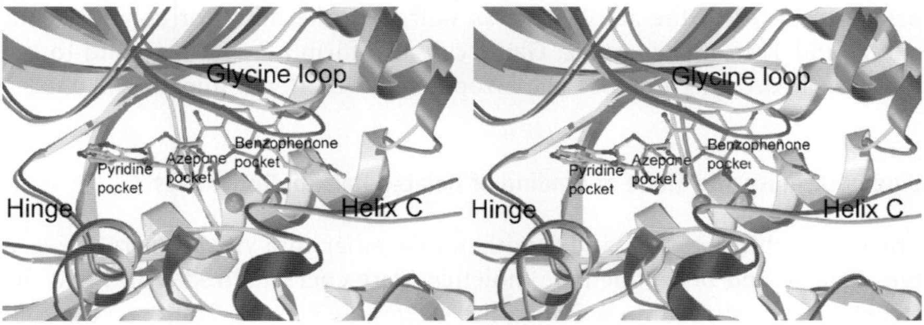

Fig. 8 Binding of a balanol derivative to the ATP binding pocket of PKA (*light grey*) superimposed with the AMP-PNP structure (*dark grey*); [1CDK (Bossemeyer et al. 1993)]

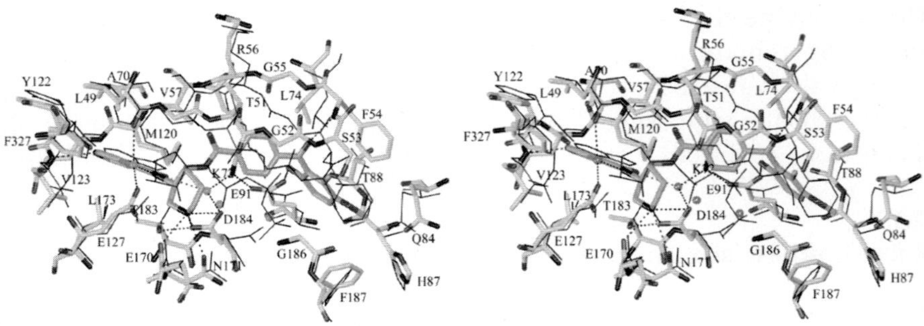

Fig. 9 Binding of a balanol derivative to the ATP binding pocket of PKA in structural detail

apparently critical for tight-binding inhibitors. Two H-bonds exist from the amide group to two water molecules that bridge polar contacts between the amide NH and Glu127 and Leu49 and between the amides CO to Lys72 and Asp184.

The azepane pocket—stretching over the ribose subsite—contains the azepane and the ester part of the molecule. This pocket is bounded by residues from the glycine loop (Gly50, Thr51, Gly52, Val57), β-sheet 3 (Lys72), the catalytic loop (Glu170, Asn171) and Asp184 from the beginning of the activation loop. The protonated azepane nitrogen forms H-bonds to Asn171 and Asp184.

The benzophenone pocket is bounded on one side by the flexible glycine loop, which is displaced compared to the AMP-PNP PKA complex (see Fig. 8). Consequently, VDW contacts exist to glycine loop residues (Ser53, Phe54, Gly55, Arg56), and also to residue Leu74 from the β-sheet 3, to several residues from helix C (Gln84, His87, Thr88, Glu91), as well as to Gly186 and Phe187 from the activation loop.

The carbonyl oxygen of the benzophenone is involved in hydrogen bonds to the backbone amide nitrogen Phe54 at the tip of the glycine loop.

Glu91, which is essential for catalysis (Schneider 2002), forms a salt bridge to Lys72 in the active state as well as in the inhibitor complex with compound 1. In this complex, Glu91 can also form a hydrogen bond to the inhibitor hydroxyl group of the benzophenone (Breitenlechner et al. 2004).

2.3.3
Binding Affinity and Mode of Binding of Related Balanol Derivatives

The other inhibitors 4, 5, and 8, with amide, ether, and vinyl linkers between the azepane and benzophenone moieties, were cocrystallized with PKA; the structures are superimposed with the ester 1 in Fig. 10. The crystal structures confirm that the bound conformations are unperturbed by the modifications. The conformation of the linker for which the torsional angle is *an-*

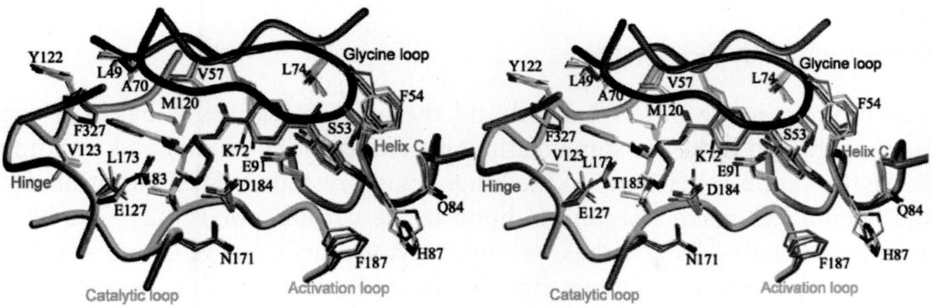

Fig. 10 Intermolecular bonding contacts in the complex between PKA and the balanol derivative. (Breitenlechner et al. 2004)

tiperiplanar in all molecules is *trans* with respect to azepane and benzophenone. This conformation is required because it orients the azepane and the benzophenone towards their binding pockets. Therefore, molecules which are preorganized in aqueous solution in the *trans* conformations should have higher binding affinities [which is in agreement with the biochemical data (Table 3)]. And indeed, ester 1 and amide 4 show tight binding (IC_{50}=5 nM or 4 nM, respectively), similar to (−)-balanol.

In the complex between the double amide 4 and PKA, there is a rearrangement of the sidechains of Asp184, Thr183 and Lys72 compared to the complex of the ester with PKA. The sidechain of Asp184 is rotated towards the amide linker and makes an H-bond to the amide nitrogen in addition to the H-bond to the azepane nitrogen; Lys72 forms an additional H-bond to the inhibitor hydroxyl group of the benzophenone, and Thr183 H-bonds to

Table 3 Properties of balanol derivatives

Inhibitor	X–YZ	Linker	Half-life[a]	IC_{50} (PKB)[a]	IC_{50} (PKA)[a]
1	O–C=O	Ester	<1 min	5 nM	5 nM
4	NH–C=O	Amide	69 h	4 nM	2 nM
5	O–CH_2	Ether	29 h	355 nM	39 nM
8	CH=CH	Vinyl		160 nM	360 nM

[a] Breitenlechner et al. 2004.

the amide next to the pyridine. In the cocrystal structure of the ether and vinyl compounds, the orientation of Asp184 corresponds to the complex of the ester with PKA, whereas the conformation of the sidechains of Thr183 and Lys72 are similar to the amide cocrystal structure (Breitenlechner et al. 2004).

2.3.4
Comparison to the (−)-Balanol

The binding mode of (−)-balanol and the new derivatives is basically the same, although there are some distinct differences. The phenol and pyridine share the canonical H-bond to the hinge region residue Val123. Additionally, the phenol can make a second H-bond to the carbonyl of Tyr122. The benzophenone in (−)-balanol has two hydroxyl groups on ring C and one hydroxyl and one carboxylate on ring D. These highly hydrophilic substituents are involved in extensive H-bonds (see above). The derivatives have substituents only on ring D, the hydroxyl group, a fluor substituent in the position of the carboxylate group and an additional methoxy group. The fluor substituent points in a similar direction as the carboxylate (towards Ser53), but is unable to make an H-bond. The hydroxyl substituent has hydrophilic contacts or H-bonds to Glu91 and Lys72 that are similar in all structures. The methoxy group extends deeper into another pocket, towards Phe187, Gln84 and His87, which is not occupied by the (−)-balanol. Asp184 of the conserved DFG motif that initiates the activation loop deserves special attention. It is probably the most flexible residue in the ATP pocket, with the greatest degree of ligand-induced motions: its sidechain points away from the pocket when it coordinates with the manganese atoms in the AMP-PNP structure (PDB-code 1CDK), or the hydroxyl group on the benzophenone ring (C) in the (−)-balanol complex, and also in the presence of ligands such as H-1152P, Y-27632, H89 and H7, but it points into the pocket with ligands such as H8 or HA-1077 and the azepane derivatives. In the latter case it forms an H-bond to the azepane nitrogen, except for the double amide 4, where the H-bond is made to the amide nitrogen of the linker. Thr183 and Leu173 seem also to be flexible, and their sidechain orientation varies. Thus the hydroxyl group of Thr183 makes H-bonds either to a conserved water molecule or to the inhibitor.

2.4
Structure of PKA with Staurosporine

Amongst the potentially therapeutic inhibitors of natural origin are the indolocarbazoles, such as staurosporine, and the bisindolylmaleimides. Staurosporine, a potent but nonselective protein kinase inhibitor, is a microbial alkaloid from *Streptomyces* sp. It inhibits PKA with a K_i of about 10 nM, along with many other kinases. Staurosporine is rather unselective against some kinases such as CK1 and CK2, with inhibitory kinetics in the micromolar range, a fact that has been connected to the existence of relatively bulky sidechains in the ATP pocket of these kinases (Meggio et al. 1995). Again, its widespread use in signalling research and as a lead compound for potential therapeutics was triggered by its efficient inhibitory activity

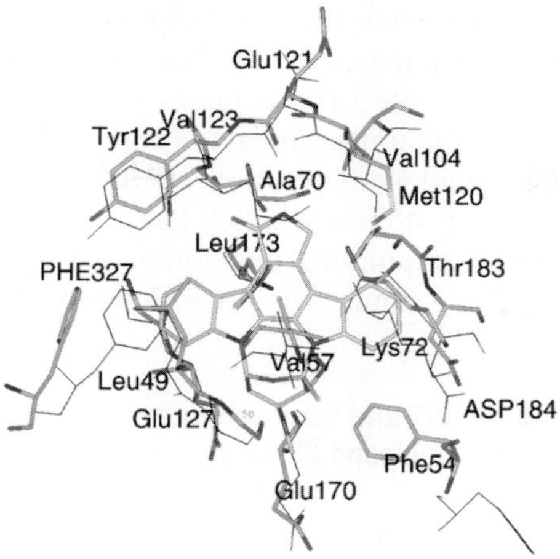

Fig. 11 Induced fit movements of enzyme residues in the vicinity of staurosporine upon binding of staurosporine to PKA (Prade et al. 1997). Residues rendered as *stick models* are from the 1STC structure, residues from 1CDK are represented as *lines*

against PKC. Staurosporine shows similar binding modes with different protein kinases. Cocrystal structures were solved from staurosporine in complex with inactive CDK2 (PDB-code 1AQ1) (Lawrie et al. 1997) and with active PKA (1STC) (Prade et al. 1997; Toledo and Lydon 1997), with CSK (1BYG) (Lamers et al. 1999), Chk1 (1NVR) (Zhao et al. 2002), MapKap kinase 2 (1NXK) (Underwood et al. 2003), Gsk3β (1Q3D) (Bertrand et al. 2003), Lck (1QPJ) (Zhu et al. 1999), and with the AGC kinase PDK1 (Komander et al. 2003). The molecule binds to PKA with two hinge region H-bonds, one to Val123 amide and the other to the Glu121 carbonyl group. Both hydrogen bonds are conserved adenine contacts, and established in all other staurosporine structures in an identical manner. Also comparable to ATP, the staurosporine methylamino group makes contacts to both the carbonyl of Glu170 (seen also with all H-inhibitors except H-1152P) and to the sidechain of Glu127. The latter contact was also made by fasudil, but not by other H-inhibitors cocrystallized with PKA. In addition to these four hydrogen bonds, staurosporine makes a large number of VDW contacts with the enzyme, possibly because the kinase undergoes induced fit movements upon binding of the inhibitor. In order to accommodate the large staurosporine, most sidechains in the contact area of the inhibitor, the peptide backbone in the region of Val104 and Thr183, and the C-terminal stretch including residue Phe327, move by up to almost 5 Å and expand the ATP pocket (Fig. 11). Phe327, however, makes favourable edge-to-plane contacts with one of the staurosporine indoles. None of the other kinases that have been cocrystallized with staurosporine, including PDK1, possesses a residue corresponding to Phe327, which is conserved amongst most AGC kinases. Another aromatic residue that undergoes a conformational change to contact staurosporine is Phe54 at the tip of the glycine-rich loop. Phe54 bends inwards towards the inhibitor and makes favourable VDW contacts with the methyl group at the staurosporine sugar ring. A similar contact is observed in Chk1, where a tyrosine residue in the homologous position interacts with the methyl group of the staurosporine sugar. Although Cdk2, Csk, Gsk3β and Lck have a Tyr or Phe residue at the corresponding position at the tip of the glycine-rich loop, none of them makes a similar contact with this aromat.

2.5 Structures of PDK1 with UCN01 and Staurosporine: Role of a Glutamine Switch in Ligand Binding

2.5.1 3-Phosphoinositide-Dependent Protein Kinase 1

The cellular integration of growth factor signals via membrane receptors results in the activation of the phosphatidylinositol 3-kinase (PI3 K), which in turn generates the membrane-bound second messengers phosphatidylinositol 3,4-diphosphate [PI (3,4)P2] and PI(3,4,5)P3. These second messengers recruit PKB/Akt via a mechanism that involves 3-phosphoinositide-dependent kinase 1 (PDK1), resulting in insulin regulation, cell growth and cell survival (Vanhaesebroeck and Alessi 2000). The PDK1 kinase activity was purified first from rabbit skeletal muscle (Alessi et al. 1997b) and rat brain (Stokoe et al. 1997). Human PDK1 is a polypeptide of 556 amino acids (63.1 kDa) with at least three domains (Alessi et al. 1997a): an AGC-Ser-Thr kinase domain that spans residues 84–341; a pleckstrin homology domain (PH) at the C-terminus (residues 450–550), which binds to the PtdIns(3,4,5)P3 and PtdIns(3,4)P2; and the N-domain (first 50 residues) with yet-unclear function. Phosphorylation sites in this domain for various protein kinases are assumed to play a role in PDK1 activity (Park et al. 2001; Wick et al. 2002; Kim et al. 2003; Taniyama et al. 2003).

Originally described as a PKB kinase, PDK1 can also phosphorylate and activate many Ser-Thr kinases, all of them members of the AGC subfamily. Reports to date include the phosphorylation and activation of the p70-kDa ribosomal S6 kinase (S6 K) (Alessi and Cohen 1998; Pullen et al. 1998); possibly the cAMP-dependent protein kinase (PKA) (Cheng et al. 1998); the serum- and glucocorticoid-regulated protein kinase (SGK) (Kobayashi and Cohen 1999); the p90-kDa ribosomal S6 kinase (RSK1) (Jensen et al. 1999; Richards et al. 1999) and its isoform RSK2 (Frodin et al. 2000); PKC (Le Good et al. 1998) and protein kinase C-related kinase (PRK) (Flynn et al. 2000) by PDK1.

In two-hybrid screening it was found that PDK1 interacts with a 24-amino acid fragment called PIF (PDK1-interacting fragment) (Balendran et al.

1999) corresponding to the C-terminus of PRK2. PIF is characteristic for most AGC kinases, always located downstream of the catalytic domain, and corresponds to the hydrophobic motif (HM) with the consensus sequence FXXFS/TY. Atypical PKCs and PRK isoforms have an acidic residue (Asp or Glu) instead of Ser or Thr, in the case of PKA the motif is truncated (FSEF-COOH), while PDK1 itself has no hydrophobic motif (Vanhaesebroeck and Alessi 2000). Typically, PDK1 interacts with the HM of its substrates when the HM is phosphorylated. This interaction through the phosphorylated HM is essential for the activation of RSK2 (Frodin et al. 2000), PKC (Gao et al. 2001), PRK (Balendran et al. 2000), S6 K and GSK (Biondi et al. 2001). The PIF-binding pocket of PDK1 is located in the catalytic domain, first determined by comparison with the structure of PKA and verified by the crystal structure of PDK1 (Biondi et al. 2000; Biondi et al. 2002). Further modelling studies determined that a PIF-binding pocket and a phosphate pocket are present in PDK1 and most other AGC kinases (Frodin et al. 2002).

The activation of PKB by PDK1 (through phosphorylation of the activation loop Thr308) and the presence of PI(3,4,5)P3 is rather the result of a recruitment and colocalization of both enzymes at the membrane than of the activation of either enzyme directly by the phosphatidylinositides. Consequently, the activation loop phosphorylation of the other AGC kinases by PDK1 is not enhanced by the presence of PI(3,4,5)P3. These other kinases recruit PDK1 rather via the phosphorylated hydrophobic motif. However, the regulation of the prerequisite phosphorylation of the hydrophobic motif often appears to be dependent on PI(3,4,5)P3. PDK1, in contrast to the other AGC kinases, lacks such a hydrophobic motif, but has instead a hydrophobic pocket similar to the binding site for the FXXF C-terminal hydrophobic motif of PKA (Frodin et al. 2000).

In summary, there are two models for PDK1 activation. One is for PKB, which consists of the recruitment of both kinases to the membrane by phosphatidylinositol phosphate through their respective PH domains. The proximity of both kinases facilitates the activation. The other model, valid for the rest of AGC kinases, consists of a two-step activation process. An HM kinase first phosphorylates the hydrophobic motif that is then recognized by PDK1, which in turn transfers the activating phosphate to the activation loop.

A significant number of human cancers correlate with enhanced levels of PI(3,4,5,)P3 that lead to activation of PKB and S6 K and result in enhanced cell proliferation and tumour cell survival. Thus, PDK1 as the activating upstream kinase may be a promising target for small molecule drugs that target either the hydrophobic pocket of the kinase or the ATP binding site. PDK1 has been cocrystallized with staurosporine and UCN01 (Komander et al. 2003).

UCN01 (or 7-hydroxystaurosporine) is a derivate of staurosporine with an additional hydroxyl group on the lactam ring. UCN01 was isolated, as staurosporine, from *Streptomyces* sp. and was originally believed to be selective for PKC, but in fact inhibits several other kinases (Davies et al. 2000; Gescher 2000). UCN01 is undergoing clinical trials because of its property to inhibit growth and induce apoptosis of cancer cells. Staurosporine and UCN01 bind to PDK1 very much as staurosporine binds to PKA. Both form the corresponding hydrogen contacts from the lactam ring to the hinge backbone, and both make contacts from the methylamino group to Glu166 (Glu127 in PKA) and to the backbone carbonyl of Glu209 (Glu170 in PKA). In contrast to PKA, the Phe93 (Phe54 in PKA) does not bend inwards to contact the staurosporine hydroxyl group. The reason may be again the exchange of the Gly55 homologue to serine (Ser94) in PDK1.

2.5.2 PDK1 Cocrystals with Staurosporine and UCN01

The inhibitory profile of UCN01 across a panel of several protein kinases is different from that of staurosporine. Since the binding modes of both inhibitors is identical in PDK1 and in Chk1 (PDB-code 1NVQ) (Zhao et al. 2002), selectivity must be defined by the environment of the 7-hydroxy group of UCN01. This group makes a direct hydrogen bond to Thr222 (Thr183 in PKA), usually reserved for a contact of the ATP N7. The kinases that are inhibited most strongly by UCN01 have a corresponding Thr or Ser residue, either in this position or in the position of Val 143 (Val104 in PKA), which could make a similar contact to the 7-hydroxy group. It is assumed that kinases which are inhibited more potently by staurosporine than by UCN01 appear to have bulkier sidechains in the environment of the 7-hydroxy group (Johnson et al. 2002b), such as Met120 in PKA or Phe80 in CDK2.

In addition, the 7-hydroxy group binds via water to the sidechain of a glutamine residue (Gln220), which changes its conformation towards the ATP pocket in order to establish this interaction. This rotamer change of this glutamine residue in association with the occupation of the binding site is especially noteworthy because it was previously observed in a mutant of PKA (Gaßel et al. 2003). In the attempt to design a surrogate kinase for PKB based on PKA, Val123 (the hinge region residue that is involved in almost all inhibitor, enzyme backbone contacts) was mutated to alanine, and Leu173 to methionine. Unexpectedly, the mutant showed defects (tenfold reduction in affinity) in binding of ATP and inhibitors not explained by these two conservative sidechain exchanges. In a crystal structure of the mutant apoenzyme, the reason for the kinetic defects became clear: Gln181, located close to the hinge region but in the wild-type enzyme, is directed outwards towards the surface of the enzyme and adopts a different rotamer and occupies the space freed by the exchange of Val123 to alanine, partly obstructing the adenosine pocket. In a cocrystal structure with MgATP, the residue adopts its normal conformation again. The conformational change, however, apparently costs energy, as ligand binding is weakened. An additional mutation of this Gln181 to lysine, conserved in most other kinases, restores the basic situation, with the lysine adopting the orientation of Gln181 in wild-type PKA or the corresponding lysine in Chk1 or PKB. Interestingly, PDK1 is the only kinase which has a glutamine residue in the 181 position as PKA, and an alanine sidechain in the Val123 position as PKB, which might lead to the expectation of a possible similar conformational change of the glutamine sidechain towards the adenosine pocket as observed in the PKA-to-PKB mutant. As the structure with UCN01 confirms, this is indeed the case. Although an in vivo relevance of this situation is not clear, such a behaviour in principle offers a way to communicate the occupation of the ATP binding site to the surface of the enzyme (Gaßel et al. 2003) and represents an unexpected mechanism for inhibitor selectivity. In a possible analogy, a glutamine residue in the allosteric site of glycogen phosphorylase is known to change its conformation upon phosphorylation of the enzyme and to hinder access of glucose-6-phosphate (Sprang et al. 1988).

2.6 PKA Cocrystal Structures with Bisindolylmaleimide Inhibitors Selective for PKC

2.6.1 Protein Kinase C

Discovered in 1977 (Inoue et al. 1977; Kishimoto et al. 1977), PKC is one of the most intensely studied subjects in signalling research. In humans, 10 PKC isoforms are present, confirmed by the analysis of the human genome (Manning et al. 2002). Besides the catalytic core domain, which is conserved among PKA, PKB and PKC with more than 40% identity, the PKC isoforms have additional domains, which allow the interaction with a number of activity-modulating substances.

Three distinct subfamilies of PKC isoforms can be defined according to their essential activators: (1) conventional PKCs (α, βI/II, γ), which require phosphatidylserine (PS), diacylglycerol (DAG) and Ca^{2+}; (2) novel PKCs (δ, ϵ, η, θ), which need PS and DAG but they are insensitive towards Ca^{2+}; and (3) atypical PKCs (ζ,ι), which are insensitive to both DAG and Ca^{2+}, although PS regulates activity (for reviews see Way et al. 2000; Newton 2003 and citations therein). Furthermore, additional lipid mediators, like fatty acids and lysophospholipids, have been shown to influence the catalytic activity of PKCs (Nishizuka 1995). Interaction of PKCs with the activators leads to phosphorylation of a threonine residue on the activation loop of all PKC isoforms and additionally of a serine or threonine residue in the hydrophobic motif of the conventional and novel PKCs. The atypical PKCs possess a glutamate at the hydrophobic motif phosphorylation position that performs the activation function (for reviews see Newton 2001, 2003). PKCs are involved in the signal transduction cascades that regulate proliferation, apoptosis, contraction, migration, hypertrophy, secretion and further growth factor-dependent processes (for review see Dempsey et al. 2000). PKCα, for example, is involved in regulation of proliferation, apoptosis, differentiation, cell migration and adhesion, among other cellular and pathogenic processes (for a review see Nakashima 2002). Consistent with its prominent role in different signal transduction pathways, PKC is implicated in different diseases. The earliest studies associated PKC with cancer via the influence of the tumour-promoting phorbol esters (Nishizuka 1984; Castagna et al. 1982). The effects of PKCs in the field of cancer are manifold (for review see Hofmann 2001); for example, whereas PKCα, PKCβII, PKCϵ and the atypical PKC isoforms appear to be antiapoptotic, the PKCδ isoform is activated by caspase-induced proteolysis and may serve to amplify downstream processes in the apoptotic pathway (for review see Dempsey et al. 2000). Many molecules with PKC-modulatory activity have been developed to elucidate PKC signalling in cancer and other diseases. Early compounds have often been naturally occurring substances (e.g. staurosporine from *Streptomyces* sp.), whereas the more recent ones have been developed with an increased selectivity. Three classes of protein kinase C modulators have been developed so far, grouped by their mode of action:

a. ATP-competitive inhibitors which bind in the catalytic site of protein kinases (e.g. indolocarbazoles, bisindolylmaleimides, balanols, flavonoids and phenylaminopyrimidines)
b. Inhibitors that that bind to one of the regulatory domains of an PKC isoform (e. g. phospholipid and sphingolipid analogues, lactones and antiestrogens)
c. An antisense oligonucleotide that binds to the mRNA (for review see Tamm et al. 2001)

The antisense oligonucleotide ISIS3521 binds isoenzyme specific to the messenger RNA of PKCα and shows antitumour activity in human glioblastoma, breast and lung xenograft models (Tamm et al. 2001; Swannie and Kaye 2002). The most important inhibitor with the ability to bind to regulatory domains of a PKC isoform is bryostatin, which belongs to the group of macrocyclic lactones derived from the marine bryozoan *Bugula neritina* (Pettit et al. 1970). The binding of bryostatin leads after an initial activation to a down-regulation of PKC activity (for review see Hofmann 2001) and is in clinical trials against various cancers (e.g. melanoma, non-Hodgkin's lymphoma, colorectal, renal) both as a single agent and in combination with chemotherapy (for review see Swannie and Kaye 2002).

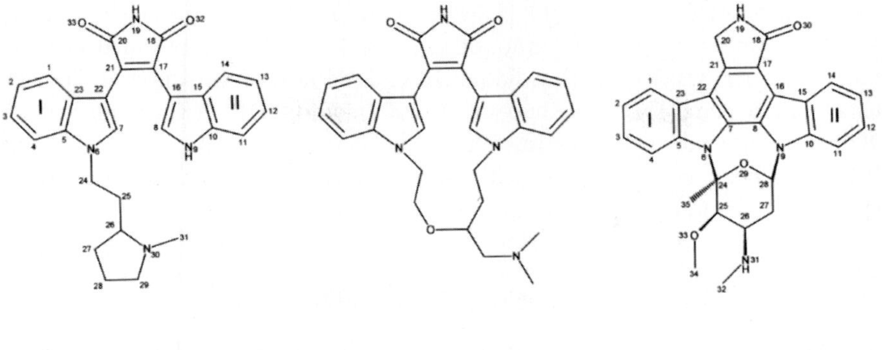

Bisindolylmaleimide 2 (Bim2) LY333531 Staurosporine

Fig. 12 Cognates of the bisindolylmaleimide/indolocarbozole group of protein kinase inhibitors. Bisindolylmaleimide 2 (BIM2) has been cocrystallized with a PKA mutant and with PDK1 (Gaßel et al. 2004; Komander et al. 2004); LY333531 (ruboxistaurin) has been cocrystallized with PDK1 (Komander et al. 2004); staurosporine has been cocrystallized with several kinases including PKA [(Prade et al. 1997) PDB code 1STC]

Besides these interesting compounds, a number of ATP-competitive inhibitors have been shown to down-regulate PKC activity. The earliest members of this group are the indolocarbazole staurosporine, which binds with high affinity to PKC, and the flavonoid quercetin with a low-affinity binding mode. Both exhibit a broad spectrum of interacting protein kinases and other enzymes. The staurosporine derivative PKC412 (*N*-benzoyl-staurosporine, CGP41251) originally designed as a PKC inhibiter, is indeed more specific than staurosporine but has significant activity against various other kinases, including KDR (kinase insert domain containing receptor), vascular endothelial growth factor (VEGF)-R2, platelet-derived growth factor (PDGF) and c-Kit. PKC412 shows in vitro and in vivo antiproliferative activity accompanied by a cell-cycle arrest at the G2/M state and polyploidy (Fabbro et al. 2000). Furthermore, PKC412 modulates the P-glycoprotein-mediated drug resistance (Ganeshaguru et al. 2002) via PKC inhibition and shows antiangiogenic action, which is related to its activity towards VEGF (Fabbro et al. 2002). It is in clinical trials for treatment of neovascular retinopathy and different kind of cancers. Although broad unspecificity is probably a pharmacological disadvantage, some crystal structure complexes with these compounds have been solved. However, no PKC crystal structure has been reported to date, despite the fact that PKC has been known as an interesting pharmacological target for years. Available cocrystal structures of PKC inhibitors with a related kinase are those of staurosporine and its closely related derivative UCN01 (see above) and the bisindolylmaleimides (see below) (Fig. 12). Besides cocrystallization with PKA (PDB code 1STC) (Prade et al. 1997), the extended and rigid planar staurosporine has been crystallized with Cdk2 (PDB code 1AQ1) (Lawrie et al. 1997) Src kinase (PDB code 1BYG) (Lamers et al. 1999) and others. UCN01 (7-hydroxystaurosporine) has been cocrystallized with Cdk2 (PDB code 1PKD) (Johnson et al. 2002b), Chk1 (PDB code 1NVQ) (Zhao et al. 2002), and PDK1 (Komander et al. 2003). Furthermore, quercetin, which shows a weak inhibitory effect on PKC, has been cocrystallized with the Src kinase Hck (PDB-code 2HCK) (Sicheri et al. 1997).

2.6.2
Cocrystal Structures of PKA with Bisindolylmaleimides

Recently, we were able to solve the structure of a flexible derivative of staurosporine, namely bisindolylmaleimide 2 (BIM2) in complex with PKA (PDB-code 1SZM) (Gaßel et al. 2004) (Fig. 12). The bisindolylmaleimide class of PKC inhibitors is derived from staurosporine by elimination of a single bond. This converts the extended planar aromatic group into the three aromats described in the compound name, with corresponding additional degrees of freedom. The resulting dimer shows unusual conformations of the kinase as well as of the inhibitor. The kinase molecule A of the dimer is in general comparable to the kinase structure of 1STC (Prade et al. 1997), with two major differences: (1) the whole turn region including residues Gly52, Ser53, Phe54 and Gly55 of the glycine loop (and not merely the sidechain of Phe54) is turned down, probably to enable a contact between the methyl group of the pyrrolidine-tail of BIM2 and phe54 of the glycine loop; (2) the linker region around Phe327 is flexible (not resolved in the electron density) in the BIM2 structure, possibly due to lesser interaction with the inhibitor compared to staurosporine and all other inhibitors crystallized with PKA so far (Fig. 13). In contrast to the planar and rigid molecule staurosporine, the twisted conformation of the indole rings limits the number of possible VDW contacts to residues Val57 and Leu49 from the glycine-rich loop. While the methylamino group of staurosporine mimics the interaction of the ATP–ribose hydroxyl groups with the backbone carbonyl of Glu170 and the sidechain of Glu127, the pyrrolidine moiety of BIM2 does not establish these interactions. In the presence of BIM2, both residues adopt different rotamers: Glu127 to avoid a steric conflict with the pyrrolidine group, which prevents any H-bond contact with the inhibitors, and Glu170 to establish a sidechain contact to the amino group the pyrrolidine ring. Both residues are key residues for recognition of the substrate consensus sequence of PKA and probably other AGC kinases such as PKC also.

The molecule B of the dimer is in the most open conformation so far described for PKA. In addition to the common opening hinge movement around amino acid residue 125 (Olah et al. 1993) of PKA structures in open conformations such as 1STC (Prade et al. 1997), or the apoenzyme structures (1CTP) (Karlsson et al. 1993) and 1J3H (Akamine et al. 2003), the ki-

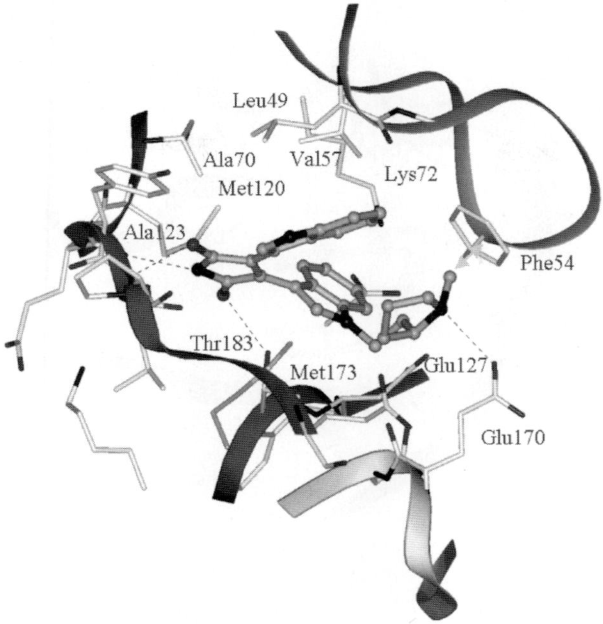

Fig. 13 Binding pattern of BIM2 in PKA molecule A (intermediate open conformation of the enzyme). Inhibitor-interacting residues are indicated. The hinge region H-bonds Ala123:N-O32 and Glu121:O–N19 are supplemented by Thr183OG1—O33 (Gaßel et al. 2004). Conserved parts of the backbone are indicated as *ribbon*: the hinge region, the metal binding loop, and the catalytic loop

nase in molecule B shows a rotation or twist of its N- and C-lobe by 15 degrees when compared with molecule A of 1J3H. This rotation is clockwise for the N-lobe when looking from above the N-lobe towards the C-lobe. The axis of this rotation goes through the centre of both N- and C-lobes. Furthermore, the hinge region is displaced by up to 5 Å out of this common position. These considerable movements of the kinase domains in molecule B are induced by the reversed binding of BIM2, which is possible because of the symmetrical nature of the maleimide head group (Fig. 14). The binding of BIM2 in molecule A and molecule B is similar with respect to the hinge contacts of the maleimide groups, and the VDW contacts to Ala70, a conserved residue from β-strand 3. An H-bond from the maleimide carbonyl to the sidechain of Thr183 is established only in molecule A. Although the bisindolylmaleimide scaffold itself is apparently symmetric, the pyrrolidine substitution on indole I breaks the symmetry and defines an overall orientation. Thus, while the hydrogen bonding pattern of the maleimide and hinge loop remains the same between the two binding modes, the hinge hydrogen bond acceptor of the inhibitor is alternately the oxygen distal or proximal to the substituted indole I in molecules A and B, respectively. This upsidedown

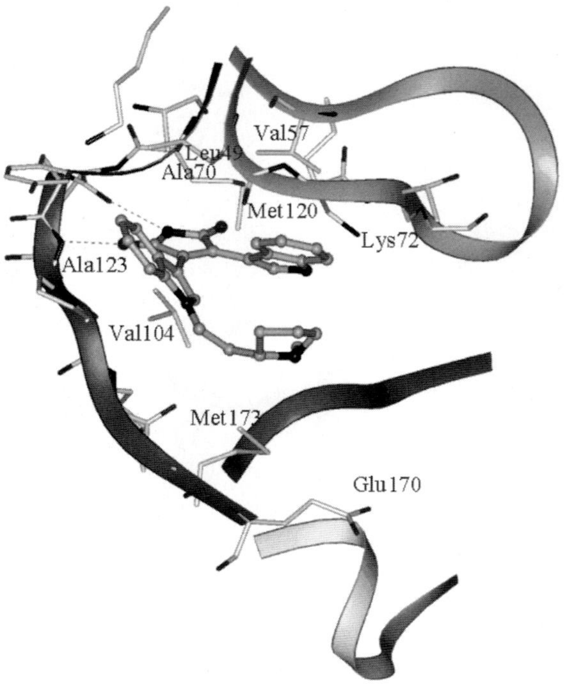

Fig. 14 Binding pattern of BIM2 in PKA molecule B (open conformation). Inhibitor interacting residues are indicated. The C-terminal lobe residues Glu127, Glu170 and Met173 are not in contact with the inhibitor. Hinge region H-bonds exist between Ala123:N–O33 and Glu121:O–N19 (Gaßel et al. 2004). Different parts of the backbone are indicated as *ribbons*: the hinge region, the metal binding loop, and the catalytic loop

orientation of the maleimide affects the relative orientations of the indole moieties by the means of the different interacting residues of the kinase. An exception is Val57, which is, in both orientations of the inhibitor, one of the coordinating residues of the inwards-rotated indole II. The orientation of the pyrrolidine is in both cases parallel, in a VDW-contact distance to the indole I. The pyrrolidine of BIM2 in molecule B seems to be coordinated only by this intramolecular interaction, because no contacts to the kinase are established. As a result, BIM2 adopts two very different conformations, with different rotamers for the pyrrolidine-tethered indole I (delta chi 90°) and the untethered indole II (delta chi 30°). In PKA, BIM2 is bound to the same kinase under identical conditions in two different inhibitor conformations to two different conformations of the protein, possible because of the symmetric nature of the maleimide head group. This apparent directing effect of the maleimide group on the overall binding pattern might be a useful feature to explore in future inhibitor design.

2.6.3
Structures of PDK1 with Bisindolylmaleimides and LY333531

Bisindolylmaleimides were also cocrystallized with PDK1 (PDB-codes 1UU7, 1UU8, 1UU9, 1UVR) (Komander et al. 2004). The structure obtained with PDK1 and BIM2 is very similar to the molecule A of our structure of PKA and BIM2, but an alternative conformation comparable to the molecule B structure of PKA with BIM2 was not observed in the case of PDK1. The hinge region contacts of the bisindolylmaleimides are conserved between the two kinases. As in PKA, BIM2 in PDK1 also shows the inwards rotation of the untethered indole. As one of the rare AGC kinase without a comparable residue to Phe327, the PDK1 structure also lacks these contacts between the inhibitor and the kinase, in this respect similar to the structure of PKA, where the corresponding peptide stretch is mobile and not resolved. As a striking difference between the two BIM2 kinase complexes, the glycine-rich loop in PDK1 shows no conformational change similar to that in PKA, and no contact between the Phe54 homologue in PDK1 is made to the pyrrolidine-attached methyl group of BIM2. A possible reason is the exchange of Gly52 (PKA) to serine in PDK1, which reduces the flexibility of the glycine flap and might cause steric problems. As in the less-pronounced case of the Phe54 interaction with the staurosporine sugar methyl group in PKA, where other kinases that possess the corresponding residue and still do not make the contact, the real reasons for the presence or absence of this interaction may be different.

The presence of a PKA molecule which contains an upsidedown-oriented BIM2 inhibitor, in contrast to PDK1, may be facilitated by Pro124 in PKA. In the B molecule in PKA, BIM2 is wedged between Val57 from the N-lobe, and Pro124, which makes one-sixth of all VDW contacts to the inhibitor.

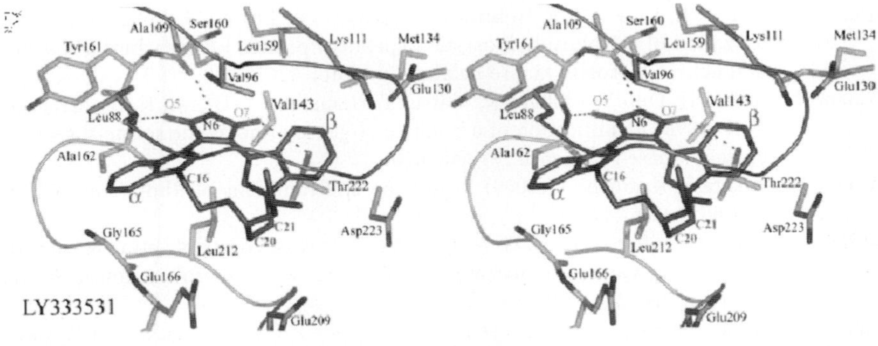

Fig. 15 Stereo representation of LY333531 interactions within the ATP binding pocket of PDK1. Ligand carbon atoms are in *dark grey* and protein carbon atoms in *light grey*. Hydrogen bonds are indicated by *black dotted lines*. A *grey ribbon* indicates the protein backbone. (Komander et al. 2004)

The corresponding residue is a lysine in PDK1, which would not be suitable for similar interactions.

Another PKC inhibitor of the bisindolylmaleimide class, LY333531 or ruboxistaurin, has also been cocrystallized in complex with PDK1 (PDB-code 1UU3) (Komander et al. 2004) (Fig. 15). LY333531 shows PKC isoform specificity (e.g. 80- and 60-fold selectivity for PKCβI and PKCβII over PKCα (Jirousek et al. 1996) and is in phase III clinical trials for diabetic retinopathy and diabetic macular oedema (Frank 2002 and citations therein). LY333531 shares much of the flexibility of BIM2, except that the cyclic connection of both N-atoms of the indoles with a 6-atom ether linker prevents a comparable inwards rotation of one indole as seen with bisindolylmaleimide 2 (Fig. 12). Komander et al. explain the higher binding affinity of inhibitors such as staurosporine, UCN01 and LY333531 in contrast to bisindolylmaleimides by a preference of PDK1 for carbon atoms at specific positions which are satisfied by the indolocarbazoles and LY333531 but not by the bisindolylmaleimides. Mutagenesis of PDK1 and sequence comparisons, however, did not explain the selectivity of the bisindolylmaleimides and LY333531 for the PKC isoforms.

References

Akamine P, Madhusudan Wu J, Xuong NH, Ten Eyck LF, Taylor SS (2003) Dynamic features of cAMP-dependent protein kinase revealed by apoenzyme crystal structure. J Mol Biol 327:159–171

Alessi DR, Cohen P (1998) Mechanism of activation and function of protein kinase B. Curr Opin Genet Dev 8:55–62

Alessi DR, Deak M, Casamayor A, Caudwell FB, Morrice N, Norman DG, Gaffney P, Reese CB, MacDougall CN, Harbison D, Ashworth A, Bownes M (1997a) 3-Phosphoinositide-dependent protein kinase-1 (PDK1): structural and functional homology with the Drosophila DSTPK61 kinase. Curr Biol 7:776–789

Alessi DR, James SR, Downes CP, Holmes AB, Gaffney PR, Reese CB, Cohen P (1997b) Characterization of a 3-phosphoinositide-dependent protein kinase which phosphorylates and activates protein kinase Balpha. Curr Biol 7:261–269

Amano M, Mukai H, Ono Y, Chihara K, Matsui T, Hamajima Y, Okawa K, Iwamatsu A, Kaibuchi K (1996) Identification of a putative target for Rho as the serine-threonine kinase protein kinase N. Science 271:648–650

Amano M, Fukata Y, Kaibuchi K (2000) Regulation and functions of Rho-associated kinase. Exp Cell Res 261:44–51

Aubol BE, Nolen B, Shaffer J, Ghosh G, Adams JA (2003) Novel destabilization of nucleotide binding by the gamma phosphate of ATP in the yeast SR protein kinase Sky1p. Biochemistry 42:12813–12820

Balendran A, Casamayor A, Deak M, Paterson A, Gaffney P, Currie R, Downes CP, Alessi DR (1999) PDK1 acquires PDK2 activity in the presence of a synthetic peptide derived from the carboxyl terminus of PRK2. Curr Biol 9:393–404

Balendran A, Biondi RM, Cheung PCF, Casamayor A, Deak M, Alessi DR (2000) A 3-phosphoinositide-dependent protein kinase-1 (PDK1) docking site is required for the phosphorylation of protein kinase C zeta (PKC zeta) and PKC-related kinase 2 by PDK1. J Biol Chem 275:20806–20813

Barbier P, Huber I, Schneider F, Stadlwieser J, Taylor S (1995) Preparation of 3-amino/hydroxy-4-[4-benzoylphenylcarboxylamino/oxy]azepine and homolog protein kinase inhibitors. (F.Hoffmann-La Roche Ag:Switz [663393]: pp 1–47 EP663393

Barbier P, Stadlwieser J, Taylor S (1997) Novel azepanes and their ring homologs for therapy and prophylaxis of protein kinase mediated diseases. (F. Hoffmann-La Roche Ag:Switz [9702249]:pp 1–43 WO9702249

Battistutta R, De Moliner E, Sarno S, Zanotti G, Pinna LA (2001) Structural features underlying selective inhibition of protein kinase CK2 by ATP site-directed tetrabromo-2-benzotriazole. Protein Sci 10:2200–2206

Bayliss R, Sardon T, Vernos I, Conti E (2003) Structural basis of aurora-A activation by TPX2 at the mitotic spindle. Mol Cell 12:851–862

Bertrand JA, Thieffine S, Vulpetti A, Cristiani C, Valsasina B, Knapp S, Kalisz HM, Flocco M (2003) Structural characterization of the GSK-3beta active site using selective and non-selective ATP-mimetic inhibitors. J Mol Biol 333:393–407

Biondi RM, Cheung PCF, Casamayor A, Deak M, Currie RA, Alessi DR (2000) Identification of a pocket in the PDK1 kinase domain that interacts with PIF and the C-terminal residues of PKA. EMBO J 19:979–988

Biondi RM, Kieloch A, Currie RA, Deak M, Alessi DR (2001) The PIF-binding pocket in PDK1 is essential for activation of S6 K and SGK, but not PKB. EMBO J 20:4380–4390

Biondi RM, Komander D, Thomas CC, Lizcano JM, Deak M, Alessi DR, van Aalten DMF (2002) High resolution crystal structure of the human PDK1 catalytic domain defines the regulatory phosphopeptide docking site. EMBO J 21:4219–4228

Bossemeyer D (1994) The glycine-rich sequence of protein kinases: a multifunctional element. Trends Biochem Sci 19:201–205

Bossemeyer D, Engh RA, Kinzel V, Ponstingl H, Huber R (1993) Phosphotransferase and substrate binding mechanism of the cAMP-dependent protein-kinase catalytic subunit from porcine heart as deduced from the 2.0 angstrom structure of the complex with Mn2+ adenylyl imidodiphosphate and inhibitor peptide Pki(5–24). EMBO J 12:849–859

Breitenlechner CB, Wegge T, Berillon L, Graul K, Marzenell K, Friebe W-G, Thomas U, Schumacher R, Huber R, Engh RA, Masjost B (2004) Structure-based optimization of novel azepane derivatives as PKB inhibitors. J Med Chem 47:1375–1390

Breitenlechner CB, Gaßel M, Hidaka H, Kinzel V, Huber R, Engh RA, Bossemeyer D (2003) Protein Kinase A in complex with Rho kinase inhibitors Y-27632, fasudil (HA-1077) and H-1152P: structural basis of selectivity. Structure 11:1595–1607

Chen HX, Marshall JL, Ness E, Martin RR, Dvorchik B, Rizvi N, Marquis J, McKinlay M, Dahut W, et al (2000) A safety and pharmacokinetic study of a mixed-backbone oligonucleotide (GEM231) targeting the type I protein kinase A by two-hour infusions in patients with refractory solid tumors. Clin Cancer Res 6:1259–1266

Cheng XD, Ma Y, Moore M, Hemmings BA, Taylor SS (1998) Phosphorylation and activation of cAMP-dependent protein kinase by phosphoinositide-dependent protein kinase. Proc Natl Acad Sci U S A 95:9849–9854

Davies SP, Reddy H, Caivano M, Cohen P (2000) Specificity and mechanism of action of some commonly used protein kinase inhibitors. BioChem J 351:95–105

De Azevedo WF, Jr, Mueller-Dieckmann HJ, Schulze-Gahmen U, Worland PJ, Sausville E, Kim SH (1996) Structural basis for specificity and potency of a flavonoid inhibitor of human CDK2, a cell cycle kinase. Proc Natl Acad Sci U S A 93:2735–2740

De Moliner E, Brown NR, Johnson LN (2003) Alternative binding modes of an inhibitor to two different kinases. Eur J Biochem 270:3174–3181

Dempsey EC, Newton AC, Mochly-Rosen D, Fields AP, Reyland ME, Insel PA, Messing RO (2000) Protein kinase C isozymes and the regulation of diverse cell responses. Am J Physiol Lung Cell Mol Physiol 279:L429–L438

Engh RA, Bossemeyer D (2001) The protein kinase activity modulation sites: mechanisms for cellular regulation—targets for therapeutic intervention. Adv Enzym Regul 41:121–149

Engh RA, Bossemeyer D (2002) Structural aspects of protein kinase control—role of conformational flexibility. Pharmacol Ther 93:99–111

Engh RA, Girod A, Kinzel V, Huber R, Bossemeyer D (1996) Crystal structures of catalytic subunit of cAMP-dependent protein kinase in complex with isoquinolinesulfonyl protein kinase inhibitors H7, H8, and H89. Structural implications for selectivity. J Biol Chem 271:26157–26164

Fabbro D, Ruetz S, Bodis S, Pruschy M, Csermak K, Man A, Campochiaro P, Wood J, O'Reilly T, Meyer T (2000) PKC412—a protein kinase inhibitor with a broad therapeutic potential. Anticancer Drug Des 15:17–28

Fabbro D, Ruetz S, Buchdunger E, Cowan-Jacob SW, Fendrich G, Liebetanz J, Mestan J, O'Reilly T, Traxler P, Chaudhuri B, Fretz H, Zimmermann J, Meyer T, Caravatti G, Furet P, Manley PW (2002) Protein kinases as targets for anticancer agents: from inhibitors to useful drugs. Pharmacol Ther 93:79–98

Flynn P, Mellor H, Casamassima A, Parker PJ (2000) Rho GTPase control of protein kinase C-related protein kinase activation by 3-phosphoinositide-dependent protein kinase. J Biol Chem 275:11064–11070

Fox T, Coll JT, Xie XL, Ford PJ, Germann UA, Porter MD, Pazhanisamy S, Fleming MA, Galullo V, Su MSS, Wilson KP (1998) A single amino acid substitution makes ERK2 susceptible to pyridinyl imidazole inhibitors of p38 MAP kinase. Protein Sci 7:2249–2255

Frank RN (2002) Potential new medical therapies for diabetic retinopathy: protein kinase C inhibitors. Am J Ophthalmol 133:693–698

Frodin M, Jensen CJ, Merienne K, Gammeltoft S (2000) A phosphoserine-regulated docking site in the protein kinase RSK2 that recruits and activates PDK1. EMBO J 19:2924–2934

Frodin M, Antal TL, Dummler BA, Jensen CJ, Deak M, Gammeltoft S, Biondi RM (2002) A phosphoserine/threonine-binding pocket in AGC kinases and PDK1 mediates activation by hydrophobic motif phosphorylation. EMBO J 21:5396–5407

Fukata Y, Amano M, Kaibuchi K (2001) Rho-Rho kinase pathway in smooth muscle contraction and cytoskeletal reorganization of non-muscle cells. Trends Pharmacol Sci 22:32–39

Ganeshaguru K, Wickremasinghe RG, Jones DT, Gordon M, Hart SM, Virchis AE, Prentice HG, Hoffbrand AV, Man A, Champain K, Csermak K, Mehta AB (2002) Actions of the selective protein kinase C inhibitor PKC412 on B-chronic lymphocytic leukemia cells in vitro. Haematologica 87:167–176

Gao T, Toker A, Newton AC (2001) The carboxyl terminus of protein kinase C provides a switch to regulate its interaction with the phosphoinositide-dependent kinase, PDK-1. J Biol Chem 276:19588–19596

Gaßel M, Breitenlechner CB, König N, Huber R, Engh RA, Bossemeyer D (2004) The protein kinase C inhibitor bisindolyl-maleimide II binds with reversed orientations to different conformations of PKA. J Biol Chem (in press)

Gaßel M, Breitenlechner CB, Ruger P, Jucknischke U, Schneider T, Huber R, Bossemeyer D, Engh RA (2003) Mutants of protein kinase A that mimic the ATP-binding site of protein kinase B (AKT). J Mol Biol 329:1021–1034

Gescher A (2000) Staurosporine analogues—pharmacological toys or useful antitumour agents? Crit Rev Oncol Hematol 34:127–135

Gibbs CS, Knighton DR, Sowadski JM, Taylor SS, Zoller MJ (1992) Systematic mutational analysis of cAMP-dependent protein kinase identifies unregulated catalytic subunits and defines regions important for the recognition of the regulatory subunit. J Biol Chem 267:4806–4814

Gustafsson AB, Brunton LL (1999) Differential and selective inhibition of protein kinase A and protein kinase C in intact cells by balanol congeners. Mol Pharmacol 56:377–82

Hall SE, Ballas LM, Kulanthaivel P, et al (1994) Preparation of balanoids as protein kinase C inhibitors. (Nichols:Gina M USA Sphinx Pharmaceuticals Corporation [9420062]):pp 1–559 WO9420062

Hanks SK, Quinn AM (1991) Protein kinase catalytic domain sequence database: identification of conserved features of primary structure and classification of family members. Methods Enzymol 200:38–62

Hofmann J (2001) Modulation of protein kinase C in antitumor treatment. Rev Physiol Biochem Pharmacol 142:1–96

Hu H, Jagdmann EG Jr, Mendoza JS (1995) Preparation of substituted fused and bridged bicyclic compound protein kinase C inhibitors. (Lilly:Eli Co USA [9530640]:pp 1–84 1995 WO9530640

Hubbard SR (1997) Crystal structure of the activated insulin receptor tyrosine kinase in complex with peptide substrate and ATP analog. EMBO J 16:5572–5581

Hunenberger PH, Helms V, Narayana N, Taylor SS, McCammon JA (1999) Determinants of ligand binding to cAMP-dependent protein kinase. Biochemistry 38:2358–2366

Huse M, Kuriyan J (2002) The conformational plasticity of protein kinases. Cell 109:275–282

Ikenoya M, Hidaka H, Hosoya T, Suzuki M, Yamamoto N, Sasaki Y (2002) Inhibition of Rho kinase-induced myristoylated alanine-rich C kinase substrate (MARCKS) phosphorylation in human neuronal cells by H-1152, a novel and specific Rho kinase inhibitor. J Neurochem 81:9–16

Inoue M, Kishimoto A, Takai Y, Nishizuka Y (1977) Studies on a cyclic nucleotide-independent protein kinase and its proenzyme in mammalian tissues. II Proenzyme and its activation by calcium-dependent protease from rat brain. J Biol Chem 252:7610–7616

Ishizaki T, Uehata M, Tamechika I, Keel J, Nonomura K, Maekawa M, Narumiya S (2000) Pharmacological properties of Y-27632, a specific inhibitor of Rho-associated kinases. Mol Pharmacol 57:976–983

Itoh K, Yoshioka K, Akedo H, Uehata M, Ishizaki T, Narumiya S (1999) An essential part for Rho-associated kinase in the transcellular invasion of tumor cells. Nat Med 5:221–225

Jagdmann GE, Defauw JM, Lampe JW, Darges JW, Kalter K (1996) Potent and selective PKC inhibitory 5-membered ring analogs of balanol with replacement of the carboxamide moiety. Bioorg Med Chem Lett 6:1759–1764

Jensen CJ, Buch MB, Krag TO, Hemmings BA, Gammeltoft S, Frodin M (1999) 90-kDa ribosomal S6 kinase is phosphorylated and activated by 3-phosphoinositide-dependent protein kinase-1. J Biol Chem 274:27168–27176

Jirousek MR, Gillig JR, Gonzalez CM, Heath WF, McDonald JH, III Neel DA, Rito CJ, Singh U, Stramm LE, Melikian-Badalian A, Baevsky M, Ballas LM, Hall SE, Winneroski LL, Faul MM (1996) (S)-13-[(dimethylamino)methyl]-10,11,14,15-tetrahydro-4,9:16, 21-dimetheno-1H, 13H-dibenzo[e,k]pyrrolo[3,4-h][1,4,13]oxadiazacyclohexadecene-1,3(2H)-d ione (LY333531) and related analogues: isozyme selective inhibitors of protein kinase C beta. J Med Chem 39:2664–2671

Johnson DA, Li F, Gangal M, Juliano C, Gorfain E, Taylor SS (2002a) Domain closure, segmental flexibility, and the catalytic cycle of A-kinase. Biophys J 82:1624

Johnson LN, De Moliner E, Brown NR, Song H, Barford D, Endicott JA, Noble MEM (2002b) Structural studies with inhibitors of the cell cycle regulatory kinase cyclin-dependent protein kinase 2. Pharmacol Ther 93:113–124

Karlsson R, Zheng JH, Xuong NH, Taylor SS, Sowadski JM (1993) Structure of the mammalian catalytic subunit of cAMP-dependent protein-kinase and an inhibitor peptide displays an open conformation. Acta Crystallogr D Biol Crystallogr 49:381–388

Kim DW, Hwang JH, Suh JM, Kim H, Song JH, Hwang ES, Hwang IY, Park KC, Chung HK, Kim JM, Park J, Hemmings BA, Shong M (2003) RET/PTC (rearranged in transformation/papillary thyroid carcinomas) tyrosine kinase phosphorylates and activates phosphoinositide-dependent kinase 1 (PDK1): an alternative phosphatidylinositol 3-kinase-independent pathway to activate PDK1. Mol Endocrinol 17:1382–1394

Kinzel V, Kubler D (1976) Single step purification of the catalytic subunit(s) of cyclic 3', 5'-adenosine monophosphate-dependent protein kinase(s) from rat muscle. Biochem Biophys Res Commun 71:257–264

Kishimoto A, Takai Y, Nishizuka Y (1977) Activation of glycogen phosphorylase kinase by a calcium-activated, cyclic nucleotide-independent protein kinase system. J Biol Chem 252:7449–7452

Knighton DR, Zheng JH, Ten Eyck LF, Ashford VA, Xuong NH, Taylor SS, Sowadski JM (1991) Crystal structure of the catalytic subunit of cyclic adenosine monophosphate-dependent protein kinase [see comments]. Science 253:407–414

Kobayashi T, Cohen P (1999) Activation of serum- and glucocorticoid-regulated protein kinase by agonists that activate phosphatidylinositide 3-kinase is mediated by 3-phosphoinositide-dependent protein kinase-1 (PDK1) and PDK2. Biochem J 339:319–328

Koide K, Bunnage ME, Gomez Paloma L, Kanter JR, Taylor SS, Brunton LL, Nicolaou KC (1995) Molecular design and biological activity of potent and selective protein kinase inhibitors related to balanol. Chem Biol 2:601–8

Komander D, Kular GS, Bain J, Elliott M, Alessi DR, van Aalten DMF (2003) Structural basis for UCN-01 (7-hydroxystaurosporine) specificity and PDK1 (3-phosphoinositide-dependent protein kinase-1) inhibition. BioChem J 375:255–262

Komander D, Kular GS, Schüttelkopf AW, Deak M, Prakash KRC, Bain J, Elliott M, Garrido-'Franko M, Kozikowski AP, Alessi DR, van Aalten DMF (2004) Interactions of LY333531 and other bisindolyl maleimide inhibitors with PDK1. Structure 12:215–226

Kubler D, Gagelmann M, Pyerin W, Kinzel V (1979) Isolation of the catalytic subunits of cyclic AMP-dependent protein kinases from different mammalian tissues on the basis of charge differences of their subunits. Hoppe Seylers Z Physiol Chem 360:1421–1431

Kulanthaivel P, Hallock Y, Boros C, Hamilton SM, Janzen WP, Ballas LM, Loomis CR, Jiang JB, Katz JB, Steiner JR, Clardy J (1993) Balanol: a novel and potent inhibitor of protein kinase C from the fungus *Verticillium balanoides*. J Am Chem Soc 115:6452–6453

Lamers MB, Antson AA, Hubbard RE, Scott RK, Williams DH (1999) Structure of the protein tyrosine kinase domain of C-terminal Src kinase (CSK) in complex with staurosporine. J Mol Biol 285:713–725

Lampe JW, Biggers CK, Defauw JM, Foglesong RJ, Hall SE, Heerding JM, Hollinshead SP, Hu H, Hughes PF, Jagdmann GE, Jr, Johnson MG, Lai YS, Lowden CT, Lynch MP, Mendoza JS, Murphy MM, Wilson JW, Ballas LM, Carter K, Darges JW, Davis JE, Hubbard FR, Stamper ML (2002) Synthesis and protein kinase inhibitory activity of balanol analogues with modified benzophenone subunits. J Med Chem 45:2624–43

Lawrie AM, Noble ME, Tunnah P, Brown NR, Johnson LN, Endicott JA (1997) Protein kinase inhibition by staurosporine revealed in details of the molecular interaction with CDK2 [letter]. Nat Struct Biol 4:796–801

Le Good JA, Ziegler WH, Parekh DB, Alessi DR, Cohen P, Parker PJ (1998) Protein kinase C isotypes controlled by phosphoinositide 3-kinase through the protein kinase PDK1. Science 281:2042–2045

Leung T, Manser E, Tan L, Lim L (1995) A novel serine/threonine kinase binding the Ras-related RhoA GTPase which translocates the kinase to peripheral membranes. J Biol Chem 270:29051–29054

Lodowski DT, Pitcher JA, Capel WD, Lefkowitz RJ, Tesmer JJG (2003) Keeping G proteins at bay: a complex between G protein-coupled receptor kinase 2 and Gbetagamma. Science 300:1256–1262

Madhusudan Akamine P, Xuong NH, Taylor SS (2002) Crystal structure of a transition state mimic of the catalytic subunit of cAMP-dependent protein kinase. Nat Struct Biol 9:273–277

Manning G, Whyte DB, Martinez R, Hunter T, Sudarsanam S (2002) The protein kinase complement of the human genome. Science 298:1912–1934

Marambaud P, Ancolio K, Alves da Costa C, Checler F (1999) Effect of protein kinase A inhibitors on the production of Abeta40 and Abeta42 by human cells expressing normal and Alzheimer's disease-linked mutated betaAPP and presenilin 1. Br J Pharmacol 126:1186–1190

Matsui T, Amano M, Yamamoto T, Chihara K, Nakafuku M, Ito M, Nakano T, Okawa K, Iwamatsu A, Kaibuchi K (1996) Rho-associated kinase, a novel serine threonine kinase, as a putative target for the small GTP binding protein Rho. EMBO J 15:2208–2216

Meggio F, Donella DA, Ruzzene M, et al (1995) Different susceptibility of protein kinases to staurosporine inhibition. Kinetic studies and molecular bases for the resistance of protein kinase CK2. Eur J Biochem 234:317–322

Montminy M (1997) Transcriptional regulation by cyclic AMP. Annu Rev Biochem 66:807–822

Nakashima S (2002) Protein kinase C alpha (PKC alpha): regulation and biological function. J Biochem (Tokyo) 132:669–675

Narayana N, Diller TC, Koide K, Bunnage ME, Nicolaou KC, Brunton LL, Xuong NH, Ten Eyck LF, Taylor SS (1999) Crystal structure of the potent natural product inhibitor balanol in complex with the catalytic subunit of cAMP-dependent protein kinase. Biochemistry 38:2367–2376

Narumiya S, Ishizaki T, Uehata M (2000) Use and properties of ROCK-specific inhibitor Y-27632. Methods Enzymol 325:273–284

Nelson NC, Taylor SS (1981) Differential labeling and identification of the cysteine- containing tryptic peptides of catalytic subunit from porcine heart cAMP-dependent protein kinase. J Biol Chem 256:3743–3750

Newton AC (2001) Protein kinase C: structural and spatial regulation by phosphorylation, cofactors, and macromolecular interactions. Chem Rev 101:2353–2364
Newton AC (2003) Regulation of the ABC kinases by phosphorylation: protein kinase C as a paradigm. BioChem J 370:361–371
Nishizuka Y (1984) The role of protein kinase C in cell surface signal transduction and tumour promotion. Nature 308:693–698
Nishizuka Y (1995) Protein kinase C and lipid signaling for sustained cellular responses. FASEB J 9:484–496
Nolen B, Ngo J, Chakrabarti S, Vu D, Adams JA, Ghosh G (2003) Nucleotide-induced conformational changes in the Saccharomyces cerevisiae SR protein kinase, Sky1p, revealed by X-ray crystallography. Biochemistry 42:9575–9585
Ohshima S, Yanagisawa M, Katoh A, Fujii T, Sano T, Matsukuma S, Furumai T, Fujiu M, Watanabe K, Yokose K, et al (1994) Fusarium merismoides Corda NR 6356, the source of the protein kinase C inhibitor, azepinostatin. Taxonomy, yield improvement, fermentation and biological activity. J Antibiot (Tokyo) 47:639–47
Olah GA, Mitchell RD, Sosnick TR, Walsh DA, Trewhella J (1993) Solution structure of the cAMP-dependent protein kinase catalytic subunit and its contraction upon binding the protein kinase inhibitor peptide. Biochemistry 32:3649–3657
Ono-Saito N, Niki I, Hidaka H (1999) H-series protein kinase inhibitors and potential clinical applications. Pharmacol Ther 82:123–131
Orellana SA, Amieux PS, Zhao X, McKnight GS (1993) Mutations in the catalytic subunit of the cAMP-dependent protein kinase interfere with holoenzyme formation without disrupting inhibition by protein kinase inhibitor. J Biol Chem 268:6843–6846
Pargellis C, Tong L, Churchill L, Cirillo PF, et al (2002) Inhibition of p38 MAP kinase by utilizing a novel allosteric binding site. Nat Struct Biol 9:268–272
Park J, Hill MM, Hess D, Brazil DP, Hofsteenge J, Hemmings BA (2001) Identification of tyrosine phosphorylation sites on 3-phosphoinositide-dependent protein kinase-1 and their role in regulating kinase activity. J Biol Chem 276:37459–37471
Pettit GR, Day JF, Hartwell JL, Wood HB (1970) Antineoplastic components of marine animals. Nature 227:962–963
Prade L, Engh RA, Girod A, Kinzel V, Huber R, Bossemeyer D (1997) Staurosporine-induced conformational changes of cAMP-dependent protein kinase catalytic subunit explain inhibitory potential. Structure 5:1627–1637
Pullen N, Dennis PB, Andjelkovic M, Dufner A, Kozma SC, Hemmings BA, Thomas G (1998) Phosphorylation and activation of p70s6 k by PDK1. Science 279:707–710
Richards SA, Fu J, Romanelli A, Shimamura A, Blenis J (1999) Ribosomal S6 kinase 1 (RSK1) activation requires signals dependent on and independent of the MAP kinase ERK. Curr Biol 9:810–820
Russo AA, Jeffrey PD, Pavletich NP (1996) Structural basis of cyclin-dependent kinase activation by phosphorylation. Nat Struct Biol 3:696–700
Sasaki Y, Suzuki M, Hidaka H (2002) The novel and specific Rho kinase inhibitor (S)-(+)-2-methyl-1- [(4-methyl-5-isoquinoline)sulfonyl]-homopiperazine as a probing molecule for Rho kinase-involved pathway. Pharmacol Ther 93:225–232
Schneider T (2002) Kinetische und strukturelle Untersuchungen zur Funktion ausgewählter konservierter Aminosäurereste der katalytischen Untereinheit Ca der Proteinkinase A. Universität Bielefeld
Schulze Gahmen U, Brandsen J, Jones HD, Morgan DO, Meijer L, Vesely J, Kim SH (1995) Multiple modes of ligand recognition: crystal structures of cyclin-dependent protein kinase 2 in complex with ATP and two inhibitors, olomoucine and isopentenyladenine. Proteins 22:378–391

Setyawan J, Koide K, Diller TC, Bunnage ME, Taylor SS, Nicolaou KC, Brunton LL (1999) Inhibition of protein kinases by balanol: Specificity within the serine/threonine protein kinase subfamily. Mol Pharmacol 56:370–376

Shimokawa H, Iinuma H, Kishida H, Nakashima M, Kato K (2001) Antianginal effect of fasudil, a Rho kinase inhibitor, in patients with stable effort angina: a multicenter study. Circulation 104:2843

Sicheri F, Moarefi I, Kuriyan J (1997) Crystal structure of the Src family tyrosine kinase Hck [see comments]. Nature 385:602–609

Sinnett-Smith J, Lunn JA, Leopoldt D, Rozengurt E (2001) Y-27632, an inhibitor of Rho-associated kinases, prevents tyrosine phosphorylation of focal adhesion kinase and paxillin induced by bombesin: dissociation from tyrosine phosphorylation of p130(CAS). Exp Cell Res 266:292–302

Sprang SR, Acharya KR, Goldsmith EJ, Stuart DI, Varvill K, Fletterick RJ, Madsen NB, Johnson LN (1988) Structural changes in glycogen phosphorylase induced by phosphorylation. Nature 336:215–221

Stokoe D, Stephens LR, Copeland T, Gaffney PR, Reese CB, Painter GF, Holmes AB, McCormick F, Hawkins PT (1997) Dual role of phosphatidylinositol-3,4,5-trisphosphate in the activation of protein kinase B. Science 277:567–570

Swannie HC, Kaye SB (2002) Protein kinase C inhibitors. Curr Oncol Rep 4:37–46

Takemoto M, Sun JX, Hiroki J, Shimokawa H, Liao JK (2002) Rho kinase mediates hypoxia-induced downregulation of endothelial nitric oxide synthase. Circulation 106:57–62

Tamm I, Dorken B, Hartmann G (2001) Antisense therapy in oncology: new hope for an old idea? Lancet 358:489–497

Tanaka H, Ohshima N, Takagi M, Komeima K, Hidaka H (1998) Novel vascular relaxant, Hmn-1152—its molecular mechanism of action. Naunyn Schmiedebergs Arch Pharmakol 358:P3740

Taniyama Y, Weber DS, Rocic P, Hilenski L, Akers ML, Park J, Hemmings BA, Alexander RW, Griendling KK (2003) Pyk2-dependent tyrosine phosphorylation of PDK1 mediates cell spreading. FASEB J 17:A1351

Toledo LM, Lydon NB (1997) Structures of staurosporine bound to CDK2 and cAPK—new tools for structure-based design of protein kinase inhibitors. Structure 5:1551–1556

Trauger JW, Lin FF, Turner MS, Stephens J, LoGrasso PV (2002) Kinetic mechanism for human Rho-kinase II (ROCK-II). Biochemistry 41:8948–8953

Traxler P (2003) Tyrosine kinases as targets in cancer therapy—successes and failures. Expert Opin Ther Targets 7:215–234

Uehata M, Ishizaki T, Satoh H, Ono T, Kawahara T, Morishita T, Tamakawa H, Yamagami K, Inui J, Maekawa M, Narumiya S (1997) Calcium sensitization of smooth muscle mediated by a Rho- associated protein kinase in hypertension. Nature 389:990–994

Underwood KW, Parris KD, Federico E, et al (2003) Catalytically active MAP KAP kinase 2 structures in complex with staurosporine and ADP reveal differences with the autoinhibited enzyme. Structure 11:627–636

Vanhaesebroeck B, Alessi DR (2000) The P13K-PDK1 connection: more than just a road to PKB. BioChem J 346:561–576

Walsh DA, Perkins JP, Krebs EG (1968) An adenosine 3',5'-monophosphate-dependant protein kinase from rabbit skeletal muscle. J Biol Chem 243:3763–3765

Way KJ, Chou E, King GL (2000) Identification of PKC-isoform-specific biological actions using pharmacological approaches. Trends Pharmacol Sci 21:181–187

Wick MJ, Wick KR, Chen H, He H, Dong LQ, Quon MJ, Liu F (2002) Substitution of the autophosphorylation site Thr516 with a negatively charged residue confers constitutive activity to mouse 3-phosphoinositide-dependent protein kinase-1 in cells. J Biol Chem 277:16632–16638

Wong CF, Hunenberger PH, Akamine P, Narayana N, Diller T, McCammon JA, Taylor S, Xuong NH (2001) Computational analysis of PKA-balanol interactions. J Med Chem 44:1530–1539

Xu R-M, Carmel G, Kuret J, Cheng X (1996) Structural basis for selectivity of the isoquinoline sulfonamide family of protein kinase inhibitors. Proc Natl Acad Sci U S A 93:6308–6313

Yang J, Cron P, Good VM, Thompson V, Hemmings BA, Barford D (2002) Crystal structure of an activated Akt/protein kinase B ternary complex with GSK3-peptide and AMP-PNP. Nat Struct Biol 9:940–944

Zhao B, Bower MJ, McDevitt PJ, Zhao HZ, Davis ST, Johanson KO, Green SM, Concha NO, Zhou BBS (2002) Structural basis for Chk1 inhibition by UCN-01. J Biol Chem 277:46609–46615

Zheng J, Knighton DR, Ten Eyck LF, Karlsson R, Xuong N, Taylor SS, Sowadski JM (1993) Crystal structure of the catalytic subunit of cAMP-dependent protein kinase complexed with MgATP and peptide inhibitor. Biochemistry 32:2154–2161

Zhu X, Kim JL, Newcomb JR, Rose PE, Stover DR, Toledo LM, Zhao H, Morgenstern KA (1999) Structural analysis of the lymphocyte-specific kinase Lck in complex with non-selective and Src family selective kinase inhibitors. Structure Fold Des 7:651–661

HEP (2005) 167:125–155

Inhibitors of Protein Kinase CK2: Structural Aspects

R. Battistutta[1] · S. Sarno[2] · G. Zanotti[1] (✉)

[1] Chemistry Department, University of Padova,
Venetian Institute of Molecular Medicine (VIMM), Padova, Italy
giuseppe.zanotti@unipd.it
[2] Biological Chemistry Department, University of Padova,
Venetian Institute of Molecular Medicine (VIMM), Padova, Italy

Abstract Protein kinase CK2 is one of the most challenging members of the kinase superfamily. Although this protein has been the subject of intensive studies over the last 50 years, very little is known about its precise biological function and mode of regulation. The CK2 holoenzyme is composed of two catalytic α- and two regulatory β-subunits and is classified as an acidophilic Ser/Thr kinase. Unique properties of the catalytic α-subunit are its intrinsic activity and high pleiotropicity. CK2 is supposed to be involved in many fundamental aspects of the normal cell life as well as in degenerative processes that can lead to cancer or tumor pathologies. This makes CK2 an interesting target for the development of inhibitors with pharmacological perspectives. The inhibitors studied are directed to the CK2 ATP-binding site that, among the known kinases, carries some distinctive features as indicated by its ability to use both ATP and GTP as co-substrates and the low susceptiveness to staurosporine inhibition. On the basis of three-dimensional crystal structures, we describe and discuss the effects of the binding to CK2 of inhibitors with a potency in the low micromolar range belonging to different chemical families, i.e., benzotriazoles, anthraquinones, and quinazolinones. The overall structure of the protein is poorly affected by the binding of these small molecules. In the proximity of the binding site, the most affected residues are Asn118, His160, Met163, and those of the glycine-rich loop. Two of the inhibitors, namely tetrabromo-2-benzotriazolo (TBB) and the indoloquinazolinone IQA, display a significant selectivity among panels of tens of different kinases. An important common energetic contribution to the inhibitors' binding is ascribed to the hydrophobic interaction with the apolar surface region of the CK2 binding cleft. The shape and the reduced dimension of the CK2 active site in comparison with other kinases are essential in explaining the selectivity of these inhibitors as well as the anomalous low potency of staurosporine.

Keywords CK2 · Kinase inhibitors · Complexes · Crystal structure · Anthraquinones · Benzotriazoles · Quinazolinones

1 Protein Kinase CK2

One of the first members of the protein kinase superfamily ever discovered is CK2, formerly known as "casein kinase 2." The first report, dated 1954 by Burnett and Kennedy, described this enzyme isolated from liver extracts along with protein kinase CK1 (Burnett and Kennedy 1954). For their experiments, the authors utilized casein as an artificial substrate, and this is the reason for the early name casein kinase 2 (indeed, since casein is not a natural substrate for the enzyme, and since the real ones are still undefined, the name was moved to the more generic "CK2").

Protein kinase CK2 is an eukaryotic acidophilic Ser/Thr protein kinase. This ubiquitous enzyme is well conserved throughout evolution and, based on a recent classification of the human kinome (Manning et al. 2002b; see also the web-site at http://kinase.com/kinbase/), the catalytic subunit belongs to the so-called other kinase group, i.e., without strong similarities to other groups, giving origin to the CK2 family. Among the nearest relatives are the cyclin-dependent kinases, belonging to the CMGC group.

The holoenzyme comprises a tetrameric assembly formed by two catalytic (α) and two regulatory (β) subunits. Depending on the species, several catalytic and regulatory paralogs have been identified; in humans, two catalytic (α- and α') subunits and one regulatory (β) subunit are known.

Owing to some peculiar properties, CK2 is considered a quite anomalous protein kinase (Pinna 2002): (a) it is highly pleiotropic, (b) it can use ATP and guanosine triphosphate (GTP) as co-substrates, (c) the target serine or threonine must be surrounded by acidic residues and (d) the α-catalytic subunit is intrinsically active. Finally, most importantly, the precise function of this enzyme has not been deciphered. For recent reviews on the subject, see references (Pinna 2002; Litchfield 2003; Meggio and Pinna 2003).

2
Substrate Pleiotropicity and Function

To date, more than 300 substrates are known for CK2 (Meggio and Pinna 2003). Although most of these substrates are phosphorylated on serine or threonine residues, and consequently CK2 is classified as a Ser/Thr kinase, some examples of tyrosine phosphorylation are also documented (Chardot et al. 1995; Marin et al. 1999). In this respect, evidence was presented that indeed both the α- and α'-catalytic subunits of CK2 undergo an intermolecular autocatalytic event on a tyrosine placed in the activation loop, very likely Tyr182 (Donella-Deana et al. 2001). The high pleiotropicity is a distinctive feature of this kinase. Looking at the classes of proteins that are phosphorylated, it has been assumed that CK2 is involved in many aspects of cell cycle regulation, cell growth and differentiation, embryogenesis, and, recently, apoptosis. Abnormally high levels of the enzyme detected in transgenic mouse lymphomas (Seldin and Leder 1995) and in solid tumors (Guerra and Issinger 1999) have suggested the involvement of CK2 in tumorigenesis phenomena (Tawfic et al. 2001). Nevertheless, while both CK2 catalytic and regulatory subunits have been demonstrated essential for cell viability in *Saccharomyces cerevisiae* (Padmanabha et al. 1990), in *Caenorhabditis elegans* (Fraser et al. 2000), and in mice (Buchou et al. 2003), the precise functions of this enzyme are not well understood. Recently, it has been proposed that CK2 also has a crucial role in the transduction of survival signals, protecting the cell against stress events (Ahmed et al. 2002).

3
Constitutive Activity and Lack of Regulatory Mechanisms

Mechanisms regulating the catalytic activity of most protein kinases that have been recognized to date include the control by additional subunits or domains and phosphorylation and dephosphorylation events (Johnson et al. 1996; Huse and Kuriyan 2002). In the regulation of most, but not all, protein kinases, also a (auto)phosphorylation process takes place in the activation loop, often at a residue corresponding to the threonine-197 in cAMP-dependent protein kinase (cAPK) [for instance in cdc2 and mitogen-activated protein kinase (MAPK)]. Despite CK2's discovery almost 50 years ago and the numerous studies that followed, the regulatory mechanism is still the subject of intense discussion, and none of the aforementioned regulations looks to be appropriate.

The catalytic subunit of this enzyme is intrinsically active, even in absence of the regulatory segment; once the holoenzyme is formed, its activity can increase or decrease, depending on the substrate involved. It was suggested (Pinna 2002) that, unlike many other kinases that are usually inactive in the cell and are activated only transiently, CK2 is regulated in the opposite manner; i.e., when present, it is normally active and is regulated by inactivation. To make the scenario even more complicate, recently it has been proved that the dimeric β-subunit can indeed interact with several partners other than the CK2 α-subunit, suggesting for the β-subunit a more complicated role (Litchfield 2003). Evidence of possible distinctive roles for the isolated catalytic and regulatory subunits has led to the hypothesis that a balance in the expression of the two subunits together with their different specific localization in the cell compartments can contribute to the regulation of CK2 functions (Faust and Montenarh 2000).

The constitutive activity of CK2 has also been postulated to be responsible for the exploitation of this kinase by an increasing number of viral agents for the phosphorylation of proteins essential for their cell cycle.

4
General Structural Features of Ser/Thr Protein Kinases Catalytic Domain

Ser/Thr protein kinase catalytic domains are structurally well conserved throughout evolution, from prokaryotes to mammals, while their amino acid sequences show a much lower degree of similarity (Manning et al. 2002a; Young et al. 2003). Nevertheless, residues essential for the function of the enzyme are conserved in all kinases that invariably share some characteristic properties (Hanks and Hunter 1995). Figure 1 shows an alignment between the sequences of cAPK, that is often considered as the reference prototype kinase, and the CK2 catalytic α-subunit from human and *Zea mays*, with the most important residues highlighted.

The overall three-dimensional structure comprises both β-strands and α-helices, with a large predominance of the former in the N-terminal lobe and of the latter in the C-terminal one (Fig. 2).

Between the two lobes an essentially hydrophobic deep cleft is formed, where the co-substrate (ATP or, less frequently, GTP) can bind. The two lobes are connected by a segment known as the hinge region, where the adenine moiety of ATP can be anchored by means of some hydrogen bonds.

In order to be active, the conformation of a kinase must guarantee the access of cosubstrate and substrate to the catalytic zone and the correct arrangement of the catalytic and binding residues; in particular, the proper orientation of ATP is crucial for catalysis. The binding of the ATP phosphate tail to the enzyme is favored by two metal ions, usually magnesium, that are coordinated by an asparagine residue of the so-called catalytic loop (Asn161 in CK2, 171 in cAPK) and an aspartate at the beginning of the activation segment (Asp175 in CK2, 184 in cAPK).

Two other structurally conserved important zones in kinases are the Gly-rich loop, or p-loop, and the helix αC (Fig. 2); the Gly-rich loop contributes

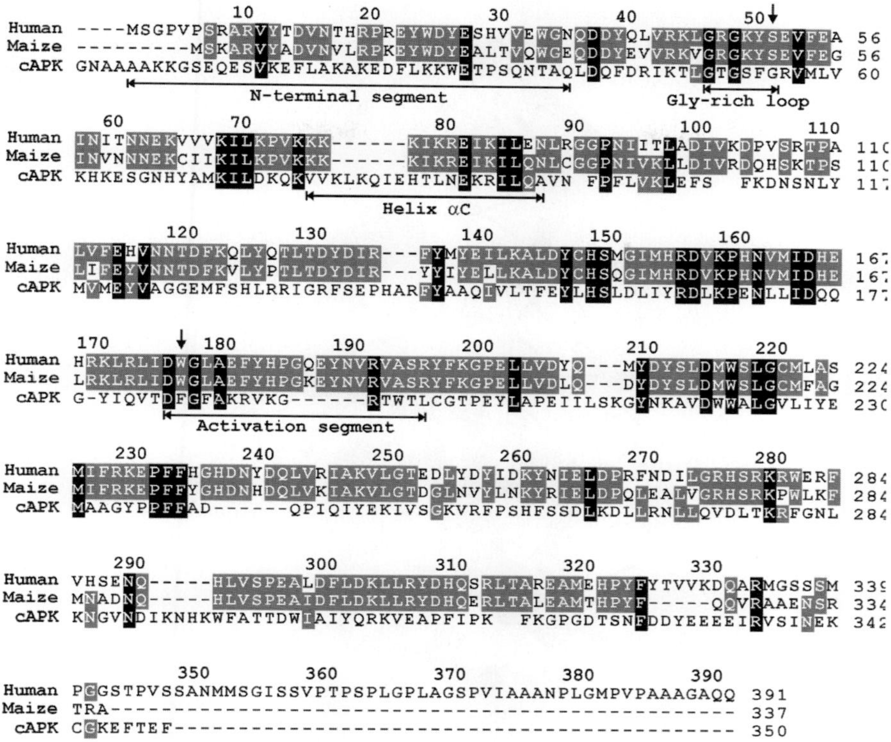

Fig. 1 Sequence alignment of cAPK and CK2 catalytic α-subunits from human and maize. *Vertical arrows* mark important residues not conserved between cAPK and CK2, as discussed in the text. The structurally and functionally important regions of CK2 are indicated. *Numbering in the upper line* refers to human CK2 sequence. *Black background*, residues identical in all three sequences; *gray background*, residues identical in only two sequences

to strengthen the ATP anchoring, while the orientation of the αC helix is essential for the activity of the enzyme. In Ser/Thr kinases that present inactive and active forms, as in the case of cAPK or CDK2, helix αC has been found with an orientation substantially different in the two arrangements (Jeffrey et al. 1995). So, when a transition from an inactive to an active structure occurs, there is usually a rearrangement of the relative orientation of the two lobes, to properly position essential residues of the catalytic site (for instance those corresponding to Lys72 and Asp166 in CDK2) and a concomitant correct positioning of the αC helix in the N-terminal domain. Another important structural change occurring for the activation is represented by the displacement of the activation segment, a long loop in the C-terminal domain, that moves away from the close position of the inactive form to an open one (Fig. 2), allowing the binding of the substrate and co-substrate to

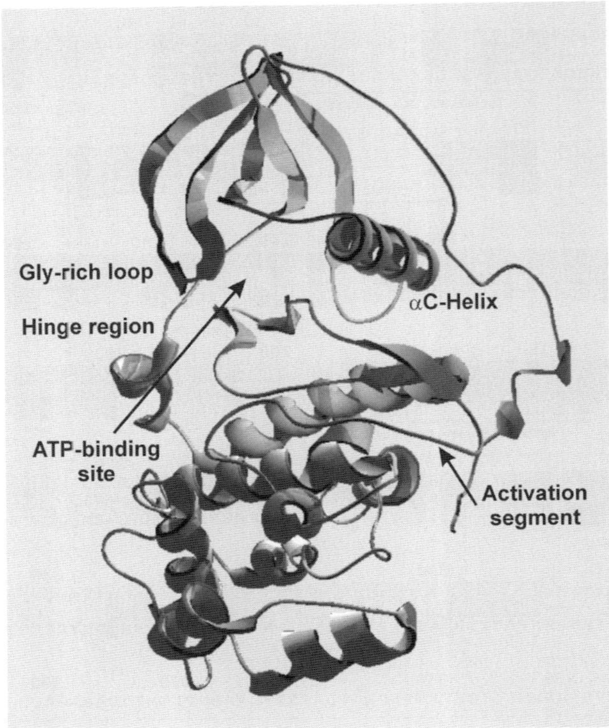

Fig. 2 Three-dimensional structure of Apo-CK2. Regions important in all Ser/Thr kinases are indicated. The N-terminal region (*upper part*) is rich in β-sheets while the C-terminal one (*lower part*) is rich in α-helical structure. ATP binds in the cleft between the two lobes, adjacent to the Gly-rich loop and the hinge region. The activation segment adopts an open active conformation

the enzyme (Johnson et al. 1996). This movement can be caused by a phosphorylation event, as in the case of cAPK when Thr197 is phosphorylated, sometimes coupled with an interaction with e regulatory subunit, as in the case of CDK2 with cyclin. The activation segment displacement is made possible principally by a rotation of a short stretch of three amino acids positioned at the beginning of the loop; this tripeptide, Asp-Phe-Gly, is highly conserved in kinases but not in CK2, where the phenylalanine is substituted by a tryptophan at position 176 (indicated by a vertical arrow in Fig. 1). The C-terminal end of the activation segment, the p+1 loop, is responsible for substrate recognition and binding.

It must be noted, however, that not all kinases show a dramatic transition from an active to an inactive form as exhibited by CDK2 and cAPK. As already mentioned, CK2 is one of the few examples being found solely in the active form.

5 Three-Dimensional Structure of CK2 Catalytic α-Subunit

The first three-dimensional structure of a catalytic subunit of CK2 is that from *Zea mays*, appeared in 1998 (Niefind et al. 1998). Due to the high degree of identity with the human enzyme, CK2 from maize has been considered a suitable model for all the subsequent inhibition studies. This hypothesis has been validated by the recent determination of the crystal structure of the human holoenzyme (Niefind et al. 2001) and by those of the human catalytic subunit and a mutant independently determined by two different groups (Ermakova et al. 2003; Pechkcova et al. 2003). In all these structures the α-subunit shows essentially the same features of that from maize, particularly as far as the active site is concerned.

The CK2 catalytic subunit bears most of the sequence and structural features common to all Ser/Thr kinase. Regarding the primary structure, two notable exceptions are: (a) in the Gly-rich loop (residues 46–51 in CK2) the third glycine (indicated by a vertical arrow in Fig. 1) in the consensus sequence GXGXøG is missing (ø is usually a tyrosine, as in CK2, or a phenylalanine); (b) at the beginning of the activation segment a tryptophan (residue 176 in CK2) substitutes a phenylalanine in the otherwise conserved three-peptide Asp-Phe-Gly (Fig. 1).

Another distinctive feature of CK2 is the presence of a basic cluster at the beginning of helix αC (residues 74–80), where 6 out of 7 consecutive amino acids are basic (5 lysines and one arginine). The presence of this basic cluster, also known as a substrate recognition site, is supposed to be in relation with the attitude of CK2 to phosphorylate highly acidic substrates with the minimal consensus sequence Ser/Thr-X-X-Asp/Glu (Meggio et al. 1994). Other basic amino acids present in the p+1 loop at the C-terminal end of the activation segment, namely Arg191, Arg195 and Lys198, have been found relevant for substrate recognition (Sarno et al. 1996).

The elucidation of the three-dimensional structure of the catalytic domain of CK2 has unveiled the origin of the intrinsic activity of the enzyme (Niefind et al. 1998), showing that CK2 bears all the same structural properties responsible for the active state of cAPK, taken as the prototype of an active Ser/Thr kinase (Engh and Bossemeyer 2002). In CK2 many of the N-terminal thirty residues make several hydrophobic and polar interactions with some other important regions of the protein, located both in the N-terminal and C-terminal domains, contributing to the stabilization of the active conformation. Of particular interest are the interactions with the activation segment, which consequently is constrained in an open active state (Fig. 2). These interactions are unique among the protein kinases whose structure is known, and indeed they occur between residues highly conserved in CK2 s from different species but not among other kinases.

The presence of the tryptophan-176 instead of a phenylalanine, distinctive of CK2, contributes to block the activation segment in the open active conformation; that because a hydrogen bond between the nitrogen of the tryptophan indole ring and the backbone carbonyl of Leu173 hampers the possibility of the rotation necessary for the transition from an inactive to an active conformation, possible if a phenylalanine is present instead.

The active conformation of the enzyme is granted also by the exact relative orientation of the N- and C-terminal lobes, by the proper position of the substrate and co-substrate anchoring and catalytic residues of the active site and by the correct orientation of the αC helix, spanning residues from 74 to 89. In particular, Glu81 contributes, through an ionic interaction, to orient Lys68 in the optimal position for the proper alignment of the ATP phosphates for catalysis. The importance of Lys68 and Glu81 (numbering is referred to CK2 sequence) is underlined by their conservation in all kinase sequences known to date.

In the hinge region of CK2, three are the residues involved in the nucleotides binding: Glu114, Val116 and Asn118. In the case of ATP, two hydrogen bonds between N1 and N6 of adenosine and backbone carbonyl of Glu114 and amide of Val116 are present; these interactions are typical of many kinases. In the case of GTP, atoms N1 and O6 of the purine moiety are hydrogen bound to the amide and the carbonyl of the backbone of Val116. Asparagine 118 is involved in the coordination of both co-substrates, ATP and GTP, also with the involvement of a water molecule mediating the interaction with the co-substrates. The dual co-substrate specificity is achieved by means of two well-structured water molecules that allow the switching between the different coordination modes of ATP and GTP through an hydrogen bond frame shift (Niefind et al. 1999).

6
CK2 Tetrameric Assembly

In vivo, human CK2 is found mainly, although not exclusively, in a tetrameric assembly, composed of two catalytic α- (or α') and two regulatory β-subunits. Evidence has accumulating that these subunits can exist in vivo also in isolated forms, with specific functions (Pinna and Meggio 1997). While the catalytic subunit, when isolated, is found in a monomeric state, the regulatory subunits have a strong tendency to form dimers, due to the presence of a zinc-finger motif (Chantalat et al. 1999). This dimeric state is spontaneously formed in solution and is thought to be responsible for the recruitment of the two catalytic subunits in order to assemble the final tetramer (Graham and Litchfield 2000).

The three-dimensional structure of the human holoenzyme, carrying α-subunits lacking of the C-terminal tail, was determined at 3.1 Å resolution

(Niefind et al. 2001). Even if the quality of the final model at this resolution is limited, nevertheless it clearly indicates that the catalytic subunit is poorly affected by the presence of the regulatory one. In other words, the inclusion in the tetramer does not significantly modify the structure of the isolated human catalytic subunit. The overall structure of the holoenzyme shows a "butterfly" shape, where the regulatory dimer, whose structure is very similar to that in the isolated form, binds two α-subunits that do not interact with each other. The surfaces of interaction between the subunits are not extensive, and this is somewhat unexpected due to the remarkable resistance to the action of denaturing agents showed by the holoenzyme. The interpretation of the large amount of biochemical and functional data accumulated in the years is not always straightforward in terms of the structural properties unveiled by the three-dimensional structure of the holoenzyme. This analysis is currently underway and is subject of debate in the field.

7 Protein Kinase Inhibitors

Interest in the development of protein kinase inhibitors has grown so enormously in the last decade, both in academic and industrial laboratories, that now the protein kinase family is the second most important drug target (Cohen 2002). This is mainly due to the involvement of the superfamily of protein kinases in many key functions of cell life, including cell cycle regulation, development, proliferation, signal transmission, and apoptosis. Abnormalities in the natural roles of this class of enzyme are often associated with human diseases, especially cancer and tumor pathologies, whose treatment has so far been restricted to cytotoxic and hormonal agents (Goel et al. 2002). Even though the application of kinase inhibitors as drugs is a very challenging task, mostly because of the conservation of structural features within the ATP-binding clefts, now many kinase inhibitors are in clinical trials or even in the market, the majority of them as anti-tumor drugs (Cohen 2002).

The estimate that at least 500 different protein kinases are encoded in the human genome makes really challenging the design of molecules that specifically target a single protein without affecting closely related kinases. The targeting of the ATP-binding site has the obvious drawbacks of the existence of other ATP-utilizing proteins and the high intracellular concentrations of ATP. Although peptide inhibitors directed to the substrate binding site may in principle offer a higher degree of specificity, they have their own set of problems that includes low affinity and potential bioavailability issues.

One of the first kinase inhibitors discovered has been staurosporine, that shows a large activity spectrum and therefore a low selectivity. Most protein kinases are inhibited by staurosporine with IC_{50} in the low nanomolar range. Interestingly, CK2, as well as a few other kinases, is less affected by this inhibitor, with IC_{50} in the micromolar range. This trait, together with the quite unique ability of CK2 to utilize both ATP and GTP as phosphate donor, suggests an appreciable difference in the structural properties of the active site that potentially can be exploited in the inhibitors optimization process.

The most common chemical scaffolds used as ATP site-directed kinase inhibitors are derivatives of heterocyclic compounds, such as quinazolines, phenylamino- or pyrido- or pyrrolo- or pyrimido- or pyrazolo-pyrimidines, pyrrolo-pyridines, indolin-2-ones, purines, pyridinyl- or pyrimidinyl-imidazoles, and phthalazines. Some other building blocks are derived from natural products, such as alkaloids, flavonoids, and the aforementioned staurosporine (Garcia-Echeverria et al. 2000).

Recently, an insulin receptor tyrosine kinase bisubstrate inhibitor competitive against both nucleotide and peptide substrates has been designed (Parang et al. 2001). The crystal structure of its complex with the protein tyrosine kinase (PTK) has confirmed the double anchoring scheme of target binding. This bisubstrate inhibitor could be a precursor of a new interesting class of anticancer therapeutic agents, allowing the possibility to take advantage of the small differences in the various kinase binding sites to improve the selectivity of the inhibition (Parang and Cole 2002).

The availability of an increasing number of three-dimensional structures of inhibitor/kinases complexes are helping in clarifying the atomic basis for the different selectivity and potency (Toledo et al. 1999). These crystal structures are often the starting point for the optimization of additional analogs through rational drug design approaches. A representative case is that of CDK2, whose crystal structures in complex with a number of key inhibitors has been used to explain the observed structure–activity relationships within the compound series and to guide the design of more potent inhibitors (Gray et al. 1998; Davis et al. 2001; Hardcastle et al. 2002). Nowadays, the first step in the research of a new promising chemical scaffolds is often the running of a virtual screen of a huge amount of chemical compounds utilizing as a target the three-dimensional structure of the protein kinase in complex with some inhibitor (Stahura et al. 1999). A similar approach has been successful in the case of different tyrosine kinases such as epidermal growth factor receptor (EGFR)/ErbB2 kinases, Flt-1 kinase, and Abl kinase (Traxler et al. 2001).

Probably the most exciting result in the field of kinase inhibitors concerns chronic myelogenous leukemia (CML), due to a translocation involving chromosome 8 and 22 that generates the BCR-Abl fusion protein. In normal cells, c-Abl is found in the nucleus as a negative regulator of cell growth, while BCR-Abl behaves as a fully cytoplasmic intrinsically active Tyr-kinase, giving rise to the development of this cancer. Recently, a very potent and selective inhibitor of BCR-Abl, Gleevec (or Glivec or STI-571 or CPG 57148B), a phenylamino-pyrimidine derivative, has come into the market in the treatment of CML, with very low or even null side effects. An important step in the comprehension of the mechanism of inhibition has been the elucidation of the crystal structure of the Abl domain in complex with STI-571.

8
CK2 Inhibition

The oncogenic potential of CK2 and its involvement in virally mediated pathologies has led to an increasing number of studies aimed at the discovery of selective inhibitors. These molecules could constitute not only lead compounds for drug development, but also useful tools for the clarification of the protein function in vivo.

An important aspect of CK2 that could simplify the drug design process is that this enzyme is always active and does not undergo the relevant conformational changes typical of most protein kinases. This circumstance allows us to overcome the difficulty that sometimes arises in correlating biochemical inhibition data, often obtained with activated kinases, with structural data derived from inhibitors bound to the inactive form of the enzyme. Moreover, it is not always possible to crystallize protein kinases in their active state. In the case of complexes with the inactive form of kinases, caution must be used in the straightforward interpretation of the inhibition data in terms of structural details that can represent a situation slightly but significantly different from that occurring in the biochemical experiments. However, there are examples, as with the Abl kinase, where the structure of the complex between an inhibitor, Gleevec in this case, bound to an inactive state of the enzyme could help in the interpretation of the biochemical data.

Two characteristics of CK2 must be considered in the development of highly specific inhibitors: (a) the active site can utilize both ATP and GTP as co-substrates and this feature is quite unique among kinases that usually are specific for ATP; (b) staurosporine is a well-known, potent inhibitor of protein kinases, with a really broad spectrum of activity, but it is only marginally efficient on CK2 (Meggio et al. 1995). These two features indicate that the catalytic site of CK2 has some unique characteristics that can be exploited to design inhibitors with a high degree of specificity. The determination of the three-dimensional structure of CK2 in complex with different inhibitors is an essential step in the elucidation of the critical properties of the active site.

In recent years we have determined the crystal structure of several complexes between the α-catalytic subunit of CK2 from *Zea mays* and ATP site-directed inhibitors. In particular, we have studied four members of the anthraquinone-related compounds, one halogenated benzotriazole and an indoloquinazolinone derivative.

To date, the best-characterized classes of CK2 inhibitor are the following: (a) hydroxylated polycyclic aromatic compounds with anthraquinone/xanthenone or fluorenone or flavone scaffolds; (b) halogenated benzimidazoles or benzotriazoles; (c) indole derivatives of quinazolinone.

9 Common Features of Inhibitor-CK2 Complexes

The close structural similarities between the *Zea mays* and the human α-catalytic subunits strongly support the decision to work with the maize enzyme in structural inhibition studies: this enzyme has a higher tendency to produce good diffracting crystals, and this is the reason why it has been preferred to the human enzyme.

Like the majority of the kinase inhibitors, those crystallized in complex with maize CK2 also bind to the catalytic site of the enzyme in the position normally occupied by an ATP (or GTP) molecule that acts as phosphate donor (Fig. 3).

Since the crystal structure of the apo-form of CK2 is known (Battistutta et al. 2001), an evaluation of the effect of the different inhibitors on the enzyme structure is possible.

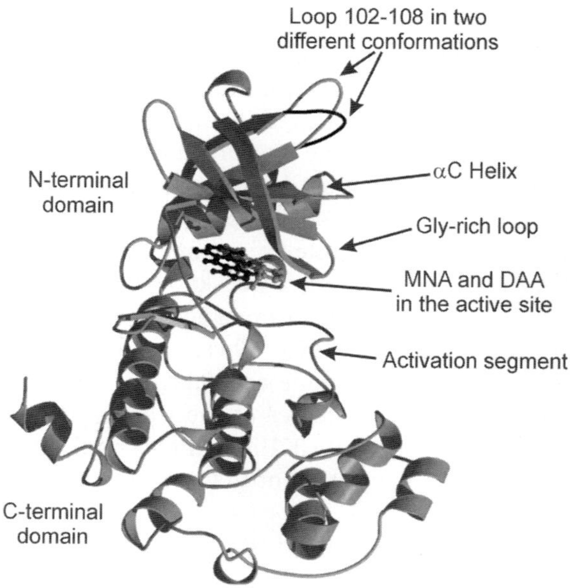

Fig. 3 Crystal structure of maize CK2 in complex with two inhibitors of the anthraquinone family. The positions of MNA and DAA in the active site are indicated. Note the different conformations of loop 102–108 (see text for discussion)

In general, the structure of the protein is poorly affected by the binding of a small molecule, either a co-substrate, such as ATP or GTP, or an inhibitor. The C-terminal lobe of the protein, conventionally considered starting with asparagine 118 and extending to the C-terminal end, is practically unaffected by the formation of the complex. The superposition of the different structures indicates a remarkable rigidity, with the exception of few residues facing the catalytic site, mainly Asn118, His160, and Met163. The N-terminal lobe shows a higher degree of flexibility than the C-terminal one, although the changes are in any case limited. The β-strands present in the N-terminal domain have the ability to "fine tune" their position to better accommodate ligands with different properties. Near the active site, in the glycine-rich loop and in the hinge region, some residues can be found with different conformations depending on the bound molecule. As reported in the following sections, the Gly-rich loop backbone has shown a significant flexibility, as indicated by the ability to move "up" or "down" depending on the ligand (Fig. 4). A functional relevance was recently attributed to this flexibility noted in the inhibitors/CK2 complexes. It has been suggested that in the holoenzyme the β-subunit can contribute to block and stabilize this region from behind the catalytic subunit (back-stabilization) and that this can destabilize a possible closed inactive conformation of the CK2 activation segment (Ermakova et al. 2003).

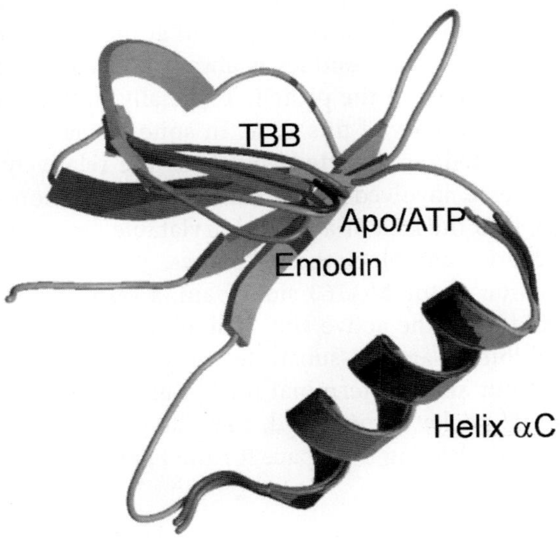

Fig. 4 Superposition of the Gly-rich zone and the αC helix of CK2 in the Apo form and in complex with emodin, tetrabromo-2-benzotriazolo (*TBB*), and ATP. The position of the αC-helix is very well conserved in all CK2 structures. The Gly-rich loop shows a higher degree of variation depending on the occupancy of the ATP-binding site

In many kinases the presence of an inhibitor in the active site alters the conformation of the flexible Gly-rich loop, often by means of an interaction with the aromatic residue preceding the third glycine (Huse and Kuriyan 2002). In CK2 a similar interaction has never been observed.

Comparing the crystal structures of several CK2 α-subunits from *Zea mays*, changes were noted in the external loop spanning residues 102–108, found in two different conformations (Fig. 3 and Table I; De Moliner et al. 2003). These changes have been attributed to crystallization and/or freezing condition rather than to ligand-binding effects, since they are reflected on small but significant variations in some parameters of the crystallographic unit cell. The recent independent determination of the crystallographic structures of the human α-subunit alone and of a mutant showed this region in the same conformation, defined as "closed," while in the holoenzyme the "open" conformation has been detected. Whether this variation is only a crystallographic artifact, as formerly suggested (De Moliner et al. 2003), or has a functional relevance, as subsequently proposed (Ermakova et al. 2003), remains an open question.

The position of the helix in the N-terminal domain, helix αC, is particularly well conserved in all the three-dimensional structures of CK2 known to date (Fig. 4). As reported above, the correct position of this helix is one of the most striking properties of active protein kinases. The maintenance of the position of helix αC is therefore well in accordance with the notion of the constitutive activity of CK2, as well as the overall rigidity of the enzyme.

The stretch of residues whose conformation is less characterized is that spanning from Leu70 to Lys76, just before and at the beginning of helix αC. The electron density of these residues is always worse defined compared to that of the remaining part of the protein, especially in the side chains, indicating an intrinsic flexibility of this zone. In spite of that, the orientation of helix αC is not affected, as reported above. As the relatively mobile 70–76 segment is considered involved in the substrate recognition, this flexibility is probably related to the lack of a phosphorylatable amino acid stretch that can eventually interact and block these residues.

The conformation of the Met163 side chain, a residue distinctive of CK2 located in the middle of the active site, is significantly affected by the presence of both inhibitors and co-substrate. In apo-CK2α, the side chain of Met163 stretches out and the terminal methyl group points into the cavity. When the catalytic pocket is occupied, the side chain is folded away from the center of the cleft, leaving free space for the ligand.

10 Anthraquinones Inhibitors

Anthraquinones are compounds able to interact with the nucleotide-binding sites of enzymes such as dehydrogenases, kinases, and ATPases, due to their structural similarities with adenine nucleotides such as ATP, adenosine diphosphate (ADP), and nicotinamide adenine dinucleotide (NAD). Anthraquinones and xanthones from natural sources have several potential therapeutic applications, for instance as antiviral, antimicrobial, or anti-cancer drugs (Ali et al. 2000). The extended planar structure of these compounds possibly makes them cytotoxic in that they are able to act as DNA intercalators. Even if that makes questionable the employment of this class of compounds in clinical practice, one might take advantage of them as chemical tools to elucidate the different cellular functions and regulations of CK2 for the optimization of highly specific and selective inhibitors.

Several anthraquinones and related xanthones have been tested with in vitro phosphorylation assays as potential inhibitors for CK2 (Sarno et al. 2002). Emodin (1,3,8-trihydroxy-6-methyl-antraquinone), previously reported as a tyrosine kinase inhibitor (Chan et al. 1993), was the first member of the anthraquinone family to be discovered that was also able to inhibit CK2 (Yim et al. 1999). The chemical formula and the inhibition potency (inhibitory constant, K_i) for emodin as well for other anthraquinones is reported in Fig. 5. Starting from this parent compound, a large number of anthraquinones and xanthone derivatives have been screened on CK2, allowing the identification of some interesting compounds with lower IC_{50} (or K_i) values. The most promsising ones have been submitted to crystallization trials, and for those that have generated good diffracting crystals (Fig. 5), the

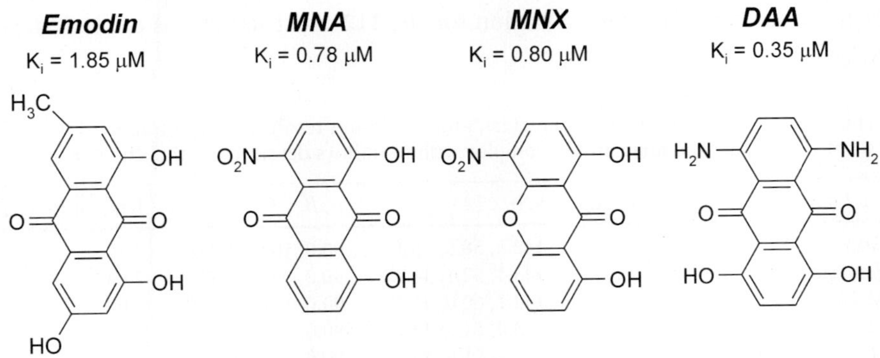

Fig. 5 Chemical formulae and inhibition potencies for the four anthraquinones crystallized in complex with CK2. *Emodin*, 1,3,8-trihydroxy-6-methyl-antraquinone; *MNA*, 1,8-dihydroxy-4-nitro-anthraquinone; *MNX*, 1,8-dihydroxy-4-nitro-xanthen-9-one; *DAA*, 1,4-diamino-5,8-dihydroxy-anthraquinone

three-dimensional structures have been determined. The inhibitory constant K_i for the four compounds crystallized is in the micromolar range, from 1.85 μM for emodin to 0.35 μM for DAA.

Emodin is the first anthraquinone derivative crystallized in complex with *Zea mays* CK2 as an ATP site-directed competitive inhibitor. This natural compound is extracted from the rhizomes of *Rheum palmatum* and is used as anti-inflammatory and anti-cancer drug, especially in the Asian continent (Yim et al. 1999). Emodin has an inhibitory constant (K_i) of 1.85 μM for CK2, while it is poorly effective on other Ser/Thr protein kinases. This compound is able to inhibit also some Tyr-kinases, although with a lower efficiency (Jayasuriya et al. 1992). For instance, the receptor Tyr-kinase Her-2 neu is inhibited with a K_i value of 21 μM (Zhang et al. 1998), an order of magnitude higher than that for CK2.

Crystals of the emodin/CK2 complex were obtained by the soaking method (Battistutta et al. 2000). As emodin is poorly soluble in aqueous media, crystals of the maize CK2 catalytic subunit in the apo-form have been soaked for several hours with a saturated solution of emodin, which results in red for the presence of the inhibitor. The formation of the complex was evident because, within a few hours, the red coloring concentrated in the crystals, whereas the surrounding solution changed to pale orange. These crystals are isomorphous with those of maize CK2 grown in the presence of co-substrates ATP and GTP and also with those of the other anthraquinones complexes obtained with co-crystallization procedures (see below); all belongs to the C2 space group, with cell parameters reported in Table 1.

The co-substrate-competitive inhibitory activity of emodin is due to its ability to bind to the active site of CK2. Although the binding of the inhibitor poorly influences the overall architecture of the protein that remains in a structurally (but obviously not functional) active state, some regions of the catalytic subunit undergo appreciable structural changes, especially in the N-terminal lobe. The rms deviation for the 112 α-carbon atoms of the N-ter-

Table 1 Space group, unit cell parameters, and maximum resolution of diffraction for crystals of CK2 in the Apo form and in complex with inhibitors described in this chapter

CK2 complexes	Space group	a, b, c (Å)	α, β, γ (°)	Resolution (Å)
Apo-CK2	C2	142.8, 58.5, 45.1[a]	90.0, 102.6, 90.0[a]	2.10
Emodin	C2	143.1, 52.1, 44.9[b]	90.0, 99.3, 90.0[b]	2.63
MNA	C2	142.1, 60.6, 45.0[a]	90.0, 102.8, 90.0[a]	2.00
MNX	C2	143.0, 51.7, 44.7[b]	90.0, 99.3, 90.0[b]	1.79
DAA	C2	143.1, 51.8, 44.7[b]	90.0, 99.7, 90.0[b]	1.70
TBB	P1	48.3, 55.9, 60.3	89.8, 102.5, 99.3	2.19
IQA	C2	141.5, 60.3, 44.4[a]	90.0, 102.6, 90.0[a]	1.68

[a,b] Different cell parameters corresponding to the two conformations of loop 102–108 (see text for discussion).

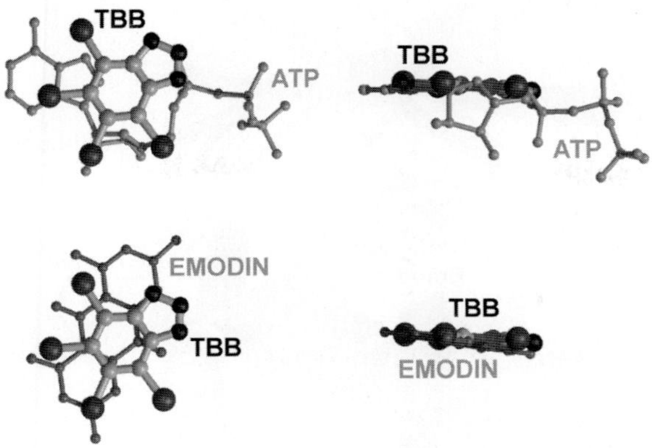

Fig. 6 Superposition of TBB and ATP (*upper panel*) and emodin (*lower panel*) in the active site of CK2. A "top" view" on the *left* and a "side" view (90° rotation) on the *right* are shown. TBB is chosen as reference

minal lobe, from positions 7 to 118, is 1.29 Å, while the rms deviation drops to 0.40 Å for the 215 α-carbon atoms of the C-terminal domains, from position 119 to 333.

The two most variable regions are the Gly-rich loop from residue 58 to 63 and the exposed loop from residue 102 to 108. The electron density of this second long loop is poorly defined, indicating a remarkable flexibility of this zone. For other anthraquinone complexes, crystals of better diffracting quality and higher resolution have been obtained with co-crystallization methods. In these cases, the electron density of the loop 102–108 is better defined, allowing the detection of the two possible conformations of this loop, the "open" and the "closed" ones (Fig. 3).

The emodin inhibitor is inserted into the active site cavity deeper than the ATP or GTP molecules, with only two out of three rings roughly superimposable to the nucleotide base (Fig. 6). As a result, the inhibitor occupies a hydrophobic zone of the CK2 active site that shows a certain degree of variability among protein kinases (Scapin 2002), and this can be responsible for the limited selectivity of this inhibitor.

Among the anthraquinone derivatives studied so far, emodin causes the larger variations in the conformation of the residues belonging to the active site. Around the binding site, significant differences in the position of amino acid Asn118, of the side chain of His160, and of the triplet Arg47-Gly48-Lys49 have been detected (Fig. 7). In particular, the backbone segment from Arg47 to Lys49, which is part of the Gly-rich loop, is found shifted toward the interior of the active site, in a position that entraps emodin inside. Emodin is kept in the active site between the two lobes of the protein mainly by hydrophobic contacts involving residues Val45, Val53, Ile66, Leu85, Val95, Leu111, Phe113, Val116, Met163, and Ile174. The release of the inhibitor

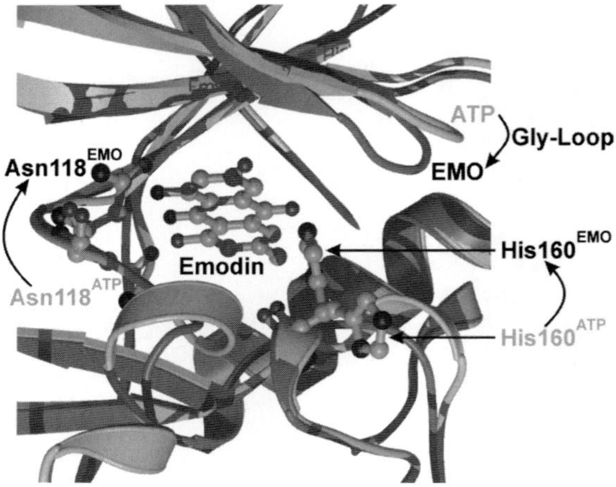

Fig. 7 Movements caused by emodin (*EMO*) binding. The different positions of Asn118, Gly-rich loop, and His160 of CK2 in complex with ATP (*gray labels*) and with emodin (*black labels*) are illustrated. A portion of the αC-helix can be distinguished behind His160

from the cavity is hampered both by the 46–50 segment and by residues His160 and Asn118 (Fig. 7), whose α-carbon moves about 1.2 Å from its original position. The orientation of the side chain of Asn118 contributes to the enclosure of the cavity, as well as the imidazole ring of His160, which is able to form a new H-bond with the carbonyl oxygen of Arg47.

The presence of hydroxyls at positions 6 and 8 of emodin seems relevant for an optimal inhibitory potential (Jayasuriya et al. 1992). In our structure, no clear polar interactions have been found between the inhibitor and the protein. The hydroxyl group in position 6 is 3.40 Å away from the backbone carbonyl of Val45, 3.70 Å from the amide nitrogen of Arg47, and 3.98 Å from the imidazole nitrogen of His160, while that in position 8 is 3.99 Å away from the side chain carbonyl of Asn118. These interactions are too loose to be considered hydrogen bond-like, but the relatively low resolution of 2.63 Å of the model does not completely rule out the possibility of polar interactions between the inhibitor and the protein. In this respect, it can be relevant to notice that emodin does not completely fill in the cavity, whose actual volume is slightly larger than that of the inhibitor. The quality of the electron density of emodin is to some extent poorer than that of the surrounding residues, suggesting that emodin could maintain some degree of freedom once encapsulated into the pocket. The higher mean value of the emodin thermal B factor of 58 $Å^2$ compared to that of the backbone atoms of the enzyme of 50 $Å^2$ is consistent with these observations. On the other hand, another possible or complementary explanation of the effect of the hydroxyl functions is that they increase the solubility of emodin in an aqueous environment.

Emodin shows a slightly higher inhibition constant against CK1 than against CK2. This observation can be explained with the conservation of the main requirements for the inhibitor binding in the two kinases. On the other hand, cAMP-dependent protein kinase (cAPK) is inhibited by emodin with a constant two orders of magnitude higher, and this corresponds to a higher variation in the active sites characteristics. Residues Val66, Ile174, and Phe113 in CK2 are replaced by Ala70, Thr183, and Met120 in cAPK, with the latter two closer together (only 3.80 Å apart). A comparison of the molecular models of CK2 and cAPK indicates that emodin cannot interact in the same way with the two proteins, unless a large rearrangement of residues Thr183 and Met12 of cAPK takes place.

Crystals of CK2 complexes with other anthraquinones, namely MNA (a mono-nitro derivative, 1,8-dihydroxy-4-nitro-anthraquinone), MNX (a mono-nitro xanthenone, 1,8-dihydroxy-4-nitro-xanthen-9-one), and DAA, (a di-amino derivative, 1,4-diamino-5,8-dihydroxy-anthraquinone), have been obtained by co-crystallization techniques. This approach has allowed for the achievement of better resolutions (up to 1.70 Å) with respect to soaking methods used in the case of emodin and TBB (Table 1). The poor solubility in water of the inhibitors has been overcome by dissolving them at high concentration in dimethylsulfoxide (DMSO) and then incubating the protein with the solution obtained for a final maximum concentration of the organic solvent equal to 5%.

Among these three inhibitors, MNX is the one that causes the greatest variation in the N-terminal domain of the enzyme, at the level of the backbone from residues 72 to 75 and of the Gly-rich loop (residues 45–51). The latter "collapses" into the co-substrate binding cavity, in a manner similar to that displayed by the emodin complex. In the case of MNX, this displacement is not coupled with a rotation of the His160 and Asn118 side chains.

MNA and MNX, whose positions in the active site are fully superimposable (Fig. 8), orient the nitro group toward the hinge region, with the result that the hydroxyl groups can make contacts with Lys68 (Fig. 9). Besides hydrophobic and van der Waals interactions, in comparison with emodin and TBB (see next paragraph), MNX and MNA are able to form further polar interactions with the active site of the enzyme. These additional interactions contribute both to increase the affinity for the enzyme, as indicated by the lower K_i values, and to orient the molecules in a different way inside the active site.

In the MNA/CK2 complex, the nitro group of MNA is found lying in a plane roughly perpendicular to that of the aromatic rings (Fig. 8), as expected for the steric hindrance of the adjacent carbonyl group (*ortho* effect). In the crystal, MNA is present in the active site in a double conformation, with the nitro group oriented toward the external portion of the ATP-binding cavity in the higher occupancy conformation (67%). MNA forms four hydrogen bonds: the two hydroxyl groups and the carbonyl oxygen located on the

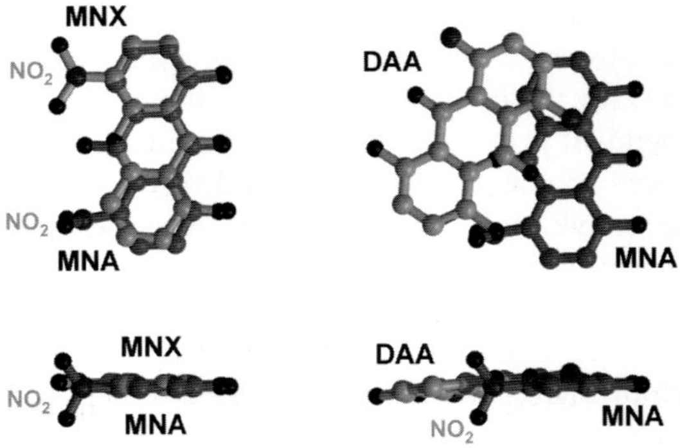

Fig. 8 Superposition of the three anthraquinones MNA (taken as reference), MNX, and DAA in the active site of CK2. Note that the nitro group of MNA is not co-planar with the aromatic rings as in the case of MNX

same side of the inhibitor interact with side chains of Asp175, Lys68, and a solvent molecule (Fig. 9). Similarly to the cases of the MNX/CK2 and DAA/CK2 complexes, this solvent molecule interacts also with Glu81 and Trp176.

In MNX, the central carbonyl function is absent and, therefore, in the crystal structure the nitro group is co-planar with the aromatic plane

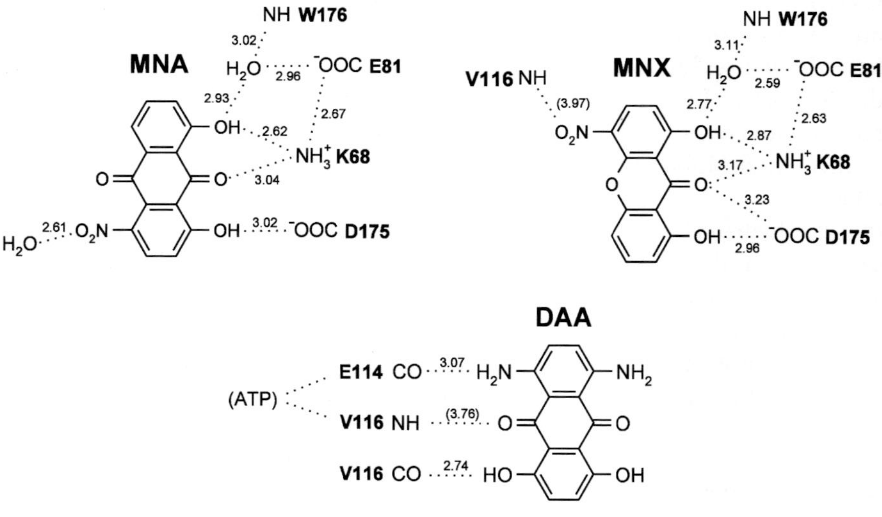

Fig. 9 Polar interactions between CK2 and anthraquinone inhibitors. Hydrogen bonds and salt bridges are indicated by *dotted lines*; distances are reported in Ångstroms. For DAA, the distance to the NH of Val116 is reported for comparison with ATP binding (ATP is hydrogen bound to backbone CO of Glu114 and backbone NH of Val116 in the hinge region)

(Fig. 8). MNX interacts with the protein in a way similar to MNA, but it enters the active site in one single orientation, with the nitro group in the deeper position inside the cavity.

The importance of the nitro function in MNA and MNX is outlined by the observation that, if missing as in 1,8-dihydroxy-anthraquinone and 1,8-dihydroxy-xanthen-9-one, the inhibitory constants (K_i) rise to values higher than 40 μM. However, in our models there are no direct chemical interactions between the nitro groups and the protein. This leads to the hypothesis that the effect of the NO_2 group is related to the electron-withdrawing property of this substituent, which is able to increase the dissociation constant of the phenolic hydroxyl group in the *para* position. As a result, this becomes more acidic, as confirmed both by theoretical analyses and experimental data. The resulting partially negatively charged oxygen can provide a better anchor for Lys68, with which it is interacting at distances typical for hydrogen bonds formation.

The third inhibitor of the series, DAA, that lacks the nitro group, binds to the active site in a different way if compared to MNA and MNX. DAA prefers a position inside the cleft near the hinge region, where it can interact with backbone carbonyls of Glu114 and Val116 via two hydrogen bonds (Fig. 9). This particular mode of interaction confers to DAA one of the highest inhibition potency (K_i value of 0.35 μM) among the anthraquinones studied so far.

Taken together, the four crystal structures of CK2 in complex with anthraquinone derivatives revealed three different modes of binding to the ATP-binding site. In spite of their common scaffold, anthraquinones can anchor to the hinge region, as DAA does in a way similar to the adenine moiety of ATP, or they can interact with Lys68 and Asp175, although with different orientations (MNA and MNX), or, finally, they can sit deeply inside the cavity with no strong polar interactions with the protein (emodin).

11 Tetrabromo-2-Benzotriazole

4,5,6,7-tetrabromo-benzotriazole (TBB or tetrabromo-2-azabenzimidazole) is a CK2 inhibitor developed starting from the 5,6-dichloro-1-(β-d-ribofuranosyl)benzimidazole (DRB) parent molecule. DRB was found inhibiting CK2 with a relatively high inhibitory constant, (K_i=24 μM) and a rather low specificity (Zandomeni et al. 1986). After several modifications (Fig. 10), namely the replacement of two chlorine atoms with four bromine ones, the depletion of the sugar moiety, and the substitution of the imidazole ring with a triazole, the final compound not only shows a lower K_i (0.2–0.6 μM), but also a higher selectivity for CK2 (Szyszka et al. 1995; Shugar 1999). At variance with the precursor, TBB is also able to discriminate between CK1

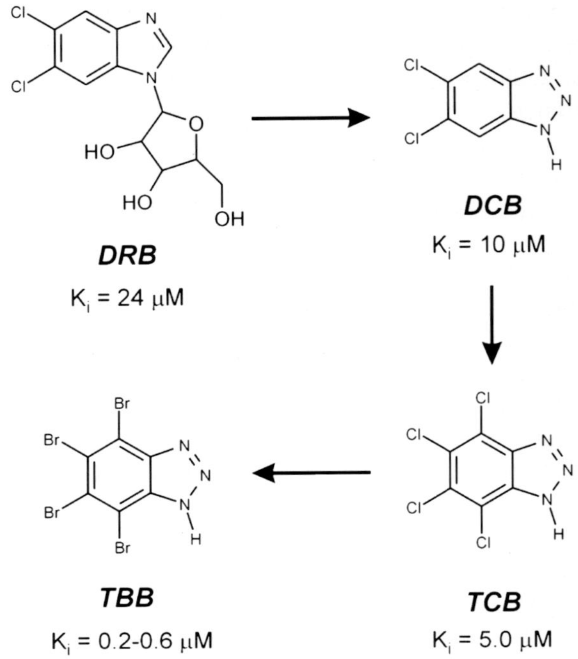

Fig. 10 Scheme of the chemical modifications that have led to the development of TBB starting from DRB (see text for details). The K_i for the four compounds is reported

and CK2 (Sarno et al. 2001) and is one of the most selective CK2 inhibitor now known.

Crystals of the complex CK2/TBB belong to the P1 space group (Battistutta et al. 2001), while all crystals of the catalytic subunit of CK2 from *Zea mays*, either in the apo form or in complex with co-substrates or inhibitors, belong to space group C2 (Table 1). The reason for this variation in the crystal parameters is not fully understood.

As in the case of the anthraquinones, the N-terminus domain shows a more noticeable variation than the structurally more conserved C-terminus one, with the remarkable exception of helix αC. Again, regions from residue 102 to 108 and from 70 to 74, immediately upward the αC helix, show a less defined electron density and a higher flexibility, as indicated by the higher B-factor values. TBB binds to the active site essentially by means of hydrophobic interactions involving residues Val45, Val53, Ile66, Val95, Phe113, Val116, Met163, and Ile174. Due to the bulkiness of the four bromine atoms, TBB fills almost perfectly the active site cleft (Fig. 11) and this appears to be the main reason for the potency and selectivity of the inhibitor. This hypothesis is corroborated by the lower activity of two TBB analogs, where bromine atoms are substituted by the less bulky chlorines. The inhibitory constants of tetrachlorobenzotriazole (TCB) and dichlorobenzotriazole

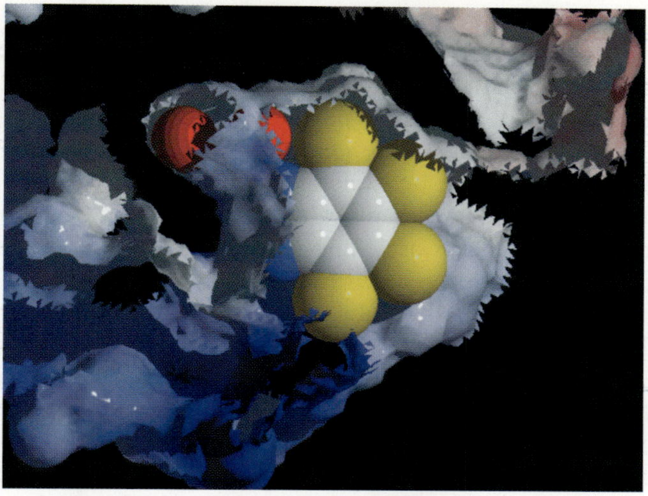

Fig. 11 Full spheres (CPK) model of TBB in the active site of CK2. A portion of the surface of the ATP-binding site is shown colored according to the electrostatic potential (positive charges in *blue*, negative charges in *red*). TBB atoms colors: carbon in *white*, nitrogen in *blue*, bromines in *yellow*. The two water molecules that connect TBB to Trp176 and Glu81 are represented as *red spheres*

(DCB) are 5 and 10 μM respectively (Fig. 10), one order of magnitude higher than that of TBB (Shugar 1999).

Nitrogen N1 of TBB is linked to Oϵ2 of Glu81 via two water molecules that make a bridge between the two atoms (Figs. 11 and 12). This is the only po-

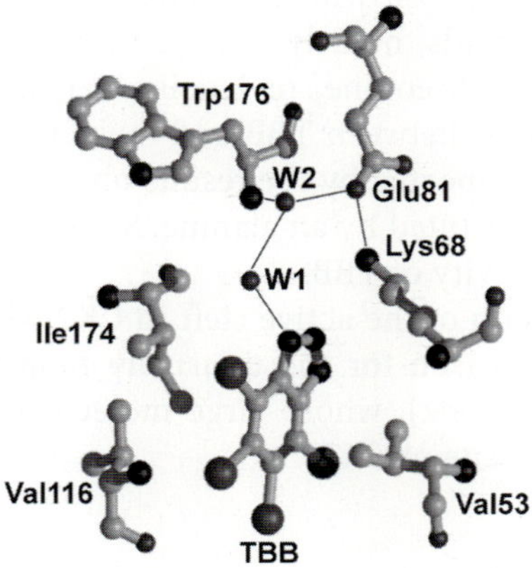

Fig. 12 Ball-and-stick models of TBB and some of the interacting residues. Polar interactions are indicated by *continuous lines*. Water molecules (W1 and W2) are represented as *isolated spheres*. Carbons in *gray*, nitrogens, oxygens, and bromines (*larger spheres*) in *black*. Residues 53, 116, 174 are part of the hydrophobic surface that surrounds TBB

lar interaction present in the complex. The structural importance of one of these two water molecules (W2 in Fig. 12) is testified by its presence in almost all the CK2 crystal structures now determined. This solvent molecule is tightly bound to the deeper portion of the active site where polar side chains are present, for instance the well-conserved Lys68 and Glu81. As seen for several inhibitors, it can be exploited by ligands as hydrogen bond anchoring sites. Two other important water molecules have been identified in the ATP and GTP complexes of CK2 (Niefind et al. 1999) as responsible for the unique "dual-co-substrate specificity" of CK2. All these water molecules seem to play a specific role in modulating the ligand/protein interaction inside the ATP-binding site.

In the CK2/TBB complex, histidine-160 side chain adopts the same orientation as in the presence of emodin. In the presence of TBB, however, the Gly-rich loop is shifted away from His160, probably owing to the large size of the bromines, with the consequence that the H-bond between the His160 side chain and Arg47 backbone cannot take place. This highlights once more the flexibility of the glycine loop, capable to adjust itself to the type of ligand bound in the cavity. In fact, the Gly-rich loop has a very similar conformation in the apo-CK2 and when the enzyme is bound to ATP or GTP, whereas in the presence of emodin and TBB it moves toward or away from the N-terminal lobe, respectively (Fig. 4).

In the attempt to rationalize the selectivity of TBB toward CK2 on a wide panel of different kinases (Sarno et al. 2001), the active sites of the kinases whose structure is known have been compared to that of CK2. From this analysis it emerges that CK2 bears an ATP-binding site invariably smaller in size, due to some characteristic bulky side chains which in CK2 reduce the space available to cofactors or inhibitors. These typical residues are Ile(Val)66, Met163, and Ile174, which in most protein kinases are replaced with less bulky amino acids, namely alanine versus Ile66, leucine or valine versus Met163, alanine, threonine, or leucine versus Ile174. This suggests that a perfect fit in shape between TBB and the active site is crucial for the selectivity and is also supported by the results obtained with a mutant where Ile(Val)66 has been substituted by an alanine. Such a mutant is less susceptible to the inhibitory activity of TBB.

The smaller dimension of the active cleft in CK2 with respect to other kinases can also be the reason for the unusually modest sensitivity to staurosporine (Sarno et al. 2002), whose large molecular size may hamper the entrance into the active site of CK2.

12 Indoloquinazolinones

To identify new inhibitors, a virtual screening analysis among the in-house collection of chemical compounds has recently been performed by researchers of Novartis Pharma against a human CK2 three-dimensional model (Vangrevelinghe et al. 2003). This analysis has led to the discovery of a new class of potent and selective inhibitors of CK2, the indoloquinazolinones. The most promising compound, IQA [(5-oxo-5,6-dihydro-indolo(1,2-a)quinazolin-7-yl)acetic acid], with a K_i of 0.17 μM, has been co-crystallized in complex with CK2 (Table 1) and the final three-dimensional structure at 1.68 Å resolution has been recently reported (Sarno et al. 2003).

IQA lays inside the catalytic pocket of CK2 on the same plane occupied by the ATP purine moiety. The hydrophobic side of IQA faces the hinge region of the protein, while the polar side is oriented toward Lys68. IQA is found in the ATP-binding site in two different orientations, differing for a rotation of the acetate function (Fig. 13). The two alternative conformations have been refined with final occupancies of 50%. In the first conformation, the carboxylic function makes an internal hydrogen bond with the lactam nitrogen, closing a six-member ring, and interacts with the hydroxyl oxygen of Ser51. This conformation is largely favored in solution (Fig. 14), as confirmed by nuclear magnetic resonance (NMR) spectroscopy analysis. Therefore, it has to be assumed that the second conformation is stabilized when bound to the CK2 active site, where it is found as abundant as the first one. In fact, in the second conformation the carboxylate group is involved in

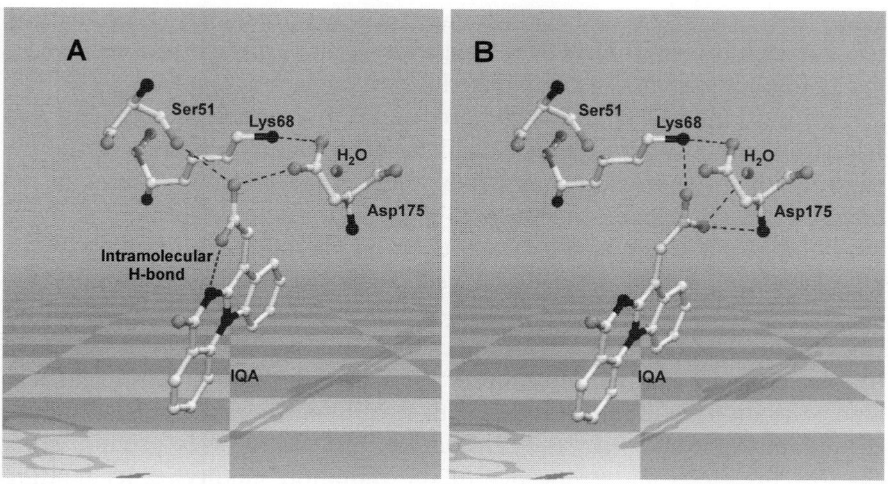

Fig. 13A, B Polar interactions of IQA with Ser51, Lys68, and Asp175 of CK2. IQA binds to CK2 in two conformations, shown in **A** and **B**

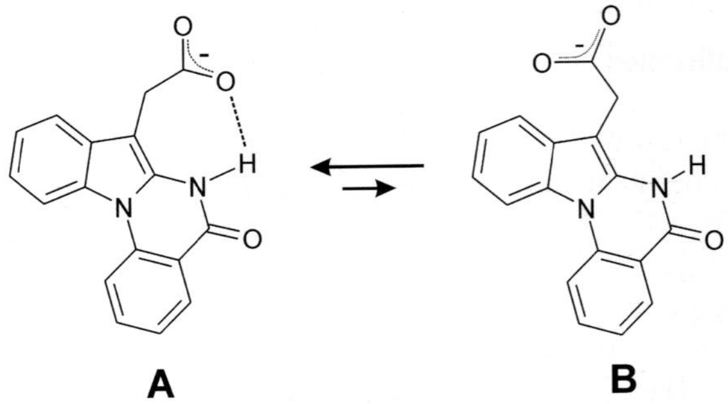

Fig. 14A, B Equilibrium between the two conformations of IQA present in solution. As evidenced by nuclear magnetic resonance (NMR) analysis, the species with the internal hydrogen bond is predominant in solution (species **A** on the *left*)

three hydrogen bonds, one with the amine function of Lys68, one with the backbone nitrogen of Asp175, and one with a water molecule in turn connected to the backbone amide of Trp176 (Fig. 13). This water molecule is the same found in all CK2 structures solved to date, with the exception of the emodin complex, as already mentioned.

For both conformations, the major contribution to the binding comes from the hydrophobic interaction with non-polar residues in the binding site, i.e., Val45, Val53, Ile66, Lys68, Val95, Phe113, Val116, Met163, and Ile174. In this respect, it is remarkable that the total buried surface upon inhibitor binding is quite large, about 730 $Å^2$. The importance of the hydrophobic interactions in the binding of IQA is supported by the considerable decrease of the inhibitory efficiency observed in the cases of Val66Ala and Ile174Ala mutants. In fact, mutation of Ser51 with a glycine does not significantly affect the K_i value. This is in agreement with the observation that the two different orientations of IQA bind with similar affinity, since they share the hydrophobic contacts, while they differ in the interaction with Ser51.

The best inhibitor of CK2 discovered so far, IQA, albeit more potent and selective than those previously available, is not yet totally specific for the enzyme. With the increasing number of three-dimensional structures of inhibitors/CK2 complexes, it should be possible to improve the selectivity of inhibitors using a structure-based drug design method. Anyhow, this task is not straightforward, since we have seen from the previous examples that compounds extremely similar to one another, like MNA, MNX, DAA, and emodin, bind to the active site of the enzyme in a significantly different way. In practice, a limited modification of the structure of the inhibitor, for example the addition of a substituent with the aim of increasing the number of H-bond interactions (like the addition of an OH or NH_2 group), often changes the electronic properties of the inhibitor, modifying its binding mode. In the case of CK2 inhibitors, this is probably worsened by the relatively limited complexity of the small molecules used. A more extended surface of interaction between the inhibitor and the enzyme could help not only to decrease the K_i, but also to stabilize its binding mode.

Another point about computer-aided drug design has to be stressed. In the in silico procedure for the identification and characterization of the indoloquinazolinone derivatives, such as CK2 inhibitors, a model of IQA bound to the enzyme has been proposed (Vangrevelinghe et al. 2003). In this model, the acetate group of IQA faces the hinge region and interacts with arginine-43, with a orientation opposite to that found in the experimental crystal structure. In this case, it comes out that while virtual screening protocols could usefully select some interesting compounds among a large database, the docking procedures have been unable to correctly position the inhibitor in the enzyme active site. For the correct detailed description of the interactions between IQA and CK2, the determination of the crystal structure of the complex was an unavoidable step.

13
Concluding Remarks

In this chapter we have described the binding modes of some CK2 inhibitors that target the ATP-binding site. These inhibitors belong to different chemical families and have inhibitory constants in the low micromolar range. Two of them, namely TBB and IQA, display a significant selectivity among panels of tens of different kinases, and can be considered an encouraging starting point for the development of compounds of potential pharmacological interest.

For all the inhibitors here described, the main energetic contribution to the binding is attributed to hydrophobic interaction with the apolar surface region of the CK2 binding cleft. In this respect, the shape and the reduced dimension of the CK2 active site in comparison with other kinases are essential in explaining the selectivity of these inhibitors as well as the anomalous low potency of staurosporine. In particular, isoleucine/valine-66 and isoleucine-174, residues unique to CK2, play an important role as demonstrated by mutagenesis studies. The aromatic nature of the inhibitors can be considered a key characteristic of these compounds, providing the main energetic contribution to the binding.

In general, the ATP-binding sites of kinases present both polar and hydrophobic portions. While the characteristics of the polar moiety are quite conserved among the family, as, for instance, some key residues in the hinge regions, in the phosphate anchor region, or other residues like lysine-68, glutamate-81, and aspartate-175 (CK2 numbering), the hydrophobic ones have a higher degree of variability in the amino acid composition. Consequently, the selectivity is ensured by targeting the hydrophobic portion of the binding site while the presence of polar interactions (hydrogen bonds, salt bridges) enhances the potency of the inhibitor. The inhibitors here described can be considered more selective than potent, and this is in agreement with the above considerations in that they bind to the enzyme mainly through hydrophobic interactions. As noticed for the four anthraquinones, the presence of polar interactions is essential to increase the binding potency; in this respect, the interactions with the hinge region seem more effective (see the case of DAA in comparison with emodin). To produce inhibitors in the nanomolar range, as would be desirable, our aim is now concentrated in the increase of the number and strength of the polar interactions between the inhibitors and the enzyme, without depleting the hydrophobic interactions. Other important points are the increase of the solubility of these compounds in water and the analysis of their potential pharmacological properties.

The estimate of the selectivity of a kinase inhibitor is always a difficult task; in fact, while the number of kinases has been estimated around 500 from the human genome, the enzymes really available for inhibition assays are only a fraction of that (around some tens). The development of enzyme mutants resistant to the inhibitory activity of a specific compound but with a catalytic activity similar to the wild-type protein [i.e., mutants Ile66Ala and Ile174Ala for CK2 (Sarno et al. 2002)] can be very useful in the analysis of its selectivity. In fact, the recovery of the original kinase activity by means of such mutants in the presence of the specific inhibitor in in vivo assays can be considered a validation of the involvement of just that kinase in the process under study.

References

Ahmed K, Gerber DA, Cochet C (2002) Joining the cell survival squad: an emerging role for protein kinase CK2. Trends Cell Biol 12:226–230

Ali AM, Ismail NH, Mackeen MM, Yazan LS, Mohamed SM, Ho ASH, Lajis NH (2000) Antiviral, cytotoxic and antimicrobial activities of anthraquinones isolated from the roots of Morinda elliptica. Pharm Biol 38:298–301

Battistutta R, Sarno S, De Moliner E, Papinutto E, Zanotti G, Pinna LA (2000) The replacement of ATP by the competitive inhibitor emodin induces conformational modifications in the catalytic site of protein kinase CK2. J Biol Chem 275:29618–29622

Battistutta R, De Moliner E, Sarno S, Zanotti G, Pinna LA (2001) Structural features underlying selective inhibition of protein kinase CK2 by ATP site-directed tetrabromo-2-benzotriazole. Protein Sci 10:2200–2206

Buchou T, Vernet M, Blond O, Jensen HH, Pointu H, Olsen BB, Cochet C, Issinger OG, Boldyreff B (2003) Disruption of the regulatory beta subunit of protein kinase CK2 in mice leads to a cell-autonomous defect and early embryonic lethality. Mol Cell Biol 23:908–915

Burnett G, Kennedy EP (1954) The enzymatic phosphorylation of proteins. J Biol Chem 211:969–980

Chan TC, Chang CJ, Koonchanok NM, Geahlen RL (1993) Selective inhibition of the growth of ras-transformed human bronchial epithelial cells by emodin, a protein-tyrosine kinase inhibitor. Biochem Biophys Res Commun 193:1152–1158

Chantalat L, Leroy D, Filhol O, Nueda A, Benitez MJ, Chambaz EM, Cochet C, Dideberg O (1999) Crystal structure of the human protein kinase CK2 regulatory subunit reveals its zinc finger-mediated dimerization. EMBO J 18:2930–2940

Chardot T, Shen H, Meunier JC (1995) Dual specificity of casein kinase II from the yeast Yarrowia lipolytica. C R Acad Sci III 318:937–942

Cohen P (2002) Protein kinases: the major drug targets of the twenty-first century? Nat Rev Drug Discov 1:309–315

Davis ST, Benson BG, Bramson HN, Chapman DE, Dickerson SH, Dold KM, Eberwein DJ, Edelstein M, Frye SV, Gampe Jr RT, Griffin RJ, Harris PA, Hassell AM, Holmes WD, Hunter RN, Knick VB, Lackey K, Lovejoy B, Luzzio MJ, Murray D, Parker P, Rocque WJ, Shewchuk L, Veal JM, Walker DH, Kuyper LF (2001) Prevention of chemotherapy-induced alopecia in rats by CDK inhibitors. Science 291:134–137

De Moliner E, Moro S, Sarno S, Zagotto G, Zanotti G, Pinna LA, Battistutta R (2003) Inhibition of protein kinase CK2 by anthraquinone-related compounds. A structural insight. J Biol Chem 278:1831–1836

Donella-Deana A, Cesaro L, Sarno S, Brunati AM, Ruzzene M, Pinna LA (2001) Autocatalytic tyrosine-phosphorylation of protein kinase CK2 alpha and alpha' subunits: implication of Tyr182. Biochem J 357:563–567

Engh RA, Bossemeyer D (2002) Structural aspects of protein kinase control-role of conformational flexibility. Pharmacol Ther 93:99–111

Ermakova I, Boldyreff B, Issinger OG, Niefind K (2003) Crystal structure of a C-terminal deletion mutant of human protein kinase CK2 catalytic subunit. J Mol Biol 330:925–934

Faust M, Montenarh M (2000) Subcellular localization of protein kinase CK2. A key to its function? Cell Tissue Res 301:329–340

Fraser AG, Kamath RS, Zipperlen P, Martinez-Campos M, Sohrmann M, Ahringer J (2000) Functional genomic analysis of *C. elegans* chromosome I by systematic RNA interference. Nature 408:325–330

Fredenhagen A, Mett H, Meyer T, Buchdunger E, Regenass U, Roggo BE, Petersen F (1995) Protein tyrosine kinase and protein kinase C inhibition by fungal anthraquinones related to emodin. J Antibiot Tokyo 48:1355–1358

Garcia-Echeverria C, Traxler P, Evans DB (2000) ATP site-directed competitive and irreversible inhibitors of protein kinases. Med Res Rev 20:28–57

Goel S, Mani S, Perez Soler R (2002) Tyrosine kinase inhibitors: a clinical perspective. Curr Oncol Rep 4:9–19

Graham KC, Litchfield DW (2000) The regulatory beta subunit of protein kinase CK2 mediates formation of tetrameric CK2 complexes. J Biol Chem 275:5003–5010

Gray NS, Wodicka L, Thunnissen AM, Norman TC, Kwon S, Espinoza FH, Morgan DO, Barnes G, LeClerc S, Meijer L, Kim SH, Lockhart DJ, Schultz PG (1998) Exploiting chemical libraries, structure, and genomics in the search for kinase inhibitors. Science 281:533–538

Guerra B, Issinger OG (1999) Protein kinase CK2 and its role in cellular proliferation, development and pathology. Electrophoresis 20:391–408

Hanks SK, Hunter T (1995) Protein kinases 6. The eukaryotic protein kinase superfamily: kinase (catalytic) domain structure and classification. FASEB J 9:576–596

Hardcastle IR, Golding BT, Griffin RJ (2002) Designing inhibitors of cyclin-dependent kinases. Annu Rev Pharmacol Toxicol 42:325–348

Huse M, Kuriyan J (2002) The conformational plasticity of protein kinases. Cell 109:275–282

Jayasuriya H, Koonchanok NM, Geahlen RL, McLaughlin JL, Chang CJ (1992) Emodin, a protein tyrosine kinase inhibitor from Polygonum cuspidatum. J Nat Prod 55:696–698

Jeffrey PD, Russo AA, Polyak K, Gibbs E, Hurwitz J, Massague J, Pavletich NP (1995) Mechanism of CDK activation revealed by the structure of a cyclinA-CDK2 complex. Nature 376:313–320

Johnson LN, Noble ME, Owen DJ (1996) Active and inactive protein kinases: structural basis for regulation. Cell 85:149–158

Litchfield DW (2003) Protein kinase CK2: structure, regulation and role in cellular decisions of life and death. Biochem J 369:1–15

Manning G, Plowman GD, Hunter T, Sudarsanam S (2002a) Evolution of protein kinase signaling from yeast to man. Trends Biochem Sci 27:514–520

Manning G, Whyte DB, Martinez R, Hunter T, Sudarsanam S (2002b) The protein kinase complement of the human genome. Science 298:1912–1934

Marin O, Meggio F, Sarno S, Cesaro L, Pagano MA, Pinna LA (1999) Tyrosine versus serine/threonine phosphorylation by protein kinase casein kinase-2. A study with peptide substrates derived from immunophilin Fpr3. J Biol Chem 274:29260–29265

Meggio F, Marin O, Pinna LA (1994) Substrate specificity of protein kinase CK2. Cell Mol Biol Res 40:401–409

Meggio F, Donella Deana A, Ruzzene M, Brunati AM, Cesaro L, Guerra B, Meyer T, Mett H, Fabbro D, Furet P, Dobrowolska G, Pinna LA (1995) Different susceptibility of protein kinases to staurosporine inhibition. Kinetic studies and molecular bases for the resistance of protein kinase CK2. Eur J Biochem 234:317–322

Meggio F, Pinna LA (2003) One-thousand-and-one substrates of protein kinase CK2? FASEB J 17:349–368

Niefind K, Guerra B, Pinna LA, Issinger OG, Schomburg D (1998) Crystal structure of the catalytic subunit of protein kinase CK2 from *Zea mays* at 2.1 Å resolution. EMBO J 17:2451–2462

Niefind K, Putter M, Guerra B, Issinger OG, Schomburg D (1999) GTP plus water mimic ATP in the active site of protein kinase CK2. Nat Struct Biol 6:1100–1103

Niefind K, Guerra B, Ermakowa I, Issinger OG (2001) Crystal structure of human protein kinase CK2: insights into basic properties of the CK2 holoenzyme. EMBO J 20:5320–5331

Padmanabha R, Chen Wu JL, Hanna DE, Glover CV (1990) Isolation, sequencing, and disruption of the yeast CKA2 gene: casein kinase II is essential for viability in Saccharomyces cerevisiae. Mol Cell Biol 10:4089–4099

Parang K, Cole PA (2002) Designing bisubstrate analog inhibitors for protein kinases. Pharmacol Ther 93:145–157

Parang K, Till JH, Ablooglu AJ, Kohanski RA, Hubbard SR, Cole PA (2001) Mechanism-based design of a protein kinase inhibitor. Nat Struct Biol 8:37–41

Pechkova E, Zanotti G, Nicolini C (2003) Three-dimensional atomic structure of a catalytic subunit mutant of human protein kinase CK2. Acta Cryst D 59:2133–2139

Pinna LA (2002) Protein kinase CK2: a challenge to canons. J Cell Sci 115:3873–3878

Pinna LA, Meggio F (1997) Protein kinase CK2 ("casein kinase-2") and its implication in cell division and proliferation. Prog Cell Cycle Res 3:77–97

Sarno S, Vaglio P, Meggio F, Issinger OG, Pinna LA (1996) Protein kinase CK2 mutants defective in substrate recognition. Purification and kinetic analysis. J Biol Chem 271:10595–10601

Sarno S, Moro S, Meggio F, Zagotto G, Dal Ben D, Ghisellini P, Battistutta R, Zanotti G, Pinna LA (2002) Toward the rational design of protein kinase casein kinase-2 inhibitors. Pharmacol Ther 93:159–168

Sarno S, De Moliner E, Ruzzene M, Pagano MA, Battistutta R, Bain J, Fabbro D, Schoepfer J, Elliott M, Furet P, Meggio F, Zanotti G, Pinna LA (2003) Biochemical and 3D-structural data on the specific inhibition of protein kinase CK2 by (5-oxo-5,6-dihydro-indolo(1,2-a)quinazolin-7-yl)acetic acid (IQA). Biochem J 374:639–646

Sarno S, Reddy H, Meggio F, Ruzzene M, Davies SP, Donella Deana A, Shugar D, Pinna LA (2001) Selectivity of 4,5,6,7-tetrabromobenzotriazole, an ATP site-directed inhibitor of protein kinase CK2 ('casein kinase-2'). FEBS Lett 496:44–48

Scapin G (2002) Structural biology in drug design: selective protein kinase inhibitors. Drug Discov Today 7:601–611

Seldin DC, Leder P (1995) Casein kinase II alpha transgene-induced murine lymphoma: relation to theileriosis in cattle [see comments]. Science 267:894–897

Shugar D (1999) Viral and host-cell protein kinases: enticing antiviral targets and relevance of nucleoside, and viral thymidine, kinases. Pharmacol Ther 82:315–335

Stahura FL, Xue L, Godden JW, Bajorath J (1999) Molecular scaffold-based design and comparison of combinatorial libraries focused on the ATP-binding site of protein kinases. J Mol Graph Model 17:1–9:51–52

Szyszka R, Grankowski N, Felczak K, Shugar D (1995) Halogenated benzimidazoles and benzotriazoles as selective inhibitors of protein kinases CK I and CK II from Saccharomyces cerevisiae and other sources. Biochem Biophys Res Commun 208:418–424

Tawfic S, Yu S, Wang H, Faust R, Davis A, Ahmed K (2001) Protein kinase CK2 signal in neoplasia. Histol histopathol 16:573–582

Toledo LM, Lydon NB, Elbaum D (1999) The structure-based design of ATP-site directed protein kinase inhibitors. Curr Med Chem 6:775–805

Traxler P, Bold G, Buchdunger E, Caravatti G, Furet P, Manley P, O'Reilly T, Wood J, Zimmermann J (2001) Tyrosine kinase inhibitors: from rational design to clinical trials. Med Res Rev 21:499–512

Vangrevelinghe E, Zimmermann K, Schoepfer J, Portmann R, Fabbro D, Furet P (2003) Discovery of a potent and selective protein kinase CK2 inhibitor by high-throughput docking. J Med Chem 46:2656–2662

Yim H, Lee YH, Lee CH, Lee SK (1999) Emodin, an anthraquinone derivative isolated from the rhizomes of Rheum palmatum, selectively inhibits the activity of casein kinase II as a competitive inhibitor. Planta Med 65:9–13

Young TA, Delagoutte B, Endrizzi JA, Falick AM, Alber T (2003) Structure of Mycobacterium tuberculosis PknB supports a universal activation mechanism for Ser/Thr protein kinases. Nat Struct Biol 10:168–174

Zandomeni R, Zandomeni MC, Shugar D, Weinmann R (1986) Casein kinase type II is involved in the inhibition by 5,6-dichloro-1-beta-D-ribofuranosylbenzimidazole of specific RNA polymerase II transcription. J Biol Chem 261:3414–3419

Zhang L, Lau YK, Xi L, Hong RL, Kim DS, Chen CF, Hortobagyi GN, Chang C, Hung MC (1998) Tyrosine kinase inhibitors, emodin and its derivative repress HER-2/neu-induced cellular transformation and metastasis-associated properties. Oncogene 16:2855–2863

HEP (2005) 167:157–188

Aminoglycoside Kinases and Antibiotic Resistance

D. H. Fong[1] · D. L. Burk[1] · A. M. Berghuis[2] (✉)

[1] Department of Biochemistry, McGill University, 740 Dr. Penfield Avenue, Montreal, QC, H3A 1A4, Canada

[2] Departments of Biochemistry and Microbiology & Immunology, McGill University, 740 Dr. Penfield Avenue, Rm 5202, Montreal, QC, H3A 1A4, Canada
Albert.berghuis@mcgill.ca

Abstract The evolution of antibiotic-resistant bacteria represents a serious public health concern. The appearance of strains with resistance to multiple antibiotics threatens to render some infections untreatable by existing drugs. As a result, there is considerable interest in understanding the mechanisms of antibiotic resistance and in identifying ways in which antibiotic resistance can be overcome. Aminoglycoside antibiotics are broad-spectrum bactericidal compounds that are commonly used in the treatment of serious nosocomial infections. They exert their activity by binding to the A-site of the bacterial 30S ribosomal subunit where they impair the fidelity of protein translation. A number of bacterial strains have developed resistance to many aminoglycosides as a result of their acquisition of aminoglycoside-modifying enzymes that inactivate the antibiotic by reducing its affinity for the bacterial ribosome. These modifying enzymes can be classified into three groups according to the identity of the group used to modify the antibiotic substrate—aminoglycoside acetyltransferases, aminoglycoside phosphotransferases (kinases) and aminoglycoside nucleotidyltransferases. One of the best-understood aminoglycoside-modifying enzymes is aminoglycoside 3′-phosphotransferase type IIIa [APH (3′)-IIIa]. This enzyme catalyses the transfer of a phosphate moiety from ATP to a range of aminoglycoside substrates. Surprisingly, when the three-dimensional atomic structure of APH (3′)-IIIa was determined, it was found to possess striking similarity to eukaryotic protein kinases. Strategies to overcome resistance to aminoglycoside antibiotics are multifaceted and include: (1) novel aminoglycosides that are either not modified, or have low affinity for modifying enzymes, (2) mechanism-based inhibitors that exploit the enzyme's activity, (3) inhibitors of eukaryotic protein kinases that bind in the nucleotide-binding pocket, (4) bridged molecules that interact with both the nucleotide and aminoglycoside binding sites and (5) cationic peptides that resemble protein kinase inhibitors. By pursuing these leads, it is hoped that compounds will be developed that will allow aminoglycoside antibiotics to remain useful components of the physician's armamentarium.

Keywords Aminoglycoside · Protein kinase · Antibiotic resistance · Inhibitor design

1 Introduction

Advances in the development of antibiotics are being compromised by bacterial populations exhibiting multiple antibiotic resistance and a number of antibiotics have been rendered clinically obsolete. The development of multidrug-resistant strains of bacteria creates the potential for epidemics of infections that are either untreatable or which can only be treated by one or a few antibiotics.

Aminoglycosides are a class of antibiotics used in the treatment of serious infections caused by gram-negative organisms. Some infections that resist treatment by other antibiotics have retained susceptibility to one or more aminoglycosides. However, the clinical effectiveness of this class of antibiotics has been seriously compromised by the emergence of strains of bacteria that are resistant to their effects.

2 Aminoglycosides and Aminoglycoside Resistance

2.1 Aminoglycoside Antibiotics

The first aminoglycoside, streptomycin, was isolated from the soil bacterium *Streptomyces griseus* in 1944 (Schatz et al. 1944). Streptomycin proved to be the first successful drug against *Mycobacterium tuberculosis* and became widely popular in the 1940s and 1950s. The impact of streptomycin was of such significance that Selman A. Waksman was awarded the Nobel Prize in Medicine in 1952 for its discovery. While streptomycin continues to be an integral part of modern chemotherapy for tuberculosis since its clinical introduction over 50 years ago, a variety of natural and semisynthetic aminoglycosides with broad antimicrobial spectra have also been discovered and developed. Despite their toxic effects on the kidney and the inner ear (Forge and Schacht 2000), aminoglycosides are among the most commonly used antibiotics due to their low cost and high efficacy against both gram-positive and gram-negative bacteria, and in some cases, protozoal infections (Berman and Fleckenstein 1991).

From a chemical perspective, aminoglycosides are a group of structurally diverse, water soluble, polycationic molecules. They contain an aminocyclitol nucleus and two or three aminosugar rings linked to the nucleus via glycosidic bonds. They can be grouped into two main categories based on the structure of the central aminocyclitol ring. The first group, which includes streptomycin, contains a streptidine derivative; the second, larger group, which includes neomycin and kanamycin, contains a 2-deoxystreptamine ring derivatized at either the 4- and 5-positions or the 4- and 6-positions (Fig. 1). Conventionally, the numbering of the 6-aminohexose ring linked to the 4-position of the 2-deoxystreptamine is designated by prime (′), and the pentose or hexose ring linked to the 5- or 6-position is denoted by double prime (″).

Unlike many other antibiotics, aminoglycosides are bactericidal compounds. The primary target of these drugs in the bacterial cell is the 30S ribosomal RNA, as shown by chemical footprinting experiments (Moazed and Noller 1987), and more recently, evidence from crystallographic studies (Carter et al. 2000). Nonetheless, some details concerning the uptake and action of aminoglycosides remain elusive. Existing evidence indicates that the first step of aminoglycoside uptake involves an energy-requiring transport across the cell membrane (Wright et al. 1998). Once inside the cell, the aminoglycosides bind to the A-site (the decoding site) of the 16S ribosomal RNA (Moazed and Noller 1987) and trigger certain conformational changes in the A-site that normally occur only when there is a correct interaction between cognate tRNA and mRNA (Pape et al. 2000; Ogle et al. 2002; Rodnina et al. 2002). As a result, the stability of the binding of near-cognate aminoacyl-tRNA to this site is increased and the ribosome is unable to discriminate between cognate and near- or non-cognate tRNA–mRNA complexes, and the production of defective proteins ensues. Subsequently, the faulty proteins are presumably inserted into the cytoplasmic membrane, leading to the loss of membrane integrity. Additional aminoglycosides are then rapidly transported across the damaged membrane, leading to the accumulation of the drug in the cytoplasm, saturation of all ribosomes and ultimately cell death (Wright et al. 1998).

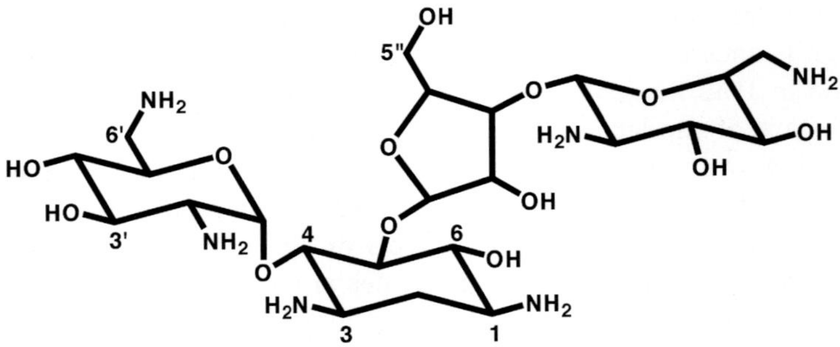

Neomycin B
(4,5-disubstituted 2-deoxystreptamine)

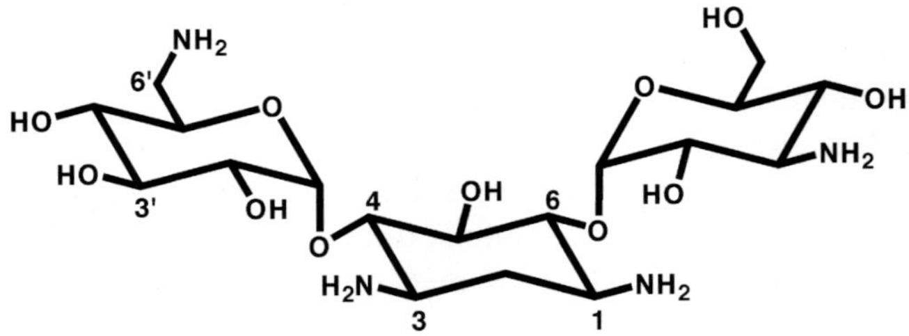

Kanamycin A
(4,6-disubstituted 2-deoxystreptamine)

Fig. 1 Examples of two aminoglycoside antibiotics based on 2-deoxystreptamine. Neomycin B is derivatized at the 4- and 5-positions of the central 2-deoxystreptamine ring, while kanamycin A is derivatized a the 4- and 6-positions

2.2 Resistance to Aminoglycosides

There are three principal mechanisms of bacterial resistance to antibiotics. First, the bacteria can prevent accumulation of antibiotics inside the cell either via changes in membrane permeability or via efflux pumps that export the drug from the cell. Second, the bacteria could also alter, by mutation or chemical modification (Thompson et al. 1985; Cundliffe 1989) the target of the antibiotic (such as the ribosome) to preclude the effects of the antibiotic. Last, antibiotics that manage to enter the cell can be enzymatically modified such that they have reduced affinity for their target and, therefore, can no longer exert their antimicrobial effects (Llano-Sotelo et al. 2002). This last mechanism is the most prevalent means of resistance to aminoglycosides in

Table 1 Aminoglycoside-modifying enzymes

AAC		APH		ANT	
AAC(2′)	Ia, Ib, Ic, Id, Ie	APH(3′)	Ia, Ib, Ic	ANT(4′)	Ia
-	IIa, IIb	-	IIa, IIb	-	IIa
AAC(6′)	Ia-In, Ip-Ix, Iz	-	IIIa	ANT(6)	Ia
-	IIa, IIb	-	IVa	ANT(9)	Ia
AAC(1)	Ia	-	Va	-	Ib
AAC(3)	Ia, Ib	-	VIa	ANT(2″)	Ia
-	IIa, IIb, IIc	-	VIIa	ANT(3″)	Ia
-	IIIa, IIIb, IIIc	APH(4)	Ia, Ib	-	-
-	IVa	APH(6)	Ia, Ib, Ic, Id	-	-
-	VIa	APH(9)	Ia, Ib	-	-
-	VIIa	APH(2″)	Ia, Ib, Ic, Id	-	-
-	VIIIa	APH(3″)	Ia, Ib	-	-
-	IXa	APH(7″)	Ia	-	-
-	Xa	-	-	-	-

clinical isolates (Davies 1991). Three families of aminoglycoside-modifying enzymes have been identified. They are aminoglycoside *N*-acetyltransferases (AACs), aminoglycoside *O*-phosphotransferases (APHs) and aminoglycoside *O*-nucleotidyltransferases (ANTs). They render aminoglycoside antibiotics inactive by catalysing the transfer of an acetyl group (from acetyl CoA), a phosphate group or an adenyl group (both from ATP) to the aminoglycoside. Over 50 aminoglycoside-modifying enzymes have been identified (Table 1) and they are named using nomenclature proposed by Shaw (Shaw et al. 1993). First, each enzyme is designated by the reaction they carry out: AAC for acetylation, APH for phosphorylation, and ANT for adenylation. This is followed by the regiospecificity of the group transferred, designated in parentheses. Next follows a Roman numeral, which specifies the unique aminoglycoside substrate profile. A final lower case letter identifies the distinct genes which confer identical resistance phenotypes.

2.3 Aminoglycoside Phosphotransferases

Although many aminoglycoside-modifying enzymes are capable of conferring a resistant phenotype, generally only APHs yield high levels of resistance (Vakulenko and Mobashery 2003). APHs constitute the second largest group of aminoglycoside-modifying enzymes carrying out the phosphorylation of specific hydroxyl groups of aminoglycosides using ATP as a cofactor. Over 20 distinct aminoglycoside kinases have been identified, and they show significant sequence similarity (Nurizzo et al. 2003). APHs are classified into seven types (Table 1) (Shaw et al. 1993) and among them, APH(3′) enzymes make up the largest group, comprising seven sub-classes [APH(3′)-I to

Table 2 Substrate profiles of selected aminoglycoside-modifying enzymes

Enzyme	Profile	Reference(s)
APH(3′)-Ia	Kanamycin, neomycin, lividomycin, paromomycin, ribostamycin	Oka et al. 1981
APH(3′)-IIa	Kanamycin, neomycin, butirosin, paromomycin, ribostamycin	Beck et al. 1982
APH(3′)-IIIa	Kanamycin, amikacin, isepamicin, gentamicin B, butirosin, lividomycin, paromomycin, ribostamycin,	Gray and Fitch 1983; Trieu-Cuot and Courvalin 1983
APH(2″)-Ia (bifunctional enzyme)	Kanamycin, amikacin, tobramycin, dibekacin, gentamicin, isepamicin, sisomicin, netilmicin, neomycin, butirosin, lividomycin, paromomycin, ribostamycin, neamine	Daigle et al. 1999a; Ferretti et al. 1986

APH(3′)-VII]. They have been isolated from both gram-positive and gram-negative bacteria, including aminoglycoside-producing organisms (Shaw et al. 1993).

APH(3′)-IIIa is the best-studied aminoglycoside kinase. It was originally isolated from *Streptococcus faecalis* (Trieu-Cuot and Courvalin 1983) and *Staphylococcus aureus* (Gray and Fitch 1983). Subsequently, the gene was detected in *Campylobacter coli*, which became a precedent for the transfer of antibiotic resistance gene transfer between gram-positive and gram-negative bacteria (Papadopoulou and Courvalin 1988; Taylor et al. 1988). The *aph(3′)-IIIa* gene from *Enterococcus faecalis* has been cloned and the protein expressed and purified from *Escherichia coli* (McKay et al. 1994a). APH(3′)-IIIa has one of the broadest substrate ranges among all single-function aminoglycoside-modifying enzymes (Table 2). As its name implies, APH(3′)-IIIa catalyses the transfer of a phosphate group to the 3′-hydroxyl of the antibiotic substrate. Interestingly, it is also able to transfer a phosphate group from ATP to the 5″ hydroxyl of neomycin-type aminoglycosides (McKay et al. 1994a; Thompson et al. 1996b). Hence, aminoglycosides which lack the 3′-hydroxyl, such as lividomycin, are also substrates for APH(3′)-IIIa, since they can be modified at the 5″-position. In this sense, it should be named more appropriately as APH(3′)(5″)-IIIa. The enzyme is 264 amino acid residues in size, with a molecular mass of 31,000 Da. The phosphorylation reaction catalysed by APH(3′)-IIIa has been shown to follow a Theorell–Chance mechanism where ATP binds to the enzyme first, followed by the aminoglycoside; phosphorylated aminoglycoside is then quickly released, followed by the rate-limiting step—the release of ADP. Evidence suggests that the phosphoryl transfer occurs through direct attack of the 3′-hydroxyl group of the aminoglycoside on the γ-phosphate of ATP (Thompson et al. 1996a). APH(3′)-IIIa is the first aminoglycoside kinase to be structurally characterized. The three-dimensional atomic structure of the enzyme complexed with

ADP was determined to 2.2 Å by X-ray crystallography (Hon et al. 1997) (see Sect. 3). Subsequently, structures of APH(3′)-IIIa in the apoenzyme form (i.e. no substrates), in complex with the non-hydrolyzable ATP analogue adenosine 5′-(β,γ-imino)triphosphate, AMPPNP (Burk et al. 2001), as well as APH(3′)-IIIa bound with ADP and kanamycin A or neomycin B (Fong and Berghuis 2002), have been determined.

Two other APH(3′) enzymes, APH(3′)-Ia and APH(3′)-IIa, have also been extensively characterized. The amino acid sequences of APH(3′)-Ia, APH(3′)-IIa and APH(3′)-IIIa enzymes share approximately 30% identity. APH(3′)-Ia is the most commonly disseminated APH in gram-negative bacteria. The *aph(3′)-Ia* gene was discovered on transposon Tn*903* in *E. coli* (Oka et al. 1981), encoding an enzyme that is able to phosphorylate a range of clinically useful aminoglycoside antibiotics (Table 2) (Shaw et al. 1993). Steady-state kinetic studies of APH(3′)-Ia indicate that the phosphorylation reaction occurs via a rapid equilibrium random mechanism and, like APH(3′)-IIIa, the phosphoryl group is believed to be transferred in a direct displacement manner (Siregar et al. 1995).

Although APH(3′)-IIa is rarely found in clinical isolates, it is still a well-known APH. The *aph(3′)-IIa* gene, encoded on transposon Tn*5* (Beck et al. 1982) is widely used in molecular biology as a selectable marker in both eukaryotic and prokaryotic studies. APH(3′)-Ia and APH(3′)-IIa have almost identical substrate spectra (Table 2). Recently, the crystal structure of APH(3′)-IIa complexed with kanamycin has been solved (Nurizzo et al. 2003). It is essentially identical to the structure of APH(3′)-IIIa with root mean square (rms) deviation for Cα atoms of about 1.7 Å.

Another important resistance factor in gram-positive pathogens is APH(2″)-Ia. The gene *aph(2″)-Ia* is downstream of *aac(6′)-Ie*, and they are conjointly expressed as one enzyme with two reaction centres. This bifunctional enzyme is capable of inactivating essentially all clinically available aminoglycosides containing a 2-deoxystreptamine ring (Ferretti et al. 1986; Leclercq et al. 1992) (Table 2) and is most prevalent in methicillin-resistant *S. aureus* (MRSA) isolates in many parts of the world (Schmitz et al. 1999; Udo and Dashti 2000; Ida et al. 2001). The regiospecificity of AAC(6′)-Ie-APH(2″)-Ia is not very stringent. In addition to acetylating the amino group at the 6′-position, the AAC domain can also acetylate the 6′-hydroxyl of lividomycin and paromomycin. Whereas APH(2″) denotes the transfer of a phosphate group to the 2″-hydroxyl of the drug, phosphorylation at the 3′- and 3″-positions of most 4,5-disubstituted aminoglycosides, and the 5″-position of lividomycin, has also been observed (Daigle et al. 1999a). The phosphorylation reaction of APH(2″)-Ia proceeds through a random rapid equilibrium mechanism (Martel et al. 1983). The amino acid sequence of APH(2″)-Ia is about 15% identical to that of APH(3′)-IIIa.

3
3′-Aminoglycoside *O*-Phosphotransferase-IIIa Structure and Similarity to Eukaryotic Protein Kinases

APH(3′)-IIIa from enterococci and staphylococci is perhaps the best understood of the aminoglycoside-modifying enzymes. Experiments have revealed much about the kinetic properties, mechanism and structure of this enzyme. As a result, APH(3′)-IIIa has become a useful model for the study of aminoglycoside kinases.

3.1
Tertiary Structure

The APH(3′)-IIIa enzyme is composed of two lobes, a 94-residue N-terminal lobe and a larger 157-residue C-terminal lobe. The two lobes are joined by a 12-residue linker region containing a short β-strand and α-helix. The N-terminal lobe consists of a five-stranded antiparallel β-sheet, with an α-helix located between two β-strands and a short 3_{10} helix preceding the first β-strand. The architecture of the N-terminal lobe of APH(3′)-IIIa is similar to that observed in eukaryotic protein kinases (ePKs) such as the catalytic subunits of cyclic AMP (cAMP)-dependant protein kinase (cAPK), casein kinase (CsK) and phosphorylase kinase (PhK) (Owen et al. 1995; Xu et al. 1995; Knighton et al. 1991). For structurally conserved main-chain atoms in the N-terminal lobe, the rms deviation in atomic position is only 1.8 Å between APH(3′)-IIIa and cAPK. This is remarkable, given the fact that the sequence identity between the two enzymes is less than 6% for these residues.

The 12-residue linker that connects the N- and C-terminal lobes of APH(3′)-IIIa is also structurally similar to the equivalent region in the structures of protein kinases such as cAPK. The linker consists of a short α-helix flanked by sections of random coil. The C-terminal lobe of APH(3′)-IIIa can be divided into three sections: (1) a central core composed of two α-helices and a long hairpin-shaped loop incorporating two short sections of antiparallel β-sheet, (2) an insert region composed of two α-helices connected by long loop and (3) a C-terminal region composed of two α-helices.

There are four areas in which APH(3′)-IIIa differs significantly from ePKs such as cAPK (Fig. 2). First, in APH(3′)-IIIa, the loop between β-strands 1 and 2 contains a one-residue insertion and adopts a different conformation than that observed in ePKs (*red*). While this loop is the location of the conserved GXGXXG motif in protein kinases, the motif is not observed in APH(3′)-IIIa. Second, as a consequence of differences in the C-terminal lobes of APH(3′)-IIIa and the protein kinases, the location of the α-helix in the linker region is shifted in APH(3′)-IIIa with respect to where it is usually located in the protein kinases (*yellow*). Third, APH(3′)-IIIa has a 60-residue insert in its C-terminal lobe (*blue*). Consisting of two α-helices and a 19-res-

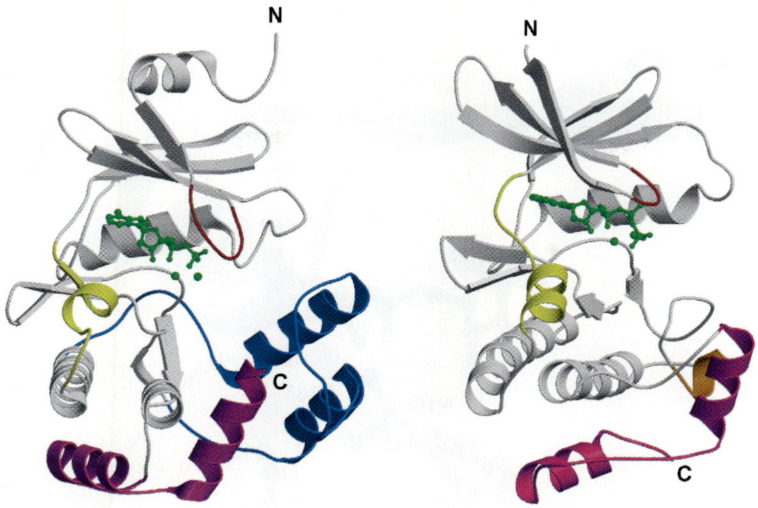

Fig. 2 A comparison of the structures of APH(3′)-IIIa (*left*) and cAPK (*right*) highlighting, in colour, the areas with significant differences. These areas include: (1) the loop between strands $\beta 1$ and $\beta 2$ (*red*), (2) the linker region between the N- and C-terminal domains (*yellow*), (3) a 60-residue insert in APH(3′)-IIIa (*blue*), (4) a smaller insertion found in ePK's (*orange*) and (5) the last two α-helices of the C-terminal domain (*magenta*). The ATP cofactor and its associated magnesium ions are depicted as *green balls-and-sticks*

idue loop, this insertion occupies the space of a smaller section of polypeptide found in ePKs (*orange*). The latter has a distinctly different conformation from that seen in APH(3′)-IIIa and has been identified as important in substrate selectivity and specificity (Taylor et al. 1992; Madhusudan et al. 1994). This section of the ePK sequence also corresponds to the activation segment in some protein kinases, containing sites of phosphorylation that switch the enzyme from an inactive to an active conformation (Johnson et al. 1996; Yamaguchi and Hendrickson 1996). Lastly, the positions of the two α-helices at the end of the C-terminal lobes are significantly different in the APH(3′)-IIIa and ePK structures (*magenta*).

3.2 ATP-Binding Site

The binding site for ATP and its associated magnesium ions in APH(3′)-IIIa is located in the deep cleft between the N- and C-terminal lobes. Of the four absolutely conserved residues in both eukaryotic protein kinases and aminoglycoside phosphotransferases, three are located in the ATP-binding pocket where they interact with the cofactor and its associated magnesium ions—Asp190, Asn195 and Asp208 (Fig. 3). Two additional highly conserved residues, Lys44 and Glu60, are also found in the active site.

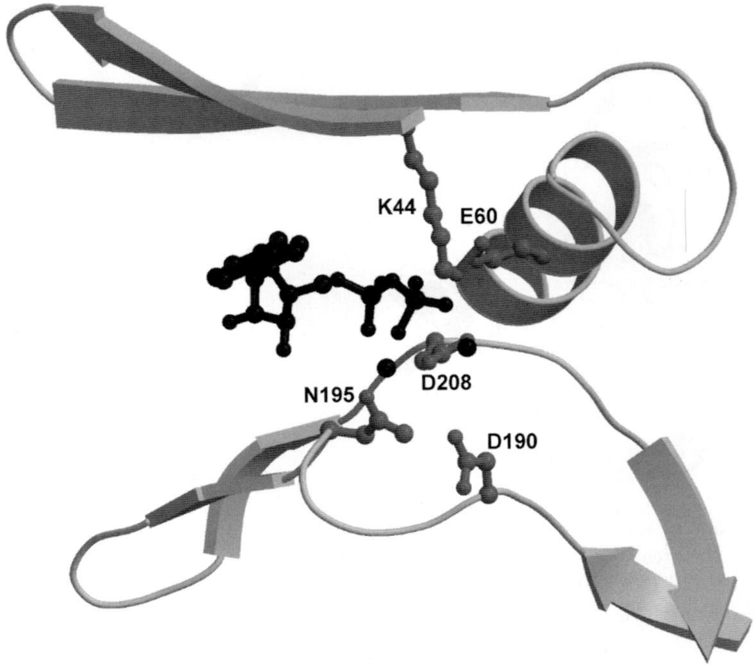

Fig. 3 The nucleotide-binding pocket of APH(3′)-IIIa. The backbone is shown as *ribbon* and conserved residues are drawn as *balls-and-sticks*, both in *light grey*. ATP and its associated magnesium ions are drawn as *balls-and-sticks in black*

Lys44 is positioned over the binding site, interacting with the α- and β-phosphates of the cofactor. Evidence from mutagenesis studies suggests that Lys44 influences the K_m for ATP and thus makes an important contribution to ATP binding (Hon et al. 1997). The analogous lysine residue in the protein kinase family is also positioned to interact with the α- and β-phosphates of ATP. Glu60 is positioned in such a way that it hydrogen bonds to the side chain of Lys44, orienting it so that it interacts with the α- and β-phosphates of ATP.

In protein kinases, the residue corresponding to Asp190 has been proposed as a general base assisting in substrate deprotonation (Madhusudan et al. 1994). Although mutagenesis of Asp190 in APH(3′)-IIIa results in drastically lower activity, supporting a role for this residue in catalysis, its role in catalysis has not been definitively identified (Hon et al. 1997; Zhou and Adams 1997). The function of Asp190 may be limited to positioning of the substrate hydroxyl group during phosphoryl transfer (Boehr et al. 2001b).

Mutagenesis studies of Asn195 indicated that this residue was important for ATP binding. Since Asn195 interacts with ATP via a magnesium ion, it has been suggested that the decrease in ATP affinity is the result of a non-optimally coordinated metal ion (Boehr et al. 2001b). Asp208 is a ligand of both active site metal ions, and an Asp208Ala mutation results in a protein without detectable aminoglycoside kinase activity (Boehr et al. 2001b). Thus, Asp208 appears to be critical for catalysis in APH(3′)-IIIa, facilitating the generation or stabilization of the transition state.

3.3 Aminoglycoside-Binding Site

The three-dimensional atomic structures of APH(3′)-IIIa in complex with ADP and either the 4,6-disubstituted aminoglycoside kanamycin A or the 4,5-disubstituted aminoglycoside neomycin B have recently been determined (Fong and Berghuis 2002). Comparison of these structures with those of the apo, ADP and AMPPNP complexes of APH(3′)-IIIa shows that most of the enzyme is rather rigid, with no evidence of gross domain movements associated with aminoglycoside binding. The most significant conformational change observed is a shift in the C-terminal insertion known as the aminoglycoside-binding loop. The loop folds over towards the antibiotic

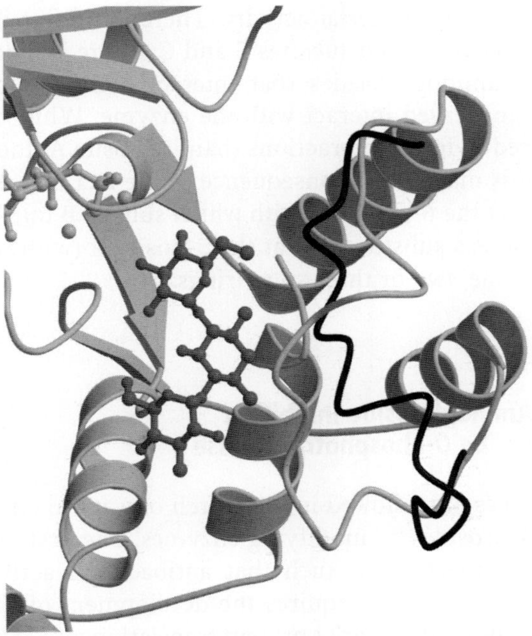

Fig. 4 An illustration of the APH(3′)-IIIa aminoglycoside-binding pocket showing the conformational changes that occur upon aminoglycoside binding. The backbone of the kanamycin ternary structure of APH(3′)-IIIa is shown as *ribbon* and the nucleotide cofactor and magnesium ions are drawn in *balls-and-sticks*, both in *light grey*. Kanamycin is shown as *balls-and-sticks in grey*. The antibiotic binding loop of the APH(3′)-IIIa-ADP complex without bound aminoglycoside has been overlaid and coloured *black*. The movement of this loop is the largest conformational difference between the ternary and binary complexes

substrate, interacts with the aminoglycoside and completes the binding pocket (Fig. 4). The majority of the residues that line the aminoglycoside-binding pocket are acidic, and consequently the pocket is negatively charged. Thus, the binding pocket complements the aminoglycoside substrates, which are invariably positively charged.

The aminoglycoside-binding site of APH(3′)-IIIa can be considered to be composed of three distinct binding subsites. The first of these, subsite A, interacts with the central 2-deoxystreptamine ring of the aminoglycoside and the hexose substituted at the 4-position of this central ring (the prime ring). The second subsite (subsite B) interacts with groups substituted at the 6-position of the 2-deoxystreptamine ring (the double prime ring). Consequently, this subsite is involved in binding only those substrates that have this type of modification, i.e. 4,6-disubstituted aminoglycosides. In contrast, the third subsite (subsite C) interacts with groups substituted at the 5-position of the central ring of 4,5-disubstituted aminoglycoside substrates.

Most of the hydrogen bond interactions observed between the aminoglycoside substrate and the APH(3′)-IIIa enzyme are via subsite A. The central 2-deoxystrpetamine and prime rings that interact here are common to most aminoglycoside substrates and have been found to be the minimum essential components for antibacterial activity. There are fewer interactions between the aminoglycoside and subsites B and C. There is more variability in the parts of the aminoglycosides that interact here, and only functional groups that are conserved interact with the enzyme. While both subsites B and C are involved in fewer interactions than is subsite A, they differ significantly in size. This may be the consequence of the fact that the aminoglycoside substituents at the 6-position (with which subsite B interacts) are single hexose rings, whereas substitutions at the 5-position (with which subsite C interacts) can be one, two or three sugar rings.

4 Circumventing Aminoglycoside Inhibition by 3′-Aminoglycoside *O*-Phosphotransferase

Two main principles are followed in the search of ways to circumvent inactivation of aminoglycosides by modifying enzymes. The first involves abolishing the resistance mechanism such that antibacterial activity can be restored. The second approach requires the development of compounds that are effective inhibitors of bacterial protein translation and can also evade resistant mechanisms. Most of these studies have been done with the phosphotransferase class of enzyme due to the amount of information available. Many compounds were developed based on the binding properties of the aminoglycosides, as well as on the kinetic mechanism of the aminoglycoside-modifying enzymes. Additionally, structural information has added much insight in the development of aminoglycoside derivatives and inhibitors targeted at the cofactor binding site or the whole binding cleft.

4.1
Targeting the Aminoglycosides and Their Binding Pocket

Most studies of strategies to circumvent the effects of resistance factors have focussed on aminoglycoside binding. The advantage of such an approach is that since the compound would necessarily mimic features of an aminoglycoside, it could be a universal inhibitor for all three classes of aminoglycoside-modifying enzymes.

4.1.1
Removing the Target Functional Group

There have been some successes in modifying existing aminoglycoside antibiotics to generate new compounds that bind, but are not inactivated

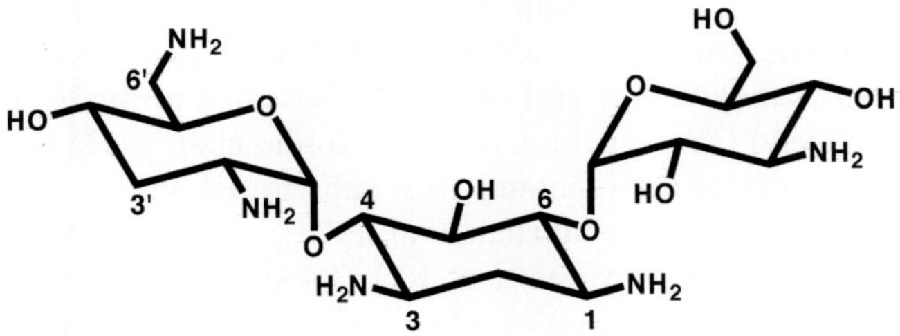

Tobramycin
(3'-deoxykanamycin B)

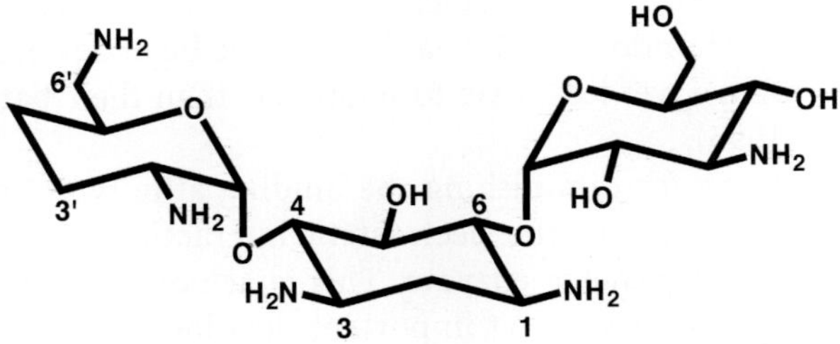

dibekacin
(3',4'-dideoxykanamycin B)

Fig. 5 Structures of the aminoglycosides tobramycin (*top*) and dibekacin (*bottom*). Both molecules lack a 3′-hydroxyl group, making them resistant to modification by APH(3′)-IIIa

by, resistance enzymes. For example, tobramycin (3′-deoxykanamycin B) (Umezawa et al. 1971b) and dibekacin (3′,4′-dideoxykanamycin B) (Umezawa et al. 1971a), both lacking the 3′-hydroxyl, are competitive inhibitors for APH(3′)s (McKay and Wright 1995) (Fig. 5). Both molecules evade modification by the APH(3′) enzymes. However, they can be deactivated by other classes of aminoglycoside-modifying enzymes.

4.1.2 Reducing the Binding Affinity

Another approach involves modifying the antibiotic in such a way that it can no longer bind to the aminoglycoside-modifying enzymes. This strategy is based on the observation that the naturally occurring butirosins, which possess a 4-amino-2-hydroxybutyryl (AHB) group on the amine at the 1-position of the 2-deoxystreptamine ring, are resistant to many inactivating enzymes, yet retain their bactericidal properties (Tsukiura et al. 1973) (Fig. 6a). It is thought that the AHB and other side chains at the 1-amino position hinder binding to the aminoglycoside-modifying enzyme (Kondo and Hotta 1999). This observation led to the development of second generation semisynthetic aminoglycoside antibiotics such as amikacin (Fig. 6b) and arbekacin (kanamycin A and dibekacin derivated at the N1 by an AHB group, respectively) (Kawaguchi et al. 1972; Kondo et al. 1973a,b; Holm et al. 1983), isepamicin (Fig. 6c) (gentamicin B substituted with a 4-amino-2-hydroxypropionyl at N1) (Nagabhushan et al. 1978), as well as netilmicin (sisomicin with ethyl group introduced at N1) (Wright 1976). They have been shown to be clinically useful, especially arbekacin, which is effective against MRSA infections (Kondo and Hotta 1999) and whose antibiotic activity is unaffected by 2′- and 3″-acetylation (Hotta et al. 1996, 1998). Unfortunately, some level of resistance has been noted, chiefly as a consequence of inactivation by the bifunctional enzyme AAC(6′)-Ie-APH(2″)-Ia (Kondo et al. 1993b; Fujimura et al. 1998; Fujimura et al. 2000). Subsequently, two derivatives of arbekacin, 2″-amino-2″-deoxyarbekacin and 2″-amino-5,2″-dideoxy-5-epiaminoarbekacin (Kondo et al. 1993a, 1994), have been developed and shown to be active in vivo, yet less toxic to mammals than their parent compound (Inouye et al. 1996).

Another scheme for diminishing the binding affinity of aminoglycosides for APHs is by minimizing the electrostatic interactions between the aminoglycoside and the resistance enzyme. This is achieved through the deletion of amino or hydroxyl groups at important positions on neamine and kanamycin B (Roestamadji et al. 1995a; McKay et al. 1996). These modified drugs retain their antibacterial activity but have a significantly reduced rate of phosphorylation and affinity for APH(3′)-Ia and APH(3′)-IIa, probably due to the removal of specific ionic and hydrogen bond interactions between the

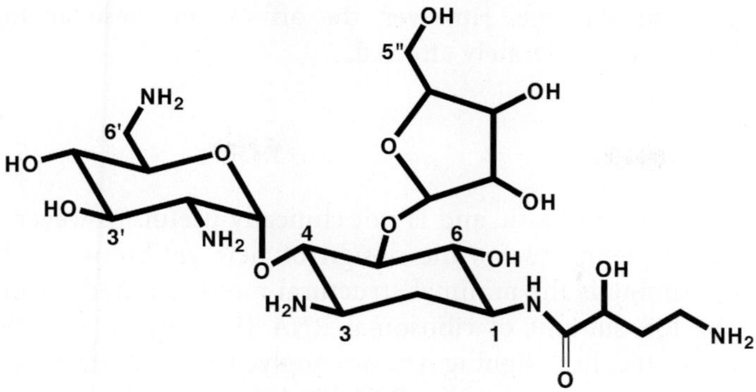

Butirosin

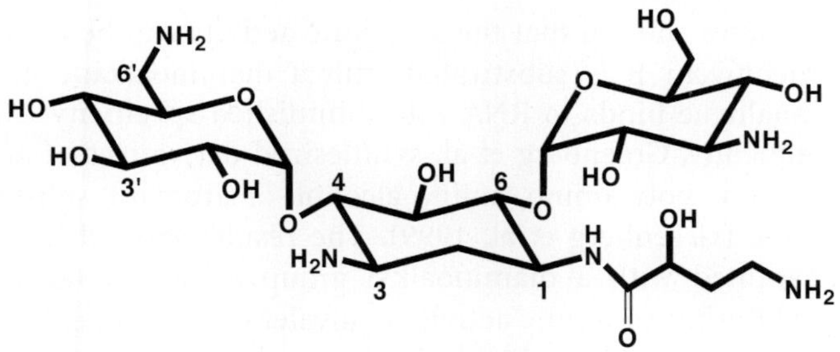

Amikacin
(Kanamycin A derivative)

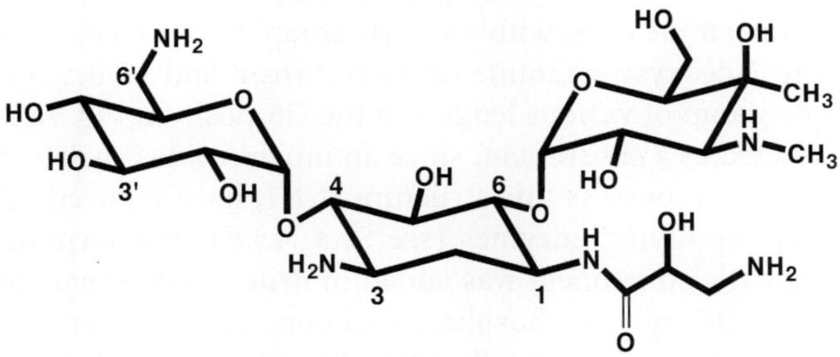

Isepamicin
(Gentamicin B derivative)

Fig. 6 Three aminoglycosides with substitutions at the 1-amino group of the central 2-deoxystreptamine ring. Butirosin is naturally occurring, while amikacin and isepamicin are semisynthetic aminoglycosides. The 1-amino substitutions are believed to hinder binding to aminoglycoside-modifying enzymes, making these compounds resistant to inactivation

substrate and the enzyme. However, the affinity of these analogues for APH(3′)-IIIa is only moderately affected.

4.1.3 Neamine Derivatives

Neamine is a poor antibiotic and is not clinically useful. However, it serves as an invaluable template for the design of new antibiotics. It has been shown that neamine is the minimal structural motif required for binding to the A-site of 16S subunit of ribosomal RNA (Fourmy et al. 1996, 1998). Hence, it is sensible, in designing new aminoglycosides, to preserve the minimum structural motif required for RNA binding and antibiotic activity, but to deviate from typical aminoglycoside structures, in order to elude the various modifying enzymes.

Previous studies showed that the antibiotic activity can be retained when ring IV of neomycin B is substituted with a diaminoalkane group, even though the analogue binds to RNA with diminished specificity (Alper et al. 1998). Subsequently, Greenberg et al. synthesized derivatives of neamine by appending various poly amino, amino alcohol, or aromatic substitutions at the O5-position (Greenberg et al. 1999). The results showed that the compounds substituted with a diaminoalkyl group enhanced the binding to RNA while exhibiting antibiotic activity equivalent to neamine.

More recently, several neamine derivatives were synthesized based on the interactions observed in the nuclear magnetic resonance (NMR) solution structure of paromomycin bound to an A-site rRNA template, as well as extensive searches in the Cambridge Structural Database and the National Cancer Institute 3-D Database (Haddad et al. 2002). These compounds are composed of a neamine core, with an AHB group or its analogue at the N1-position of the 2-deoxystreptamine (as in butirosin and amikacin), plus an diaminoalkane group of various lengths at the O6-position Fig. 7a). An AHB group was selected as a substituent, since aminoglycosides such as butirosin and amikacin, which possess this structure at N1, have reduced affinity for aminoglycoside-modifying enzymes (see Sect. 4.1.2). The terminal amine-containing aliphatic component was added in order to improve the interaction between the O6 and the phosphate backbone of the target rRNA. Many of the designed compounds were shown to be capable of binding to a fragment modelling the A-site of the *E. coli* rRNA, and demonstrated broad spectrum antibiotic activity that is much higher than their parent compound or equal to that of other commonly used aminoglycosides. Some of these designed antibiotics were shown to be poor substrates of APH(3′)-Ia and AAC(6′)-Ie-APH(2″)-Ia, the bifunctional enzyme. The crystal structure of the A-site rRNA template in complex with a designer neamine derivative of high antibiotic activity has recently been reported (Russell et al. 2003). The structure showed that the binding mode of the designer compound is essentially identical to that of paromomycin (Carter et al. 2000). Comparison

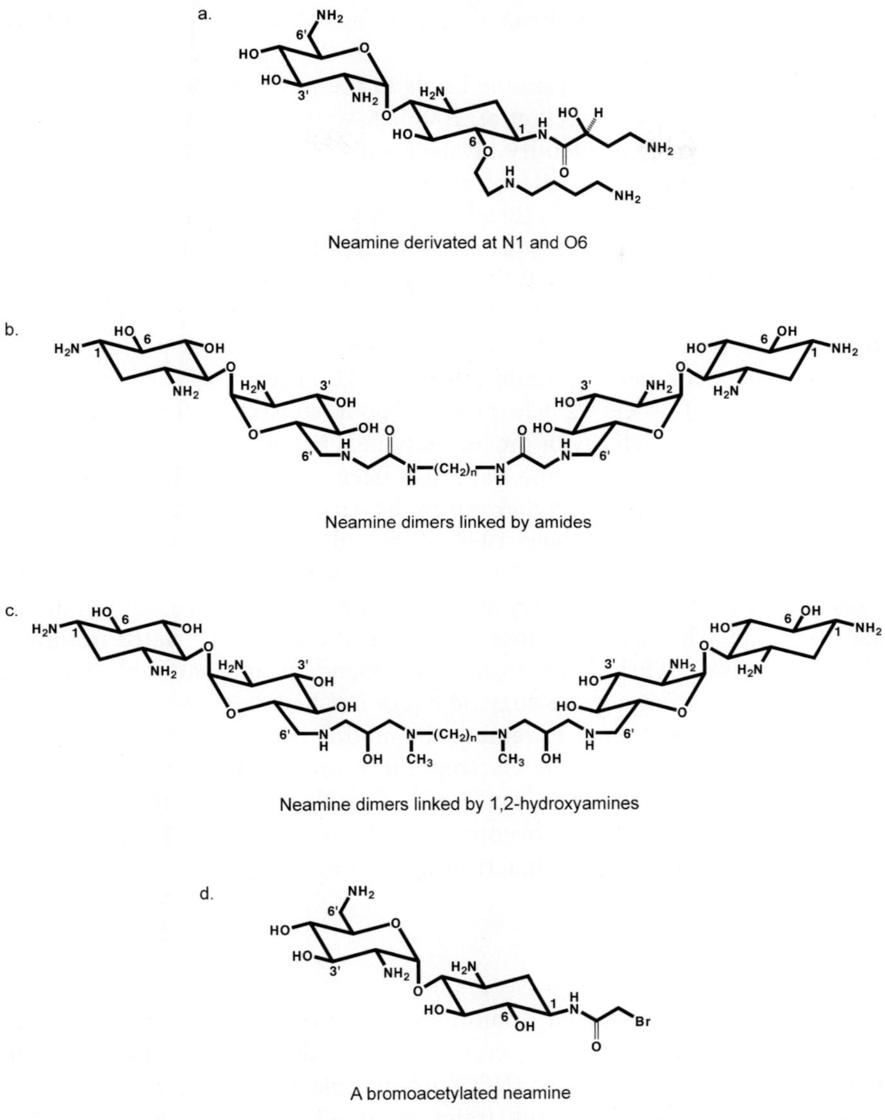

Fig. 7a–d Four synthetic aminoglycosides based on the structure of neamine, the minimal structure required for binding to the bacterial ribosome. **a** A neamine derivative with AHB and diaminoalkane substitutions at the N1 and O6 positions, respectively. **b** Amine-linked neamine dimers. **c** 1,2-hydroxyamine-linked neamine dimers. **d** A bromoacetylated neamine

of neamine derivatives to the kanamycin A bound to APH(3′)-IIIa (Fong and Berghuis 2002) also explains the basis of the designer molecules' ability to elude inactivation by aminoglycoside-modifying enzymes. The AHB moiety at the N1-position forms steric clashes with the antibiotic binding loop of

APH(3′)-IIIa, impeding the formation of an active ternary complex (Russell et al. 2003).

It has been shown that neamine binds to the A-site model of prokaryotic rRNA in a 2:1 ratio (Sucheck et al. 2000). A series of neamine dimers were constructed in order to identify bivalent aminoglycosides that would interact with the model target site of aminoglycosides in bacteria, and at the same time resist modification by aminoglycoside-modifying enzymes due to its dramatically altered and unusual structure. Two neamine molecules are joined by either amides or 1,2-hydroxyamine with methylene bridges of variable lengths (Fig. 7b,c). These compounds were found to possess antibiotic activity that is comparable or even superior to that of neamine. They are also potent competitive inhibitors of APH(2″) activity of the bifunctional enzyme AAC(6′)-Ie-APH(2″)-Ia and are poor substrates for APH(3′)-IIIa and the AAC(6′)-Ie activity of the bifunctional enzyme.

Four derivatives of neamine have also been synthesized by regiospecifically appending a bromoacetyl group to the various amines of the antibiotic (Roestamadji and Mobashery 1998) (Fig. 7d). The affinity of the bromoacetylated compounds for APH(3′)-IIa is significantly reduced. In the presence of ATP, the phosphorylation reaction would proceed but at an attenuated rate, whereas in the absence of ATP, the bromoacetylated neamines would inactivate APH(3′)-IIa in a time-dependent and saturable manner. Moreover, the activity of the enzyme could not be recovered despite extensive dialysis, in an attempt to remove the modified neamine molecules. This observation suggests that the electrophilic bromoacetyl group could form covalent bonds with different nucleophilic residues in the active site. As a result, the modified neamine becomes irreversibly bound to the enzyme and prevents it from binding and inactivating aminoglycosides.

4.1.4
Mechanism-Based Inhibition

The first mechanism-based inhibitors of APH(3′)s were described by Roestamadji et al. (1995b). The compounds are derivatives of neamine and kanamycin B, in which a nitro (NO_2) group replaces the amine at the 2′-position (Fig. 8). These suicide substrates are excellent substrates for APH(3′)s but poor antibiotics. Upon phosphorylation by APH(3′) enzymes at the 3′-hydroxyl, the phosphoryl group, being an excellent leaving group, is

Fig. 8 Proposed mechanism of aminoglycoside kinase inhibition by 2′-nitro aminoglycoside derivatives. Spontaneous loss of phosphate from a phospho-aminoglycoside yields an electrophilic nitroalkene. Trapping of a nucleophilic active site residue (*Nuc*) produces an inactivated enzyme

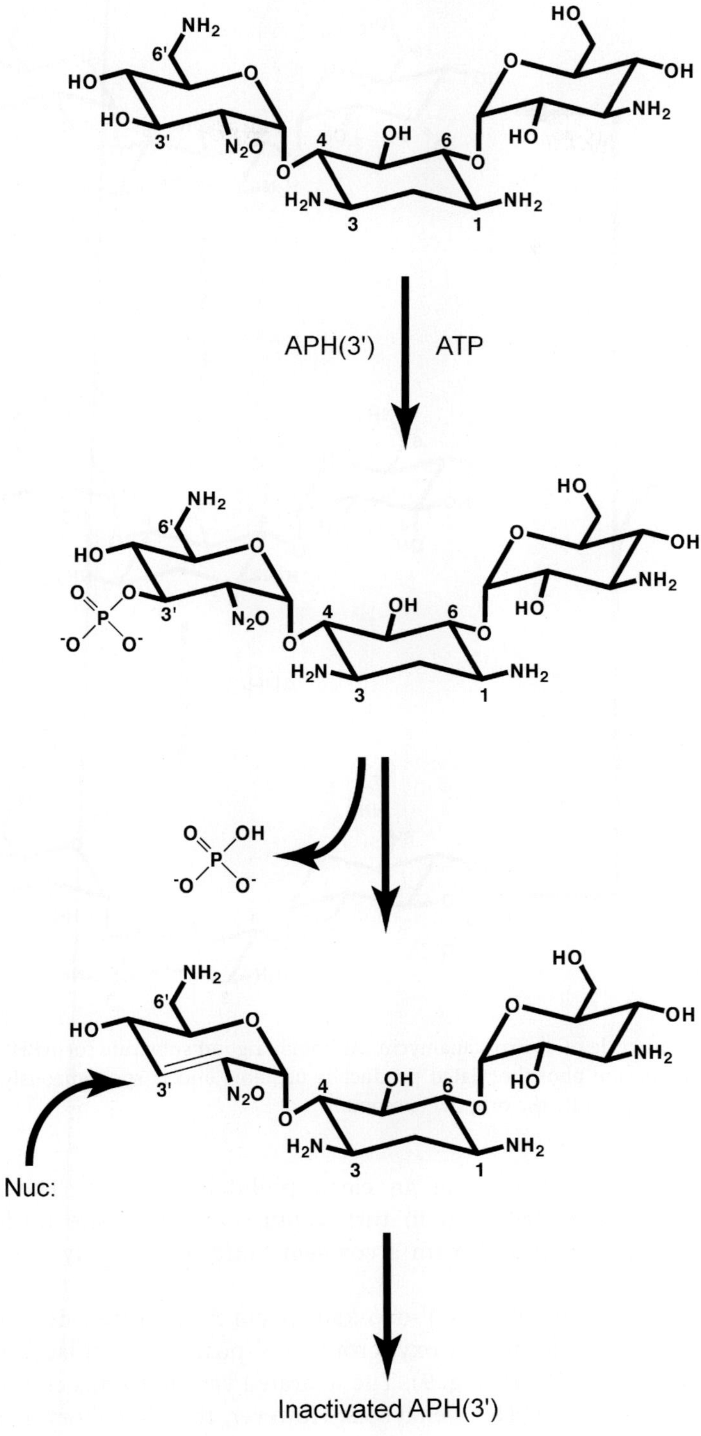
APH(3')
ATP
Nuc:
Inactivated APH(3')

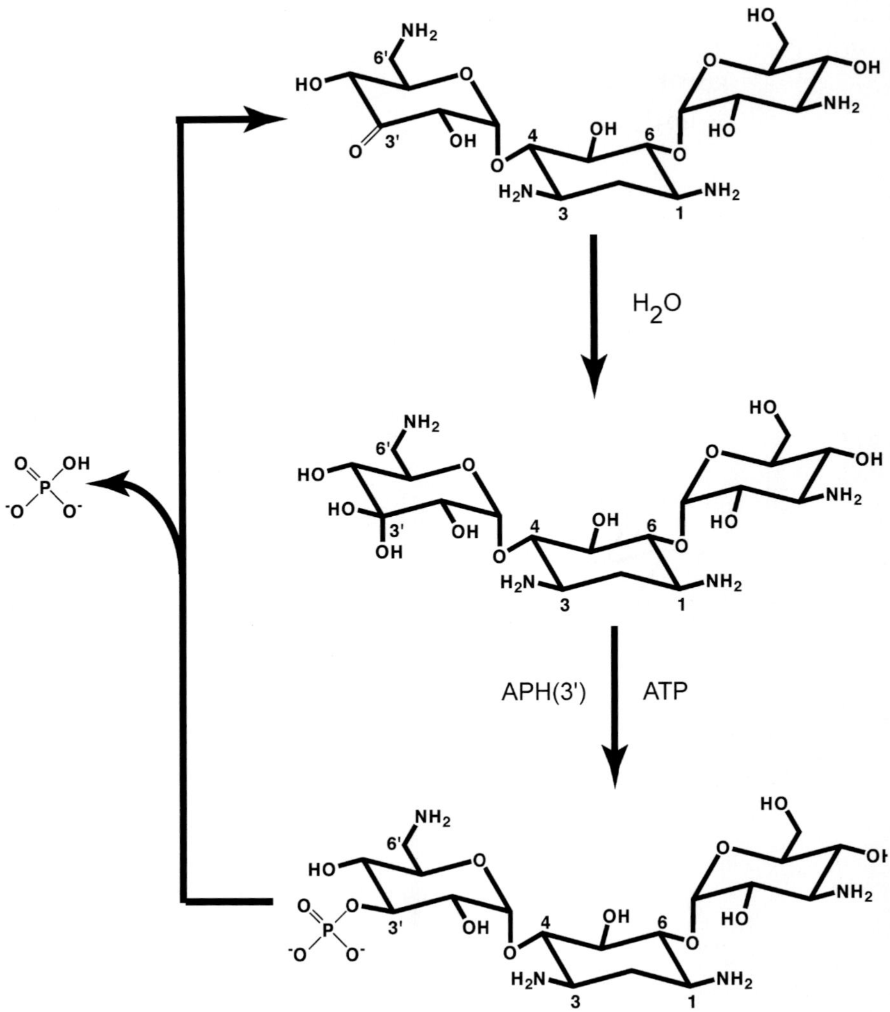

Fig. 9 Reaction cycle of 3′-oxo-kanamycin. Although a good substrate for APH(3′) phosphotransferases, the phosphorylated product is unstable and is spontaneously dephosphorylated to regenerate the original compound

rapidly eliminated, generating an electrophilic nitroalkene. The reactive electrophilic intermediate can in turn capture an active-site nucleophilic amino acid side chain and form a covalent bond, irreversibly inactivating the enzymes.

A more recent derivative is 3′-oxo-kanamycin A, a self-regenerating aminoglycoside, in which the hydroxyl group at 3′-position is replaced by a ketone (Haddad et al. 1999) (Fig. 9). The hydrated variant of this compound is a good substrate for APH(3′) enzymes. However, the phosphorylated product is unstable and releases the inorganic phosphate in a spontaneous non-enzymatic way, regenerating the parent compound. The antibiotic is therefore not inactivated, making the resistance enzymes obsolete.

The molecular recognition of aminoglycosides in both the ribosomal A-site and all three classes of resistance enzymes is accomplished in analogous ways. In the case of APH(3′) enzymes, this is illustrated by comparing the binding of paromomycin I to the 16S ribosomal RNA (Carter et al. 2000) and neomycin B to APH(3′)-IIIa (Fong and Berghuis 2002). The crystal structure of the 30S ribosome in complex with different aminoglycosides (including paromomycin I) has been solved (Carter et al. 2000). Paromomycin I is a 4,5-disubstituted 2-deoxystreptamine aminoglycoside that can be inactivated by many APH(3′) enzymes. The structure of paromomycin I closely resembles that of neomycin B; the only difference is in the functional group at the 6′-position, where paromomycin I has a hydroxyl and neomycin B an amino group. Comparison of the binding of neomycin B to APH(3′)-IIIa and paromomycin I to the A-site of the bacterial ribosome reveals that the conformation of the aminoglycosides and the hydrogen bond network between the aminoglycoside and their respective targets are essentially identical. However, the two complexes differ considerably in their van der Waals interactions. The face of the aminoglycoside that makes most of the van der Waals interactions with APH(3′)-IIIa is opposite to that which interacts with the bacterial ribosome (Fong and Berghuis 2002) (Fig. 10). The similarities in aminoglycoside binding to the two targets explain the effectiveness of APH(3′)-IIIa as a resistance factor, but more importantly, the differences in binding mechanism can be exploited in the design strategies of inhibitors

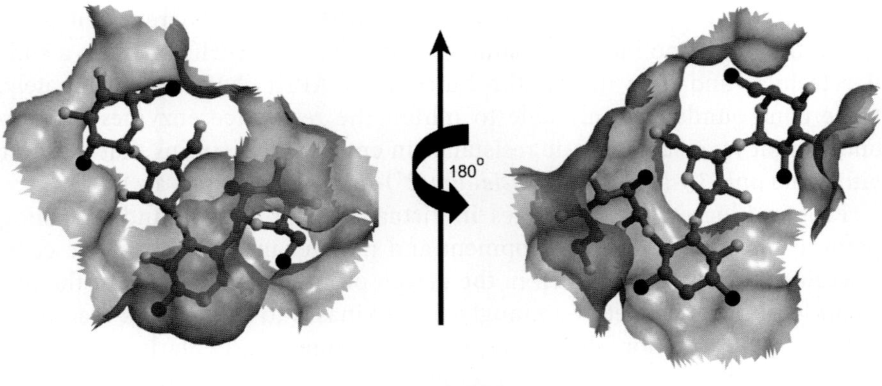

Fig. 10 The van der Waals surface of the aminoglycoside binding site of APH(3′)-IIIa (*left*) and the bacterial ribosome (*right*). APH(3′)-IIIa is shown with bound neomycin B, while the ribosome structure has bound paromomycin I. Atoms of the ball-and-stick illustrations of the aminoglycoside are colour coded as follows: oxygen, *light grey*; carbon, *grey*; nitrogen, *black*

and novel aminoglycoside variants. For example, the binding of aminoglycoside derivatives can be blocked by modifying the corresponding face with bulky chemical moieties (Fong and Berghuis 2002; Vicens and Westhof 2003).

4.2 Targeting the Nucleotide-Binding Pocket

Studies on aminoglycoside kinase inhibitors that target the nucleotide binding site were prompted by the elucidation of the three-dimensional structure of APH(3′)-IIIa. As discussed above, the overall structure of APH(3′)-IIIa is remarkably similar to that of eukaryotic protein kinases, especially in the ATP binding domain (see Sect. 3). This finding led to the survey of the effectiveness of a wide range of ePK inhibitors such as the indole carbazoles, the flavonoids, and the isoquinolinesulphonamides (which are all competitive inhibitors of ATP) against aminoglycoside kinases (Daigle et al. 1997). The basis of this study was that molecules that target the nucleotide-binding site would prevent the binding of ATP and thus disrupt the enzyme function. One limitation of this approach of inhibitor design is that only those aminoglycoside-modifying enzymes that use ATP cofactors would be inhibited. Of the three classes of ePK inhibitors tested, the isoquinolinesulphonamides (Fig. 11a) have been found to be good competitive inhibitors of ATP for both APH(3′)-IIIa and the bifunctional enzyme, AAC(6′)-Ie-APH(2″)-Ia. Structural studies reveal that these inhibitors bind to the active site of protein kinases by forming a hydrogen bond between the nitrogen of the isoquinoline and the main chain amide hydrogen of the linker peptide that joins the N- and the C-terminal domains (Engh et al. 1996; Xu et al. 1996). An analogous hydrogen bond is also observed between the N1 of the purine ring in ADP or AMPPNP and the linker of APH(3′)-IIIa. Therefore, it is inferred that isoquinolinesulphonamides would bind to APH(3′)-IIIa in a similar fashion and thus inhibit the function of APH(3′)-IIIa. Unfortunately, these compounds are only able to inhibit the resistance enzymes in vitro and cannot reverse antibiotic resistance in enterococcal strains that harbour either the *aph(3′)-IIIa* or *aac(6′)-Ie-aph(2″)-Ia* gene (Daigle et al. 1997).

Protein kinases play key roles in virtually every activity and signalling pathway involved in the development and maintenance of eukaryotic cells. Therefore, care must be taken in the design of inhibitors directed at the nucleotide-binding pocket of aminoglycoside kinases to avoid cross-reactivity. Structural information about the proteins becomes particularly valuable in this respect. By examining the structures of APHs and ePKs, it is possible to identify distinguishing features that might be utilized in the development of compounds that would selectively inhibit APHs without affecting host protein kinases (Boehr et al. 2002). For example, the crystal structure of APH(3′)-IIIa showed that Tyr42 is located near the nucleotide binding site

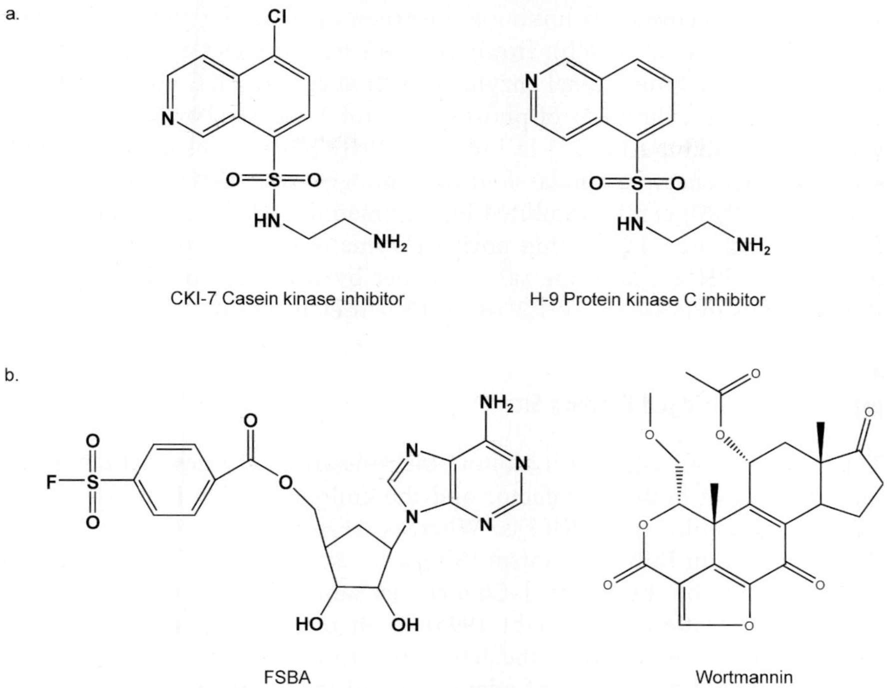

Fig. 11 **a** Structures of two isoquinolinesulphonamide inhibitors of protein kinases. **b.** Structures of FSBA (*left*) and wortmannin (*right*), protein kinase inhibitors that target the nucleotide-binding site

and that its aromatic ring side chain forms stacking interactions with the adenine moiety of ATP. This residue is highly conserved as either a tyrosine or phenylalanine among APH(3′) enzymes, but it is predominantly an alanine in protein kinases (Burk et al. 2001). The orientation of the adenine ring in protein kinases and APH(3′)-IIIa also differs by a rotation of about 40° due to the difference in electrostatic interactions in the nucleotide binding site (Burk et al. 2001; Burk and Berghuis 2002). It is possible that such a difference could be exploited to produce an inhibitor specific to APHs, eluding the problem of protein kinase inhibition by APH inhibitors.

Another complication to overcome in the development of broad spectrum antibiotics that target the nucleotide binding site are the differences in the active sites between various APHs. As described earlier in this section, APH(3′)-IIIa and AAC(6′)-Ie-APH(2″)-Ia display definite selectivity towards one specific class of protein kinase inhibitor, implying that the nucleotide binding sites have critical differences (Boehr et al. 2001a). This issue was further illustrated by Wright et al. using 5′-[*p*-(fluorosulfonyl)benzoyl]adenosine (FSBA) and wortmannin (Fig. 11b) (Boehr et al. 2001a). Previous experiments showed that FSBA, a hydrophilic ATP analogue, inactivates

APH(3′)-IIIa by covalently linking to invariant Lys44 in the nucleotide-binding site (McKay et al. 1994b). However, FSBA has no effect on the APH(2″)-Ia portion of the bifunctional enzyme (Boehr et al. 2001a). Conversely, wortmannin, a potent inhibitor of phosphoinositol 3-kinase (Powis et al. 1994), was able to inhibit APH(2″)-Ia but not APH(3′)-IIIa. Phosphatidylinositol kinase, which shares a similar fold as aminoglycoside and protein kinases (Rao et al. 1998), can be inhibited by wortmannin, which covalently modifies Lys802 in the ATP-binding pocket (Wymann et al. 1996). Wortmannin inactivates APH(2″)-Ia in the same manner by covalently binding to Lys52 [homologous to Lys44 in APH(3′)-IIIa] (Boehr et al. 2001a).

4.3 Exploiting the Bridged Binding Site

The feasibility of designing inhibitors for resistance enzymes that target the binding sites of both the cofactor and the aminoglycoside is based on the enzyme mechanism of APH(3′)s. Whereas APH(3′)-Ia functions by a random equilibrium BiBi mechanism (Siregar et al. 1995), APH(3′)-IIIa catalyses its reaction by the Theorell–Chance mechanism, a form of ordered BiBi mechanism (McKay and Wright 1995). Both mechanisms require that all substrates must be present in the active site prior to catalysis. Using this approach, tethered derivatives of adenosine and the aminoglycoside neamine have been synthesized (Liu et al. 2000). These bisubstrate analogues are made by covalently linking the 5′-hydroxyl of adenosine to the 3′-hydroxyl of neamine via methylene linkers of various lengths (Fig. 12). Appropriate linker lengths that very nearly span the distance between the ATP and the aminoglycoside binding sites should manifest themselves by showing strong inhibition of the resistance enzyme. When tested against the APH(3′)-Ia and APH(3′)-IIIa, compounds with linkers of 6–7 carbons in length were found to be the most potent competitive inhibitors of both ATP and kanamycin A.

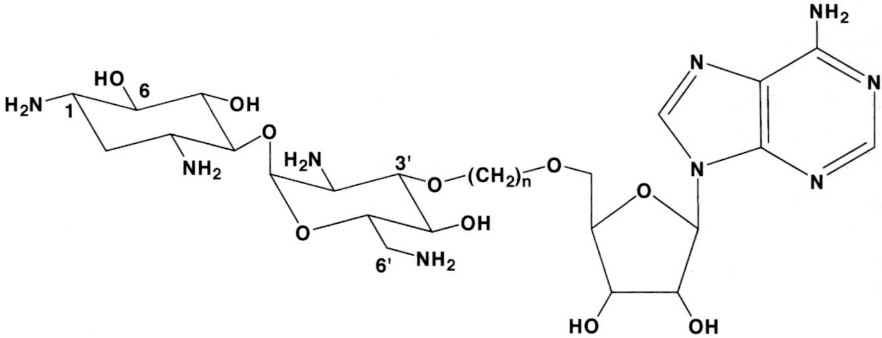

Fig. 12 A tethered derivative of adenosine and neamine that targets both the nucleotide- and substrate-binding sites of aminoglycoside-modifying enzymes

These bisubstrate inhibitors must contain many elements required for binding both regions of the active site of aminoglycoside kinases. The specificity of the molecule is increased and the problem of cross-reactivity with host protein kinases can be circumvented. Nevertheless, the breadth of activity of these molecules is reduced, since they are able to bind only those resistance factors that utilize ATP. In addition, the requirement for sufficient specificity in both binding pockets means that compounds that are developed to meet these conditions are likely to be large. Such compounds are unlikely to be effective therapeutic agents, due to issues associated with membrane transport of large molecules (Burk and Berghuis 2002).

4.4
Alternative Strategies for Circumventing Antibiotic Resistances

In addition to the investigation of the inhibition of APHs using ePK inhibitors that target ATP binding, the discovery of the structural similarities between aminoglycoside and protein kinases also led to the examination of the ability of APHs to phosphorylate protein kinase substrates (Daigle et al. 1999b). APH(3′)-IIIa and APH(2″)-Ia (of the bifunctional enzyme) were shown to be capable of phosphorylating peptide substrates, but at a much slower rate than the phosphorylation of aminoglycosides. The binding modes of peptide substrates were examined by modelling studies using the structure of APH(3′)-IIa. The crystal structure of APH(3′)-IIa in complex with kanamycin A is the newest addition to the array of structural information on aminoglycoside-modifying enzymes (Nurizzo et al. 2003). The cAMP kinase inhibitor PKI in the conformation observed in the crystal structure of cAMP-dependent protein kinase (Zheng et al. 1993) was modelled into the active site of APH(3′)-IIa (Smith and Baker 2002). The peptide can be readily accommodated in the binding site of APH(3′)-IIa with very few steric hindrances detected between the inhibitor and the resistance enzyme.

The possibility of using cationic peptides as starting molecules for the development of broad-spectrum inhibitors of resistance enzyme activities was therefore examined (Boehr et al. 2003). Due to the large number of negatively charged residues in the binding pockets of aminoglycoside-modifying enzymes, positively charged peptides are the preferred substrates. Both APH(3′)-IIIa and APH(2″)-Ia were inhibited by protegrin, indolicidin and its analogue, CP10A, in a non-competitive manner with both ATP and kanamycin. The inhibition patterns demonstrate that the peptides bind to both the free enzyme and to enzyme-substrate complexes. Together, these results suggest that the peptide inhibitors have multiple binding modes and may span both the ATP and aminoglycoside binding sites. Furthermore, the modelling study of cAMP kinase PKI and APH(3′)-IIa corroborated the inhibition kinetics experiments that showed that PKI fully occupied the aminoglycoside binding site as well as a large portion of the putative ATP binding site (Smith and Baker 2002). Although some antimicrobial peptides are able to penetrate the cytoplasm of the bacterium, many are known to act on the cytoplasmic membrane (Wu et al. 1999). Unfortunately, none of the peptides that inhibited resistance enzymes in vitro displayed synergistic antimicrobial properties with aminoglycosides in organisms harbouring resistance genes (Boehr et al. 2003).

5 Conclusions

Despite the tremendous success of antibiotics over the past 50 years, infectious diseases remain a serious problem for public health due to the prevalence of antibiotic-resistant pathogens. Aminoglycoside resistance is no longer restricted to the hospital environment, but now represents a problem for communities in both developing and developed worlds. To date, there is no known inhibitor of aminoglycoside-modifying enzymes that can be used in combination with existing aminoglycosides in a clinical setting. Ideally, a single inhibitor would be designed that would block the function of all the aminoglycoside-modifying enzymes. However, the design of a molecule that would bind effectively to binding sites of all three classes of enzymes would be extremely difficult. Although the negatively charged aminoglycoside-binding sites are a common feature in all three classes of resistant enzymes, differing ranges of substrate specificity and regiospecificity give rise to distinct features in the various classes of enzymes. However, it is plausible to develop a compound which would effectively block the activity of one family of enzymes, despite subtle differences between enzymes within each family. The design of new antibacterial agents that bind to the A-site of the bacterial ribosome is also equally challenging. A newly designed molecule has to fulfill an array of prerequisites before it can be considered as a drug candidate. It will have to be taken up into the bacterial cell, bind to the bacterial ribosome, interfere with protein translation and be a poor substrate for resistance enzymes. Given the findings on aminoglycoside inhibition by APHs described here and as more mechanistic and structural information on aminoglycoside-modifying enzymes becomes available, it is possible that the restoration of current aminoglycosides as well as the development of new aminoglycoside and nucleotide derivatives with antibacterial activity may indeed be possible in the future.

References

Alper PB, Hendrix M, Sears P, Wong C-H (1998) Probing the specificity of aminoglycoside-ribosomal RNA interactions with designed synthetic analogs. J Am Chem Soc 120:1965–1978

Beck E, Ludwig G, Auerswald EA, Reiss B, Schaller H (1982) Nucleotide sequence and exact localization of the neomycin phosphotransferase gene from transposon Tn5. Gene 19:327–36

Berman JD, Fleckenstein L (1991) Pharmacokinetic justification of antiprotozoal therapy. A US perspective. Clin Pharmacokinet 21:479–493

Boehr DD, Draker K, Koteva K, Bains M, Hancock RE, Wright GD (2003) Broad-spectrum peptide inhibitors of aminoglycoside antibiotic resistance enzymes. Chem Biol 10:189–96

Boehr DD, Lane WS, Wright GD (2001a) Active site labeling of the gentamicin resistance enzyme AAC(6′)-APH(2″) by the lipid kinase inhibitor wortmannin. Chem Biol 8:791–800

Boehr DD, Thompson PR, Wright GD (2001b) Molecular mechanism of aminoglycoside antibiotic kinase APH(3′)-IIIa: roles of conserved active site residues. J Biol Chem 276:23929–36

Boehr DD, Farley AR, Wright GD, Cox JR (2002) Analysis of the pi-pi stacking interactions between the aminoglycoside antibiotic kinase APH(3′)-IIIa and its nucleotide ligands. Chem Biol 9:1209–17

Burk DL, Berghuis AM (2002) Protein kinase inhibitors and antibiotic resistance. Pharmacol Ther 93:283–92

Burk DL, Hon WC, Leung AK-W, Berghuis AM (2001) Structural analyses of nucleotide binding to an aminoglycoside phosphotransferase. Biochemistry 40:8756–8764

Carter AP, Clemons WM, Brodersen DE, Morgan-Warren RJ, Wimberly BT, Ramakrishnan V (2000) Functional insights from the structure of the 30S ribosomal subunit and its interactions with antibiotics. Nature 407:340–348

Cundliffe E (1989) How antibiotic-producing organisms avoid suicide. Annu Rev Microbiol 43:207–33

Daigle DM, McKay GA, Wright GD (1997) Inhibition of aminoglycoside antibiotic resistance enzymes by protein kinase inhibitors. J Biol Chem 272:24755–8

Daigle DM, Hughes DW, Wright GD (1999a) Prodigious substrate specificity of AAC(6′)-APH(2″), an aminoglycoside antibiotic resistance determinant in enterococci and staphylococci. Chem Biol 6:99–110

Daigle DM, McKay GA, Thompson PR, Wright GD (1999b) Aminoglycoside antibiotic phosphotransferases are also serine protein kinases. Chem Biol 6:11–8

Davies JE (1991) Aminoglycoside-aminocyclitol antibiotics and their modifying enzymes. In: Lorian V (ed) Antibiotics in laboratory medicine. Williams & Wilkins, Baltimore, pp 691–713

Engh RA, Girod A, Kinzel V, Huber R, Bossemeyer D (1996) Crystal structures of catalytic subunit of cAMP-dependent protein kinase in complex with isoquinolinesulfonyl protein kinase inhibitors H7, H8, and H89. Structural implications for selectivity. J Biol Chem 271:26157–64

Ferretti JJ, Gilmore KS, Courvalin P (1986) Nucleotide sequence analysis of the gene specifying the bifunctional 6′-aminoglycoside acetyltransferase 2″-aminoglycoside phosphotransferase enzyme in Streptococcus faecalis and identification and cloning of gene regions specifying the two activities. J Bacteriol 167:631–8

Fong DH, Berghuis AM (2002) Substrate promiscuity of an aminoglycoside antibiotic resistance enzyme via target mimicry. EMBO J 21:2323–2331
Forge A, Schacht J (2000) Aminoglycoside antibiotics. Audiol Neurootol 5:3-22
Fourmy D, Recht MI, Blanchard SC, Puglisi JD (1996) Structure of the A site of Escherichia coli 16S ribosomal RNA complexed with an aminoglycoside antibiotic. Science 274:1367–71
Fourmy D, Recht MI, Puglisi JD (1998) Binding of neomycin-class aminoglycoside antibiotics to the A-site of 16 S rRNA. J Mol Biol 277:347–62
Fujimura S, Tokue Y, Takahashi H, Nukiwa T, Hisamichi K, Mikami T, Watanabe A (1998) A newly recognized acetylated metabolite of arbekacin in arbekacin-resistant strains of methicillin-resistant Staphylococcus aureus. J Antimicrob Chemother 41:495–7
Fujimura S, Tokue Y, Takahashi H, Kobayashi T, Gomi K, Abe T, Nukiwa T, Watanabe A (2000) Novel arbekacin- and amikacin-modifying enzyme of methicillin-resistant Staphylococcus aureus. FEMS Microbiol Lett 190:299–303
Gray GS, Fitch WM (1983) Evolution of antibiotic resistance genes: the DNA sequence of a kanamycin resistance gene from Staphylococcus aureus. Mol Biol Evol 1:57–66
Greenberg WA, Priestley ES, Sears PS, Alper PB, Rosenbohm C, Hendrix M, Hung S-C, Wong C-H (1999) Design and synthesis of new aminoglycoside antibiotics containing neamine as an optimal core structure: correlation of antibiotic activity with in vitro inhibition of translation. J Am Chem Soc 121:6527–6541
Haddad J, Vakulenko S, Mobashery S (1999) An antibiotic cloaked by its own resistance enzyme. J Am Chem Soc 121:11922–11923
Haddad J, Kotra LP, Llano-Sotelo B, Kim C, Azucena EF Jr, Liu M, Vakulenko SB, Chow CS, Mobashery S (2002) Design of novel antibiotics that bind to the ribosomal acyltransfer site. J Am Chem Soc 124:3229–37
Holm SE, Hill B, Lowestad A, Maller R, Vikerfors T (1983) A prospective, randomized study of amikacin and gentamicin in serious infections with focus on efficacy, toxicity and duration of serum levels above the MIC. J Antimicrob Chemother 12:393–402
Hon WC, McKay GA, Thompson PR, Sweet RM, Yang DS, Wright GD, Berghuis AM (1997) Structure of an enzyme required for aminoglycoside antibiotic resistance reveals homology to eukaryotic protein kinases. Cell 89:887–95
Hotta K, Zhu CB, Ogata T, Sunada A, Ishikawa J, Mizuno S, Ikeda Y, Kondo S (1996) Enzymatic 2′-N-acetylation of arbekacin and antibiotic activity of its product. J Antibiot (Tokyo) 49:458–64
Hotta K, Sunada A, Ishikawa J, Mizuno S, Ikeda Y, Kondo S (1998) The novel enzymatic 3″-N-acetylation of arbekacin by an aminoglycoside 3-N-acetyltransferase of Streptomyces origin and the resulting activity. J Antibiot (Tokyo) 51:735–42
Ida T, Okamoto R, Shimauchi C, Okubo T, Kuga A, Inoue M (2001) Identification of aminoglycoside-modifying enzymes by susceptibility testing: epidemiology of methicillin-resistant Staphylococcus aureus in Japan. J Clin Microbiol 39:3115–21
Inouye S, Tamura A, Niizato T, Takeuchi T, Hamada M, Kondo S (1996) Antibacterial activity and nephrotoxicity of two novel 2″-amino derivatives of arbekacin. J Infect Chemother 2:84–89
Johnson LN, Noble ME, Owen DJ (1996) Active and inactive protein kinases: structural basis for regulation. Cell 85:149–58
Kawaguchi H, Naito T, Nakagawa S, Fujisawa KI (1972) BB-K 8, a new semisynthetic aminoglycoside antibiotic. J Antibiot (Tokyo) 25:695–708
Knighton DR, Zheng JH, Ten Eyck LF, Ashford VA, Xuong NH, Taylor SS, Sowadski JM (1991) Crystal structure of the catalytic subunit of cyclic adenosine monophosphate-dependent protein kinase. Science 253:407–14

Kondo S, Iinuma K, Yamamoto H, Ikeda Y, Maeda K (1973a) Letter: Synthesis of (S)-4-amino-2-hydroxybutyryl derivatives of 3′,4′-dideoxykanamycin B and their antibacterial activities. J Antibiot (Tokyo) 26:705–7

Kondo S, Iinuma K, Yamamoto H, Maeda K, Umezawa H (1973b) Letter: Syntheses of 1-n-(S)-4-amino-2-hydroxybutyryl)-kanamycin B and −3′, 4′-dideoxykanamycin B active against kanamycin-resistant bacteria. J Antibiot (Tokyo) 26:412–5

Kondo S, Shibahara S, Usui T, Kudo T, Tamura A, Gomi S, Ikeda Y, Ikeda D, Takeuchi T (1993a) New 2″-amino derivatives of arbekacin, potent aminoglycoside antibiotics against methicillin-resistant Staphylococcus aureus. J Antibiot (Tokyo) 46:531–4

Kondo S, Tamura A, Gomi S, Ikeda Y, Takeuchi T, Mitsuhashi S (1993b) Structures of enzymatically modified products of arbekacin by methicillin-resistant. Staphylococcus aureus. J Antibiot (Tokyo) 46:310–5

Kondo S, Ikeda Y, Ikeda D, Takeuchi T, Usui T, Ishii M, Kudo T, Gomi S, Shibahara S (1994) Synthesis of 2″-amino-2″-deoxyarbekacin and its analogs having potent activity against methicillin-resistant Staphylococcus aureus. J Antibiot (Tokyo) 47:821–32

Kondo S, Hotta K (1999) Semisynthetic aminoglycoside antibiotics: Development and enzymatic modifications. J Infect Chemother 5:1-9

Leclercq R, Dutka-Malen S, Brisson-Noel A, Molinas C, Derlot E, Arthur M, Duval J, Courvalin P (1992) Resistance of enterococci to aminoglycosides and glycopeptides. Clin Infect Dis 15:495–501

Liu M, Haddad J, Azucena E, Kotra LP, Kirzhner M, Mobashery S (2000) Tethered bisubstrate derivatives as probes for mechanism and as inhibitors of aminoglycoside 3′-phosphotransferases. J Org Chem 65:7422–31

Llano-Sotelo B, Azucena EF Jr, Kotra LP, Mobashery S, Chow CS (2002) Aminoglycosides modified by resistance enzymes display diminished binding to the bacterial ribosomal aminoacyl-tRNA site. Chem Biol 9:455–63

Madhusudan, Trafny EA, Xuong NH, Adams JA, Ten Eyck LF, Taylor SS, Sowadski JM (1994) cAMP-dependent protein kinase: crystallographic insights into substrate recognition and phosphotransfer. Protein Sci 3:176–87

Martel A, Masson M, Moreau N, Le Goffic F (1983) Kinetic studies of aminoglycoside acetyltransferase and phosphotransferase from Staphylococcus aureus RPAL. Relationship between the two activities. Eur J Biochem 133:515–21

McKay G, Thompson P, Wright G (1994a) Broad spectrum aminoglycoside phosphotransferase type III from Enterococcus: overexpression, purification, and substrate specificity. Biochemistry 33:6936–6944

McKay GA, Robinson RA, Lane WS, Wright GD (1994b) Active-site labeling of an aminoglycoside antibiotic phosphotransferase (APH(3′)-IIIa). Biochemistry 33:14115–20

McKay GA, Wright GD (1995) Kinetic mechanism of aminoglycoside phosphotransferase type IIIa. Evidence for a Theorell-Chance mechanism. J Biol Chem 270:24686–92

McKay GA, Roestamadji J, Mobashery S, Wright GD (1996) Recognition of aminoglycoside antibiotics by enterococcal-staphylococcal aminoglycoside 3′-phosphotransferase type IIIa: role of substrate amino groups. Antimicrob Agents Chemother 40:2648–50

Moazed D, Noller HF (1987) Interaction of antibiotics with functional sites in 16S ribosomal RNA. Nature 327:389–94

Nagabhushan TL, Cooper AB, Tsai H, Daniels PJ, Miller GH (1978) The syntheses and biological properties of 1-N-(S-4-amino-2-hydroxybutyryl)-gentamicin B and 1-N-(S-3-amino-2-hydroxypropionyl)-gentamicin B. J Antibiot (Tokyo) 31:681–7

Nurizzo D, Shewry SC, Perlin MH, Brown SA, Dholakia JN, Fuchs RL, Deva T, Baker EN, Smith CA (2003) The crystal structure of aminoglycoside-3′-phosphotransferase-IIa, an enzyme responsible for antibiotic resistance. J Mol Biol 327:491–506

Ogle JM, Murphy FV, Tarry MJ, Ramakrishnan V (2002) Selection of tRNA by the ribosome requires a transition from an open to a closed form. Cell 111:721–32

Oka A, Sugisaki H, Takanami M (1981) Nucleotide sequence of the kanamycin resistance transposon Tn903. J Mol Biol 147:217–26

Owen DJ, Noble ME, Garman EF, Papageorgiou AC, Johnson LN (1995) Two structures of the catalytic domain of phosphorylase kinase: an active protein kinase complexed with substrate analogue and product. Structure 3:467–82

Papadopoulou B, Courvalin P (1988) Dispersal in Campylobacter spp. of aphA-3, a kanamycin resistance determinant from gram-positive cocci. Antimicrob Agents Chemother 32:945–8

Pape T, Wintermeyer W, Rodnina MV (2000) Conformational switch in the decoding region of 16S rRNA during aminoacyl-tRNA selection on the ribosome. Nat Struct Biol 7:104–7

Powis G, Bonjouklian R, Berggren MM, Gallegos A, Abraham R, Ashendel C, Zalkow L, Matter WF, Dodge J, Grindey G, et al (1994) Wortmannin, a potent and selective inhibitor of phosphatidylinositol-3-kinase. Cancer Res 54:2419–23

Rao VD, Misra S, Boronenkov IV, Anderson RA, Hurley JH (1998) Structure of type IIbeta phosphatidylinositol phosphate kinase: a protein kinase fold flattened for interfacial phosphorylation. Cell 94:829–39

Rodnina MV, Daviter T, Gromadski K, Wintermeyer W (2002) Structural dynamics of ribosomal RNA during decoding on the ribosome. Biochimie 84:745–54

Roestamadji J, Mobashery S (1998) The use of neamine as a molecular template: inactivation of bacterial antibiotic resistance enzyme aminoglycoside 3′-phosphotransferase type IIa. Bioorg Med Chem Lett 8:3483–3486

Roestamadji J, Grapsas I, Mobashery S (1995a) Loss of individual electrostatic interactions between aminoglycoside antibiotics and resistance enzymes as an effective means to overcoming bacterial drug resistance. J Am Chem Soc 117:11060–11069

Roestamadji J, Grapsas I, Mobashery S (1995b) Mechanism-based inactivation of bacterial aminoglycoside 3′-phosphotransferases. J Am Chem Soc 117:80–84

Russell RJ, Murray JB, Lentzen G, Haddad J, Mobashery S (2003) The complex of a designer antibiotic with a model aminoacyl site of the 30S ribosomal subunit revealed by X-ray crystallography. J Am Chem Soc 125:3410–1

Schatz A, Bugie E, Waksman SA (1944) Streptomycin, a substance exhibiting antibiotic activity against gram-positive and gram-negative bacteria. Proc Soc Exp Biol Med 55:66–69

Schmitz FJ, Fluit AC, Gondolf M, Beyrau R, Lindenlauf E, Verhoef J, Heinz HP, Jones ME (1999) The prevalence of aminoglycoside resistance and corresponding resistance genes in clinical isolates of staphylococci from 19 European hospitals. J Antimicrob Chemother 43:253–9

Shaw KJ, Rather PN, Hare RS, Miller GH (1993) Molecular genetics of aminoglycoside resistance genes and familial relationships of the aminoglycoside-modifying enzymes. Microbiol Rev 57:138–163

Siregar JJ, Miroshnikov K, Mobashery S (1995) Purification, characterization, and investigation of the mechanism of aminoglycoside 3′-phosphotransferase type Ia. Biochemistry 34:12681–8

Smith CA, Baker EN (2002) Aminoglycoside antibiotic resistance by enzymatic deactivation. Curr Drug Targets Infect Disord 2:143–60

Sucheck SJ, Wong AL, Koeller KM, Boehr DD, Draker K-a, Sears P, Wright GD, Wong C-H (2000) Design of bifunctional antibiotics that target bacterial rRNA and inhibit resistance-causing enzymes. J Am Chem Soc 122:5230–5231

Taylor DE, Yan W, Ng LK, Manavathu EK, Courvalin P (1988) Genetic characterization of kanamycin resistance in Campylobacter coli. Ann Inst Pasteur Microbiol 139:665–76

Taylor SS, Knighton DR, Zheng J, Ten Eyck LF, Sowadski JM (1992) Structural framework for the protein kinase family. Annu Rev Cell Biol 8:429–62

Thompson J, Skeggs PA, Cundliffe E (1985) Methylation of 16S ribosomal RNA and resistance to the aminoglycoside antibiotics gentamicin and kanamycin determined by DNA from the gentamicin-producer, Micromonospora purpurea. Mol Gen Genet 201:168–73

Thompson PR, Hughes DW, Wright GD (1996a) Mechanism of aminoglycoside 3′-phosphotransferase type IIIa: His188 is not a phosphate-accepting residue. Chem Biol 3:747–55

Thompson PR, Hughes DW, Wright GD (1996b) Regiospecificity of aminoglycoside phosphotransferase from Enterococci and Staphylococci (APH(3′)-IIIa). Biochemistry 35:8686–8695

Trieu-Cuot P, Courvalin P (1983) Nucleotide sequence of the Streptococcus faecalis plasmid gene encoding the 3′5″-aminoglycoside phosphotransferase type III. Gene 23:331–41

Tsukiura H, Saito K, Kobaru S, Konishi M, Kawaguchi H (1973) Aminoglycoside antibiotics. IV. BU-1709 E1 and E2, new aminoglycoside antibiotics related to the butirosins. J Antibiot (Tokyo) 26:386–8

Udo EE, Dashti AA (2000) Detection of genes encoding aminoglycoside-modifying enzymes in staphylococci by polymerase chain reaction and dot blot hybridization. Int J Antimicrob Agents 13:273–9

Umezawa H, Umezawa S, Tsuchiya T, Okazaki Y (1971a) 3′,4′-dideoxy-kanamycin B active against kanamycin-resistant Escherichia coli and Pseudomonas aeruginosa. J Antibiot (Tokyo) 24:485–7

Umezawa S, Tsuchiya T, Muto R, Nishimura Y, Umezawa H (1971b) Synthesis of 3′-deoxykanamycin effective against kanamycin-resistant Escherichia coli and Pseudomonas aeruginosa. J Antibiot (Tokyo) 24:274–6

Vakulenko SB, Mobashery S (2003) Versatility of aminoglycosides and prospects for their future. Clin Microbiol Rev 16:430–50

Vicens Q, Westhof E (2003) Molecular recognition of aminoglycoside antibiotics by ribosomal RNA and resistance enzymes: an analysis of x-ray crystal structures. Biopolymers 70:42–57

Wright GD, Berghuis AM, Mobashery S (1998) Aminoglycoside antibiotics. Structures, functions, and resistance. Adv Exp Med Biol 456:27–69

Wright JJ (1976) Synthesis of 1-*N*-ethylsisomicin: a broad-spectrum semisynthetic aminoglycoside antibiotic. J Chem Soc Chem Commun 6:206–208

Wu M, Maier E, Benz R, Hancock RE (1999) Mechanism of interaction of different classes of cationic antimicrobial peptides with planar bilayers and with the cytoplasmic membrane of Escherichia coli. Biochemistry 38:7235–42

Wymann MP, Bulgarelli-Leva G, Zvelebil MJ, Pirola L, Vanhaesebroeck B, Waterfield MD, Panayotou G (1996) Wortmannin inactivates phosphoinositide 3-kinase by covalent modification of Lys-802, a residue involved in the phosphate transfer reaction. Mol Cell Biol 16:1722–33

Xu RM, Carmel G, Sweet RM, Kuret J, Cheng X (1995) Crystal structure of casein kinase-1, a phosphate-directed protein kinase. EMBO J 14:1015–23

Xu RM, Carmel G, Kuret J, Cheng X (1996) Structural basis for selectivity of the isoquinoline sulfonamide family of protein kinase inhibitors. Proc Natl Acad Sci U S A 93:6308–13

Yamaguchi H, Hendrickson WA (1996) Structural basis for activation of human lymphocyte kinase Lck upon tyrosine phosphorylation. Nature 384:484–9

Zheng J, Knighton DR, ten Eyck LF, Karlsson R, Xuong N, Taylor SS, Sowadski JM (1993) Crystal structure of the catalytic subunit of cAMP-dependent protein kinase complexed with MgATP and peptide inhibitor. Biochemistry 32:2154–61

Zhou J, Adams JA (1997) Is there a catalytic base in the active site of cAMP-dependent protein kinase? Biochemistry 36:2977–84

Part III

Pharmacological Potential and Inhibitors of Individual Classes of Protein Phosphatases

HEP (2005) 167:191–214

Protein Tyrosine Phosphatases as Therapeutic Targets

A. Cheng · N. Uetani · C. Lampron · M. L. Tremblay (✉)

McGill Cancer Centre and Department of Biochemistry, McGill University,
3655 Promenade Sir William Osler, Montreal, QC, H3G 1Y6, Canada
michel.tremblay@mcgill.ca

Abstract The protein tyrosine phosphatases (PTPs) are a family of regulatory enzymes that are critical for a wide variety of cellular functions. During the last decade, the interest and findings on the role of PTPs in signal transduction have increased tremendously. Initially, these enzymes were viewed as negative regulators of signaling cascades triggered by protein tyrosine kinases (PTKs). It is now well established that several members of the PTP family are also positive regulators of several signaling pathways. Compelling evidence from biochemical, cell biology, and gene-targeting studies has implicated PTPs in multiple processes that include metabolism, development, immunity, and cancer. Indeed, mutations in several PTP genes are associated with human disorders. Moreover, many pathological organisms have acquired specific PTPs or target host cell PTPs to increase virulence and promote their own propagation. Taken together, these findings identified specific PTPs as significant targets for the therapeutic intervention in human diseases. For instance, the discovery that PTP1B is a negative regulator of insulin signaling revealed that this molecule is an attractive target for the treatment of insulin-resistant diseased states like type 2 diabetes mellitus and obesity. At the other end of the spectrum, the phosphatases of the CDC25 subfamily, which are key regulators of the cell cycle, are currently targeted for the treatment of cancers. These are just two examples that are discussed in this review. Although, we are still in the infancy in understanding PTP function, several of these enzymes are currently intensely investigated for their potential therapeutic values.

Keywords Protein tyrosine phosphatase · Tyrosine phosphorylation · Signal transduction · Microbial phosphatase · Therapeutic targets

1 Introduction

1.1 Background

Reversible phosphorylation on tyrosine residues represents an important means by which cells regulate signal transduction. Tyrosine phosphorylation is known to alter protein conformation, modulate enzymatic activity, and also create binding sites for the recruitment of signaling proteins involved in the regulation of many basic biological processes such as cell proliferation, differentiation, migration, apoptosis, and embryogenesis (Blume-Jensen and Hunter 2001). The control of intracellular tyrosine phosphorylation levels depends on the coordinated action of two opposing enzymes, the protein tyrosine kinases (PTKs) and the protein tyrosine phosphatases (PTPs). To date, most studies have focused on PTKs, and, subsequently, much remains to be discovered concerning the physiological functions of PTPs. Nevertheless, several enzymes within this family have recently received much attention as attractive targets for the treatment of several diseases, including diabetes and cancer.

1.2 PTPs and Impact on Public Health

In the last 5 years, the PTP field has rapidly gained special interest with particular emphasis on PTP1B. Gene targeting studies in mice strongly supported that PTP1B is involved in the insulin resistance associated with type 2 diabetes mellitus (Elchebly et al. 1999a; Klaman et al. 2000a). This disease and associated disorders are becoming a serious threat to human health with a global figure of about 150 million people affected. Moreover, mutations in genes coding for different members of the PTP family have been associated with various congenital diseases (Minassian et al. 1998; Serratosa et al. 1999; Digilio et al. 2002; Legius et al. 2002; Tartaglia et al. 2002). Overexpression of several PTPs has also been observed in several human cancers, including breast and colon cancers (Tabiti et al. 1995; Lee et al. 2000; Pestell et al. 2000; Saha et al. 2001). These observations together indicate that PTPs are key factors of many different diseases with a wide impact on public health. PTPs are also critical factors for several pathogens that cause a large spectrum of diseases worldwide, amongst which typhoid fever is still responsible for 600,000 deaths annually (Pang et al. 1998) and *Helicobacter pylori*, which is responsible for gastric ulcer and malignancy, infects about half of the world population (Rothenbacher and Brenner 2003). Thus, selected PTPs may also represent novel targets against particular infectious diseases. In this review, we will describe the recent findings demonstrating the implication of PTPs in human diseases and health care. We will also discuss the therapeutic potential of targeting various members of the PTP family.

2 Review

2.1 PTP Family

Members of the PTP superfamily of structurally related enzymes are defined by a highly conserved catalytic domain. Within this 250 amino acid region, the active site signature sequence [HCXXGXXR] contains the invariant cysteine residue that is critical for PTP activity (Tonks and Neel 2001). Sequence data from the human genome and recent estimates from the literature predict the existence of 117 members for the PTP family (see the Gene Ontology Consortium at http://www.geneontology.org/ and http://science.novonordisk.com/ptp/). Based on their sequences, structures, and functions we divided the PTP family into three categories: (1) the low molecular weight PTPs (LMW PTPs), (2) the dual-specific phosphatase (DSP), and (3) the phosphotyrosine-specific enzymes (classical PTPs).

LMW PTPs represent a small group of 18-kDa enzymes with broad tissue expression (Raugei et al. 2002). Overexpression of LMW PTPs in cells has been shown to dephosphorylate the platelet-derived growth factor receptor (PDGFR) (Chiarugi et al. 1995), p190RhoGTPase-activating protein (p190RhoGAP) (Chiarugi et al. 2000), as well as the epinephrineA2 (EphA2) kinase (Kikawa et al. 2002). These studies link LMW PTPs to both growth factor and adhesion signaling, suggesting that they may be important for many cellular processes, including mitogenesis and transformation. Recently, LMW PTP was also proposed to play a positive role in T cell receptor signaling similar to the one proposed for CD45 (Bottini et al. 2002). However, the physiological functions of these enzymes remain unclear.

DSPs have the ability to dephosphorylate both tyrosine and serine/threonine residues. The most prominent members include the Vaccinia virus phosphatase-related enzymes, cell division cycle 25 (CDC25), and the mitogen-activated protein kinase (MAPK) phosphatases (MKPs). The best-characterized functions of these examples involve the regulation of the MAPK pathway and cell cycle progression (Keyse 2000; Lyon et al. 2002). Another interesting group of DSPs include the PTEN (phosphatase and tensin homolog deleted on chromosome 10) and myotubularin phosphatases (Maehama et al. 2001). Although the sequence of their catalytic domains is similar to other DSPs, both PTEN and myotubularin act primarily as phosphoinositide phosphatases. In contrast, their activity on protein substrates remains in doubt. Nevertheless, the importance of these two enzymes is highlighted by the presence of mutations that are responsible for severe human diseases, including cancer and muscular development.

The classical PTPs—the major group of the PTP family—comprise two groups, the intracellular and transmembrane (receptor type) enzymes, from which 17 subtypes were derived based upon their sequence similarity among catalytic PTP domains (Andersen et al. 2001). The receptor type PTPs generally contain an extra-cellular segment with putative ligand-binding domains, a single transmembrane region and one or two cytoplasmic catalytic domains, where the first domain contains most if not all catalytic activity. The intracellular PTPs have a single catalytic domain and varying amino- or carboxy-terminal extensions containing protein-binding domains that are believed to have targeting or regulatory functions (Tonks and Neel 2001).

Despite the large heterogeneity in all the PTP subgroups, the crystal structure of several members (mostly catalytic domains) revealed that they all display a similar core folding feature (Barford 1999; Andersen et al. 2001). Thus, this common active site structure suggests that these enzymes use a similar mechanism for catalysis (Zhang 1998; Li and Dixon 2000; Kolmodin and Aqvist 2001).

2.2 Enzyme/Substrate Specificity

The above observations raise questions as to how enzyme/substrate specificity can be achieved despite common active site structure. Although binding affinity is primarily dependent on the catalytic site, the specificity is mainly achieved by a substrate-induced conformational change through specific interactions involving contacts outside the catalytic site that favor catalysis (Barford 2001; Zhang et al. 2002). In the case of the classical PTPs the situation is not as clear and was recently reviewed (Ostman and Bohmer 2001; Tonks and Neel 2001). A likely model is that, in vivo, individual PTPs act against a limited number of cellular targets and that a given cellular target is probably regulated by more than one PTP. However, it appears that each PTP performs a unique interaction with a substrate, indicating that intrinsic catalytic domain specificity exists (Tonks and Neel 2001). Recent studies on the DSP Cdc14 elegantly demonstrate how this can occur (Gray et al. 2003).

A variety of protein interacting domains have been described for PTPs, including Src homology 2 (SH2) domains, proline-rich motifs (interacting with SH3 domains), PDZ domains, and band 4.1 homology domains (Li and Dixon 2000; Ostman and Bohmer 2001; Tonks and Neel 2001; Raugei et al. 2002). Targeting signals to the nucleus or the endoplasmic reticulum have also been identified in some PTPs. Post-translational isoprenylation of members of the PTP4A subfamily was suggested to help direct these molecules to the plasma membrane (Cates et al. 1996) Therefore, substrate selectivity is dependent to some extent on the protein interacting motifs and targeting signals contained in each intracellular PTP. Following these lines, it is evident that several mechanisms such as structural properties, subcellular localization, associated proteins, and others, concur to restrict the PTP members to their corresponding substrates and thereby specifying their physiological roles.

2.3 Regulation of PTP Action

Temporal activation of PTPs is another important factor in the regulation of PTP action. Activation can be regulated at the transcriptional level, or by post-translational mechanisms such as phosphorylation on serine/threonine residues (Draetta and Eckstein 1997; Digilio et al. 2002; Zheng et al. 2002), or on tyrosine residues (Ostman and Bohmer 2001; Raugei et al. 2002). Furthermore, enzymatic activity can be inhibited rapidly and reversibly by oxidation of the essential catalytic cysteine residue (Mahadev et al. 2001; Meng et al. 2002; Raugei et al. 2002). Intramolecular interactions, such as disulfide bonds (Caselli et al. 1994; Caselli et al. 1998) and blockade of the catalytic site by SH2 domains (Hof et al. 1998), have also been suggested to be important mechanisms to inhibit PTP activity. For receptor type PTPs, ligand-induced dimerization can result in inhibition of phosphatase activity of some enzymes like PTP-α, CD45 (Majeti et al. 1998), and possibly PTP-β/ζ (Deuel et al. 2002). Activation and alteration of subcellular localization patterns following calpain-mediated proteolytic cleavage is yet another means of regulation for intracellular PTP1B (Frangioni et al. 1993; Rock et al. 1997), PTPMEG (Gu and Majerus 1996; Pasquet et al. 1998), and more recently for the receptor type PTP-α and PTP-ϵ (Gil-Henn et al. 2001).

		Name	Related Human diseases/therapeutic targets/physiological roles
LMW		LMW PTP	positively regulates growth factor and adhesion signaling
DSP		Cdc25	various cancers, positively regulates cell cycle
DSP		PTEN	hamartoma-neoplasia syndrome
pTyr-specific (Classical) PTPs	Cytosolic	PTP1B	diabetes, obesity, breast and ovarian cancers
		TCPTP	diabetes, macrophage activation, cytokine signaling
		SHP-1	leukemias, breast, ovarian, prostate and pancreatic cancers
		SHP-2	Noonan and Leopard syndromes, myeloid leukemias
		PTP-PEST	PAPA syndrome (autoinflammatory disease)
	Receptor Type	CD45	severe combined immunodeficiency disease (SCID), autoimmune diseases, antibody-based therapy
		PTPα	colon cancer, diabetes, positively regulates signaling via Src
		PTPε	positively regulates signaling via Src phosphorylation
		LAR	diabetes, neuronal development and regeneration
		PTPσ	neuronal development and regeneration
		PTPδ	learning and memory, neurite outgrowth
		DEP1	p120(ctn) and beta-catenin regulation, vascular development
		PTPβ	neuronal migration, neurite outgrowth, gliogenesis

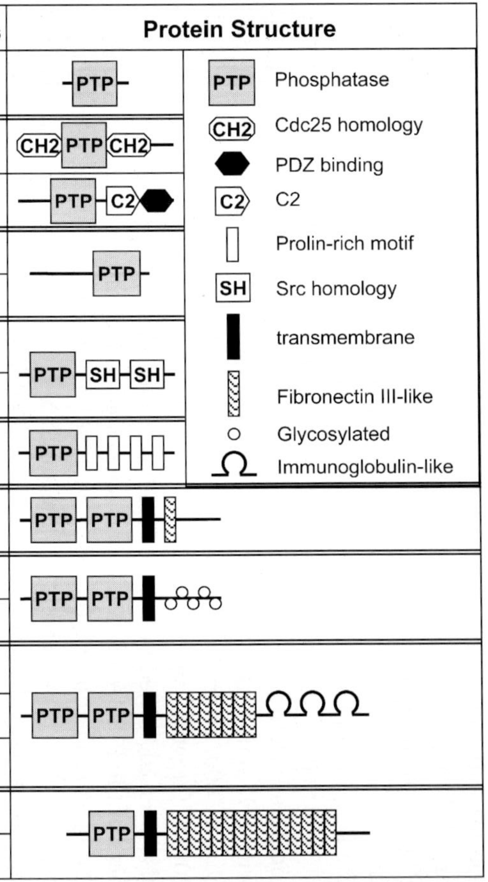

Fig. 1 Summary of the PTP family members that are involved in human diseases. These are potential therapeutic targets

2.4
Involvement of PTP in Human Diseases

The physiological functions of PTPs have primarily been derived from gene-targeting studies in mice or genetic studies involving human diseases (Li and Dixon 2000). It is easily noted that PTPs are involved in a variety of biological functions that include embryonic development, hematopoiesis, immunity, metabolism, and others (Fig. 1). It stands to reason that although PTPs are affected in several genetic and metabolic diseases, not all can serve as therapeutic targets. For example, those diseases that are caused by a loss of function may mainly be targeted using gene therapy approaches (i.e., PTEN and SHP-1, see below). A caveat would be that in dominant-negative mutations, gene therapy would unlikely be usable. Other approaches that could specifically target the mutated PTPs, such as antisense or siRNA, could then serve as potential therapeutic treatment.

First, we discuss below PTP1B in diabetes and obesity as a paradigm, and the following will summarize recent findings that demonstrate a relevant role of various PTPs in specific human disease applications. For some, we will also reveal their current state as therapeutic targets either for PTP candidates for pharmaceutical inhibition or as potential targets for gene therapies.

2.4.1
Metabolic Diseases

2.4.1.1
PTP1B

Undeniably, PTP1B has been the most studied PTP to date as judged by the recent numerous publications and its potential impact in the diabetes field. The intense focus on PTP1B is primarily based on the observation that PTP1B is a negative regulator of insulin and leptin signal transduction (Cheng et al. 2002a; Cook and Unger 2002). Indeed, PTP1B-deficient mice display both increased insulin (Elchebly et al. 1999a; Klaman et al. 2000b) and leptin signaling (Cheng et al. 2002b; Zabolotny et al. 2002). Furthermore, PTP1B may also modulate the metabolic functions of growth hormone (Gu et al. 2003). Importantly, these mice are resistant to diabetes obesity.

The direct implication of PTP1B in these human diseases is further fortified by the identification of associated mutations and polymorphisms in the human PTP1B gene. The PTP1B locus maps to human chromosome 20 in the region q13.1-q13.2 (Brown-Shimer et al. 1990) and its mouse ortholog to the syntenic H2-H3 region of chromosome 2 (Forsell et al. 2000). Interestingly, this region was also identified as a quantitative trait loci (QTL) linked to insulin and obesity (Lembertas et al. 1997). Consistent with a role for PTP1B in human insulin resistance, single nucleotide polymorphisms have been found within the coding region (Echwald et al. 2002; Mok et al. 2002) or the 3′ untranslated region (UTR) (Di Paola et al. 2002), both of which are associated with diabetic parameters.

The identification of PTP1B as a critical regulator of insulin action has led to an explosive motivational force to generate PTP1B inhibitors. It is not surprising that there exist a number of approaches for developing anti-PTP compounds. Such ongoing programs are presently examining the efficacy of small-molecule inhibitors directed against the catalytic site, antisense oligonucleotides, monoclonal antibodies and gene therapy. It is now accepted that inhibition of PTP1B represents the best paradigm for the development of PTP inhibitors in the treatment of type 2 diabetes and obesity. Considerable efforts to derive small chemical inhibitors of PTP1B guided by the information acquired on structural biology were initiated with some successes (reviewed in Johnson et al. 2002 and the chapter by Møller et al. in this volume).

One of the driving forces in the PTP field stems from the early observations that vanadate, a competitive inhibitor of PTPs, possesses insulin-mimetic properties. However, vanadate is non-specific in its action towards PTPs, and it presents toxic effects as it accumulates in the body. Novel PTP1B inhibitors have been designed using multiple approaches, and include both phosphorus and non-phosphorus derivatives. To date, the most potent PTP1B inhibitor published possesses a K_i of 2.4 nM (Zhang et al. 2002). This compound has also been shown to increase insulin receptor (IR) phosphorylation of hepatoma cells when used at the micromolar range. Currently, the major challenge in developing specific PTP1B small-molecule inhibitors is to find selectivity against T cell (TC)-PTP, the most closely related PTP, and the identification of suitable physico-chemical properties for oral delivery.

An alternative approach to small molecule inhibitors is the technology of antisense oligonucleotides (ASO). As a proof-of-concept demonstration, Abbott Laboratories and ISIS pharmaceuticals recently utilized PTP1B ASO in mouse models. The injection of a PTP1B ASO (ISIS-113715) in hyperglycemic obese mice was recently reported to improve insulin sensitivity (Zinker et al. 2002) and to modulate fat storage and lipogenesis in adipose tissue (Rondinone et al. 2002). Administration of their ASO was able to decrease PTP1B expression in both adipose and liver tissue. The resulting treated mice displayed increased insulin sensitivity and reduction in adiposity. Phase I clinical trials were announced last spring (2003).

Although PTP1B clearly plays a negative role in insulin signaling, its effects seem to be tissue specific. In particular, IR phosphorylation in adipose tissue seems unperturbed in PTP1B-deficient mice. This raises the possibility that other PTPs such as PTP-$\alpha$and leukocyte antigen-related PTP (LAR), may participate in this process (Cheng et al. 2002a). For example, LAR knockout mice exhibit alterations in glucose metabolism, albeit with only modest increases in IR phosphorylation (Ren et al. 1998). In contrast, muscle-specific transgenic expression of LAR in mice does seem to suggest that this enzyme may play a causative role in insulin resistance that is observed in diabetes (Zabolotny et al. 2001). In recent reports, TC-PTP has also been found to dephosphorylate the IR (Galic et al. 2003). Confirmation of this finding in animal studies is ongoing.

2.4.2 Cancer

Intuitively, since the majority of oncogenes are tyrosine kinases, it was previously thought that PTPs might act as tumor suppressors. However, it is now clear that PTPs may act negatively or positively in modulating signaling pathways. In the past 5 years several examples of both type of action by PTPs in cancer have been reported, leading to the possible validation of some of those PTPs as genuine targets in cancer treatment. The following are some of the most obvious examples.

2.4.2.1 CDC25

The dual-specific phosphatase CDC25 members, CDC25A, -B and -C, are all known to act as positive regulators at distinct phases of the mammalian cell cycle through their ability to dephosphorylate and activate cyclin-dependent kinases (CDKs) (Nilsson and Hoffmann 2000). CDC25A is likely to be important for G1/S phase transition, in preserving genomic integrity and initiation of mitosis, while CDC25B and CDC25C act on the G2/M transition phase (Lazo et al. 2002). CDC25A and CDC25B possess oncogenic properties (Galaktionov et al. 1995), are transcriptional targets of the c-myc proto-oncogene (Galaktionov et al. 1996), and are overexpressed in various human tumors (Cangi et al. 2000; Pestell et al. 2000). Already, they have been reported to be important genes in prognostic studies, where expression of both CDC25A and CDC25B correlate with survival in patients suffering from ovarian cancers (Broggini et al. 2000). On the other hand, despite the biochemical evidence that implicates CDC25C in proliferation and transformation, CDC25C-deficient mice do not display an overt phenotype (Chen et al. 2001). Perhaps functional redundancy exists among the three family members.

One attractive aspect of CDC25 inhibitor development lies in the unique structural features of these enzymes compared to other PTPs. The crystal structures of CDC25A and CDC25B have both been solved, and show that most of the similarity to other PTPs is found in the active site loop containing the PTP signature motif. Focusing on diverging motifs may facilitate the design of specific inhibitors of the CDC25 PTPs. Furthermore, very little similarity exists between the three family members, and this may allow for an additional level of specificity.

Most CDC25 inhibitory compounds reported to date have been derived from both synthetic and natural products (Pestell et al. 2000). In particular, a vitamin K analog (a quinine derivative) has recently been shown to be a potent CDC25 inhibitor, and possesses anti-proliferative properties when administered to breast cancer and hepatoma cell lines (Kar and Carr 2000; Kar et al. 2003). This compound acts in the micromolar range, and thus more studies will likely be needed to increase effectiveness.

2.4.2.2 PTEN

PTEN (also called MMAC1 or TEP1) is a member of the dual-specific PTPs. PTEN was originally identified as a candidate tumor suppressor gene located on human chromosome 10q23. Recent studies have demonstrated that somatic mutations in PTEN are responsible for hamartoma-neoplasia syndrome such as Cowden, Bannayan-Zonana, and Lhermitte-Duclos diseases (Wishart and Dixon 2002). Although PTEN possesses both protein and lipid phosphatase activities, it preferentially dephosphorylates phospholipids. It is also its lipid phosphatase activity that is essential for PTEN tumor suppression (Maehama et al. 2001). Among D3-phosphorylated inositol phospholipids, PtdIns(3,4,5)P3 has been shown as the principal physiological substrate of PTEN, which regulates Akt and PDK1 activity.

2.4.2.3 Other PTPs Involved in Cancer Development

One promising target reported in the PTP family is the dual phosphatase PRL-3 and its closely related homolog PRL-1. These PTPs have been shown to promote invasiveness of cancer cells in vitro, and PRL3 was also found in metastatic human liver tumors (Saha et al. 2001; Zeng et al. 2003). Thus, targeting of PRL3 may provide an excellent means to prevent the development of metastasis.

SHP-1 is a SH2 domain-containing cytoplasmic PTP, and it is predominantly expressed in hematopoietic cells. SHP-1 has been suggested as a tumor suppressor and its expression is dramatically decreased in most lymphocytic-related cancers, as well as in breast, ovarian, prostate, and pancreatic cancers (Wu et al. 2003). SHP-2 is a close relative of SHP-1 and may also play an important role in cancer. Mutations in this gene are found in myeloid leukemias such as non-syndromic juvenile myelomonocytic leukemia (Tartaglia et al. 2003).

Unlike the PTPs mentioned above, the evidence for the role of other PTPs in malignant transformation is less substantial. However, loss of heterozygosity (LOH) for a few PTPs has been demonstrated in various types of cancers. As mentioned above, LOH for SHP-1 occurs with high frequency in lymphoblastic leukemias (Oka et al. 2002). PTP-κ, whose expression is developmentally regulated in the CNS, was recently shown to exhibit LOH in 76% of CNS lymphomas (Nakamura et al. 2003). DEP1 is a candidate for the mouse colon-cancer susceptibility locus *Scc1* and is frequently deleted in human cancers (Ruivenkamp et al. 2002).

PTP-PEST is a cytosolic enzyme that was found to modulate the actin cytoskeleton and focal adhesion turnover (Angers-Loustau et al. 1999; Garton and Tonks 1999). Following fibronectin signaling activation, a cascade of tyrosine phosphorylation events is initiated that cumulate into the tyrosine phosphorylation of the adaptor protein p130cas. From this protein, several signals branch out that promote actin polymerization to cell proliferation. By inhibiting PTP-PEST activity, one may thus block cell migration as was shown with the knockout PTP-PEST fibroblasts (Angers-Loustau et al. 1999). Hence, specific inhibitors of PTP-PEST could serve as anti-metastatic agents and anti-angiogenic agents.

On the other hand, PTPs can also play a positive role in cellular transformation. PTP-α is a receptor PTP that activates Src kinases via dephosphorylation of the C-terminal negative regulatory site. Overexpression of PTP-α causes cellular transformation of fibroblasts via activation of Src kinases (Zheng et al. 1992; den Hertog et al. 1993). Conversely, in fibroblasts lacking PTP-α, both Src and Fyn activation are diminished under resting conditions as well as during integrin signaling (Ponniah et al. 1999; Su et al. 1999). In human colon cancer, increased expression of PTP-α has been observed (Tabiti et al. 1995). PTP-ϵ, which is closely related to PTP-α, also has been suggested to activate Src kinase. It has been shown that absence of PTP-ϵ reduced Src activity and altered Src phosphorylation in neu-induced mammary tumor cells (Gil-Henn and Elson 2003). Interestingly, increased Src expression and activity are also increased in colon cancer, suggesting a possible link. On the same theme, PTP1B has been reported to similarly dephosphorylate the negative regulatory site of c-src (Arregui et al. 1998; Bjorge et al. 2000; Cheng et al. 2001). Moreover, PTP1B was reported to be increased in expression in breast and ovarian cancers (Wiener et al. 1994a,b; Zhai et al. 1993). These findings suggest that in many instances selectable inhibition of PTP activity would be a suitable means for cancer treatment.

2.4.3
Noonan Syndrome and SHP-2

SHP-2 is a widely expressed non-receptor PTP that contains two amino-terminal SH2 domains, a carboxyl-terminal catalytic domain and a C-terminal segment containing two tyrosine phosphorylation sites (Feng 1999). Several studies to delineate the function of SHP-2 in cell signaling demonstrate that it primarily acts as a positive regulator of the cellular response to growth factors, hormones, cytokines, and cell adhesion molecules, and thus it is a critical regulator of proliferation and differentiation. However, it can act as a negative regulator in some pathways. Recently, it has been shown that germline mutations in PTPN11, which encodes SHP-2, cause Noonan syndrome and the related Leopard syndrome, both sharing several clinical features such as facial dysmorphia, short stature, and cardiac defects (Tartaglia et al. 2001; Digilio et al. 2002; Legius et al. 2002; Tartaglia et al. 2002). As mentioned above, mutations in SHP-2 also can lead to myeloid leukemias (Tartaglia et al. 2003). Interestingly, these mutations are suggested to result in a gain of function of SHP-2 where the intramolecular inhibitory binding of the amino-SH2 domain would be lost, resulting in a constitutive activation of the phosphatase. SHP-2 may be also important in pathogenesis by *Helicobacter pylori* (see Sect. 2.4.6). These findings support the potential value for SHP-2 specific inhibitors as therapeutic agents. In contrast with gain of function, SHP-2 gene knockout mice show embryonic lethality at midgestation and data from SHP-2 gene knockout and SHP-2 chimeric mice clearly indicate that this PTP is essential for hematopoiesis and multiple embryonic development.

2.4.4 Neuronal Development and Nerve Regeneration

The closely related receptor type PTPs, LAR, PTP-δ and PTP-σ have been shown to play crucial roles in axon growth and guidance (Johnson and Van Vactor 2003). The extracellular segment of these proteins consists of three immunoglobulin-like repeats and four to eight type III fibronectin repeats generated by alterative splicing. These structures resemble cell adhesion molecules (CAMs) and they are specifically expressed in the CNS, suggesting cellular roles during axon guidance and synapse formation. Consistent with this notion, *Drosophila* mutants in the closely related receptor-type PTP (RPTP) (Dlar and DPTP69D) exhibit severe defects in axonal pathfinding (Johnson and Van Vactor 2003).

Genetic studies in mice have strongly implicated these enzymes in the development of the nervous system (Yeo et al. 1997; Elchebly et al. 1999; Wallace et al. 1999; Uetani et al. 2000). Recently PTP-σ has been shown as a negative modulator of neurite outgrowth, and PTP-σ knockout mice functionally recover faster than wild-type mice after facial and sciatic nerve axotomy in vivo (McLean et al. 2002; Thompson et al. 2003). By comparison, the absence of LAR delays recovery of sensory, but not of motor, nerve function following sciatic nerve injury (Xie et al. 2001). Furthermore, the extracellular domains of LAR and PTP-δ function as a homophilic ligand and promote neurite outgrowth (Wang and Bixby 1999; Yang et al. 2003). These data suggest that targeting these PTPs may achieve an improvement in nerve regeneration after neuronal injuries.

Another enzyme involved in human neuronal diseases is the DSP Laforin. Positional cloning identified this gene in Lafora's disease, an autosomal progressive myoclonus epilepsy (Minassian et al. 1998; Serratosa et al. 1999). Genetically engineered mice deficient for Laforin show most of the symptoms of Lafora's disease, and may provide a model to understand the cellular mechanisms of Lafora's disease (Ganesh et al. 2002).

2.4.5 PTPs and Immunomodulation

2.4.5.1 CD45

CD45 is the prototypical transmembrane PTP, and is highly expressed in all hematopoietic lineages (Sasaki et al. 2001). It is well established that CD45 is critical for T and B cell activation, primarily via activation of the Src kinase Lck (Thomas 1999). Under resting conditions, Lck is maintained in an inactive state via intramolecular interactions between its C-terminal phosphorylated tyrosine (Y505) and its SH2 domain. During TCR engagement, CD45 dephosphorylates Y505 on Lck, thus allowing for activation of kinase activity. Activated Lck then phosphorylates its substrates to transmit the TCR signals that ultimately lead to transcription of genes that are important for T cell function, such as interleukin-2.

Mice lacking CD45 demonstrate impaired T cell differentiation and activation as well as B cell activation and are therefore severely immunodeficient (Kishihara et al. 1993; Byth et al. 1996). Two recent descriptions of clinically relevant CD45 mutations associated with severe combined immunodeficiency disease (SCID) in humans correlate well with the phenotype reported for the CD45-deficient mice (Kung et al. 2000; Tchilian et al. 2001). In those cases, mutations of CD45 confirm that this PTP serves as a modifier gene in immunodeficiency.

As a therapeutic target, anti-CD45 antibodies have demonstrated an antileukemic effect when used either unconjugated or attached to radioactive iodine (Nemecek and Matthews 2002). For example, ^{131}I-labeled anti-CD45 antibodies have been used to deliver radiation directly to leukemic cells, because CD45 is found on cell surface isolated from most of leukemia patient samples (Countouriotis et al. 2002). Clinical trials of this antibody-based therapy using anti-CD45 antibodies are currently in phase I/II (www.clinicaltrials.gov).

CD45 is also presumed to be a good immunomodulatory molecule to promote transplantation tolerance based on its accessibility as a transmembrane protein (Fecteau et al. 2001; Ko et al. 2002; Pagel et al. 2002). Allograft rejection is a T cell-dependent process, and interference with T cell activation through T cell receptor (TCR) can induce anergy in $CD4^+$ T cell clones. Indeed, in this context, allograft rejection has been shown to be suppressed using an antibody against CD45RB isoforms (Lazarovits et al. 1996). One possible mechanism by which such an interaction induces allograft tolerance involves the upregulation of CTLA4 (cytolytic T lymphocyte-associated antigen 4) which is an important T cell down-regulatory molecule (Fecteau et al. 2001).

Very recently, it has been shown that 77 C/G mutation in the human CD45 gene, which results in increasing CD45RA isoform expression on cell surface, is linked to several autoimmune diseases such as systemic sclerosis and hepatitis (Vogel et al. 2003), suggesting CD45 inhibitors and/or antibodies are potent therapeutics for those autoimmune diseases.

2.4.5.2
Other PTPs in the Immune System

Since the discovery that loss-of-function mutations in SHP-1 are responsible for systemic autoimmunity and severe inflammation observed in both *motheaten* and *viable motheaten* mice, SHP-1 has been shown as a major negative regulator of various signaling pathways, including T and B cell antigen receptors in hematopoietic cells (Zhang et al. 2000). Although SHP-1 has been strongly suggested to associate with various cancers and infectious diseases (see also Sects. 2.4.2 and 2.4.6), further investigation of its pathogenic roles in those diseases is proposed to develop therapeutic agents for SHP-1 associated diseases.

PTP-PEST is also highly expressed in hematopoietic cells (Cote et al. 2002). Recent work by Davidson and Veillette (2001) indicates that it is an important negative modulator of lymphocyte activation. In addition, an exciting report by Wise et al. (2002) pointed to the lack of PTP-PEST association with the adaptor protein proline serine threonine phosphatase-interacting protein (PST-PIP) as the cause of pyogenic sterile arthritis, pyoderma gangrenosum, and acne (PAPA) syndrome, an autoinflammatory disorder.

2.4.6
PTPs in Infectious Diseases

Microbial pathogens are responsible for a large spectrum of diseases that are leading causes of morbidity and mortality worldwide. Of interest are the pathogens expressing virulence factors that block animal defense reactions or alter host cell function through modulating tyrosine phosphorylation to facilitate their life cycle. Several also express their own PTPs that are essential for their infectious properties. It stands to reason that focusing on inhibiting those PTP may be a new approach in blocking these infectious agents.

2.4.6.1
Salmonella

Salmonellosis has been known as a foodborne illness, and emergence of multi-drug resistant strain is threatening to become a serious public health problem. *Salmonella* expresses a DSP (named Sptp) that participates in the entry process of this pathogen into mammalian cells that are normally non-phagocytic. By inducing a phagocytic behavior, this allows the bacterium to be protected from the host immune system (Finlay and Cossart 1997). Sptp is a multidomain protein that includes a GTPase activating domain and a dual specificity PTP domain. Although little is known about the PTP domain, it seems to play a role in downregulating the MAPK pathway (Murli et al. 2001). This may act as a means to shut-off host cell functions.

2.4.6.2
Yersinia pestis

Yersinia pestis presents historical value as being responsible for the Black Plague (Fallman et al. 2002). This pathogen expresses the phosphatase YopH that contributes to block macrophage phagocytosis and slow down the onset of the inflammatory response, thus favoring pathogen survival. The activity of YopH is essential for this effect, and it suggests that dephosphorylation of host proteins participates in this mechanism. These substrates include p130Cas and Fyn binding protein. Recently, aurintricarboxylic acid has been shown as a selective YopH inhibitor, and it may be therapeutically useful (Liang et al. 2003).

2.4.6.3
Helicobacter pylori

Helicobacter pylori is a gram-negative bacterium thought to be a primary cause of gastric ulcers and cancer. Within its arsenal, the CagA and VacA proteins bind host PTPs, and these events are critical for its detrimental effects. CagA is injected into host cells and perturbs cellular functions, including the induction of morphological changes. One target of CagA has been identified as SHP-2, and disruption of this complex abolishes the effects of CagA (Higashi et al. 2002). Hence, the formation of this complex also stimulates the phosphatase activity of SHP-2. On the other hand, VacA is critical for causing massive vacuolization of the host cell, and recently this process has been shown to be dependent on its ability to bind the receptor phosphatase PTP-ζ in a ligand-like fashion (Fujikawa et al. 2003).

2.4.6.4 Other PTPs in Infectious Diseases

Leishmania donovani (Ld) is an intracellular protozoan parasite that is the causative agent of visceral leishmaniasis. Recent findings suggest that the capacity of Ld to suppress host immune responses such as macrophage phagocytosis is related to SHP-1 (Blanchette et al. 1999; Nandan et al. 2002). It has also been suggested that calpain-mediated cleavage and activation of host cell PTP1B may play a role in amebiasis caused by the protozoan *Entamoeba histolytica* (Teixeira and Mann 2002). It is well known that the transcription and replication of HIV-1 (human immunodeficiency virus 1), the causal agent of acquired immunodeficiency syndrome (AIDS), is linked to T cell activation. Interestingly, SHP-1 may act as an important host factor participating in HIV-1 long terminal repeat (LTR) transactivation (Fortin et al. 2001; Ouellet et al. 2003).

3 Conclusion

From the initial PTP studies in the early 1980s (Nelson and Branton 1984; Sparks and Brautigan 1986), to the successful purification of PTP1B (Tonks et al. 1988a,b), we have gathered an impressive knowledge on the enzymatic properties and structure of PTPs. The realization that PTP1B could potentially be an outstanding target for diabetes and obesity has launched a broad search for pharmacological inhibitors. For the past 5 years this search revealed several difficulties in finding the optimal compounds. In spite of the difficult chemistry, one may hope that these efforts will continue. As this review entails to show, a great number of other targets await the first success with PTP1B. Once an optimal compound for PTP1B is found, it would be much easier to model such a chemical(s) to the other very closely related members of the family (Andersen et al. 2001). Overall, it is clear that the PTP family holds great promise for the treatment of several human diseases, and we only need the chemistry to catch up with the outstanding biology that has been recently revealed on many of the PTP family members.

References

Andersen JN, Mortensen OH, Peters GH, Drake PG, Iversen LF, Olsen OH, Jansen PG, Andersen HS, Tonks NK, Moller NP (2001) Structural and evolutionary relationships among protein tyrosine phosphatase domains. Mol Cell Biol 21:7117–36

Angers-Loustau A, Cote JF, Charest A, Dowbenko D, Spencer S, Lasky LA, Tremblay ML (1999) Protein tyrosine phosphatase-PEST regulates focal adhesion disassembly, migration, and cytokinesis in fibroblasts. J Cell Biol 144:1019–31

Arregui CO, Balsamo J, Lilien J (1998) Impaired integrin-mediated adhesion and signaling in fibroblasts expressing a dominant-negative mutant PTP1B [published erratum appears in J Cell Biol 1998 Dec 14;143(6):1761]. J Cell Biol 143:861–73

Barford D (1999) Colworth Medal Lecture. Structural studies of reversible protein phosphorylation and protein phosphatases. Biochem Soc Trans 27:751–766

Barford D (2001) The mechanism of protein kinase regulation by protein phosphatases. Biochem Soc Trans 29:385–391

Bjorge JD, Pang A, Fujita DJ (2000) Identification of PTP1B as the major tyrosine phosphatase activity capable of dephosphorylating and activating c-Src in several human breast cancer cell lines. J Biol Chem

Blanchette J, Racette N, Faure R, Siminovitch KA, Olivier M (1999) Leishmania-induced increases in activation of macrophage SHP-1 tyrosine phosphatase are associated with impaired IFN-gamma-triggered JAK2 activation. Eur J Immunol 29:3737–44

Blume-Jensen P, Hunter T (2001) Oncogenic kinase signalling. Nature 411:355–65

Bottini N, Stefanini L, Williams S, Alonso A, Jascur T, Abraham RT, Couture C, Mustelin T (2002) Activation of ZAP-70 through specific dephosphorylation at the inhibitory Tyr-292 by the low molecular weight phosphotyrosine phosphatase (LMPTP). J Biol Chem 277:24220–24224

Broggini M, Buraggi G, Brenna A, Riva L, Codegoni AM, Torri V, Lissoni AA, Mangioni C, D'Incalci M (2000) Cell cycle-related phosphatases CDC25A and B expression correlates with survival in ovarian cancer patients. Anticancer Res 20:4835–40

Brown-Shimer S, Johnson KA, Lawrence JB, Johnson C, Bruskin A, Green NR, Hill DE (1990) Molecular cloning and chromosome mapping of the human gene encoding protein phosphotyrosyl phosphatase 1B. Proc Natl Acad Sci U S A 87:5148–52

Byth KF, Conroy LA, Howlett S, Smith AJ, May J, Alexander DR, Holmes N (1996) CD45-null transgenic mice reveal a positive regulatory role for CD45 in early thymocyte development, in the selection of CD4+CD8+ thymocytes, and B cell maturation. J Exp Med 183:1707–1718

Cangi MG, Cukor B, Soung P, Signoretti S, Moreira GJ, Ranashinge M (2000) Role of the Cdc25A phosphatase in human breast cancer. J Clin Invest 106:753–761

Caselli A, Camici G, Manao G, Moneti G, Pazzagli L, Cappugi G (1994) Nitric oxide causes inactivation of the low molecular weight phosphotyrosine protein phosphatases. J Biol Chem 269:24878–24882

Caselli A, Marzocchini R, Camici G, Manao G, Moneti G, Pieraccini G (1998) The inactivation mechanism of low molecular weight phosphotyrosine protein phosphatase by H2O2. J Biol Chem 273:32554–32560

Cates CA, Michael RL, Stayrook KR, Harvey KA, Burke YD, Randall SK, Crowell PL, Crowell DN (1996) Prenylation of oncogenic human PTP(CAAX) protein tyrosine phosphatases. Cancer Lett 110:49–55

Chen MS, Hurov J, White LS, Woodford-Thomas T, Piwnica-Worms H (2001) Absence of apparent phenotype in mice lacking Cdc25C protein phosphatase. Mol Cell Biol 21:3853–61

Cheng A, Bal GS, Kennedy BP, Tremblay ML (2001) Attenuation of adhesion-dependent signaling and cell spreading in transformed fibroblasts lacking protein tyrosine phosphatase-1B. J Biol Chem 276:25848–55

Cheng A, Dube N, Gu F, Tremblay ML (2002a) Coordinated action of protein tyrosine phosphatases in insulin signal transduction. Eur J Biochem 269:1050–1059

Cheng A, Uetani N, Simoncic PD, Chaubey VP, Lee-Loy A, McGlade CJ, Kennedy BP, Tremblay ML (2002b) Attenuation of leptin action and regulation of obesity by protein tyrosine phosphatase 1B. Dev Cell 2:497–503

Chiarugi P, Cirri P, Raugei G, Camici G, Dolfi F, Berti A, Ramponi G (1995) PDGF receptor as a specific in vivo target for low M(r) phosphotyrosine protein phosphatase. FEBS Lett 372:49–53

Chiarugi P, Cirri P, Taddei L, Giannoni E, Camici G, Manao G, Raugei G, Ramponi G (2000) The low M(r) protein-tyrosine phosphatase is involved in Rho-mediated cytoskeleton rearrangement after integrin and platelet-derived growth factor stimulation. J Biol Chem 275:4640–6

Cook WS, Unger RH (2002) Protein tyrosine phosphatase 1B: a potential leptin resistance factor of obesity. Dev Cell 2:385–7

Cote JF, Chung PL, Theberge JF, Halle M, Spencer S, Lasky LA, Tremblay ML (2002) PSTPIP is a substrate of PTP-PEST and serves as a scaffold guiding PTP-PEST toward a specific dephosphorylation of WASP. J Biol Chem 277:2973–86

Countouriotis A, Moore TB, Sakamoto KM (2002) Cell surface antigen and molecular targeting in the treatment of hematologic malignancies. Stem Cells 20:215–29

Davidson D, Veillette A (2001) PTP-PEST, a scaffold protein tyrosine phosphatase, negatively regulates lymphocyte activation by targeting a unique set of substrates. Embo J 20:3414–26

den Hertog J, Pals CE, Peppelenbosch MP, Tertoolen LG, de Laat SW, Kruijer W (1993) Receptor protein tyrosine phosphatase alpha activates pp60c-src and is involved in neuronal differentiation. Embo J 12:3789–98

Deuel TF, Zhang N, Yeh H-J, Silos-Santiago I, Wang Z-Y (2002) Pleitrophin: a cytokine with diverse functions and a novel signaling pathway. Arch Biochem Biophys 397:162–171

Di Paola R, Frittitta L, Miscio G, Bozzali M, Baratta R, Centra M, Spampinato D, Santagati MG, Ercolino T, Cisternino C, Soccio T, Mastroianno S, Tassi V, Almgren P, Pizzuti A, Vigneri R, Trischitta V (2002) A variation in 3' UTR of hPTP1B increases specific gene expression and associates with insulin resistance. Am J Hum Genet 70:806–12

Digilio MC, Conti E, Sarkozy A, Mingarelli R, Dottorini T, Marino B, Pizzuti A, Dallapiccola B (2002) Grouping of multiple-lentigines/LEOPARD and Noonan syndromes on the PTPN11 gene. Am J Hum Genet 71:389–394

Draetta G, Eckstein J (1997) Cdc25 protein phosphatases in cell proliferation. Biochim Biophys Acta 1332:M53–M63

Echwald SM, Bach H, Vestergaard H, Richelsen B, Kristensen K, Drivsholm T, Borch-Johnsen K, Hansen T, Pedersen O (2002) A P387L variant in protein tyrosine phosphatase-1B (PTP-1B) is associated with type 2 diabetes and impaired serine phosphorylation of PTP-1B in vitro. Diabetes 51:1-6

Elchebly M, Payette P, Michaliszyn E, Cromlish W, Collins S, Loy AL, Normandin D, Cheng A, Himms-Hagen J, Chan CC, Ramachandran C, Gresser MJ, Tremblay ML, Kennedy BP (1999a) Increased insulin sensitivity and obesity resistance in mice lacking the protein tyrosine phosphatase-1B gene [see comments]. Science 283:1544–8

Elchebly M, Wagner J, Kennedy TE, Lanctot C, Michaliszyn E, Itie A, Drouin J, Tremblay ML (1999b) Neuroendocrine dysplasia in mice lacking protein tyrosine phosphatase sigma. Nat Genet 21:330–3

Fallman M, Deleuil F, McGee K (2002) Resistance to phagocytosis by Yersinia. Int J Med Microbiol 291:501–9

Fecteau S, Basadonna GP, Freitas A, Ariyan C, Sayegh MH, Rothstein DM (2001) CTLA-4 up-regulation plays a role in tolerance mediated by CD45. Nat Immunol 2:58–63

Feng GS (1999) Shp-2 tyrosine phosphatase: signaling one cell or many. Exp Cell Res 253:47–54

Finlay BB, Cossart P (1997) Exploitation of mammalian host cell functions by bacterial pathogens. Science 276:718–725

Forsell PA, Boie Y, Montalibet J, Collins S, Kennedy BP (2000) Genomic characterization of the human and mouse protein tyrosine phosphatase-1B genes. Gene 260:145–53

Fortin JF, Barbeau B, Robichaud GA, Pare ME, Lemieux AM, Tremblay MJ (2001) Regulation of nuclear factor of activated T cells by phosphotyrosyl-specific phosphatase activity: a positive effect on HIV-1 long terminal repeat-driven transcription and a possible implication of SHP-1. Blood 97:2390–400

Frangioni JV, Oda A, Smith M, Salzman EW, Neel BG (1993) Calpain-catalyzed cleavage and subcellular relocation of protein phosphotyrosine phosphatase 1B (PTP-1B) in human platelets. Embo J 12:4843–56

Fujikawa A, Shirasaka D, Yamamoto S, Ota H, Yahiro K, Fukada M, Shintani T, Wada A, Aoyama N, Hirayama T, Fukamachi H, Noda M (2003) Mice deficient in protein tyrosine phosphatase receptor type Z are resistant to gastric ulcer induction by VacA of Helicobacter pylori. Nat Genet 33:375–81

Galaktionov K, Lee AK, Eckstein J, Draetta G, Meckler J, Loda M, Beach D (1995) CDC25 phosphatases as potential human oncogenes. Science 269:1575–1577

Galaktionov K, Chen X, Beach D (1996) Cdc25 cell-cycle phosphatase as a target of c-myc. Nature 382:511–517

Galic S, Klingler-Hoffmann M, Fodero-Tavoletti MT, Puryer MA, Meng TC, Tonks NK, Tiganis T (2003) Regulation of insulin receptor signaling by the protein tyrosine phosphatase TCPTP. Mol Cell Biol 23:2096–108

Ganesh S, Delgado-Escueta AV, Sakamoto T, Avila MR, Machado-Salas J, Hoshii Y, Akagi T, Gomi H, Suzuki T, Amano K, Agarwala KL, Hasegawa Y, Bai DS, Ishihara T, Hashikawa T, Itohara S, Cornford EM, Niki H, Yamakawa K (2002) Targeted disruption of the Epm2a gene causes formation of Lafora inclusion bodies, neurodegeneration, ataxia, myoclonus epilepsy and impaired behavioral response in mice. Hum Mol Genet 11:1251–1262

Garton AJ, Tonks NK (1999) Regulation of fibroblast motility by the protein tyrosine phosphatase PTP-PEST. J Biol Chem 274:3811–8

Gil-Henn H, Elson A (2003) Tyrosine phosphatase-epsilon activates Src and supports the transformed phenotype of Neu-induced mammary tumor cells. J Biol Chem 278:15579–86

Gil-Henn H, Volohonsky G, Elson A (2001) Regulation of protein-tyrosine phosphatases alpha and epsilon by calpain-mediated proteolytic cleavage. J Biol Chem 276:31772–31779

Gray CH, Good VM, Tonks NK, Barford D (2003) The structure of the cell cycle protein Cdc14 reveals a proline-directed protein phosphatase. Embo J 22:3524–35

Gu F, Dube N, Kim JW, Cheng A, Ibarra-Sanchez Mde J, Tremblay ML, Boisclair YR (2003) Protein tyrosine phosphatase 1B attenuates growth hormone-mediated JAK2-STAT signaling. Mol Cell Biol 23:3753–62

Gu M, Majerus PW (1996) The properties of the protein tyrosine phosphatase PTPMEG. J Biol Chem 271:27751–27759

Higashi H, Tsutsumi R, Muto S, Sugiyama T, Azuma T, Asaka M, Hatakeyama M (2002) SHP-2 tyrosine phosphatase as an intracellular target of Helicobacter pylori CagA protein. Science 295:683–686

Hof P, Pluskey S, Dhe-Paganon S, Eck MJ, Shoelson SE (1998) Crystal structure of the tyrosine phosphatase SHP-2. Cell 92:441–450

Johnson KG, Van Vactor D (2003) Receptor protein tyrosine phosphatases in nervous system development. Physiol Rev 83:1-24

Johnson TO, Ermolieff J, Jirousek MR (2002) Protein tyrosine phosphatase 1B inhibitors for diabetes. Nat Rev Drug Discov 1:696–709

Kar S, Carr BI (2000) Growth inhibition and protein tyrosine phosphorylation in MCF 7 breast cancer cells by a novel K vitamin. J Cell Physiol 185:386–93

Kar S, Wang M, Wilcox CS, Carr BI (2003) Antitumor and anticarcinogenic actions of Cpd 5: a new class of protein phosphatase inhibitor. Carcinogenesis 24:411–6

Keyse SM (2000) Protein phosphatases and the regulation of mitogen-activated protein kinase signalling. Curr Opin Cell Biol 12:186–92

Kikawa KD, Vidale DR, Van Etten RL, Kinch MS (2002) Regulation of the EphA2 kinase by the low molecular weight tyrosine phosphatase induces transformation. J Biol Chem 277:39274–9

Kishihara K, Penninger J, Wallace VA, Kundig TM, Kawai K, Wakeham A, Timms E, Pfeffer K, Ohashi PS, Thomas ML, et al (1993) Normal B lymphocyte development but impaired T cell maturation in CD45-exon6 protein tyrosine phosphatase-deficient mice. Cell 74:143–156

Klaman LD, Boss O, Peroni OD, Kim JK, Martino JL, Zabolotny JM, Moghal N, Lubkin M, Kim YB, Sharpe AH, Stricker-Krongrad A, Shulman GI, Neel BG, Kahn BB (2000a) Increased energy expenditure, decreased adiposity, and tissue-specific insulin sensitivity in protein-tyrosine phosphatase 1B-deficient mice. Mol Cell Biol 20:5479–5489

Klaman LD, Boss O, Peroni OD, Kim JK, Martino JL, Zabolotny JM, Moghal N, Lubkin M, Kim YB, Sharpe AH, Stricker-Krongrad A, Shulman GI, Neel BG, Kahn BB (2000b) Increased energy expenditure, decreased adiposity, and tissue-specific insulin sensitivity in protein-tyrosine phosphatase 1B-deficient mice. Mol Cell Biol 20:5479–89

Ko S, Jaeger MD, Dahlke MH, Nakajima Y, Schlitt HJ (2002) Manipulation of CD45 antigen in transplantation tolerance. Curr Mol Med 2:249–255

Kolmodin K, Aqvist J (2001) The catalytic mechanism of protein tyrosine phosphatases revisited. FEBS Lett 498:208–213

Kung C, Pingel JT, Heikinheimo M, Klemola T, Varkila K, Yoo LI, Vuopala K, Poyhonen M, Uhari M, Rogers M, Speck SH, Chatila T, Thomas ML (2000) Mutations in the tyrosine phosphatase CD45 gene in a child with severe combined immunodeficiency disease. Nat Med 6:343–345

Lazarovits AI, Poppema S, Zhang Z, Khandaker M, Le Feuvre CE, Singhal SK, Garcia BM, Ogasa N, Jevnikar AM, White MH, Singh G, Stiller CR, Zhong RZ (1996) Prevention and reversal of renal allograft rejection by antibody against CD45RB. Nature 380:717–20

Lazo JS, Nemoto K, Pestell KE, Cooley K, Southwick EC, Mitchell DA, Furey W, Gussio R, Zaharevitz DW, Joo B, Wipf P (2002) Identification of a potent and selective pharmacophore for Cdc25 dual specificity phosphatase inhibitors. Mol Pharmacol 61:720–728

Lee SW, Reimer CL, Fang L, Iruela-Arispe ML, Aaronson SA (2000) Overexpression of kinase-associated phosphatase (KAP) in breast and prostate cancer and inhibition of the transformed phenotype by antisense KAP expression. Mol Cell Biol 20:1723–1732

Legius E, Schrander-Stumpel C, Schollen E, Pulles-Heintzberger C, Gewillig M, Fryns JP (2002) PTPN11 mutations in LEOPARD syndrome. J Med Genet 39:571–574

Lembertas AV, Perusse L, Chagnon YC, Fisler JS, Warden CH, Purcell-Huynh DA, Dionne FT, Gagnon J, Nadeau A, Lusis AJ, Bouchard C (1997) Identification of an obesity quantitative trait locus on mouse chromosome 2 and evidence of linkage to body fat and insulin on the human homologous region 20q. J Clin Invest 100:1240–7

Li L, Dixon JE (2000) Form, function, and regulation of protein tyrosine phosphatases and their involvement in human diseases. Semin Immunol 12:75–84

Liang F, Huang Z, Lee SY, Liang J, Ivanov MI, Alonso A, Bliska JB, Lawrence DS, Mustelin T, Zhang ZY (2003) Aurintricarboxylic acid blocks in vitro and in vivo activity of YopH, an essential virulent factor of Yersinia pestis, the agent of plague. J Biol Chem

Lyon MA, Ducruet AP, Wipf P, Lazo JS (2002) Dual-specificity phosphatases as targets for antineoplastic agents. Nat Rev Drug Discov 1:961–76

Maehama T, Taylor GS, Dixon JE (2001) PTEN and myotubularin: novel phosphoinositide phosphatases. Annu Rev Biochem 70:247–79

Mahadev K, Zilbering A, Zhu L, Goldstein BJ (2001) Insulin-stimulated hydrogen peroxide reversibly inhibits protein- tyrosine phosphatase 1b in vivo and enhances the early insulin action cascade. J Biol Chem 276:21938–42

Majeti R, Bilwes AM, Noel JP, Hunter T, Weiss A (1998) Dimerization-induced inhibition of receptor protein tyrosine phosphatase function through an inhibitory wedge. Science 279:88–91

McLean J, Batt J, Doering LC, Rotin D, Bain JR (2002) Enhanced rate of nerve regeneration and directional errors after sciatic nerve injury in receptor protein tyrosine phosphatase sigma knock-out mice. J Neurosci 22:5481–5491

Meng TC, Fukada T, Tonks NK (2002) Reversible oxidation and inactivation of protein tyrosine phosphatases in vivo. Mol Cell 9:387–399

Minassian BA, Lee JR, Herbrick J-A, Huizenga J, Soder S, Mungall AJ, Dunham I, Gardner R (1998) Mutations in a gene encoding a novel protein tyrosine phosphatase cause progressive myoclonus epilepsy. Nat Genet 20:171–174

Mok A, Cao H, Zinman B, Hanley AJ, Harris SB, Kennedy BP, Hegele RA (2002) A single nucleotide polymorphism in protein tyrosine phosphatase PTP-1B is associated with protection from diabetes or impaired glucose tolerance in Oji-Cree. J Clin Endocrinol Metab 87:724–7

Murli S, Watson RO, Galan JE (2001) Role of tyrosine kinases and the tyrosine phosphatase SptP in the interaction of Salmonella with host cells. Cell Microbiol 3:795–810

Nakamura M, Kishi M, Sakaki T, Hashimoto H, Nakase H, Shimada K, Ishida E, Konishi N (2003) Novel tumor suppressor loci on 6q22–23 in primary central nervous system lymphomas. Cancer Res 63:737-41

Nandan D, Yi T, Lopez M, Lai C, Reiner NE (2002) Leishmania EF-1alpha activates the Src homology 2 domain containing tyrosine phosphatase SHP-1 leading to macrophage deactivation. J Biol Chem 277:50190–7

Nelson RL, Branton PE (1984) Identification, purification, and characterization of phosphotyrosine-specific protein phosphatases from cultured chicken embryo fibroblasts. Mol Cell Biol 4:1003–12

Nemecek ER, Matthews DC (2002) Antibody-based therapy of human leukemia. Curr Opin Hematol 9:316–21

Nilsson I, Hoffmann I (2000) Cell cycle regulation by the Cdc25 phosphatase family. Prog Cell Cycle Res 4:107–114

Oka T, Ouchida M, Koyama M, Ogama Y, Takada S, Nakatani Y, Tanaka T, Yoshino T, Hayashi K, Ohara N, Kondo E, Takahashi K, Tsuchiyama J, Tanimoto M, Shimizu K, Akagi T (2002) Gene silencing of the tyrosine phosphatase SHP1 gene by aberrant methylation in leukemias/lymphomas. Cancer Res 62:6390–4

Ostman A, Bohmer FD (2001) Regulation of receptor tyrosine kinase signaling by protein tyrosine phosphatases. Trends Cell Biol 11:258–66

Ouellet M, Barbeau B, Tremblay MJ (2003) Protein tyrosyl phosphatases in T cell activation: implication for human immunodeficiency virus transcriptional activity. Prog Nucleic Acid Res Mol Biol 73:69–105

Pagel JM, Matthews DC, Appelbaum FR, Bernstein ID, Press OW (2002) The use of radioimmunoconjugates in stem cell transplantation. Bone Marrow Transplant 29:807–816

Pang T, Levine MM, Ivanoff B, Wain J, Finlay BB (1998) Typhoid fever—important issues still remain. Trends Microbiol 6:131–3

Pasquet JM, Dachary-Prigent J, Nurden AT (1998) Microvesicle release is associated with extensive protein tyrosine dephosphorylation in platelets stimulated by A23187 or a mixture of thrombin and collagen. Biochem J 333:591–599

Pestell KE, Ducruet AP, Wipf P, Lazo JS (2000) Small molecule inhibitors of dual specificity protein phosphatases. Oncogene 19:6607–6612

Ponniah S, Wang DZ, Lim KL, Pallen CJ (1999) Targeted disruption of the tyrosine phosphatase PTPalpha leads to constitutive downregulation of the kinases Src and Fyn. Curr Biol 9:535–8

Raugei G, Ramponi G, Chiarugi P (2002) Low molecular weight protein tyrosine phosphatases: small, but smart. Cell Mol Life Sci 59:941–9

Ren JM, Li PM, Zhang WR, Sweet LJ, Cline G, Shulman GI, Livingston JN, Goldstein BJ (1998) Transgenic mice deficient in the LAR protein-tyrosine phosphatase exhibit profound defects in glucose homeostasis. Diabetes 47:493–7

Rock MT, Brooks WH, Roszman TL (1997) Calcium-dependent signaling pathways in T cells. Potential role of calpain, protein tyrosine phosphatase 1B, and p130Cas in integrin-mediated signaling events. J Biol Chem 272:33377–33383

Rondinone CM, Trevillyan JM, Clampit J, Gum RJ, Berg C, Kroeger P, Frost L, Zinker BA, Reilly R, Ulrich R, Butler M, Monia BP, Jirousek MR, Waring JF (2002) Protein tyrosine phosphatase 1B reduction regulates adiposity and expression of genes involved in lipogenesis. Diabetes 51:2405–11

Rothenbacher D, Brenner H (2003) Burden of Helicobacter pylori and H. pylori-related diseases in developed countries: recent developments and future implications. Microbes Infect 5:693–703

Ruivenkamp CA, van Wezel T, Zanon C, Stassen AP, Vlcek C, Csikos T, Klous AM, Tripodis N, Perrakis A, Boerrigter L, Groot PC, Lindeman J, Mooi WJ, Meijjer GA, Scholten G, Dauwerse H, Paces V, van Zandwijk N, van Ommen GJ, Demant P (2002) Ptprj is a candidate for the mouse colon-cancer susceptibility locus Scc1 and is frequently deleted in human cancers. Nat Genet 31:295–300

Saha S, Bardelli A, Buckhaults P, Velculescu VE, Rago C, St Croix B, Romans KE, Choti MA, Lengauer C, Kinzler KW, Vogelstein B (2001) A phosphatase associated with metastasis of colorectal cancer. Science 294:1343–1346

Sasaki T, Sasaki-Irie J, Penninger JM (2001) New insights into the transmembrane protein tyrosine phosphatase CD45. Int J Biochem Cell Biol 33:1041–6

Serratosa JM, Gomez-Garre P, Gallardo ME, Anta B, de Bernabe DB, Lindhout D, Augustijn PB, Tassinari CA, Malafosse RM, Topcu M, Grid D, Dravet C, Berkovic SF, de Cordoba SR (1999) A novel protein tyrosine phosphatase gene is mutated in progressive myoclonus epilepsy of the Lafora type (EPM2). Hum Mol Genet 8:345–352

Sparks JW, Brautigan DL (1986) Molecular basis for substrate specificity of protein kinases and phosphatases. Int J Biochem 18:497–504

Su J, Muranjan M, Sap J (1999) Receptor protein tyrosine phosphatase alpha activates Src-family kinases and controls integrin-mediated responses in fibroblasts. Curr Biol 9:505–11

Tabiti K, Smith DR, Goh HS, Pallen CJ (1995) Increased mRNA expression of the receptor-like protein tyrosine phosphatase alpha in late stage colon carcinomas. Cancer Lett 93:239–248

Tartaglia M, Mehler EL, Goldberg R, Zampino G, Brunner HG, Kremer H, van der Burgt I, Crosby AH, Ion A, Jeffery S, Kalidas K, Patton MA, Kucherlapati RS, Gelb BD (2001) Mutations in PTPN11, encoding the protein tyrosine phosphatase SHP-2, cause Noonan syndrome. Nat Genet 29:465–468

Tartaglia M, Kalidas K, Shaw A, Song X, Musat DL, van der Burgt I, Brunner HG, Bertola DR, Crosby A, Ion A, Kucherlapati RS, Jeffery S, Patton MA, Gelb BD (2002) PTPN11 mutations in Noonan syndrome: molecular spectrum, genotype- phenotype correlation, and phenotypic heterogeneity. Am J Hum Genet 70:1555–1563

Tartaglia M, Niemeyer CM, Fragale A, Song X, Buechner J, Jung A, Hahlen K, Hasle H, Licht JD, Gelb BD (2003) Somatic mutations in PTPN11 in juvenile myelomonocytic leukemia, myelodysplastic syndromes and acute myeloid leukemia. Nat Genet 34:148–50

Tchilian EZ, Wallace DL, Wells RS, Flower DR, Morgan G, Beverley PC (2001) A deletion in the gene encoding the CD45 antigen in a patient with SCID. J Immunol 166:1308–1313

Teixeira JE, Mann BJ (2002) Entamoeba histolytica-induced dephosphorylation in host cells. Infect Immun 70:1816–1823

Thomas ML (1999) The regulation of antigen-receptor signaling by protein tyrosine phosphatases: a hole in the story. Curr Opin Immunol 11:270–6

Thompson KM, Uetani N, Manitt C, Elchebly M, Tremblay ML, Kennedy TE (2003) Receptor protein tyrosine phosphatase sigma inhibits axonal regeneration and the rate of axon extension. Mol Cell Neurosci 23:681–692

Tonks NK, Neel BG (2001) Combinatorial control of the specificity of protein tyrosine phosphatases. Curr Opin Cell Biol 13:182–95

Tonks NK, Diltz CD, Fischer EH (1988a) Characterization of the major protein-tyrosine-phosphatases of human placenta. J Biol Chem 263:6731–7

Tonks NK, Diltz CD, Fischer EH (1988b) Purification of the major protein-tyrosine-phosphatases of human placenta. J Biol Chem 263:6722–30

Uetani N, Kato K, Ogura H, Mizuno K, Kawano K, Mikoshiba K, Yakura H, Asano M, Iwakura Y (2000) Impaired learning with enhanced hippocampal long-term potentiation in PTPdelta-deficient mice. Embo J 19:2775–85

Vogel A, Strassburg CP, Manns MP (2003) 77 C/G mutation in the tyrosine phosphatase CD45 gene and autoimmune hepatitis: evidence for a genetic link. Genes Immun 4:79–81

Wallace MJ, Batt J, Fladd CA, Henderson JT, Skarnes W, Rotin D (1999) Neuronal defects and posterior pituitary hypoplasia in mice lacking the receptor tyrosine phosphatase PTPsigma. Nat Genet 21:334–8

Wang J, Bixby JL (1999) Receptor tyrosine phosphatase-delta is a homophilic, neurite-promoting cell adhesion molecular for CNS neurons. Mol Cell Neurosci 14:370–84

Wiener JR, Hurteau JA, Kerns BJ, Whitaker RS, Conaway MR, Berchuck A, Bast RC Jr (1994a) Overexpression of the tyrosine phosphatase PTP1B is associated with human ovarian carcinomas. Am J Obstet Gynecol 170:1177–83

Wiener JR, Kerns BJ, Harvey EL, Conaway MR, Iglehart JD, Berchuck A, Bast RC Jr (1994b) Overexpression of the protein tyrosine phosphatase PTP1B in human breast cancer: association with p185c-erbB-2 protein expression. J Natl Cancer Inst 86:372–8

Wise CA, Gillum JD, Seidman CE, Lindor NM, Veile R, Bashiardes S, Lovett M (2002) Mutations in CD2BP1 disrupt binding to PTP PEST and are responsible for PAPA syndrome, an autoinflammatory disorder. Hum Mol Genet 11:961–9

Wishart MJ, Dixon JE (2002) PTEN and myotubularin phosphatases: from 3-phosphoinositide dephosphorylation to disease. Phosphatase and tensin homolog deleted on chromosome ten. Trends Cell Biol 12:579–85

Wu C, Sun M, Liu L, Zhou GW (2003) The function of the protein tyrosine phosphatase SHP-1 in cancer. Gene 306:1-12

Xie Y, Yeo TT, Zhang C, Yang T, Tisi MA, Massa SM, Longo FM (2001) The leukocyte common antigen-related protein tyrosine phosphatase receptor regulates regenerative neurite outgrowth in vivo. J Neurosci 21:5130–5138

Yang T, Bernabeu R, Xie Y, Zhang JS, Massa SM, Rempel HC, Longo FM (2003) Leukocyte antigen-related protein tyrosine phosphatase receptor: a small ectodomain isoform functions as a homophilic ligand and promotes neurite outgrowth. J Neurosci 23:3353–63

Yeo TT, Yang T, Massa SM, Zhang JS, Honkaniemi J, Butcher LL, Longo FM (1997) Deficient LAR expression decreases basal forebrain cholinergic neuronal size and hippocampal cholinergic innervation. J Neurosci Res 47:348–60

Zabolotny JM, Kim YB, Peroni OD, Kim JK, Pani MA, Boss O, Klaman LD, Kamatkar S, Shulman GI, Kahn BB, Neel BG (2001) Overexpression of the LAR (leukocyte antigen-related) protein-tyrosine phosphatase in muscle causes insulin resistance. Proc Natl Acad Sci U S A 98:5187–92

Zabolotny JM, Bence-Hanulec KK, Stricker-Krongrad A, Haj F, Wang Y, Minokoshi Y, Kim YB, Elmquist JK, Tartaglia LA, Kahn BB, Neel BG (2002) PTP1B regulates leptin signal transduction in vivo. Dev Cell 2:489–95

Zeng Q, Dong JM, Guo K, Li J, Tan HX, Koh V, Pallen CJ, Manser E, Hong W (2003) PRL-3 and PRL-1 promote cell migration, invasion, and metastasis. Cancer Res 63:2716–22

Zhai YF, Beittenmiller H, Wang B, Gould MN, Oakley C, Esselman WJ, Welsch CW (1993) Increased expression of specific protein tyrosine phosphatases in human breast epithelial cells neoplastically transformed by the neu oncogene. Cancer Res 53:2272–8

Zhang J, Somani AK, Siminovitch KA (2000) Roles of the SHP-1 tyrosine phosphatase in the negative regulation of cell signalling. Semin Immunol 12:361–378

Zhang Z-Y (1998) Protein-tyrosine phosphatases: biological function, structural characteristics, and mechanism of catalysis. Crit Rev Biochem Mol Biol 33:1-52

Zhang Z-Y, Zhou B, Xie L (2002) Modulation of protein kinase signaling by protein phosphatases and inhibitors. Pharmacol Ther 93:307–317

Zheng XM, Wang Y, Pallen CJ (1992) Cell transformation and activation of pp60c-src by overexpression of a protein tyrosine phosphatase. Nature 359:336–9

Zheng XM, Resnick RJ, Shalloway D (2002) Mitotic activation of protein-tyrosine phosphatase alpha and regulation of its Src-mediated transforming activity by its sites of protein kinase C phosphorylation. J Biol Chem 277:21922–21929

Zinker BA, Rondinone CM, Trevillyan JM, Gum RJ, Clampit JE, Waring JF (2002) PTP1B antisense oligonucleotide lowers PTP1B protein, normalizes blood glucose, and improves insulin sensitivity in diabetic mice. Proc Natl Acad Sci U S A 99:11357–11362

HEP (2005) 167:215–262

Structure-Based Design of Protein Tyrosine Phosphatase Inhibitors

N. P. H. Møller[1] (✉) · H. S. Andersen[2] · C. B. Jeppesen[3] · L. F. Iversen[4]

[1] Signal Transduction, Novo Nordisk, Building 9S2.18, 2880 Bagsværd, Denmark
nphm@novonordisk.com
[2] MedChem Research I, Novo Nordisk, Building D9.S.02, 2760 Måløv, Denmark
[3] Molecular Pharmacology, Novo Nordisk, Building C9.S.19, 2760 Måløv, Denmark
[4] Protein Science, Novo Nordisk, Building 6A1.049, 2880 Bagsværd, Denmark

Abstract Protein tyrosine phosphatases (PTPs) are a family of intracellular enzymes that remove phosphate from tyrosine phosphorylated proteins. The PTP superfamily includes tyrosine phosphate-specific classical PTPs, dual-specificity PTPs, and low-molecular-weight PTPs. PTPs and protein tyrosine kinases reversibly regulate the phosphotyrosine level in selected cellular proteins, thereby controlling many important signaling pathways in eukaryotes. Aberrant tyrosine phosphorylation levels have been associated with the development of cancer, autoimmunity, and diabetes, thus indicating that PTPs might play important etiological and pathogenic roles in these diseases. As a result, these enzymes have recently attracted much interest as potential drug targets. This is in particular due to the finding that PTP1B knockout mice show increased insulin sensitivity and resistance to diet-induced obesity, thus indicating that PTP1B is an important negative regulator of insulin and leptin action and hence a potentially important drug target for the treatment of diabetes and obesity. The development of PTP inhibitors, in particular PTP1B inhibitors, has been greatly facilitated by an impressive number of X-ray structures that have allowed structure-based design of highly selective inhibitors of PTP1B, the main focus of this review. The initial attempts to design selective PTP inhibitors were based on replacement of pTyr with non-hydrolyzable phosphotyrosyl mimetics in small, efficient PTP peptide substrates, thereby utilizing both the potency and selectivity provided by the amino acid residues. However, several groups have now shown that it is possible to synthesize highly potent and selective non-phosphorus, non-peptide inhibitors of PTP1B. At this point, these achievements to some extent seem to have been reached at the expense of appropriate pharmacokinetic properties, including cellular uptake. Therefore, the next wave within the field of PTP inhibitors is likely to be focused on improvements in this respect. In addition, several other PTPs could potentially be attractive drug targets in autoimmunity and cancer.

Keywords Protein tyrosine phosphatase · PTP1B · X-ray · Bioinformatics · Diabetes mellitus · Enzyme kinetics

1
Introduction

Protein tyrosine phosphatases (PTPs) are a family of intracellular enzymes that remove phosphate from tyrosine phosphorylated proteins. The PTP superfamily includes the following three families: (1) tyrosine phosphate-specific, classical PTPs, (2) dual-specificity PTPs and (3) low-molecular-weight PTPs. Together with tyrosine kinases that catalyze the addition of phosphate to tyrosine residues, PTPs reversibly regulate the phosphotyrosine (pTyr) level in selected cellular proteins, thereby controlling many important signaling pathways in eukaryotes. (For recent reviews, see Møller et al. 2000; Johnson et al. 2002; van Huijsduijnen et al. 2002; Tonks 2003; Zhang and Lee 2003.) In addition to protein substrates, a small number of the PTP superfamily members, including PTEN and myotubularin, dephosphorylates lipid substrates (Maehama et al. 2001; Wishart and Dixon 2002). Traditionally, the classical PTPs (Fig. 1), which are the main topic of the current review, have been classified as receptor-type (RT1–8) or non-transmembrane/intracellular (NT1–9) PTPs based on their non-catalytic domain structure and the presence or absence of a transmembrane region (Fischer et al. 1991; Tonks and Neel 2001). We have recently performed a phylogenetic classification of PTPs and shown that there is a very close relationship between PTP domain sequence similarity and functional domains in the full-length proteins (Andersen et al. 2001). Thus, receptor-type PTPs, previously classified into

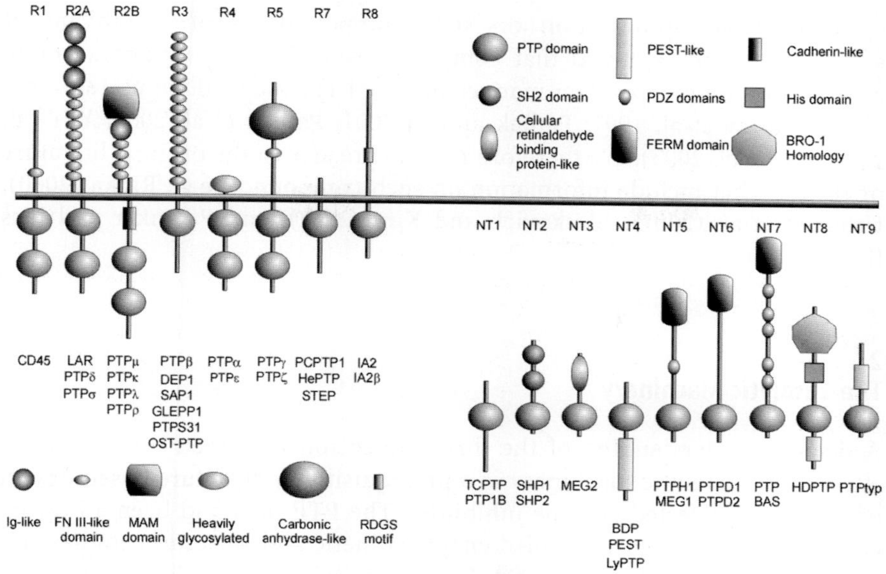

Fig. 1 Schematic representation of the classical PTP family

nine distinct subtypes, were categorized into virtually identical groups to these based on sequence homology of the catalytic domains. Similar observations and categorizations were made for intracellular PTPs.

The catalytic domains of classical PTPs consist of ~230 amino acid residues. Based on amino acid comparisons, 10 discrete and highly conserved motifs can be identified in these domains (Andersen et al. 2001). The active site sequence His-Cys-(Xxx)$_5$-Arg-Ser/Thr (residues 214–222; PTP1B numbering, which is used throughout) defines the PTP family and is often referred to as the PTP loop, the P-loop or the PTP signature motif.

Due to the critical role of PTPs in controlling cellular processes such as growth and differentiation, cell cycle, and metabolism, these enzymes have recently attracted much interest as potential drug targets. As a result, a number of laboratories both in academia and the pharmaceutical industry have devoted much energy to the discovery and development of selective inhibitors of this enzyme class. In the following we will review the most recent progress in the field and present the strategy and technological platform developed in house by the PTP inhibitor group at Novo Nordisk. From the outset it should be emphasized that we will restrict our discussion to compounds that are reversible, competitive, and time-independent PTP inhibitors and for which detailed enzyme kinetic analyses and/or structural information are provided, i.e., compounds that are suitable for structure-based design. There is a significant risk of identifying oxidizing or alkylating compounds when searching for PTP inhibitors (for details, see Sect. 8.1) and structure-based optimization on such compounds is often difficult. It should, however, be noted that compounds that irreversibly and/or more broadly in a time-dependent manner modify PTPs may still be useful in the clinic (Skorey et al. 1997; Pathak and Yi 2001; Pathak et al. 2002; Yi et al. 2002; Kar et al. 2003). We therefore refer the reader to the original literature or reviews that include information on such compounds, e.g., Ripka (2000), Urbanek et al. (2001), Blaskovich and Kim (2002), and Patankar and Jurs (2003).

2
The Catalytic Machinery

A detailed understanding of the three-dimensional geometry of the active site and the catalytic machinery is a prerequisite for structure-based design of active site-directed enzyme inhibitors. The PTP field had been advanced early on by a number of detailed enzyme kinetic and structural studies (reviewed in Burke and Zhang 1998; Denu and Dixon 1998). The X-ray structure of catalytically inactive PTP1B$_{C215S}$ mutant complexed with a synthetic tyrosine phosphorylated hexapeptide revealed the architecture of the PTP signature motif Cys-(Xxx)$_5$-Arg that forms an efficient phosphate binding site. The peptide main chain of this motif forms a half-circle with Cys215 almost in the middle, and the phosphate oxygen atoms of pTyr form a number of hydrogen bonds to the main chain nitrogens and the guanidinium group of Arg221 (Jia et al. 1995) (see Table 1 for a comprehensive list of X-ray structures of PTP1B). The binding of pTyr is further stabilized by hydrophobic and aromatic π–π interactions between the phenyl ring of pTyr and residues such as Tyr46 and Val49 in the active site pocket.

The hydrolysis of pTyr substrates is a two-step process. The consensus active site Cys215 plays an essential role in the first step. This cysteine has a low pK_a value (i.e., it is deprotonated and charged at physiological pH) and acts as a nucleophile (Pot and Dixon 1992b), which attacks phosphate leading to the formation of a cysteine–phosphate intermediate (Guan and Dixon 1991) (Fig. 2, parts 1–3). Binding of pTyr substrates to PTPs is followed by closure of the so-called WPD loop (residues 179–183) in a conformation that traps the pTyr substrate in the active site pocket. The closed WPD loop is stabilized by hydrogen bonds between the side chain of Arg221 and phosphate and the carbonyl group of Pro180 as well as by π–π interactions between Phe182 and the phenyl ring of pTyr. The closure of the WPD loop brings Asp181 into a favorable position relative to the scissile oxygen of pTyr to act as a general acid donating a proton to the leaving group (i.e., the substrate) (Zhang et al. 1994b; Denu et al. 1996; Lohse et al. 1997) (Fig. 2, parts 2 and 3). In the second step of catalysis, the thiol phosphate intermediate is attacked by a nucleophilic water molecule that is positioned optimally

Table 1 PTP1B X-ray structures

Ligand No.	PDB ID	Ligand name	Reference	Ligand No.	PDB ID	Ligand name	Reference
	1AAX	Bis(*para*-phosphophenyl)methane	Puius et al. 1997	37	1L8G	7-(1,1-Dioxo-1*H*-benzo[*d*]isothiazol-3-yloxymethyl)-2-(oxalyl-amino)-4,7-dihydro-5*H*-thieno[2,3-c]pyran-3-carboxylic acid	Iversen et al. 2001
	1BZC	4-Carbamoyl-4-{[6-(difluoro-phosphono-methyl)-naphthalene-2-carbonyl]-amino}-butyric acid	Groves et al. 1998	39	1LQF	N-Benzoyl-l-glutamyl-[4-phosphono-(difluoromethyl)]-l-phenylalanine-[4-phosphono (difluoro-methyl)]-l-phenyl-alanineamide	Asante-Appiah et al. 2002
	1BZH	Fluoromalonyl tyrosine, (2-amino-2-carbamoyl-ethylsulfanyl)-acetic acid	Groves et al. 1998	40	1N6W	N-{1-[5-(1-Carbamoyl-2-mercapto-ethylcarbamoyl)-pentylcarbamoyl]-2-[4-(difluoro-phosphono-methyl)-phenyl]-ethyl}-3-{2-[4-(difluoro-phosphono-methyl)-phenyl]-acetylamino}-succinamic acid	Sun et al. 2003
	1BZJ	6-(Difluoro-phosphono-methyl)-naphthalene-2-carboxylic acid	Groves et al. 1998	43	1NL9	2-{[4-(2-Acetylamino-2-pentylcarbamoyl-ethyl)-naphthalen-1-yl]-oxalyl-amino}-benzoic acid	Szczepan-kiewicz et al. 2003
33	1C83	6-(Oxalyl-amino)-1*H*-indole-5-carboxylic acid	Andersen et al. 2000	44	1NNY	3-({5-[(N-Acetyl-3-{4-[(carboxycarbonyl)(2-carboxyphenyl)amino]-1-naphthyl}-l-alanyl)amino]pentyl}oxy)-2-naphthoic acid	Szczepan-kiewicz et al. 2003
32	1C84	3-(Oxalyl-amino)-naphthalene-2-carboxylic acid	Andersen et al. 2000	42	1NO6	2-[(Carboxycarbonyl)(1-naphthyl)amino]-benzoic acid	Szczepan-kiewicz et al. 2003
1	1C85	2-(Oxalyl-amino)-benzoic acid	Andersen et al. 2000		1NWE	N-[4-(2-{2-[3-(2-Bromo-acetylamino)-propionylamino]-3-hydroxy-propionylamino}-ethyl)-phenyl]-oxalamic acid	Erlanson et al. 2003
36	1C86	2-(Oxalyl-amino)-4,7-dihydro-5*H*-thieno[2,3-c]pyran-3-carboxylic acid	Iversen et al. 2000	5	1NWL	3-(4-{2-[2-(2-Bromo-acetylamino)-ethyldisulfanyl]-ethylcarbamoyl}-cyclohexyl-carbamoyl)pyrazine-2-carboxylic acid	Erlanson et al. 2003
36	1C87	2-(Oxalyl-amino)-4,7-dihydro-5*H*-thieno[2,3-c]pyran-3-carboxylic acid	Iversen et al. 2000	45	1NZ7	2-[(4-{2-Acetylamino-2-[4-(1-carboxy-3-methylsulfanyl-propylcarbamoyl)-butyl-carbamoyl]-ethyl}-2-ethyl-phenyl)-oxalyl-amino]-benzoic acid	Xin et al. 2003

Table 1 (continued)

Ligand No.	PDB ID	Ligand name	Reference	Ligand No.	PDB ID	Ligand name	Reference
35	1C88	2-(Oxalyl-amino)-4,5,6,7-tetrahydro-thieno[2,3-c]pyridine-3-carboxylic acid	Iversen et al. 2000		1OEM	Apo structure (sulfenyl-amide bond between C215Sg and S216 N)	Salmeen et al. 2003
	1ECV	5-Iodo-2-(oxalyl-amino)-benzoic acid	Andersen et al. 2000		1OEO	Apo structure (C215 oxidized to cysteinesulfinic acid)	Salmeen et al. 2003
	1EEN	Phosphotyrosine, para-(benzoyl)-phenylalanine peptide, D-A-D-BPA-PTyr-l-I-P-Q-Q-G (C215S mutant)	Sarmiento et al. 2000		1OES	Apo structure (sulfenyl-amide bond between C215Sg and S216 N)	Salmeen et al. 2003
	1EEO	Phosphotyrosine peptide, L-E-L-E-F-PTyr-M-D-Y-E (C215S mutant)	Sarmiento et al. 2000		1OET	Apo structure (C215 oxidized to s-hydroxy-cysteine)	Salmeen et al. 2003
	1G1F	Phosphotyrosine peptide, Q-T-D-PTyr-PTyr-R (C215A mutant)	Salmeen et al. 2000		1OEU	Apo structure (C215 oxidized to cysteine-s-dioxide)	Salmeen et al. 2003
	1G1G	Phosphotyrosine peptide, T-D-Y-PTyr-R (C215A mutant)	Salmeen et al. 2000		1OEV	Apo structure (C215 oxidized to cysteinesulfinic acid)	Salmeen et al. 2003
	1G1H	Phosphotyrosine peptide, T-D-PTyr-PTyr-R-K-G (C215A mutant)	Salmeen et al. 2000		1ONY	2-{[2-(2-Carbamoyl-vinyl)-4-(2-methane-sulfonylamino-2-pentylcarbamoyl-ethyl)-phenyl]-oxalyl-amino}-benzoic acid	Liu et al. 2003a
15	1G7F	2-{4-[(2*S*)-2-[({[(1*S*)-1-Carboxy-2-phenyl-ethyl]amino}carbonyl)amino]-3-oxo-3-(pentylamino)propyl]phen-oxy}malonic acid	Bleasdale et al. 2001		1ONZ	2-[(7-Hydroxy-naphthalen-1-yl)-oxalyl-amino]-benzoic acid	Liu et al. 2003a
16	1G7G	2-(Carboxymethoxy)-5-[(2*S*)-2-({(2*S*)-2-[(3-carboxypropanoyl)amino]-3-phe-nyl-propanoyl}amino)-3-oxo-3-(penty-lamino)-propyl]benzoic acid	Bleasdale et al. 2001		1PH0	2-{4-[2-(*S*)-Allyloxycarbonylamino-3-{4-[(2-carboxy-phenyl)-oxalyl-amino]-phenyl}-propionylamino]-butoxy} 6-hydroxy-benzoic acid methyl ester	Liu et al. 2003c

Table 1 (continued)

Ligand No.	PDB ID	Ligand name	Reference	Ligand No.	PDB ID	Ligand name	Reference
	1GFY	2-(Oxalyl-amino)-4,7-dihydro-5*H*-thieno[2,3-c]thiopyran-3-carboxylic acid	Peters et al. 2000		1PTY	Phosphotyrosine (C215S mutant)	Puius et al. 1997
	1I57	Apo structure (C215S mutant)	Scapin et al. 2001	40	1PXH	N-{1-[5-(1-Carbamoyl-2-mercapto-ethylcarbamoyl)-pentylcarbamoyl]-2-[4-(difluoro-phosphono-methyl)-phenyl]-ethyl}-3-{2-[4-(difluoro-phosphono-methyl)-phenyl]-acetylamino}-succinamic acid	Sun et al. 2003
					1Q1M	5-{2-Fluoro-5-[3-(3-hydroxy-2-methoxy-carbonyl-phenoxy)-propenyl]-phenyl}-isoxazole-3-carboxylic acid	Liu et al. 2003b

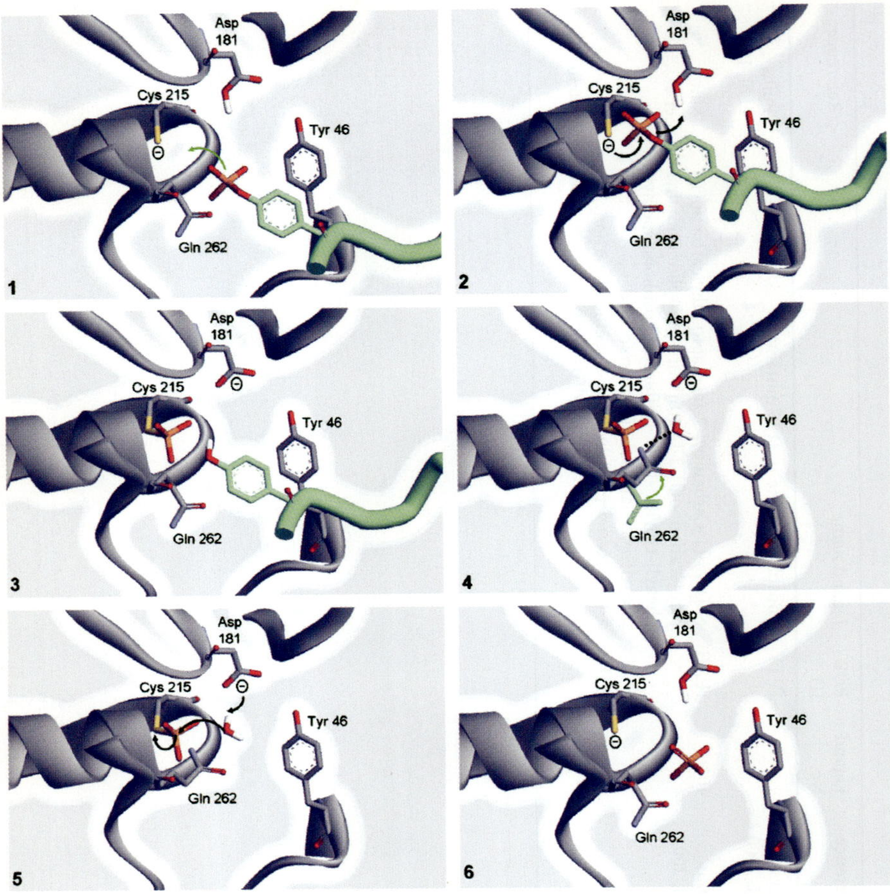

Fig. 2 Schematic representation of the catalytic mechanism of PTPs.*1–3*: Cys215 in the P-loop (PTP1B numbering used throughout) acts as a nucleophile, which attacks the phosphate leading to the formation of a cysteine-phosphate intermediate. In this first step of catalysis, Asp181 in the WPD loop acts as a general acid donating a proton to the leaving group. *4–6*: In the second step of catalysis, the thiol–phosphate intermediate is attacked by a water molecule that is positioned optimally by Gln262

by Gln262 (Pannifer et al. 1998), hence leading to the release of phosphate (Fig. 2, parts 4–6). The understanding of the catalytic machinery in PTPs has been greatly facilitated by several seminal mutational and X-ray studies (Barford et al. 1994; Stuckey et al. 1994; Jia et al. 1995; Schubert et al. 1995; Fauman et al. 1996; Pannifer et al. 1998; Sarmiento et al. 1998).

3
Bioinformatics

Bioinformatics plays an important role in modern structure-based drug design. To assist our design of selective inhibitors, we have explored the human genome for its content of PTP genes and analyzed their primary amino acid sequence in context of X-ray crystal structure information. Specifically, the degree of PTP sequence conservation was calculated from a multiple sequence alignment of 37 different PTP domains and visualized in 3D to identify unique combinations of residues in the proximity of the active site that could be addressed in structure-based design of selective inhibitors (Iversen et al. 2000; Andersen et al. 2001). Four areas seemed particularly useful, since they could be targeted by low molecular active site-directed compounds (residues by PTP1B numbering): (1) 47–48; (2) 258–259; (3) 24–254 [i.e., the second aryl phosphate binding site (Puius et al. 1997)]; and (4) 116–118 (Fig. 3). In addition, the WPD loop may offer further possibilities for obtaining both potency and selectivity. Although no single residue in these areas appears to be a unique hallmark of any PTP, the combination of the residues in these areas represents important selectivity determining regions. We have in particular concentrated our efforts around utilizing the area defined by residues 47–48 and 258–259, as will be illustrated below (Sect. 9.2).

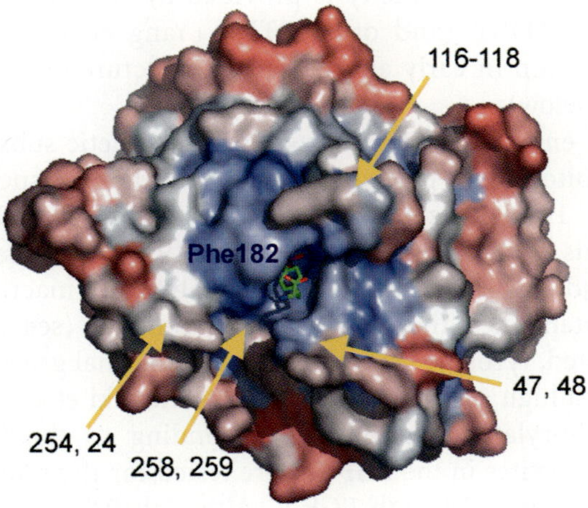

Fig. 3 Four selectivity determining regions visualized in 3D—useful for structure-based design of active site-directed inhibitors: (1) residues 47–48; (2) residues 258–259; (3) residues 24 and 254; and (4) residues 116–118. Phe182 (in the WPD loop) and a substrate (phosphotyrosine) in the active site are shown for orientation purposes. [ConSurf (http://consurf.tau.ac.il/); Glaser et al. 2003]

When developing a drug that targets an individual member of a larger protein family, it is useful to have a complete overview of all proteins in that family to avoid unintentional development of compounds that bind to non-target family members. With access to the almost finished version of the public human genome sequence (Build 33), the composition of the PTP family was recently defined. A total of 38 human classical PTP genes and 12 pseudogenes were identified, just adding one novel gene to the previously defined non-redundant database of vertebrate PTP transcripts (Andersen et al. 2001; see http://science.novonordisk.com/ptp and http://ptp.cshl.edu for a detailed analysis of the PTP family).

4 Structural Requirements for Substrate Specificity

In addition to information on the catalytic machinery, the first X-ray structures of PTP1B demonstrated a common binding mode of pTyr substrates: (1) binding of the phosphate moiety of pTyr to the P-loop (residues 214–222) and Arg221, (2) hydrophobic interactions of the phenyl ring of pTyr with the active site pocket and (3) hydrogen bonds between the main chain nitrogens of the pTyr substrate (pTyr and residue +1) and the side chain of Asp48 of PTP1B, and (4) a hydrogen bond between the main chain carbonyl of residue −2 and the main chain nitrogen of residue 47 (Jia et al. 1995; Sarmiento et al. 1998). Specificity is provided by side chain interactions of the peptide and PTP1B (and other PTPs) (Yang et al. 2000), which has served as inspiration in early approaches to structure-based design of PTP inhibitors (see below).

A number of enzyme kinetic analyses with synthetic substrates and peptide-based inhibitors have provided insight into the fine specificity of PTPs (e.g., Cho et al. 1993; Ruzzene et al. 1993; Zhang et al. 1993; Zhang et al. 1994a; Desmarais et al. 1998; Desmarais et al. 1999). In an early and elegant study, Dixon and coworkers found that a catalytically inactive [^{35}S]-labeled PTP1B$_{C215S}$ mutant, i.e., the first 'trapping mutant' (see below, Sect. 5), bound to activated, tyrosine phosphorylated epidermal growth factor receptor (EGF-R) with high affinity (K_d=100 nM) (Milarski et al. 1993). Synthetic tyrosine phosphorylated peptides corresponding to the four major autophosphorylation sites in the EGF-R were tested for their ability to displace PTP1B$_{C215S}$ from the full-length EGF-R. Although PTP1B was displaced by all four peptides, the peptides containing pTyr^{1148} or pTyr^{992} were the most potent. Peptides and peptide analogs corresponding to the EGF-R sequence around residue 992 (i.e., D-A-D-E-pY-L-I-P-Q-Q-G with pY=pTyr) have subsequently served as extremely useful tools in enzyme kinetic and structural analyses of PTP substrate specificity, and in inhibitor design, as will be discussed in the following. In a detailed analysis of the size and pTyr positioning requirements, it was found that efficient binding and catalysis was provided by Ac-D-A-D-E-pY-L-NH_2 (Zhang et al. 1994a). A structural explanation for efficient binding of substrates with acidic residues immediately N-terminal to the pTyr residue was provided by the first X-ray structures of PTP1B in complex with this EGF-R-derived peptide, demonstrating specific interactions between the acidic residues and Arg47 of PTP1B (Jia et al. 1995; Sarmiento et al. 1998). Additional support for this notion was obtained by molecular modeling of D-A-D-E-X-L-based inhibitors in CD45 and LAR (Glover and Tracey 2000).

Using 'inverse alanine scanning,' Zhang and coworkers further assessed the substrate specificity of PTP1B (Vetter et al. 2000). Separate and sequential replacement of each alanine residue in the parent peptide, Ac-AAAApYAAAA-NH_2, with the 19 other natural amino acids, identified Ac-ELEFpYMDYE-NH_2 as a highly potent PTP1B substrate. As found previously, a strong preference was observed for acidic residues. Additionally, it was noted that PTP1B could also accommodate hydrophobic and aromatic residues at the −1 position. The structural basis for this plasticity was revealed by X-ray crystallographic studies showing that accommodation of both acidic and hydrophobic residues in the −1 position was conferred by Arg47, which can adopt different conformations, thereby generating two sets of distinct binding modes (Sarmiento et al. 2000).

5 Identification of Natural Substrates: The Insulin Receptor-Regulating PTP

The above studies with synthetic peptides have advanced our understanding of the substrate specificity of PTP domains. However, in vivo PTPs act in the context of full-length folded proteins, and hence there is a need for gaining insight into the three-dimensional structural requirements for substrate specificity. Based on the understanding of the catalytic machinery (Sect. 2), Tonks and coworkers have devised an intriguing strategy by creating so-called trapping mutants, i.e., PTP mutants that are inactive or display very low activity yet retain their 3D structure intact, as well as most of the functional features needed for substrate binding and catalysis, including closure of the WPD loop (Flint et al. 1997). In particular, PTPs which are either mutated at position 215 (Cys to Ser) or at position 181 (Asp to Ala) have been used widely and have provided significant information on PTP substrate specificity in intact cells. Recently, and again based on an understanding of PTP-mediated catalysis at the molecular level, the affinity of the Asp181Ala mutant was increased considerably by introducing an alanine in position 262, i.e., the invariant glutamine that positions the nucleophilic water molecule in the second step of hydrolysis (Sect. 2). It is anticipated that this mutant, due to its higher affinity for pTyr peptides, can be used to isolate less-abundant PTP substrates (Xie et al. 2002).

The definition of the exact function of a protein requires inter- and multi-disciplinary approaches and is often based on stepwise investigations over the years. A number of approaches have been used to assist the identification of the function of specific PTPs. These studies have been reviewed in detail elsewhere, and only one example will be given to illustrate the importance of modern structural biology and the relevance of creating an intimate connection between basic science and drug discovery.

In a landmark publication, Tremblay, Kennedy, and colleagues reported that PTP1B knockout mice display increased insulin sensitivity and resistance to diet-induced obesity (Elchebly et al. 1999), a finding that was later confirmed in an independent study (Klaman et al. 2000). In the present context, it is of relevance that these studies pointed to a direct negative regulatory effect of PTP1B on the insulin receptor tyrosine kinase (IRTK). To provide a framework for the rational development of specific inhibitors of this interaction, Barford and Tonks embarked on a detailed analysis by integrating X-ray crystallography, enzyme kinetics, and peptide-binding studies, and provided strong evidence for simultaneous binding of tandem pTyr residues in the IRTK activation loop to the active site and an adjacent pTyr recognition site (Salmeen et al. 2000). The latter site, the second aryl phosphate binding site (site 2), had previously been proposed to be used for the design of specific and potent inhibitors of PTP1B (Puius et al. 1997). Further, to bind simultaneously to the active site and site 2, the substrate has to pass through (or fit in) a cleft-like part of PTP1B, which we have used in our design of selective PTP1B inhibitors (Peters et al. 2000; Iversen et al. 2001) (Sect. 9.2.5). Tonks and coworkers next used bioinformatic analyses to identify other protein kinases with tandem pTyr residues in the activation loop as potential substrates for PTP1B, and in fact evidence was provided for the notion that TYK2 and JAK2 are substrates of PTP1B (Myers et al. 2001). This is of particular interest since this might clarify part of the phenotype of the PTP1B knockout mice, i.e., resistance to diet-induced obesity, which is not easily explained by an effect of PTP1B on the IRTK-mediated anabolic signaling. Rather, such a phenotype could be due to the absence of a negative regulatory effect of PTP1B on the leptin system, which signals via JAK2. Subsequent studies of the two strains of PTP1B knockout mice provided evidence that indeed leptin signaling is increased in these mice (Cheng et al. 2002; Zabolotny et al. 2002). Together, these studies not only offer a solid biological basis for identification of PTP1B as an important drug target in diabetes and obesity, which was recently strongly supported by antisense studies in vivo (Zinker et al. 2002), but also structural inspiration for design of compounds that specifically inhibit PTP1B.

6 Nature's Regulation of PTP Activity

Aberrant tyrosine phosphorylation levels have been linked both to cancer and metabolic disease states. Hence, tight regulation and specificity of PTPs is required. Nature may achieve control of PTP activity by a number of different mechanisms, as exemplified in the following: (1) Site-specific tyrosine phosphorylation and dephosphorylation may result from inherent substrate specificity of kinases and phosphatases. (2) The interaction between PTPs and their cognate substrates may be regulated by subcellular localization which can be controlled either by targeting domains of the PTPs ('zip codes') (Mauro and Dixon 1994), alternative splicing (Shifrin and Neel 1993), or proteolytic cleavage (Frangione et al. 1993; Gil-Henn et al. 2000, 2001; Ragab et al. 2003). (3) Different isoforms of PTPs may be synthesized from the same gene due to alternative usage of isoform-specific 5′ exons and promoters (Elson and Leder 1995; Tanuma et al. 1999; Amoui et al. 2003). (4) The enzymatic activity of PTPs may further be influenced by covalent modification such as phosphorylation of specific tyrosine and serine/threonine residues (Flint et al. 1993; Moeslein et al. 1999; Ravichandran et al. 2001), or by dimerization (Bilwes et al. 1996; Majeti et al. 1998; Jiang et al. 1999; Blanchetot and Den Hertog 2000; Jiang et al. 2000; Majeti et al. 2000; Blanchetot et al. 2002a), or by oxidation of the active site cysteine (see below). (5) As with other enzymes, the cellular levels of PTPs may be further controlled by specific transcription factors (Fukada and Tonks 2003), or by the half-life of the mRNA or protein of the PTP in question.

Although most of the above principles for regulation of PTP activity and specificity could potentially be utilized for development of drugs that modulate the activity of PTPs, the most straightforward approach—and also the focus of most laboratories—is to develop active site-directed inhibitors. It should be emphasized that covalent modification of PTPs on residues in the proximity of the active site, e.g., phosphorylation of Ser50 in PTP1B (Ravichandran et al. 2001), might potentially influence the activity of inhibitors that are developed against the non-modified enzyme. It is therefore an inherent risk in a drug optimization program to rely exclusively on recombinant, non-modified proteins expressed in prokaryotic systems.

Recombinant PTPs show relatively high catalytic activity compared to protein tyrosine kinases (Denu and Dixon 1998). Therefore, it appears that there is a need for transient, reversible inactivation of PTPs to ensure proper cellular tyrosine phosphorylation levels and thereby efficient propagation of signaling. In the present context, it is of particular relevance that nature seems to regulate PTP activity by H_2O_2-mediated reversible oxidation of the active site cysteine. It took about three decades from the initial biological observations to unravel the structural basis for the effects of H_2O_2 on PTPs. In the early 1970s, Michael Czech and his colleagues made the intriguing observation that thiols mimic the action of insulin on isolated fat cells (stimulating glucose uptake and metabolism and inhibiting lipolysis) by Cu^{2+}-dependent production of H_2O_2 (Czech et al. 1974a,c). Further, it was shown that extracellular addition of H_2O_2 can mimic the action of insulin in fat cells (Czech et al. 1974c), and evidence was provided for involvement of sulfhydryl oxidation in this process (Czech et al. 1974b). The physiological relevance of these findings became apparent when it was demonstrated that insulin stimulates intracellular formation of H_2O_2 in rat epididymal fat cells (May and de Haen 1979).

A large number of other agents have also been shown to mimic the action of insulin in isolated cells, including vanadate (Dubyak and Kleinzeller 1980), which was shown to act synergistically with H_2O_2 to stimulate the insulin receptor kinase activity in intact cells in an apparently direct manner (Tamura et al. 1984; Kadota et al. 1987; Koshio et al. 1988; Heffetz et al. 1990; Heffetz and Zick 1992). However, it was not realized until 1989 that the synergistic effects of H_2O_2 and vanadate were due to the formation of "pervanadate", which increases the phosphorylation and activity of the IRTK, not directly, but by inhibiting counteracting PTP(s) (Fantus et al. 1989). This seminal publication was the first to demonstrate that perhaps it would be possible to mimic the action of insulin by inhibiting PTP(s) that negatively regulate the insulin signaling pathway. Indeed, this publication played a significant role for initiation of the PTP inhibitor drug discovery program at Novo Nordisk. In the present context, it is intriguing that recent studies have demonstrated that insulin-stimulated formation of H_2O_2 leads to reversible inhibition of PTP1B and enhancement of the insulin signaling in 3T3-L1 cells (Mahadev et al. 2001a,b).

In 1998, it was demonstrated at the biochemical level that PTPs could be negatively regulated by H_2O_2 (Denu and Tanner 1998). PTPs react rapidly with low micromolar concentrations of H_2O_2, specifically oxidizing the active site cysteine and involving a sulfenic acid intermediate. Importantly, the inactivation took place in the presence of reducing agents and it was reversible, thus providing support for the view that PTP function may be regulated in vivo by reactive oxygen species. In an attempt to determine the structure of PTP1B with the catalytic cysteine oxidized to the sulfenic acid state, Barford, Tonks, and colleagues unexpectedly observed a modification of the active site cysteine, termed "sulphenyl-amide", which was indicated by a well-defined continuous electron density between the Sγ atom of Cys215 and the main chain nitrogen atom of Ser216 in the X-ray structure (Salmeen et al. 2003). As a result, the P-loop undergoes a major conformational change (with Gly218 moving about 7 Å outwards) and the oxidized cysteine is now exposed to the reducing environment in the cell, thus facilitating the regeneration of the active state of the enzyme. Moreover, the conformational change imposed by the sulphenyl–amide bond formation results in disruption of the hydrogen bond between Ser216 and Tyr46 in the pTyr loop, and the latter tyrosine residue adopts a solvent-exposed position. Interestingly, this repositioning of Tyr46 makes PTP1B susceptible to phosphorylation by the insulin receptor, and the authors propose that such redox-dependent phosphorylation may represent an additional level of control over the signaling specificity of PTP1B. These structural studies together with the above biochemical studies provide not only a plausible novel mechanism for PTP regulation, but also a unique possibility for designing compounds that only influence signal transduction pathways that are already activated (see Sect. 10). Of note, the structural changes of PTP1B observed by addition of H_2O_2 may also be induced by addition of putative inhibitors of the enzyme (van Montfort et al. 2003; unpublished observations).

Interestingly, UV irradiation causes inactivation of PTPs and converts PTPα into a substrate-trapping mutant which can coprecipitate the platelet-derived growth factor (PDGF)-β receptor, similarly to the PTPα_{C433S} mutant (Gross et al. 1999). Further, den Hertog et al. have recently shown that H_2O_2 treatment of cells leads to rotational coupling and inactivation of PTPα dimers (Blanchetot et al. 2002b; van der Wijk et al. 2003).

Using a modified 'in-gel' PTP assay to allow visualization of oxidized PTPs, Tonks and coworkers recently provided evidence for the notion that reversible oxidation may be a general mechanism for regulation of PTP activity (Meng et al. 2002). Specifically, these authors showed that ligand-induced, transient oxidation of SHP-2 in the PDGF-R complex coincided with autophosphorylation of the receptor, thus demonstrating that PTPs not only respond to oxidative stress in the environment, but also to reactive oxygen species generated to physiological responses, as in the case of insulin signaling.

7
PTPs as Drug Targets

In the early days of PTP research, these enzymes were mainly considered as housekeeping enzymes that turned signaling processes off. A more complicated picture later emerged showing PTPs both to be negative and positive regulators of signaling pathways. Despite this, most drug discovery activities in the PTP field have so far been directed towards development of inhibitors of PTPs that negatively regulate signaling pathways, thereby intensifying and/or prolonging signaling.

In particular, the insulin signaling pathway has received much attention based on the assumption that the insulin-resistant state in type 2 diabetes could be overcome by inhibiting PTPs that negatively regulate this pathway. Based on theoretical considerations, our own efforts began back in the early 1990s by re-cloning and expression of PTP1B as a tool (Hoppe et al. 1994), searching for novel PTPs (Møller et al. 1994a,b), and by studying the tissue distribution of PTPs (Norris et al. 1997). We decided to focus on PTPs that negatively regulate upstream elements in the insulin-signaling pathway, preferentially the insulin receptor tyrosine kinase itself (Møller et al. 1995). We assumed that even the unstimulated IR had to be controlled by counteracting PTPs, i.e., potentially selective inhibitors could be used not only to treat patients with type 2 diabetes, but also type 1 diabetes. Numerous studies have since then been devoted to identification of the insulin receptor-regulating PTPs (IR-PTP) and the development of selective inhibitors thereof (reviewed in Kennedy 1999; Møller et al. 2000; Ramachandran and Kennedy 2003; Zhang and Lee 2003), namely: (1) brute force substrate trapping studies (Walchli et al. 2000); (2) in vitro studies with anti-sense oligonucleotides (Kulas et al. 1995); (3) tissue distribution analyses (Norris et al. 1997); (4) studies of the dynamics in subcellular distribution of PTPs (Calera et al. 2000); (5) insulin-based selection system analyses (Møller et al. 1995); (6) overexpression studies. As a result, several candidate PTPs have been named, including PTP1B, PTPα (Møller et al. 1995; Cong et al. 1999), and PTP-LAR (Ahmad et al. 1995; Kulas et al. 1995). As described above, PTP1B is clearly the PTP target that has been validated and addressed most in the diabetes and obesity field.

As recently pointed out by one of the key founders of the PTP field, it is important to remember that there is more to the PTP family than just PTP1B (Tonks 2003), and it should be remembered that other PTPs, in addition to PTP1B, may be involved in the negative regulation of insulin signaling. Also, other PTPs could potentially be attractive drug targets, such as CD45 in autoimmunity (Hermiston et al. 2003; Irie-Sasaki et al. 2003; Lee and Burke 2003) and SHP-1 in cancer (Wu et al. 2003). Further, other PTPs seem to be negative regulators of the immune system, by recruitment to receptor molecules with ITIMs (immunoreceptor tyrosine inhibitory motifs). It might therefore be speculated that inhibitors of such PTPs (e.g., SHP-1) enhance the activity of cells like natural killer cells (Jackson 2003). Additionally, LAR (Mooney and LeVea 2003) and PTPα (Pallen 2003) have been proposed as potential drug targets, and SHP-2 mutants are critically involved in the development of Noonan syndrome and juvenile myelomonocytic leukemia (Tartaglia et al. 2003).

In addition, PTP inhibitors may be useful for treatment of infectious diseases (reviewed in van Huijsduijnen et al. 2002). Thus, it has been found that *Helicobacter pylori*, a class I carcinogen, produces a protein, CagA, that activates SHP-2 leading to a growth factor-like response in gastric epithelial cells (Higashi et al. 2002; Hatakeyama 2003). Also, PTPζ and PTPα appear to be receptors for the *H. pylori* cytotoxin, VacA, that induces vacuolation, mitochondrial damage, cytochrome *c* release, and apoptosis of gastric epithelial cells (Yahiro et al. 1999; Yahiro et al. 2003). A number of bacterial pathogens have evolved strategies to destabilize signal transduction for their own benefit, and highly active PTPs seem to be used as such sophisticated virulence factors (Clemens et al. 1991). As an example, the *Yersinia* PTP, which has served as an excellent research tool in a number of publications, has been shown to be essential for virulence (Guan and Dixon 1990). Similarly, a PTP in *Salmonella* seems to be required for full display of virulence (Kaniga et al. 1996; Murli et al. 2001). Ullrich and coworkers recently cloned and characterized two secretory PTPs from *Mycobacterium*, one of which was proposed as a candidate virulence gene (Koul et al. 2000).

It remains to be shown if some or all of the above-mentioned PTPs will eventually prove to be good drug target candidates. Clearly, additional basic science and preclinical work will be required to validate these candidates. In any case, selective, cellularly active PTP inhibitors would be invaluable tools in such assessments.

8 Reversible, Competitive Inhibitors

8.1 Challenges

Initially, the pharmaceutical industry was reluctant to enter the PTP inhibitor field, and in particular to developing active site-directed inhibitors. The highly conserved structure of the catalytic domains of even distantly related PTPs with little primary sequence identity in combination with the expectation of a large protein family (Charbonneau and Tonks 1992; Pot and Dixon 1992a; Denu and Dixon 1998) seemed to represent insurmountable obstacles for the development of highly specific, low molecular weight inhibitors for therapeutic use (reviewed in Tonks 2003). This was also the situation in the early days in the kinase field (Cohen 2002). In the latter case, the development of a relatively specific and clinically extremely efficient kinase inhibitor, Gleevec, for the treatment of chronic myelogenous leukemia and other malignant diseases has changed the perception completely in the industry (see chapters by Cohen and Wakeling, this volume).

In our opinion, the major challenge in developing PTP inhibitors is not related to the conserved structure of PTPs as such, but rather to the very nature of the PTP catalytic machinery (Sect. 2). Indeed, we and others have demonstrated that highly selective and potent PTP inhibitors can be made (see Sect. 9). However, while the above-described low pK_a value of the catalytic cysteine in PTPs is essential for its function as a nucleophile both in the first step of catalysis and for the susceptibility to redox regulation, this same property is one of the major challenges in the identification and development of PTP inhibitors. Thus, it is a common experience among laboratories that perform high-throughput screenings to get high hit rates when searching for PTP inhibitors, in many cases caused by oxidation or alkylation of the active site cysteine (Bleasdale et al. 2001; van Montfort et al. 2003) (see below). It should be noted, however, that redox-induced conformational changes of PTPs as discussed above (Sect. 6) may represent a novel opportunity for the design of inhibitors that only influence already activated signaling pathways (Sect. 10).

Another challenge relates to the nature of the pocket of the active site of PTPs. In contrast to kinases, for which inhibitors have been developed that bind to a relatively hydrophobic pocket in the ATP binding site, the active site in PTPs is a water-molecule-filled, fairly shallow, cavity that first turns into a pocket upon closure of the WPD loop (Sect. 2). A prerequisite for this loop closure seems to be binding of the phosphate moiety of pTyr to the P-loop. Thus, many structure-based approaches are based on development of inhibitors that mimic the binding of phosphate to the P-loop. Since pTyr at neutral pH is doubly negatively charged, most competitive PTP inhibitors developed to date are similarly charged molecules. As a consequence, problems with cellular uptake, pharmacokinetic properties, and oral availability may be expected.

8.2 Identification of Chemical Lead Structures

To identify small molecule PTP lead structures, the most straightforward method is to mimic the natural substrate pTyr by making non-hydrolyzable analogs. Initial attempts in academia were very successful in developing model compounds as described below (Sect. 9.1). Since these compounds often showed poor or no cellular activity, most companies turned to high-throughput screening (HTS) in attempts to identify novel lead structures. At Novo Nordisk we used a scintillation proximity assay (SPA) with PTP1B and a biotinylated [^{33}P]-radiolabeled peptide substrate corresponding to the activation loop of the insulin receptor tyrosine kinase. A substantial number of hits were identified in the screening. However, when analyzing these hit compounds in detail, as recommended below, most were eliminated as false positives. The compound that fulfilled most of our pre-defined selection criteria (see below) was 2-(oxalylamino)-benzoic acid, OBA (compound **1**, Fig. 4; Andersen et al. 2000). This compound was found to share most of the

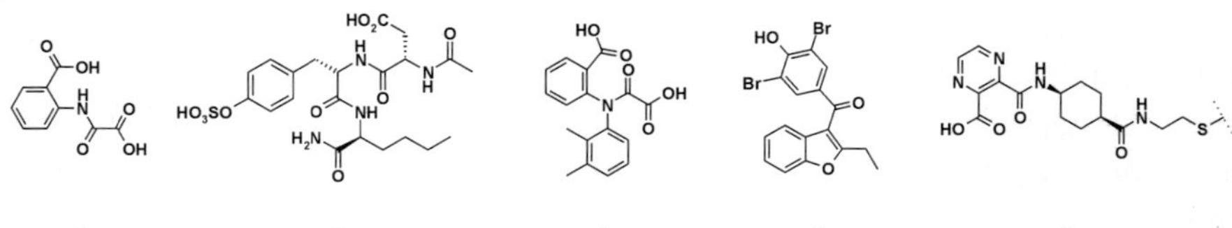

1 (1C85) 2 3 4 5 (1NWL)

Fig. 4 Chemical lead structures identified by different strategies

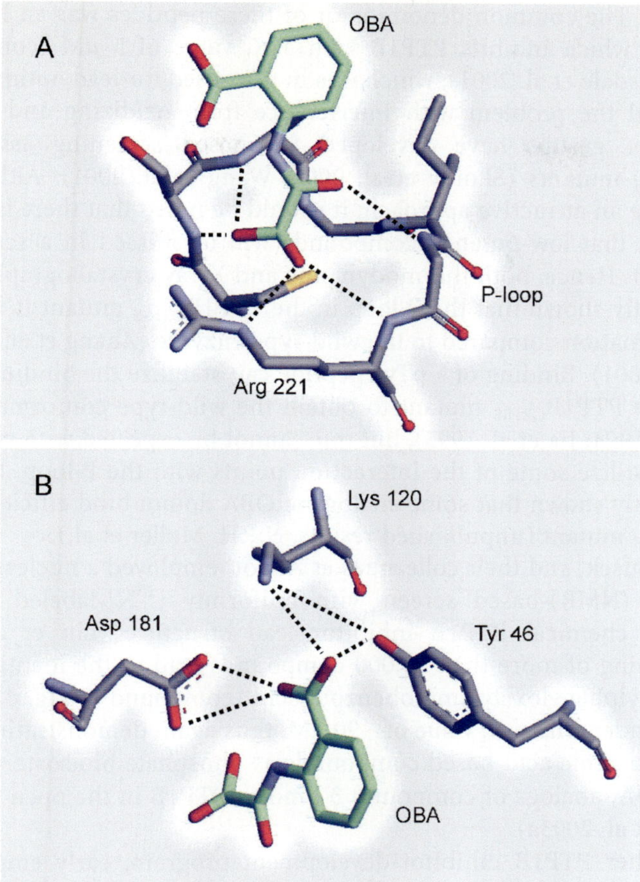

Fig. 5A, B Binding mode of OBA in PTP1B. **A** Interaction with the P-loop. **B** Unique interaction with Lys120, Asp181, and Tyr46

interaction points with the natural substrate, pTyr, and in addition showed a unique arrangement involving residues 46, 120, and 181 (pdb code 1C85– Fig. 5A and B). As will be detailed below, this simple compound has served as a basic scaffold in our development of highly potent and selective PTP inhibitors. Also, other companies have employed HTS to identify chemical leads. Initially, Bleasdale and coworkers used a broad screening strategy. However, their search for reversible, competitive inhibitors was confounded by identification of many compounds representing several chemical classes that irreversibly inhibited PTP1B by reacting with Cys215 (Bleasdale et al. 2001). Using targeted screening of a collection of compounds with suspected or known pTyr bioisosteres, these authors identified a series of relatively potent PTP1B inhibitors based on sulfotyrosyl-containing CCK-8 derived octapeptides. The common denominator of these peptides was an N-terminal tripeptide, which inhibits PTP1B with a K_i value of 5 μM (compound **2**, Fig. 4; Bleasdale et al. 2001), which was in turn used for lead optimization.

To avoid the problem with interference from oxidizing and alkylating agents, two groups have developed SPA-based screening assays using $PTP1B_{C215S}$ mutants (Skorey et al. 2001; Wang et al. 2001). Although this seems to be an attractive approach, it should be noted that there is a considerable risk that low-potency compounds will be missed in a screen using this mutant. Hence, both thermodynamic and X-ray crystallographic studies have recently shown that the P-loop in the $PTP1B_{C215S}$ mutant is in a different conformation compared to the wild-type enzyme (Zhang et al. 2000; Scapin et al. 2001). Binding of a pTyr peptide can stabilize the binding of the P-loop in the $PTP1B_{C215S}$ mutant to obtain the wild-type conformation (Barford et al. 1994; Jia et al. 1995), but this cannot be expected with compounds that only utilize some of the interaction points with the P-loop. Indeed, we have recently shown that some analogs of OBA do not bind efficiently to the $PTP1B_{C215S}$ mutant (unpublished results, N.P.H. Møller et al.).

Liu, Jirousek, and their colleagues at Abbott employed a nuclear magnetic resonance (NMR)-based screen with uniformly [^{15}N]-labeled PTP1B to identify a chemical PTP1B inhibitor lead structure (Liu et al. 2003a). The screening of more than 10,000 compounds lead to the identification of 2,3-dimethylphenyloxalylaminobenzoic acid (compound **3**, Fig. 4) as an active site binder with a K_i value of ~90 μM, thus again demonstrating the usefulness of oxamic acid-based compounds as phosphate bioisosteres. In contrast to OBA, analogs of compound **3** bind to PTP1B in the open conformation (Liu et al. 2003a).

In another PTP1B inhibitor-development program, early emphasis was given to orally availability and pharmacokinetic properties (Wrobel et al. 1999). A potent uricosuric agent benzbromarone (compound **4**, Fig. 4) that showed weak inhibition of rat PTP1B was used as a starting point for lead optimization, resulting in compounds which showed glucose lowering properties in *ob/ob* mice. One of these compounds has recently been withdrawn from phase II clinical trials, and it has been reported that the glucose-lowering effects may be attributed to PPAR-γ-activating activity of the compound (reviewed by Johnson et al. 2002).

Recently, an intriguing approach to discover novel pTyr mimetics for PTP1B was described using the 'breakaway tethering' approach (Erlanson et al. 2003). Since the active site cysteine prevents using this approach directly, a novel strategy was designed. Arg47 was mutated to a cysteine residue and labeled with an 'extender' that included an oxalic acid to protect Cys215 against alkylation. Further, an oxalic acid-based thiol was used as positive control, again demonstrating the usefulness of this moiety in the discovery of PTP inhibitors. Tether screening of 15,000 disulfide-containing fragments identified compound **5** (Fig. 4) as one of the strongest hits. Importantly, the free compound **5** displayed competitive inhibition of PTP1B, although with low potency (K_i ~4 mM). The X-ray crystal structure of compound **5** disulfide-bonded to the extender-modified $PTP1B_{R47C}$ showed several hydrogen bonds from the carboxylic acid and pyrazine moieties to the active site, and the cyclohexyl ring fits well in the hydrophobic pocket normally occupied by the phenyl ring of pTyr (pdb code 1NWL).

8.3 Recommendations and Guidelines

Our first HTS efforts at Novo Nordisk in 1996 was aimed at the identification of a general PTP inhibitor scaffold, and the number of verified hits far exceeded our initial expectations. As described above, in these screens we used a scintillation proximity assay with PTP1B and a [^{33}P]-radiolabeled peptide substrate. In these early days, the PTP(s) that negatively regulate the IR signaling pathway had not yet been identified, although several candidates had been proposed including PTP1B, LAR, and PTPα (see above). Hence, our approach was to identify a general, low molecular weight inhibitor that could be optimized for specificity against a number of different PTPs (Møller et al. 2000) (Fig. 6). These inhibitors should then in turn be used in cell-based assays to identify the PTP that negatively regulates the IR. As soon as a hit had been resynthesized and confirmed, we initiated further validation of the hit

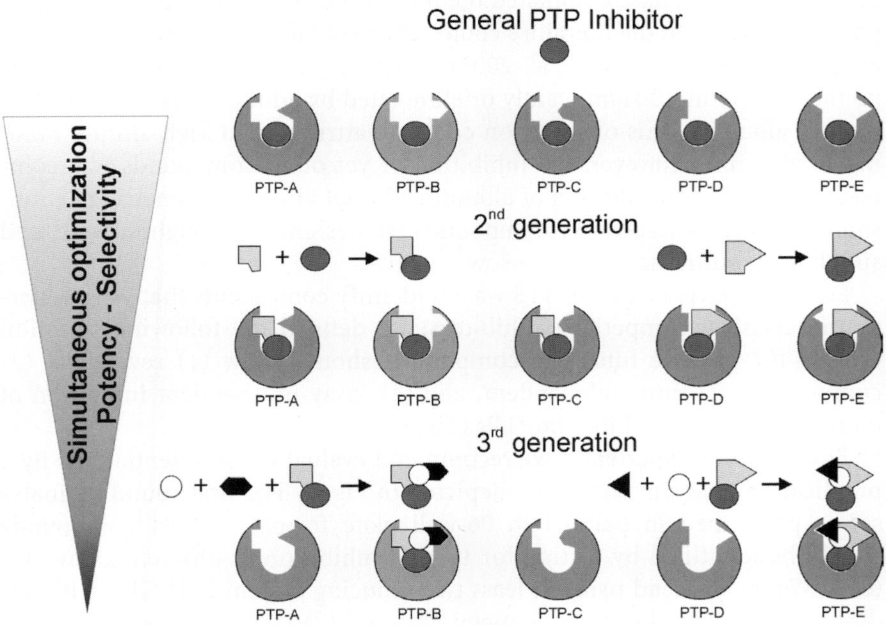

Fig. 6 Schematic representation of the Novo Nordisk lead optimization strategy

by synthesizing a number of analogs and by testing these for selectivity in biochemical assays (against other PTPs) and cell-based assays.

A variety of chemical classes were identified and several promising lead series were pursued. In particular, much attention was given to a series that included compounds that significantly induced insulin-independent glucose uptake in isolated rat soleus muscle. However, despite the synthesis of a large number of analogs within these lead series, we did not succeed in obtaining significant improvement of potency or selectivity. Indeed, rarely did we find a true structure–activity relationship (SAR). Further in-depth analyses revealed that many of these compounds showed mixed-type inhibition and, perhaps most significantly, the inhibition of PTPs depended strongly on the assay conditions, most likely because the apparent inhibition was caused by oxidation or alkylation of Cys215: (1) In some cases inhibition was abolished by using dithiothreitol (DTT at 1 mM), rather than reduced glutathione (GSH at 5 mM) as reducing agent in the assay buffer (i.e., the observed inhibition most likely was due to oxidation of the catalytic cysteine, which was prevented by the stronger reducing agent DTT). (2) On the contrary, other compounds only displayed PTP inhibitory activity in the presence of DTT, and this inhibition could be prevented by addition of ethylenediaminetetraacetate (EDTA). This type of compound most likely inhibits PTPs by a mechanism that resembles that reported for alendronate, i.e., formation of H_2O_2 by a combination of the compounds with low micromolar concentrations of DTT and trace metals (present in the buffer) (Skorey et al. 1997). In such cases, the addition of catalase eliminated the inhibition. It is likely that several compounds reported in the literature could represent false positive hits (Bleasdale et al. 2001; van Montfort et al. 2003). Further, the inhibition of some compounds was reduced significantly or eliminated by addition of carrier protein such as albumin. This observation could be attributed to high affinity binding to albumin. However, the inhibition of yet other compounds was completely abolished by addition of albumin without any stoichiometric relationship. To avoid false-positive compounds we designed a straightforward and simple test routine as detailed below.

Since the purpose of the HTS was to identify compounds that were general and classical competitive inhibitors, we defined the following selection criteria for positive hits. The compounds should show (1) reversible, (2) competitive, (3) time-independent, and (4) assay-independent inhibition of more than 3 out of 4 different PTPs (Fig. 6).

Based on our experience, we recommend evaluation of potential hits by a practical scheme similar to that depicted in Fig. 7. The first round of analyses is performed in parallel in 96-well plate format. Robust compounds should be identified by testing for type of inhibition in different assay systems. We recommend using at least two reducing systems: (1) GSH with addition of EDTA to chelate trace metal ions and (2) DTT. Further, albumin or a detergent should be added. Compounds must show similar K_i values and

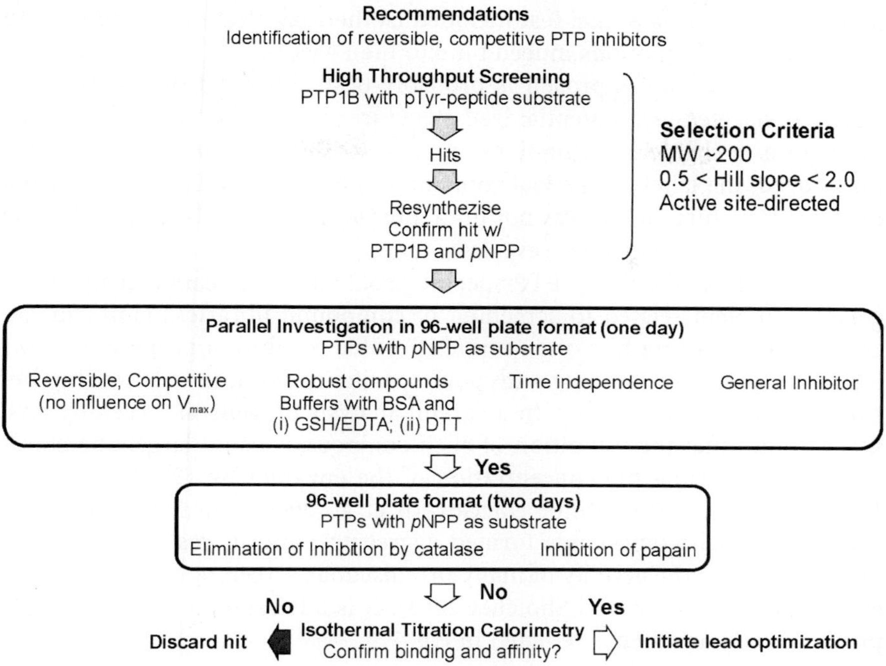

Fig. 7 Recommendations: Identification of reversible, competitive chemical leads for structure-based design of selective PTP inhibitors

competitive type of inhibition in both buffer systems (i.e., no influence of V_{max}app with increasing inhibitor concentration), and they should not be time dependent. In our case, we further require that lead compounds are general PTP inhibitors and consequently test a small battery of different PTPs. In the next round, we analyze for sensitivity to catalase (which would be an exclusion criteria) and include a specificity test by testing for activity against non-PTP enzymes with a catalytic cysteine such as papain (Fig. 8).

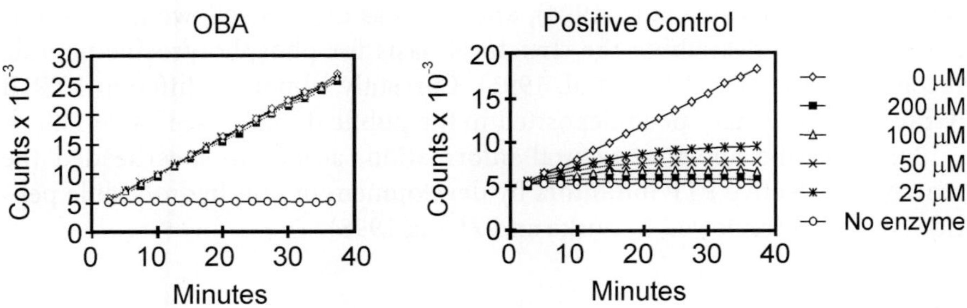

Fig. 8 Specificity check of putative PTP inhibitors in papain. OBA showing no inhibition and a non-specific PTP inhibitor demonstrating time-dependent inhibition of papain

Recently, we have as a final test included isothermal titration calorimetry to verify that the compounds indeed bind to the PTPs.

The power of our approach is probably best illustrated by the fact that OBA was selected as a potential lead structure exclusively on the basis of its behavior as a classical, textbook example of a reversible, competitive inhibitor. Indeed, the label on the vial containing the original HTS hit indicated a different structure, and it was not until after structural analysis that the true nature/structure of OBA was revealed.

In addition to the above PTP-specific problems, it appears that there is a general problem related to screening of compound libraries. Thus, further analysis of screening hits often reveals peculiar inhibition properties showing non-competitive binding with poor specificity and little relationship between structure and activity. In a careful analysis of 'general screening hits' it was found that the inhibition of such compounds could largely be eliminated by increasing the concentration of the enzymes by 10-fold despite a 1,000-fold excess of inhibitor (McGovern et al. 2002). Further analysis revealed that such compounds formed aggregates, and it was suggested this may account for the activity of many promiscuous screening hits (McGovern et al. 2002; McGovern and Shoichet 2003). It is advisable to add this simple procedure to our scheme depicted in Fig. 7.

9
Structure-Based Design—PTP1B Inhibitors

PTP1B, the first PTP to be isolated and characterized, has been leading the way in the development of PTP inhibitors (Tonks et al. 1988a, 1988b). This is partly because early studies indicated a role for PTP1B in the negative regulation of insulin signaling and hence its potential as drug target in diabetes (Sect. 7). However, the key determining factor seems to be that PTP1B and its rat ortholog, PTP1, have been used in numerous studies as model enzymes to investigate the mechanism of action of PTPs and the structural basis for substrate specificity. As early as 1994, the crystal structure of PTP1B was reported (Barford et al. 1994), and this was quickly followed by a seminal publication describing the structural basis for phosphotyrosine peptide recognition by PTP1B (Jia et al. 1995). Currently, about 40 different PTP1B X-ray structures have been deposited in the public domain (see Table 1).

Based on the above structural information, academia spearheaded the search for selective PTP inhibitors by development of non-hydrolyzable peptide mimetics (reviewed in Burke and Zhang 1998).

9.1 Peptide-Based Inhibitors—Phosphotyrosyl Mimetics

The initial attempts to design selective PTP inhibitors were based on replacement of pTyr with non-hydrolyzable phosphotyrosyl mimetics in small, efficient PTP peptide substrates, thereby utilizing both the potency and selectivity provided by the amino acid residues (reviewed in Burke and Lee 2003). The next step in inhibitor design was then planned to be modification of the peptide moiety into more drug-like compounds without losing potency or selectivity. The most straightforward solution was to replace the phosphate moiety with phosphonates, i.e., by replacing the scissile oxygen in pTyr with a non-hydrolyzable chemical group such as methylene, resulting in (phosphonomethyl)-phenylalanine (Pmp) (Domchek et al. 1992; Smyth et al. 1992). When Pmp is replacing pTyr in the Ac-D-A-D-E-pY-L-NH_2 peptide, a relatively potent inhibitor of PTP1B is obtained (i.e., K_i~10 μM—compound **6**, X=CH_2, Fig. 9) (Zhang et al. 1994a). Introduction of two fluorines at the α-methylene position in Pmp yielded F_2Pmp. Interestingly, the peptide Ac-D-A-D-E-F_2Pmp-L-NH_2 (compound **7**, Fig. 9) showed ~1,000-fold increase in affinity for the rat PTP1 compared with the Pmp peptide (Burke et al. 1994; Chen et al. 1995). This dramatic increase in affinity was due to direct interaction of the fluorines with the enzyme, rather than changes in pK_a values, as revealed at the structural level by co-crystallizing PTP1B with the non-peptidyl inhibitor [1,1-difluoro-1-1(2-naphthalenyl)-methyl]phosphonic acid (compound **18**, Fig. 11) (Burke et al. 1996b) (see below). Subsequently, it

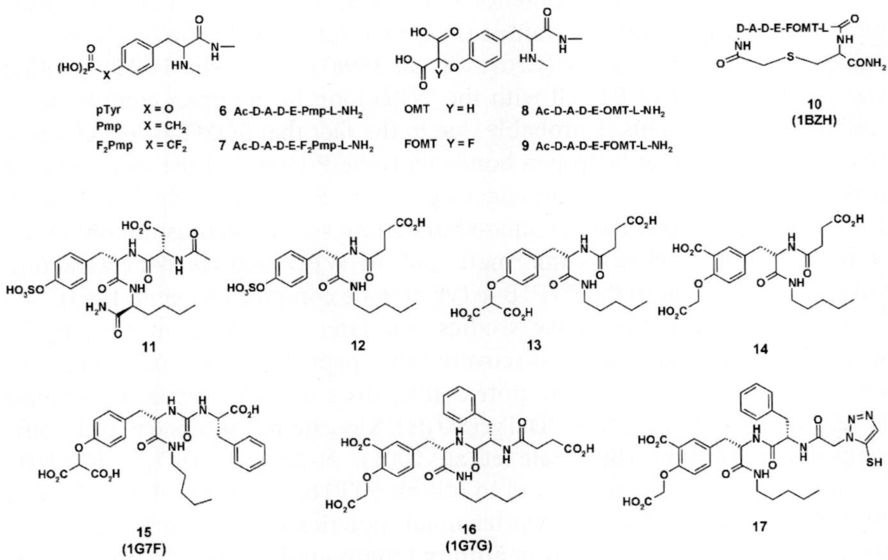

Fig. 9 Phosphotyrosyl mimetics—peptide-based inhibitors

was found that two F_2Pmp moieties in a sequence-specific manner could be used to improve the potency and selectivity of tripeptides (Desmarais et al. 1999). Thus, the tripeptide, Glu-F_2Pmp-F_2Pmp inhibited PTP1B with an IC_{50} of 40 nM, which represented more than 100-fold selectivity against CD45, PTPβ, and LAR. Interestingly, Pro-F_2Pmp-F_2Pmp is equipotent against PTP1B and PTPβ, with IC_{50} values in the 0.2–0.3 μM range.

To improve bioavailability, efforts have been directed towards the development of less-charged, non-phosphorus-containing, peptide inhibitors. One of the first steps away from peptidyl phosphonate-based inhibitors was taken by Burke and colleagues. Based on previous work (Miller et al. 1994), *L-O*-malonyltyrosine (OMT) was introduced as a relatively efficient pTyr analog in synthetic peptides used to inhibit SH2 domain interactions (Ye and Burke 1995; Ye et al. 1995). As in the above studies with F_2Pmp, OMT was introduced in parallel into the EGF receptor peptide yielding Ac-D-A-D-E-(OMT)-L-NH_2 (compound **8**, Fig. 9) that showed about a 20-fold increase in potency against PTP1B compared with Pmp (Kole et al. 1995a). Based on the experience with FPmp and F_2Pmp, these authors next incorporated fluorine in OMT yielding 4′-*O*-[2-(2-fluoromalonyl)]-l-tyrosine, FOMT, and synthesized Ac-D-A-D-E-(FOMT)-l-NH_2 (compound **9**, Fig. 9), which showed a tenfold increase in affinity for PTP1B (K_i~1 μM) compared with the unfluorinated counterpart (K_i~13 μM) (Burke et al. 1996a). When restraining the conformational flexibility of these peptides, a substantial increase in affinity for PTP1B was observed with a K_i of 0.7 μM for a cyclic OMT-based peptide (Akamatsu et al. 1997) and a K_i of 0.17 μM for the cyclic FOMT-peptide (compound **10**, Fig. 9) (Akamatsu et al. 1997).

With the above relatively potent PTP1B inhibitors at hand, Barford, Burke, and their colleagues next examined the structural basis for the inhibitory capacity of these compounds (Groves et al. 1998). The cyclic FOMT-peptide was found to bind to PTP1B with the WPD loop in the open conformation (pdb code 1BZH). This is probably due to the fact that FOMT is less efficient than pTyr in forming hydrogen bonds with the P-loop and the side chain of Arg221 and further, the aromatic ring of the FOMT peptide is displaced 1.4 Å away from the P-loop compared to natural substrate, thus not obtaining stabilization of the closed conformation of the WPD loop via π–π interaction with Phe182 as seen in the PTP1B–pTyr peptide complex (Jia et al. 1995).

The baton from the above studies was later picked up at Pharmacia, where it was serendipitously discovered that peptide analogs of cholecystokinin (CKK-8) were relatively potent inhibitors of PTP1B with a common N-terminal tripeptide, N-Ac-D-Tyr(SO_3H)-Nle-, being necessary and sufficient for inhibition (Bleasdale et al. 2001). N-Ac-D-Tyr(SO_3H)-Nle-NH_2 (compound **11**, Fig. 9) was found to inhibit PTP1B with a K_i value of 17 μM. Importantly, removal of the two terminal moieties resulted in a compound with only a twofold reduction in affinity (compound **12**—K_i=30 μM). Previously, a synthetic tris-sulfotyrosyl dodecapeptide analog of the insulin-receptor 1146-kinase domain was shown to inhibit dephosphorylation of the insulin-receptor (Liotta et al. 1994; Kole et al. 1996). Replacing the tyrosine-sulfate in the above N-terminal CCK-derived peptide with either OMT (**13**) (Kole et al. 1995a) or 2-carboxymethoxybenzoic acid (**14**), originally described by Burke and coworkers as an efficient pTyr bioisostere (Burke et al. 1998), resulted in compounds that inhibit PTP1B with K_i values of 12 and 2.8 μM, respectively (Bleasdale et al. 2001). Further development of these series led to compounds **15** (K_i=3.4 μM), **16** (K_i=0.25 μM), and **17** (K_i=0.12 μM). Prodrug analogs of compounds **16** and **17** were recently shown to enhance uptake of 2-deoxyglucose by L6 myotubes (Larsen et al. 2003).

To assist further structure-based design efforts, PTP1B was co-crystallized with compounds **15** and **16** (Bleasdale et al. 2001). The binding mode of compound **15** resembles that reported for the cyclic FOMT-based peptide (**10**) (Groves et al. 1998) with the exception that the phenyl ring of compound **15** is positioned about 1 Å closer to the P-loop, thereby causing steric hindrance contributing to the open conformation of the WPD loop. However, important hydrogen bonds to the main chain nitrogens of the P-loop are missing compared to the known PTP1B-peptide complexes. Superficially, the pTyr bioisostere in compound **16** is quite similar to OBA (**1**) (see below). However, superimposition of the crystal structures of compound **16** and OBA in complex with PTP1B reveals significant differences (Fig. 10). While OBA shares most of the interaction points of pTyr in the active site, com-

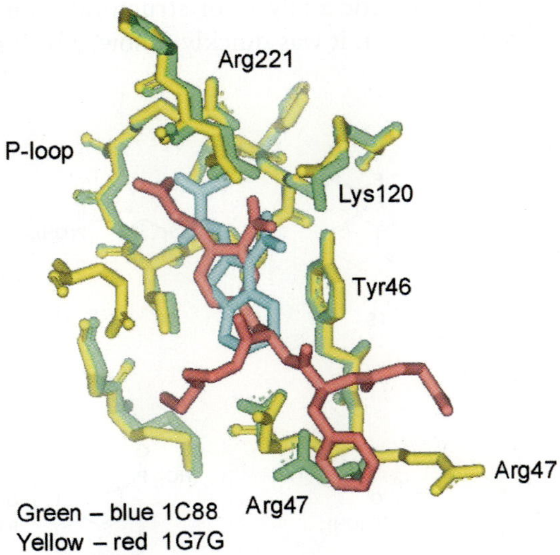

Fig. 10 Superimposition of 1C88 (PTP1B shown in *green*; OBA in *blue*) and 1G7G (PTP1B shown in *yellow*; compound **16** in *red*). OBA shares most of the interaction points of pTyr in the active site, whereas compound **16** only forms contact with Arg221 in the P-loop

pound **16** only forms contact with Arg221 in the P-loop, and the position normally taken up by the phosphate group of pTyr is essentially unoccupied by the inhibitor, but replaced with two water molecules that promote the binding between the ligand and the P-loop (Bleasdale et al. 2001). Similar to the situation with PTP1B complexed with OBA, the WPD loop is closed and the *o*-carboxy group interacts with Lys120 and Asp181. Although not reported by these authors, it is likely that the binding of compound **15** to PTP1B is pH independent, whereas the binding of compound **16**—like OBA (Andersen et al. 2000)—is pH dependent due to its interaction with Asp181.

9.2 Non-peptide Inhibitors

9.2.1 Phosphorus-Containing Inhibitors

Based on molecular modeling of several phenylalanine phosphonate analogs, Burke and colleagues took the first step towards the design of low molecular weight, non-peptide phosphatase inhibitors (Kole et al. 1995b). Fifteen different aryl-containing phosphonates were synthesized and tested for their ability to inhibit PTP1B and serine threonine phosphatases (PP1 and PP-2A). Two difluoro-naphthalene-based phosphonates [1- or 2-substitued (difluoro-naphthalen-1(2)-yl-methyl)-phosphonic acids—compounds **18** and **19**] were found to inhibit PTP1B and PP-2A equally well (Fig. 11). In contrast, the non-fluorinated counterparts are poor inhibitors (compounds **20** and **21**). Detailed enzyme kinetic analyses or structural information was not reported in this study. However, it was quickly followed by a report of the X-

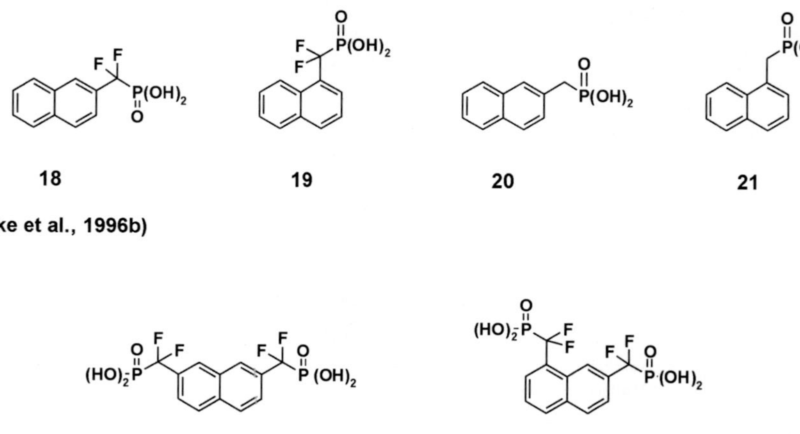

18 19 20 21

(Burke et al., 1996b)

22 23

Fig. 11 Non-peptidyl phosphorus PTP inhibitor leads

ray structure of PTP1B in complex with compound **18** (difluoro-naphthalen-2-yl-methyl)-phosphonic acid (Burke et al. 1996b; Ye and Burke 1996). Based on this structure, it was hypothesized that the addition of a hydroxyl group at the 4-position of the naphthyl ring could replace a water molecule and thereby allow H-bond formation to Tyr46 and Lys120. Indeed, addition of this hydroxyl group increased the affinity twofold, i.e., structure-based design of non-peptide PTP inhibitors was born. Further development of this concept was leading to compounds with K_i values in the low micromolar range [(Groves et al. 1998) pdb code1BZC].

At Merck-Frosst these studies were extended, and it was found that introduction of two difluoromethylenephosphonic (DFMP) groups into naphthalene-based compounds significantly increased the potency against PTP1B (Wang et al. 1998). For the first time it was demonstrated that selectivity could be obtained by different, simple substitutions. Thus, within this series one compound (**22**) was five- to sixfold more potent against PTP1B (K_i=16 μM) than CD45 and another compound (**23**) showed a fivefold preference for CD45 (K_i=9 μM) over PTP1B. Further elaborations on this approach led Zhang et al. to develop a highly selective PTP1B inhibitor with similar potency as compound **22**, i.e., K_i~1 μM (Taing et al. 1999).

9.2.2 Non-phosphorus Inhibitors

Although introduction of the DFMP group represented a significant step forward in regard to potency, it was also realized that such compounds are not cell permeable, probably due to the highly polar nature of the dianionic DFMP group (Kole et al. 1995b). The first attempt to replace phosphonate or the DFMP group in non-peptidyl inhibitors with less polar groups was reported by Burke et al. (1996a) (compounds **24** and **25**, Fig. 12). Unfortunately, the inhibitory capacity of these compounds was not reported. However, they inspired another research group to search for phosphate bioisosteres that were more effective than the malonyl and CF-malonyl groups. It was

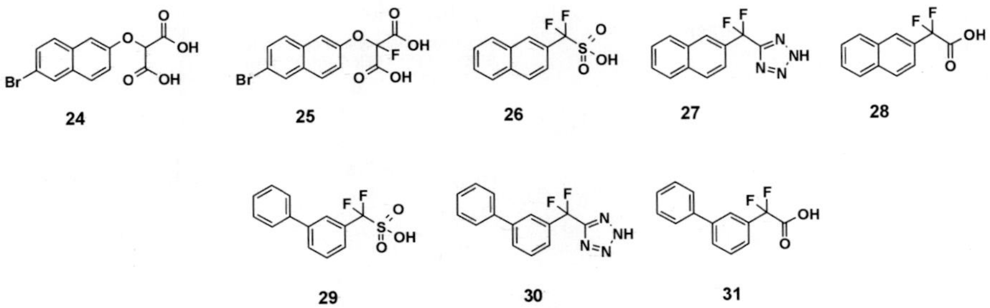

Fig. 12 Non-peptidyl, non-phosphorus PTP inhibitor leads

thus demonstrated by Taylor and coworkers that CF_2-sulfonate (**26** and **29**), CF_2-tetrazole (**27** and **30**), and CF_2-carboxylate (**28** and **31**) were more effective phosphate bioisosteres than CF-malonyl, although not as effective as DFMP (Kotoris et al. 1998) (Fig. 12). In particular, compounds **29** and **31** were investigated in more detail and found to be competitive inhibitors of PTP1B with K_i values of 49 μM and 98 μM, respectively.

9.2.3 Simultaneous Optimization Based on Bioinformatics

Our own efforts on inhibitor development started, as mentioned, with a search for a general inhibitor that potentially could be used as a synthetic scaffold or starting point for development of selective inhibitors of all PTPs (see schematic representation of this strategy in Fig. 6). OBA was identified as an active site-directed lead structure showing classical, competitive inhibition of several PTPs (Andersen et al. 2000; Sect. 8). Although negatively

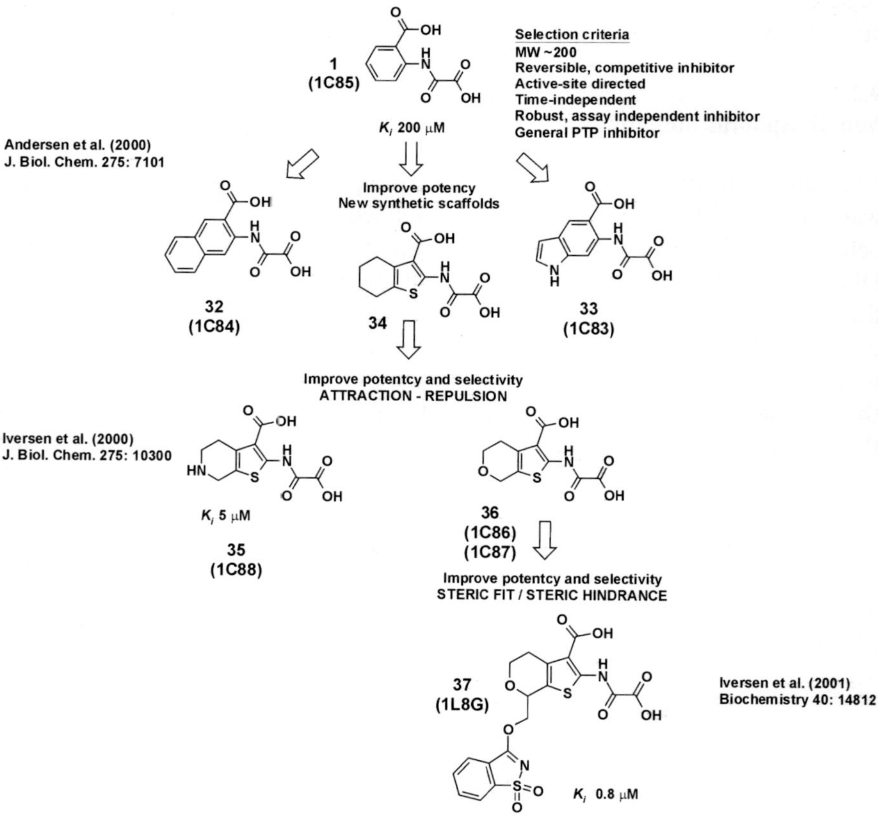

Fig. 13 Bioinformatics-based lead optimization

charged, this compound fulfilled all selection criteria with pH dependency as the only potential limitation. OBA was found to inhibit five out of six PTPs, i.e., it was indeed a general PTP inhibitor. The first step in lead optimization was to improve the general potency of OBA. Inspired by the observations with phosphonates (Sect. 9.2.1), naphthyl- (**32**) and indole-based (**33**) OBA (**1**) analogs were synthesized and found to have significantly improved affinities for several PTPs (Fig. 13). Of note, PTP-LAR, the only PTP that was not recognized by OBA, was inhibited by compound **32**, thus demonstrating that the key structural elements of OBA, i.e., the two carboxy groups bound directly, or through a carbonylamino group, to an aromatic ring represents a true, general PTP inhibitor (Andersen et al. 2000). These early studies also showed differences in inhibitor profiles of compounds **32** and **33**, thus demonstrating that subtle differences in the active site pocket can be used to obtain some selectivity. Mostly for synthetic reasons, we replaced the second aromatic ring with a saturated ring (compound **34**), which showed an almost identical inhibitory profile as that of compound 32 against a number of different PTPs (Andersen et al. 2000; Iversen et al. 2000). A number of other useful synthetic scaffolds derived from OBA were recently reported (Andersen et al. 2002).

9.2.4 Attraction—Repulsion

As described above, bioinformatic analyses revealed that residues 47, 48, 258, and 259 in combination form selectivity-determining regions. Based on modeling of compound **34** in PTP1B, we hypothesized that introduction of a basic nitrogen in this compound at position 6 would place it in an ideal distance from the acidic side chain of Asp48 to allow a salt bridge formation in PTP1B and in other PTPs, whereas with an asparagine in the equivalent position this would cause repulsion. This is an important hallmark in the approach that we have taken: simultaneous improvement of binding to the desired target (in this case by attraction) and decreased binding to non-target enzymes (repulsion). As hypothesized, compound **35** showed an about eightfold increase in potency compared to compound **34** with a K_i of ~5 μM at pH 7 and with more dramatic selectivity against most other PTPs (Iversen et al. 2000) (Fig. 13).

To validate the attraction/repulsion approach, we made reciprocal mutations in PTP1B (as representative for PTPs with an aspartic acid in position 48) and in PTPα (as representative for Asn48-PTPs). By introducing an asparagine in position 48 in PTP1B, the K_i value for compound **34** dropped about 100-fold. Conversely, the introduction of an aspartic acid in the equivalent position of PTPα resulted in significant binding, although weak compared to wild-type (wt) PTP1B. Thus, these mutants unequivocally demonstrated the importance of Asp48 in PTP1B as a selectivity-determining residue (Iversen et al. 2000). Further, by replacing the basic nitrogen in compound **35** with an oxygen atom yielding compound **36** we obtained roughly threefold increase in potency against PTP1B$_{D48\ N}$ compared to wt PTP1B and a similar decrease in potency against PTPα_{N48D}. The crystal structures finally confirmed the enzyme kinetic observations with Asp48 and Asn48 in the rotamer 3 position, 2.8 Å (i.e. hydrogen bond distance) from the basic nitrogen (wt PTP1B/compound **35**) and the pyran oxygen (PTP1B$_{D48\ N}$/compound **36**), respectively. In contrast, the wt PTP1B and comound **36** complex showed Asp48 in the rotamer 1 position, i.e. 5.8 Å away from the pyran oxygen due to repulsion. Thus, the combined analyses of these compounds and PTP mutants clearly demonstrated the importance of Asp48 in PTP1B as a selectivity-determining residue and provided further support for the simultaneous optimization strategy (Iversen et al. 2000).

9.2.5
Steric Fit—Steric Hindrance

In PTP1B, Met258 and Gly259 form the bottom of a cleft-like structure positioned between the second aryl phosphate binding site and the active site pocket. We have termed this region the 258/259 gateway, which allows easy access to the active site of PTP1B. In other PTPs with bulky side chains in position 258, the gateway is blocked. Using a number of analogs of the D-A-D-E-pY-L peptide and the reciprocal mutational approach we showed that residue 259 was a key determining residue in PTP1B and PTPα (Peters et al. 2000; pdb code 1GFY). We next decided to use this information in inhibitor design by making compounds that would bind simultaneously to the active site and the 258/259 gateway in PTP1B and TC-PTP, but not to PTPs with bulky residues in position 258. Compound **36** was used as a scaffold in these studies to allow direct evaluation of the influence of substituents on binding to the gateway. Several compounds were synthesized, and compound **37** with a saccharine-based side chain is an example of an inhibitor that efficiently address the 248/259 gateway with a K_i value of 0.6 μM and 1.1 μM against PTP1B and TC-PTP, respectively (Iversen et al. 2001) (Fig. 13). Importantly, reciprocal mutational analysis with PTP1B, and with PTPα and PTPH1 as representatives for enzymes with closed gateways, provided evidence for the general applicability of this approach. Indeed, we had simultaneously introduced a very high degree of selectivity against a broad spectrum of PTPs. Significantly, this selectivity was also found against two PTPs that contain an aspartic acid in position 48. Finally, the crystal structure of PTP1B in complex with compound **36** was used to determine the exact binding mode of the saccharine moiety (pdb code 1L8G).

9.3
Addressing Site 2: Specificity Against TC-PTP

Since the original discovery of the second aryl phosphate binding site, site 2 (Puius et al. 1997), and its potential relevance for recognition of substrates with tandem pTyr (Salmeen et al. 2000; Myers et al. 2001), several attempts have been made to design small molecule inhibitors that simultaneously address the active site and site 2 by passing through the 258/259 gateway (Fig. 14). Both peptidyl and non-peptidyl approaches have been utilized. In an extension of their studies on F_2Pmp analogs, the

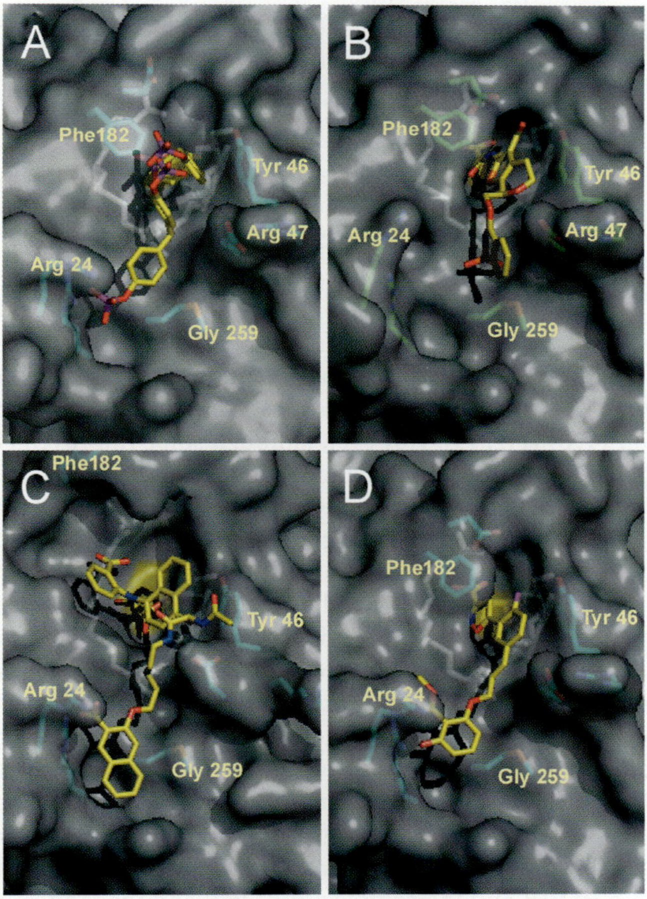

Fig. 14A–D Addressing site 2—X-ray crystallography. Moving from identification of site 2 (A—1AAX) and the 258/259 gateway (B—1L8G) to design of inhibitors that simultaneously address the active site and site 2 by passing through the gateway (C—1NNY and D—1Q1 M). The position of the WPD loop is indicated by the position of Phe182. The figures were drawn with PYMOL (see http://pymol.sourceforge.net/)

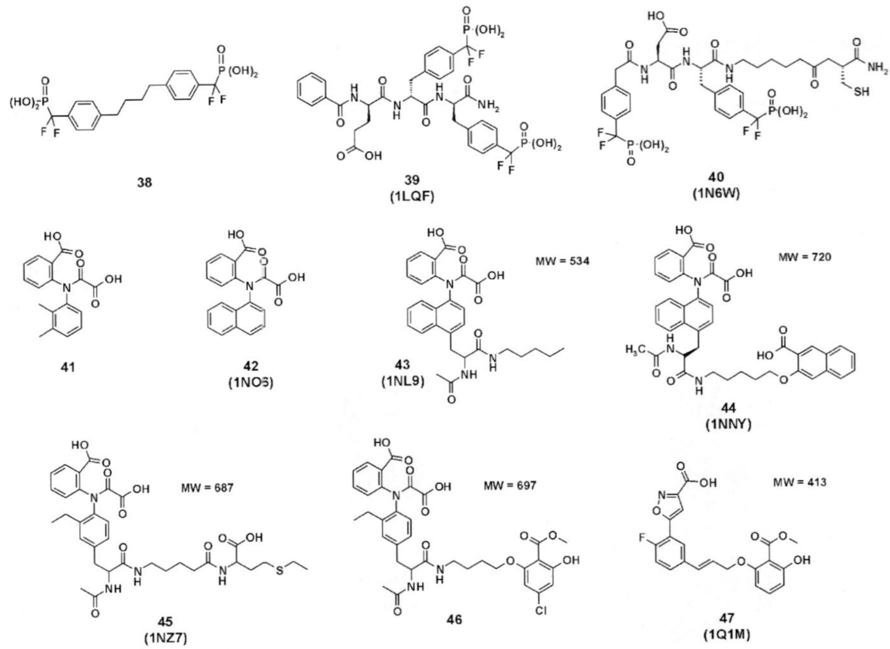

Fig. 15 Addressing site 2 chemical structures

Merck-Frosst group synthesized several compounds with different sizes of linkers connecting two F_2Pmp moieties, as exemplified with compound **38** (Taylor et al. 1998) (Fig. 15). However, although some improvement was obtained in potency, this seemed to be independent of the length of the linker, and it was therefore unlikely that the second aryl phosphate-binding region had been addressed. This was later confirmed by protein X-ray crystallographic studies that, as expected, showed binding of the proximal F_2Pmp moiety to the active site of PTP1B, whereas the distal F_2Pmp extended into the solvent and interacted with the side chain of Arg47 via a water molecule (Jia et al. 2001). The same group also used peptidyl approaches with two F_2Pmp moieties to address the second aryl phosphate-binding site in PTP1B (Desmarais et al. 1999; Asante-Appiah et al. 2001). Compound **39** is a low nanomolar, selective inhibitor of PTP1B and TC-PTP (Asante-Appiah et al. 2001), which was shown to bind to PTP1B similarly to compound **38** with interaction to Arg47. Although compound **39** does not address the second aryl phosphate binding site, a comparison of this compound in complex with PTP1B and the complex of PTP1B and the tandem phosphorylated pTyr IR peptide reveals important information regarding the structural requirements for compounds that address this site. In the PTP1B-IR peptide complex, the side chain of Arg1164 forms a cation–π interaction with the side chain of Phe182. This interaction seems to be important for orientation of the peptide substrate towards the second aryl phosphate-binding site (discussed in detail in Asante-Appiah et al. 2002). Thus, future drug design efforts might take advantage of cation–π or other interactions with the WPD loop to orientate side chains correctly through the 258–259 gateway.

The most potent and selective PTP1B inhibitor reported to date with an impressive K_i value of ~1.8 nM (compound **40**, Fig. 15) was also synthesized in an attempt to address the second aryl phosphate binding site (Shen et al. 2001). However, it was recently shown by X-ray crystallography that the distal F_2Pmp moiety of this compound does not bind to the second site but to an area defined by Lys41, Arg47, and Arg48 (Sun et al. 2003). Nonetheless, this compound represents the most potent PTP1B inhibitor and in addition exhibits roughly tenfold selectivity over TC-PTP.

A different, elegant approach was recently reported by the Abbott PTP group (Szczepankiewicz et al. 2003). Similar to our approach, this group used an oxamic acid-based compound as synthetic starting point, compound **41**, which inhibits PTP1B-mediated hydrolysis of *p*NPP with a K_i value of ~300 μM. The next step was synthesis of compound **42**, which inhibits PTP1B with a K_i value of ~40 μM. X-ray crystallography revealed that compound **42** was binding to PTP1B in the open conformation (pdb code 1NO6). Incorporation of a diamide chain at the 4-naphthyl position resulted in compound **43** (MW 533) that was about 40-fold more potent than compound **42** with a K_i value of ~1 μM. From a drug design point of view, it was important that the diamide chain was found to interact with Asp48 and that it extends into the 258/259 gateway, thus pointing towards site 2 (pdb code 1NL9). Using NMR screening with [^{13}C]-methionine-labeled PTP1B and following the resonance of Met258, several compounds were identified with weak binding affinity for site 2. One of these compounds was coupled to **43**, resulting in the potent compound **44** (K_i~20 nM—MW 719). Importantly, the naphthoic acid carboxylate group was positioned 2.6 Å from Arg254 and 2.8 Å from Arg24 (pdb code 1NNY). Although compound **44** contains features (molecular weight; three carboxy groups) that make it unlikely as a drug candidate, this is nonetheless an extremely important step forward towards structure-based design of selective PTP inhibitors. Indeed, using the same synthetic scaffold, this research group was able to synthesize potent PTP1B inhibitors (compound **45**—K_i 76 nM; compound **46**—K_i~40 nM) with about fivefold selectivity over TC-PTP (Liu et al. 2003c; Xin et al. 2003). Using the structural information obtained in these studies, the same research group set out to design selective and cell-permeable PTP1B inhibitors of smaller molecular size and with one carboxylic acid only (Liu et al. 2003b). Again, the inspiration and starting point was the oxamic acid-based inhibitors. A series of heterocycle carboxylic acids were screened with NMR for *N*-phenyloxamic acid mimetic properties. Using X-ray crystal structure-based assembly, one promising *N*-phenyloxamic acid mimetic candidate was in turn combined with a fragment that was previously found to address site 2, thus yielding compound **47**. Importantly, the molecular weight of compound **47** is only 412 Da, it is cellularly active, and it shows about 30-fold selectivity against TC-PTP. The low molecular weight should allow room for future improvement of the potency of this relatively weak PTP1B inhibitor (K_i~7 μM), while still retaining the selectivity and cellular activity.

10
Bringing It All Together: Future Challenges

During the last few years there has been significant progress in the development of PTP inhibitors. Using structure-based design approaches, several groups have shown that it is possible to synthesize highly potent and selective non-phosphorus, non-peptide inhibitors of PTP1B. However, at this point these achievements seem to have been reached at the expense of appropriate pharmacokinetic properties, including cellular uptake. Therefore, the next wave within the field of PTP inhibitors is likely to be focused on improvements in this respect.

Furthermore, although very significant progress has been achieved with respect to design of selective PTP1B inhibitors (see Sect. 9), it remains to be demonstrated that drug-like PTP1B inhibitors can be made that do not recognize TC-PTP. TC-PTP is the closest homolog to PTP1B, sharing about 74 percent identity at the amino acid level in the catalytic domains. TC-PTP exists both as a 48-kDa endoplasmic reticulum-targeted form (TC48) and a 45-kDa nuclear form (TC45). Since both PTP1B and TC48 are bound to the endoplasmic reticulum via their C-terminal extensions, it might be speculated that these two PTPs serve similar, perhaps even overlapping, functions. Indeed, in a recent publication it was suggested that TC-PTP is involved in the regulation of insulin signaling (Galic et al. 2003). However, it should be noted that TC-PTP knockout mice, in contrast to PTP1B knockout mice (Elchebly et al. 1999; Klaman et al. 2000), die a few weeks after birth, whereas heterozygous mice seem to have normal lifespan (Ibarra-Sanchez et al. 2000). At present, it is therefore unclear if PTP1B inhibitors that also recognize TC-PTP will be beneficial or harmful. To provide the structural framework for design of inhibitors that are selective for either PTP1B or TC-PTP, we have recently reported the X-ray structure of apo TC-PTP (Iversen et al. 2002). Of note, and as indicated above, two groups have provided structure-based evidence that inhibitors that are selective for PTP1B over TC-PTP are within reach (see Sect. 9.3).

Another challenge facing the PTP field is the fact that PTPs themselves seem to be regulated by covalent modifications, e.g., phosphorylation. In particular, modifications close to the active site may influence not only substrate, but also inhibitor binding. As an example, recent studies indicate that the activity of PTP1B may be influenced by phosphorylation of Ser50 (Ravichandran et al. 2001), which is positioned close to the selectivity-determining region defined by residues 47–48 and 258–259. It is quite likely that the position of the side chains of these residues will be influenced by a bulky, charged phosphate group on Ser50. Since all structure-based design activities up to this point have been carried out with catalytic domains produced in *E. coli*, it is suggested that future design efforts include testing of lead compounds either in appropriately covalently modified recombinant enzymes or in a relevant cellular context. It should also be mentioned that the activity of PTPs may be greatly influenced by domains outside the catalytic domains, and again this has to be taken into account in future PTP inhibitor development programs.

As has become apparent, almost all activities so far have been directed towards development of selective PTP1B inhibitors. However, several other classical PTPs and dual-specificity PTPs may be important novel drug targets, indicating that the focus on general PTP inhibitors may be a powerful platform for the discovery of novel therapeutics. Consistent with this concept, we have been able to use the original scaffold, OBA, as a template for synthesis of highly potent inhibitors of PTPβ with significant selectivity over PTP1B, and pharmacological characterization of such compounds may reveal new biological insights and potential clinical applications (Lund et al. 2004).

Finally, it should be, emphasized that the discovery of the transient formation of sulphenyl-amide as described in Sect. 6 may represent an exiting new avenue for structure-based design of PTP inhibitors. The significant conformational changes imposed by the sulphenyl-amide in the active site prevent binding of pTyr substrates and probably all currently known active site-dependent inhibitors. The formation of the sulphenyl-amide is reversible, and it is believed to occur in vivo after stimulation of receptor-tyrosine kinases, resulting in H_2O_2 formation. Therefore, compounds that bind to the sulphenyl-amide form of PTPs, and not to the wild-type enzymes, are expected to inhibit already-activated signaling pathways only, thereby possibly providing an additional level of specificity and limiting the risk of side effects.

Acknowledgements The authors thank (1) James G. McCormack, OSI Pharmaceuticals, Karin Bach Møller, Novo Nordisk, and Jannik N. Andersen (J.N.A.), Cold Spring Harbor Laboratory, for helpful discussions and critical reading of the manuscript; (2) J.N.A. for graphical assistance, and (3) Michael Jirousek, Gang Liu, and Cele Abad-Zapatero for sharing the coordinates of 1Q1 M with us prior to PDB release.

References

Ahmad F, Considine RV, Goldstein BJ (1995) Increased abundance of receptor-type protein-tyrosine phosphatase LAR accounts for the elevated insulin receptor dephosphorylating activity in adipose tissue of obese human subjects. J Clin Invest 95:2806–2812

Akamatsu M, Roller PP, Chen L, Zhang ZY, Ye B, Burke TR (1997) Potent inhibition of protein-tyrosine phosphatase by phosphotyrosine-mimic containing cyclic peptides. Bioorg Med Chem 5:157–163

Amoui M, Baylink DJ, Tillman JB, Lau K-HW (2003) Expression of a structurally unique osteoclastic protein-tyrosine phosphatase is driven by an alternative intronic, cell-type-specific promoter. J Biol Chem M303933200

Andersen HS, Iversen LF, Jeppesen CB, Branner S, Norris K, Møller KB, Møller NPH (2000) 2-(Oxalyl-amino)-benzoic acid is a general, competitive inhibitor of protein-tyrosine phosphatases. J Biol Chem 275:7101–7108

Andersen HS, Olsen OH, Iversen LF, Sorensen ALP, Mortensen SB, Christensen MS, Branner S, Hansen TK, Lau JF, Jeppesen L, Moran EJ, Su J, Bakir F, Judge L, Shahbaz M, Collins T, Vo T, Newman MJ, Ripka WC, Møller NPH (2002) Discovery and SAR of a novel selective and orally bioavailable nonpeptide classical competitive inhibitor class of protein-tyrosine phosphatase 1B. J Med Chem 45:4443–4459

Andersen JN, Mortensen OH, Peters GH, Drake PG, Iversen LF, Olsen OH, Jansen PG, Andersen HS, Tonks NK, Møller NPH (2001) Structural and evolutionary relationships among protein tyrosine phosphatase domains. Mol Cell Biol 21:7117–7136

Asante-Appiah E, Ball K, Bateman K, Skorey K, Friesen R, Desponts C, Payette P, Bayly C, Zamboni R, Scapin G, Ramachandran C, Kennedy BP (2001) The YRD motif is a major determinant of substrate and inhibitor specificity in T-cell protein-tyrosine phosphatase. J Biol Chem 276:26036–26043

Asante-Appiah E, Patel S, Dufresne C, Roy P, Wang QP, Patel V, Friesen RW, Ramachandran C, Becker JW, Leblanc Y, Kennedy BP, Scapin G (2002) The structure of PTP-1B in complex with a peptide inhibitor reveals an alternative binding mode for bisphosphonates. Biochemistry 41:9043–9051

Barford D, Flint AJ, Tonks NK (1994) Crystal-structure of human protein-tyrosine-phosphatase 1B. Science 263:1397–1404

Bilwes AM, Den Hertog J, Hunter T, Noel JP (1996) Structural basis for inhibition of receptor protein-tyrosine phosphatase-alpha by dimerization. Nature 382:555–559

Blanchetot C, Den Hertog J (2000) Antibody-induced dimerization of HARPTPalpha-EGFR chimera suggests a ligand dependent mechanism of regulation for RPTP alpha. FEBS Lett 484:235–240

Blanchetot C, Tertoolen LG, Overvoorde J, Den Hertog J (2002a) Intra- and intermolecular interactions between intracellular domains of receptor protein-tyrosine phosphatases. J Biol Chem 277:47263–47269

Blanchetot C, Tertoolen LGJ, Den Hertog J (2002b) Regulation of receptor protein-tyrosine phosphatase alpha by oxidative stress. EMBO J 21:493–503

Blaskovich MA, Kim HO (2002) Recent discovery and development of protein tyrosine phosphatase inhibitors. Expert Opin Ther Patents 12:871–905

Bleasdale JE, Ogg D, Palazuk BJ, Jacob CS, Swanson ML, Wang XY, Thompson DP, Conradi RA, Mathews WR, Laborde AL, Stuchly CW, Heijbel A, Bergdahl K, Bannow CA, Smith CW, Svensson C, Liljebris C, Schostarez HJ, May PD, Stevens FC, Larsen SD (2001) Small molecule peptidomimetics containing a novel phosphotyrosine bioisostere inhibit protein tyrosine phosphatase 1B and augment insulin action. Biochemistry 40:5642–5654

Burke TR Jr, Zhang Z-Y (1998) Protein-tyrosine phosphatases: structure, mechanism, and inhibitor discovery. Biopolymers 47:225–241

Burke TR, Lee K (2003) Phosphotyrosyl mimetics in the development of signal transduction inhibitors. Acc Chem Res 36:426–433

Burke TR, Kole HK, Roller PP (1994) Potent inhibition of insulin-receptor dephosphorylation by a hexamer peptide-containing the phosphotyrosyl mimetic F_2Pmp. Biochem Biophys Res Commun 204:129–134

Burke TR, Ye B, Akamatsu M, Ford H, Yan XJ, Kole HK, Wolf G, Shoelson SE, Roller PP (1996a) 4'-O-[2-(2-fluoromalonyl)]-l-tyrosine—a phosphotyrosyl mimic for the preparation of signal-transduction inhibitory peptides. J Med Chem 39:1021–1027

Burke TR, Ye B, Yan XJ, Wang SM, Jia ZC, Chen L, Zhang ZY, Barford D (1996b) Small-molecule interactions with protein-tyrosine-phosphatase ptp1b and their use in inhibitor design. Biochemistry 35:15989–15996

Burke TR Jr, Yao Z-J, Zhao H, Milne GWA, Wu L, Zhang Z-Y, Voigt JH (1998) Enantioselective synthesis of nonphosphorous-containing phosphotyrosyl mimetics and their use in the preparation of tyrosine phosphatase inhibitory peptides. Tetrahedron 54:9981–9994

Calera MR, Vallega G, Pilch PF (2000) Dynamics of protein-tyrosine phosphatases in rat adipocytes. J Biol Chem 275:6308–6312

Charbonneau H, Tonks NK (1992) 1002 Protein phosphatases. Annu Rev Cell Biol 8:463–493

Chen L, Wu L, Otaka A, Smyth MS, Roller PP, Burke TR, Denhertog J, Zhang ZY (1995) Why is phosphonodifluoromethyl phenylalanine a more potent inhibitory moiety than phosphonomethyl phenylalanine toward protein-tyrosine phosphatases. Biochem Biophys Res Commun 216:976–984

Cheng A, Uetani N, Simoncic PD, Chaubey VP, Lee-Loy A, Mcglade CJ, Kennedy BP, Tremblay ML (2002) Attenuation of leptin action and regulation of obesity by protein tyrosine phosphatase 1B. Dev Cell 2:497–503

Cho HJ, Krishnaraj R, Itoh M, Kitas E, Bannwarth W, Saito H, Walsh CT (1993) Substrate specificities of catalytic fragments of protein-tyrosine phosphatases (hPTP-β, LAR, and CD45) toward phosphotyrosylpeptide substrates and thiophosphotyrosylated peptides as inhibitors. Protein Sci 2:977–984

Clemens JC, Guan K, Bliska JB, Falkow S, Dixon JE (1991) Microbial pathogenesis and tyrosine dephosphorylation: surprising 'bedfellows'. Mol Microbiol 5:2617–2620

Cohen P (2002) Protein kinases—the major drug targets of the twenty-first century? Nat Rev Drug Discov 1:309–315

Cong LN, Chen H, Li YH, Lin CH, Sap J, Quon MJ (1999) Overexpression of protein tyrosine phosphatase-alpha (PTP- alpha) but not PTP-kappa inhibits translocation of GLUT4 in rat adipose cells. Biochem Biophys Res Commun 255:200–207

Czech MP, Lawrence JC, Lynn WS (1974a) Evidence for electron transfer reactions involved in the Cu2+ -dependent thiol activation of fat cell glucose utilization. J Biol Chem 249:1001–1006

Czech MP, Lawrence JC, Lynn WS (1974b) Evidence for the involvement of sulfhydryl oxidation in the regulation of fat cell hexose transport by insulin. Proc Natl Acad Sci USA 71:4173–4177

Czech MP, Lawrence JC, Lynn WS (1974c) Hexose transport in isolated brown fat cells. A model system for investigating insulin action on membrane transport. J Biol Chem 249:5421–5427

Denu JM, Dixon JE (1998) Protein tyrosine phosphatases: Mechanisms of catalysis and regulation. Curr Opin Chem Biol 2:633–641

Denu JM, Tanner KG (1998) Specific and reversible inactivation of protein tyrosine phosphatases by hydrogen peroxide: evidence for a sulfenic acid intermediate and implications for redox regulation. Biochemistry 37:5633–5642

Denu JM, Lohse DL, Vijayalakshmi J, Saper MA, Dixon JE (1996) Visualization of intermediate and transition-state structures in protein-tyrosine-phosphatase catalysis. Proc Natl Acad Sci USA 93:2493–2498

Desmarais S, Jia Z, Ramachandaran C (1998) Inhibition of protein tyrosine phosphatase PTP1B and CD45 by sulfotyrosyl peptides. Arch Biochem Biophys 354:225–231

Desmarais S, Friesen RW, Zamboni R, Ramachandaran C (1999) [Difluro(phosphono)methyl]phenyl-containing peptide inhibitors of protein tyrosine phosphatases. Biochem J 337:219–223

Domchek SM, Auger KR, Chatterjee S, Burke TRJ, Shoelson SE (1992) Inhibition of SH2 domain-phosphoprotein association by a nonhydrolyzable phosphonopeptide. Biochemistry 31:9865–9870

Dubyak GR, Kleinzeller A (1980) The insulin-mimetic effects of vanadate in isolated rat adipocytes. Dissociation from effects of vanadate as a (Na+-K+)ATPase inhibitor. J Biol Chem 255:5306–5312

Elchebly M, Payette P, Michaliszyn E, Cromlish W, Collins S, Loy AL, Normandin D, Cheng A, Himms-Hagen J, Chan C-C, Ramachandaran C, Gresser MJ, Tremblay ML, Kennedy BP (1999) Increased insulin sensitivity and obesity resistance in mice lacking the protein tyrosine phosphatase-1B gene. Science 283:1544–1548

Elson A, Leder P (1995) Identification of a cytoplasmic, phorbol ester-inducible isoform of protein-tyrosine-phosphatase epsilon. Proc Natl Acad Sci USA 92:12235–12239

Erlanson DA, McDowell RS, He MM, Randal M, Simmons RL, Kung J, Waight A, Hansen SK (2003) Discovery of a new phosphotyrosine mimetic for PTP1B using breakaway tethering. J Am Chem Soc 125:5602–5603

Fantus IG, Kadota S, Deragon G, Foster B, Posner BI (1989) Pervanadate [peroxide(s) of vanadate] mimics insulin action in rat adipocytes via activation of the insulin receptor tyrosine kinase. Biochemistry 28:8864–8871

Fauman EB, Yuvaniyama C, Schubert HL, Stuckey JA, Saper MA (1996) The x-ray crystal-structures of yersinia tyrosine phosphatase with bound tungstate and nitrate—mechanistic implications. J Biol Chem 271:18780–18788

Fischer EH, Charbonneau H, Tonks NK (1991) Protein tyrosine phosphatases: a diverse family of intracellular and transmembrane enzymes. Science 253:401–406

Flint AJ, Gebbink MFGB, Franza BR, Hill DE, Tonks NK (1993) Multisite phosphorylation of the protein-tyrosine phosphatase, PTB1B—identification of cell-cycle regulated and phorbol ester stimulated sites of phosphorylation. EMBO J 12:1937–1946

Flint AJ, Tiganis T, Barford D, Tonks NK (1997) Development of substrate-trapping mutants to identify physiological substrates of protein-tyrosine phosphatases. Proc Natl Acad Sci USA 94:1680–1685

Frangione JV, Oda A, Smith M, Salzman EW, Neel BG (1993) Calpain-catalyzed cleavage and subcellular relocation of protein phosphotyrosine phosphatase 1B (PTP-1B) in human platelets. EMBO J 12:4843–4856

Fukada T, Tonks NK (2003) Identification of YB-1 as a regulator of PTP1B expression: implications for regulation of insulin and cytokine signaling. EMBO J 22:479–493

Galic S, Klingler-Hoffmann M, Fodero-Tavoletti MT, Puryer MA, Meng TC, Tonks NK, Tiganis T (2003) Regulation of insulin receptor signaling by the protein tyrosine phosphatase TCPTP. Mol Cell Biol 23:2096–2108

Gil-Henn H, Volohonsky G, Toledano-Katchalski H, Gandre S, Elson A (2000) Generation of novel cytoplasmic forms of protein tyrosine phosphatase epsilon by proteolytic processing and translational control. Oncogene 19:4375–4384

Gil-Henn H, Volohonsky G, Elson A (2001) Regulation of protein-tyrosine phosphatases alpha and epsilon by calpain-mediated proteolytic cleavage. J Biol Chem 276:31772–31779

Glaser F, Pupko T, Paz I, Bell RE, Bechor-Shental D, Martz E, Ben Tal N (2003) ConSurf: identification of functional regions in proteins by surface-mapping of phylogenetic information. Bioinformatics 19:163–164

Glover NR, Tracey AS (2000) The phosphatase domains of LAR, CD45, and PTP1B: structural correlations with peptide-based inhibitors. Biochem Cell Biol 78:39–50

Gross S, Knebel A, Tenev T, Neininger A, Gaestel M, Herrlich P, Bohmer FD (1999) Inactivation of protein-tyrosine phosphatases as mechanism of UV-induced signal transduction. J Biol Chem 274:26378–26386

Groves MR, Yao Z-J, Roller PP, Burke TR, Barford D (1998) Structural basis for inhibition of the protein tyrosine phosphatase 1B by phosphotyrosine peptide mimetics. Biochemistry 37:17773–17783

Guan KL, Dixon JE (1990) Protein tyrosine phosphatase activity of an essential virulence determinant in Yersinia. Science 249:553–556

Guan KL, Dixon JE (1991) Evidence for protein-tyrosine-phosphatase catalysis proceeding via a cysteine-phosphate intermediate. J Biol Chem 266:17026–17030

Hatakeyama M (2003) Helicobacter pylori CagA–a potential bacterial oncoprotein that functionally mimics the mammalian Gab family of adaptor proteins. Microbes Infect 5:143–150

Heffetz D, Zick Y (1992) The insulinomimetic agents hydrogen peroxide and vanadate stimulate tyrosine phosphorylation of potential target proteins for the insulin- receptor kinase in intact-cells. Biochem J 288:631–635

Heffetz D, Bushkin I, Dror R, Zick Y (1990) The insulinomimetic agents H_2O_2 and vanadate stimulate protein tyrosine phosphorylation in intact cells. J Biol Chem 265:2896–2902

Hermiston ML, Xu Z, Weiss A (2003) CD45: a critical regulator of signaling thresholds in immune cells. Annu Rev Immunol 21:107–137

Higashi H, Tsutsumi R, Muto S, Sugiyama T, Azuma T, Asaka M, Hatakeyama M (2002) SHP-2 tyrosine phosphatase as an intracellular target of Helicobacter pylori CagA protein. Science 295:683–686

Hoppe E, Berne PF, Stock D, Rasmussen JS, Møller NPH, Ullrich A, Huber R (1994) Expression, purification and crystallization of human phosphotyrosine phosphatase 1B. Eur J Biochem 223:1069–1077

Ibarra-Sanchez MD, Simoncic PD, Nestel FR, Duplay P, Lapp WS, Tremblay ML (2000) The T-cell protein tyrosine phosphatase. Semin Immunol 12:379–386

Irie-Sasaki J, Sasaki T, Penninger JM (2003) CD45 regulated signaling pathways. Curr Top Med Chem 3:783–796

Iversen LF, Andersen HS, Branner S, Mortensen SB, Peters GH, Norris K, Olsen OH, Jeppesen CB, Lundt BF, Ripka W, Møller KB, Møller NPH (2000) Structure-based design of a low molecular weight, nonphosphorus, nonpeptide, and highly selective inhibitor of protein-tyrosine phosphatase 1B. J Biol Chem 275:10300–10307

Iversen LF, Andersen HS, Møller KB, Olsen OH, Peters GH, Branner S, Mortensen SB, Hansen TK, Lau J, Ge Y, Holsworth DD, Newman MJ, Møller NPH (2001) Steric hindrance as basis for structure-based design of selective inhibitors of protein-tyrosine phosphatases. Biochemistry 40:14812–14820

Iversen LF, Møller KB, Pedersen AK, Peters GH, Petersen AS, Andersen HS, Branner S, Mortensen SB, Møller NP (2002) Structure determination of T cell protein tyrosine phosphatase. J Biol Chem 277:19982–19990

Jackson DE (2003) The unfolding tale of PECAM-1. FEBS Lett 540:7–14

Jia Z, Ye Q, Dinaut AN, Wang Q, Waddleton D, Payette P, Ramachandran C, Kennedy B, Hum G, Taylor SD (2001) Structure of protein tyrosine phosphatase 1B in complex with inhibitors bearing two phosphotyrosine mimetics. J Med Chem 44:4584–4594

Jia ZC, Barford D, Flint AJ, Tonks NK (1995) Structural basis for phosphotyrosine peptide recognition by protein-tyrosine-phosphatase 1b. Science 268:1754–1758

Jiang GL, Den Hertog J, Su J, Noel J, Sap J, Hunter T (1999) Dimerization inhibits the activity of receptor-like protein-tyrosine phosphatase-alpha. Nature 401:606–610

Jiang GQ, Den Hertog J, Hunter T (2000) Receptor-like protein tyrosine phosphatase alpha homodimerizes on the cell surface. Mol Cell Biol 20:5917–5929

Johnson TO, Ermolieff J, Jirousek MR (2002) Protein tyrosine phosphatase 1B inhibitors for diabetes. Nat Rev Drug Discov 1:696–709

Kadota S, Fantus IG, Deragon G, Guyda HJ, Hersh B, Posner BI (1987) Peroxide(s) of Vanadium: a novel and potent insulin-mimetic agent which activates the insulin receptor kinase. Biochem Biophys Res Commun 14:259–266

Kaniga K, Uralil J, Bliska JB, Galan JE (1996) A secreted protein-tyrosine-phosphatase with modular effector domains in the bacterial pathogen salmonella-typhimurium. Mol Microbiol 21:633–641

Kar S, Wang MF, Wilcox CS, Carr BI (2003) Antitumor and anticarcinogenic actions of Cpd 5: a new class of protein phosphatase inhibitor. Carcinogenesis 24:411–416

Kennedy BP (1999) Role of protein tyrosine phosphatase-1B in diabetes and obesity. Biomed Pharmacother 53:466–470

Klaman LD, Boss O, Peroni OD, Kim JK, Martino JL, Zabolotny JM, Moghal N, Lubkin M, Kim YB, Sharpe AH, Stricker-Krongrad A, Shulman GI, Neel BG, Kahn BB (2000) Increased energy expenditure, decreased adiposity, and tissue-specific insulin sensitivity in protein-tyrosine phosphatase 1B-deficient mice. Mol Cell Biol 20:5479–5489

Kole HK, Akamatsu M, Ye B, Yan XJ, Barford D, Roller PP, Burke TR (1995a) Protein-tyrosine-phosphatase inhibition by a peptide-containing the phosphotyrosyl mimetic, L-O-malonyltyrosine. Biochem Biophys Res Commun 209:817–822

Kole HK, Smyth MS, Russ PL, Burke TR (1995b) Phosphonate inhibitors of protein-tyrosine and serine threonine phosphatases. Biochem J 311:1025–1031

Kole HK, Garant MJ, Kole S, Bernier M (1996) A peptide-based protein-tyrosine-phosphatase inhibitor specifically enhances insulin-receptor function in intact cells. J Biol Chem 271:14302–14307

Koshio O, Akanuma Y, Kasuga M (1988) Hydrogen peroxide stimulates tyrosine phosphorylation of the insulin receptor and its tyrosine kinase activity in intact cells. Biochem J 250:95–101

Kotoris CC, Chen M, Taylor SD (1998) Novel phosphate mimetics for the design of nonpeptidyl inhibitors of protein tyrosine phosphatases. Bioorg Med Chem Lett 8:3275–3280

Koul A, Choidas A, Treder M, Tyagi AK, Drlica K, Singh Y, Ullrich A (2000) Cloning and characterization of secretory tyrosine phosphatases of Mycobacterium tuberculosis. J Bacteriol 182:5425–5432

Kulas DT, Zhang W-R, Goldstein BJ, Furlanetto RW, Mooney RA (1995) Insulin receptor signaling is augmented by antisense inhibition of the protein tyrosine phosphatase LAR. J Biol Chem 270:2435–2438

Larsen SD, Stevens FC, Lindberg TJ, Bodnar PM, O'Sullivan TJ, Schostarez HJ, Palazuk BJ, Bleasdale JE (2003) Modification of the N-terminus of peptidomimetic protein tyrosine phosphatase 1B (PTP1B) inhibitors: Identification of analogues with cellular activity. Bioorg Med Chem Lett 13:971–975

Lee K, Burke TR (2003) CD45 protein-tyrosine phosphatase inhibitor development. Curr Top Med Chem 3:797–807

Liotta AS, Kole HK, Fales HM, Roth J, Bernier M (1994) A synthetic tris-sulfotyrosyl dodecapeptide analog of the insulin-receptor 1146-kinase domain inhibits tyrosine dephosphorylation of the insulin-receptor in-situ. J Biol Chem 269:22996–23001

Liu G, Szczepankiewicz BG, Pei ZH, Janowick DA, Xin ZL, Hajduk PJ, Abad-Zapatero C, Liang H, Hutchins CW, Fesik SW, Ballaron SJ, Stashko MA, Lubben T, Mika AK, Zinker BA, Trevillyan JM, Jirousek MR (2003a) Discovery and structure-activity relationship of oxalylarylaminobenzoic acids as inhibitors of protein tyrosine phosphatase 1B. J Med Chem 46:2093–2103

Liu G, Xin Z, Pei Z, Hajduk PJ, Abad-Zapatero C, Hutchins CW, Zhao H, Lubben TH, Ballaron SJ, Haasch DL, Kaszubska W, Rondinone CM, Trevillyan JM, Jirousek MR (2003b) Fragment screening and assembly: a highly efficient approach to a selective and cell active protein tyrosine phosphatase 1B inhibitor. J Med Chem 46:4232–4235

Liu G, Xin ZL, Liang H, Abad-Zapatero C, Hajduk PJ, Janowick DA, Szczepankiewicz BG, Pei z, Hutchins CW, Ballaron SJ, Stashko MA, Lubben TH, Berg CE, Rondinone CM, Trevillyan JM, Jirousek MR (2003c) Selective protein tyrosine phosphatase 1B inhibitors: targeting the second phosphotyrosine binding site with non-carboxylic acid-containing ligands. J Med Chem 46:3437–3440

Lohse DL, Denu JM, Santoro N, Dixon JE (1997) Roles of aspartic acid-181 and serine-222 in intermediate formation and hydrolysis of the mammalian protein-tyrosine-phosphatase PTP1. Biochemistry 36:4568–4575

Lund IK, Andersen HS, Iversen LF, Olsen OH, Møller KB, Pedersen AK, Ge Y, Holsworth DD, Newman MJ, Axe FU, and Møller NPH (2004) Structure-based Design of Selective and Potent Inhibitors of Protein-tyrosine Phosphatase beta. J Biol Chem 279:24226–24235

Maehama T, Taylor GS, Dixon JE (2001) PTEN and myotubularin: novel phosphoinositide phosphatases. Annu Rev Biochem 70:247–279

Mahadev K, Wu XD, Zilbering A, Zhu L, Lawrence JTR, Goldstein BJ (2001a) Hydrogen peroxide generated during cellular insulin stimulation is integral to activation of the distal insulin signaling cascade in 3T3-L1 adipocytes. J Biol Chem 276:48662–48669

Mahadev K, Zilbering A, Zhu L, Goldstein BJ (2001b) Insulin-stimulated hydrogen peroxide reversibly inhibits protein-tyrosine phosphatase 1B in vivo and enhances the early insulin action cascade. J Biol Chem 276:21938–21942

Majeti R, Bilwes AM, Noel JP, Hunter T, Weiss A (1998) Dimerization-induced inhibition of receptor protein-tyrosine- phosphatase function through an inhibitory wedge. Science 279:88–91

Majeti R, Xu Z, Parslow TG, Olson JL, Daikh DI, Killeen N, Weiss A (2000) An inactivating point mutation in the inhibitory wedge of CD45 causes lymphoproliferation and autoimmunity. Cell 103:1059–1070

Mauro LJ, Dixon JE (1994) 'Zip codes' direct intracellular protein tyrosine phosphatases to the correct cellular 'address'. TIBS 19:151–155

May JM, de Haen C (1979) Insulin-stimulated intracellular hydrogen peroxide production in rat epididymal fat cells. J Biol Chem 254:2214–2220

McGovern SL, Shoichet BK (2003) Kinase inhibitors: not just for kinases anymore. J Med Chem 46:1478–1483

McGovern SL, Caselli E, Grigorieff N, Shoichet BK (2002) A common mechanism underlying promiscuous inhibitors from virtual and high-throughput screening. J Med Chem 45:1712–1722

Meng TC, Fukada T, Tonks NK (2002) Reversible oxidation and inactivation of protein tyrosine phosphatases in vivo. Mol Cell 9:387–399

Milarski KL, Zhu G, Pearl CG, McNamara DJ, Dobrusin EM, MacLean D, Thieme-Sefler A, Zhang Z-Y, Sawyer T, Decker SJ, Dixon JE, Saltiel AR (1993) Sequence specificity in recognition of the epidermal growth factor receptor by protein tyrosine phosphatase 1B. J Biol Chem 268:23634–23639

Miller MJ, Bracccolino DS, Cleary DG, Ream JE, Walker MC, Sikorski JA (1994) EPSP synthase inhibitor design IV. New aromatic substrate analogs and symmetrical inhibitors containing novel 3-phosphate mimics. Bioorg Med Chem Lett 4:2605–2608

Moeslein FM, Myers MP, Landreth GE (1999) The CLK family kinases, CLK1 and CLK2, phosphorylate and activate the tyrosine phosphatase, PTP-1B. J Biol Chem 274:26697–26704

Møller NPH, Møller KB, Lammers R, Kharitonenkov A, Sures I, Ullrich A (1994a) Src kinase associates with a member of a distinct subfamily of protein-tyrosine phosphatases containing an ezrin-like domain. Proc Natl Acad Sci U S A 91:7477–7481

Møller NPH, Møller KB, Ullrich A, Møller NP (1994b) New protein tyrosine phosphatase PTP-S31 is used to develop products for treating or preventing disease associated with abnormal PTP-531, e.g., cancer or diabetes. Max Planck Ges Foerderung Wissenschaften, [WO9421800-A2], pp 9–29

Møller NPH, Møller KB, Lammers R, Kharitonenkov A, Hoppe E, Wiberg FC, Sures I, Ullrich A (1995) Selective down-regulation of the insulin receptor signal by protein-tyrosine phosphatases alpha and epsilon. J Biol Chem 270:23126–23131

Møller NPH, Iversen LF, Andersen HS, McCormack JG (2000) Protein tyrosine phosphatases (PTPs) as drug targets: inhibitors of PTP-1B for the treatment of diabetes. Curr Opin Drug Discov Devel 3:527–540

Mooney RA, LeVea CM (2003) The leukocyte common antigen-related protein LAR: candidate PTP for inhibitory targeting. Curr Top Med Chem 3:809–819

Murli S, Watson RO, Galan JE (2001) Role of tyrosine kinases and the tyrosine phosphatase SptP in the interaction of Salmonella with host cells. Cell Microbiol 3:795–810

Myers MP, Andersen JN, Cheng A, Tremblay ML, Horvath CM, Parisien JP, Salmeen A, Barford D, Tonks NK (2001) TYK2 and JAK2 are substrates of protein-tyrosine phosphatase 1B. J Biol Chem 276:47771–47774

Norris K, Norris F, Kono DH, Vestergaard H, Pedersen O, Theofilopoulos AN, Møller NPH (1997) Expression of protein-tyrosine phosphatases in the major insulin target tissues. FEBS Lett 415:243–248

Pallen CJ (2003) Protein tyrosine phosphatase alpha (PTPalpha): a Src family kinase activator and mediator of multiple biological effects. Curr Top Med Chem 3:821–835

Pannifer ADB, Flint AJ, Tonks NK, Barford D (1998) Visualization of the cysteinyl-phosphate intermediate of a protein-tyrosine phosphatase by X-ray crystallography. J Biol Chem 273:10454–10462

Patankar SJ, Jurs PC (2003) Classification of inhibitors of protein tyrosine phosphatase 1B using molecular structure based descriptors. J Chem Inf Comput Sci 43:885–899

Pathak MK, Yi TL (2001) Sodium stibogluconate is a potent inhibitor of protein tyrosine phosphatases and augments cytokine responses in hemopoietic cell lines. J Immunol 167:3391–3397

Pathak MK, Dhawan D, Lindner DJ, Borden EC, Farver C, Yi TL (2002) Pentamidine is an inhibitor of PRL phosphatases with anticancer activity. Mol Cancer Ther 1:1255–1264

Peters GH, Iversen LF, Branner S, Andersen HS, Mortensen SB, Olsen OH, Møller KB, Møller NPH (2000) Residue 259 is a key determinant of substrate specificity of protein-tyrosine phosphatases 1B and α. J Biol Chem 275:18201–18209

Pot DA, Dixon JE (1992a) A thousand and two protein tyrosine phosphatases. Biochim Biophys Acta 1136:35–43

Pot DA, Dixon JE (1992b) Active site labeling of a receptor-like protein tyrosine phosphatase. J Biol Chem 267:140–143

Puius YA, Zhao Y, Sullivan M, Lawrence DS, Almo SC, Zhang Z-Y (1997) Identification of a second aryl phosphate-binding site in protein-tyrosine phosphatase 1B: A paradigm for inhibitor design. Proc Natl Acad Sci USA 94:13420–13425

Ragab A, Bodin S, Viala C, Chap H, Payrastre B, Ragab-Thomas J (2003) The tyrosine phosphatase 1B regulates LAT phosphorylation and platelet aggregation upon Fcgamma RIIa cross-linking. J Biol Chem 278:40923–40932

Ramachandran C, Kennedy BP (2003) Protein tyrosine phosphatase 1B: a novel target for type 2 diabetes and obesity. Curr Top Med Chem 3:749–757

Ravichandran LV, Chen H, Li YH, Quon MJ (2001) Phosphorylation of PTP1B at Ser(50) by Akt impairs its ability to dephosphorylate the insulin receptor. Mol Endocrinol 15:1768–1780

Ripka WC (2000) Protein tyrosine phosphatase inhibition. Annu Rep Med Chem 35:231–250

Ruzzene M, Donella DA, Marin O, Perich JW, Ruzza P, Borin G, Calderan A, Pinna LA (1993) Specificity of T-cell protein tyrosine phosphatase toward phosphorylated synthetic peptides. Eur J Biochem 211:289–295

Salmeen A, Andersen JN, Myers MP, Tonks NK, Barford D (2000) Molecular basis for the dephosphorylation of the activation segment of the insulin receptor by protein tyrosine phosphatase 1B. Mol Cell 6:1401–1412

Salmeen A, Andersen JN, Myers MP, Meng TC, Hinks JA, Tonks NK, Barford D (2003) Redox regulation of protein tyrosine phosphatase 1B involves a sulphenyl-amide intermediate. Nature 423:769–773

Sarmiento M, Zhao Y, Gordon SJ, Zhang Z-Y (1998) Molecular-basis for substrate-specificity of protein-tyrosine-phosphatase 1B. J Biol Chem 273:26368–26374

Sarmiento M, Puius YA, Vetter SW, Keng YF, Wu L, Zhang Z-Y (2000) Structural basis of plasticity in protein tyrosine phosphatase 1B substrate recognition. Biochemistry 39:8171–8179

Scapin G, Patel S, Patel V, Kennedy B, Asante-Appiah E (2001) The structure of apo protein-tyrosine phosphatase 1B C215S mutant: more than just an S→O change. Protein Sci 10:1596–1605

Schubert HL, Fauman EB, Stuckey JA, Dixon JE, Saper MA (1995) A ligand-induced conformational change in the yersinia protein-tyrosine-phosphatase. Protein Sci 4:1904–1913

Shen K, Keng YF, Wu L, Guo XL, Lawrence DS, Zhang ZY (2001) Acquisition of a specific and potent PTP1B inhibitor from a novel combinatorial library and screening procedure. J Biol Chem 276:47311–47319

Shifrin VI, Neel BG (1993) Growth factor-inducible alternative splicing of nontransmembrane phosphotyrosine phosphatase PTP-1B premessenger rna. J Biol Chem 268:25376–25384

Skorey K, Ly HD, Kelly J, Hammond M, Ramachandran C, Huang Z, Gresser MJ, Wang QP (1997) How does alendronate inhibit protein-tyrosine phosphatases. J Biol Chem 272:22472–22480

Skorey KI, Kennedy BP, Friesen RW, Ramachandran C (2001) Development of a robust scintillation proximity assay for protein tyrosine phosphatase 1B using the catalytically inactive (C215S) mutant. Anal Biochem 291:269–278

Smyth MS, Ford H, Jr, Burke TR Jr (1992) A general-method for the preparation of benzylic alpha,alpha-difluorophosphonic acids—nonhydrolyzable mimetics of phosphotyrosine. Tetrahedron Lett 33:4137–4140

Stuckey JA, Schubert HL, Fauman EB, Zhang ZY, Dixon JE, Saper MA (1994) Crystal-structure of yersinia protein-tyrosine-phosphatase at 2. 5-angstrom and the complex with tungstate. Nature 370:571–575

Sun JP, Fedorov AA, Lee SY, Guo XL, Shen K, Lawrence DS, Almo SC, Zhang ZY (2003) Crystal structure of PTP1B complexed with a potent and selective bidentate inhibitor. J Biol Chem 278:12406–12414

Szczepankiewicz BG, Liu G, Hajduk PJ, Abad-Zapatero C, Pei ZH, Xin ZL, Lubben TH, Trevillyan JM, Stashko MA, Ballaron SJ, Liang H, Huang F, Hutchins CW, Fesik SW, Jirousek MR (2003) Discovery of a potent, selective protein tyrosine phosphatase 1B inhibitor using a linked-fragment strategy. J Am Chem Soc 125:4087–4096

Taing M, Keng YF, Shen K, Wu L, Lawrence DS, Zhang ZY (1999) Potent and highly selective inhibitors of the protein tyrosine phosphatase 1B. Biochemistry 38:3793–3803

Tamura S, Brown TA, Whipple JH, Fujita-Yamaguchi Y, Dubler RE, Cheng K, Larner J (1984) A novel mechanism for the insulin-like effect of vanadate on glycogen synthase in rat adipocytes. J Biol Chem 259:6650–6658

Tanuma N, Nakamura K, Kikuchi K (1999) Distinct promoters control transmembrane and cytosolic protein tyrosine phosphatase epsilon expression during macrophage differentiation. Eur J Biochem 259:46–54

Tartaglia M, Niemeyer CM, Fragale A, Song X, Buechner J, Jung A, Hahlen K, Hasle H, Licht JD, Gelb BD (2003) Somatic mutations in PTPN11 in juvenile myelomonocytic leukemia, myelodysplastic syndromes and acute myeloid leukemia. Nat Genet 34:148–150

Taylor SD, Kotoris CC, Dinaut AN, Wang QP, Ramachandran C, Huang Z (1998) Potent non-peptidyl inhibitors of protein-tyrosine- phosphatase 1b. Bioorg Med Chem 6:1457–1468

Tonks NK (2003) PTP1B: from the sidelines to the front lines! FEBS Lett 546:140–148

Tonks NK, Neel BG (2001) Combinatorial control of the specificity of protein tyrosine phosphatases. Curr Opin Cell Biol 13:182–195

Tonks NK, Diltz CD, Fischer EH (1988a) Characterization of the major protein-tyrosine-phosphatases of human placenta. J Biol Chem 263:6731–6737

Tonks NK, Diltz CD, Fischer EH (1988b) Purification of the major protein-tyrosine-phosphatases of human placenta. J Biol Chem 263:6722–6730

Urbanek RA, Suchard SJ, Steelman GB, Knappenberger KS, Sygowski LA, Veale CA, Chapdelaine MJ (2001) Potent reversible inhibitors of the protein tyrosine phosphatase CD45. J Med Chem 44:1777–1793

van der Wijk T, Blanchetot C, Overvoorde J, Den Hertog J (2003) Redox-regulated rotational coupling of receptor protein-tyrosine phosphatase alpha dimers. J Biol Chem 278:13968–13974

van Huijsduijnen RH, Bombrun A, Swinnen D (2002) Selecting protein tyrosine phosphatases as drug targets. Drug Discov Today 7:1013–1019 van Montfort RLM, Congreve M, Tisi D, Carr R, Jhoti H (2003) Oxidation state of the active-site cysteine in protein tyrosine phosphatase 1B. Nature 423:773–777

Vetter SW, Keng YF, Lawrence DS, Zhang ZY (2000) Assessment of protein-tyrosine phosphatase 1B substrate specificity using "inverse alanine scanning". J Biol Chem 275:2265–2268

Walchli S, Curchod ML, Gobert RP, Arkinstall S, van Huijsduijnen RH (2000) Identification of tyrosine phosphatases that dephosphorylate the insulin receptor—a brute force approach based on "substrate-trapping" mutants. J Biol Chem 275:9792–9796

Wang QP, Huang Z, Ramachandran C, Dinaut AN, Taylor SD (1998) Naphthalenebis[alpha,alpha-difluoromethylenephosphonates] as potent inhibitors of protein-tyrosine phosphatases. Bioorg Med Chem Lett 8:345–350

Wang XY, Bergdahl K, Heijbel A, Liljebris C, Bleasdale JE (2001) Analysis of in vitro interactions of protein tyrosine phosphatase 1B with insulin receptors. Mol Cell Endocrinol 173:109–120

Wishart MJ, Dixon JE (2002) PTEN and myotubularin phosphatases: from 3-phosphoinositide dephosphorylation to disease. Trends Cell Biol 12:579–585

Wrobel J, Sredy J, Moxham C, Dietrich A, Li ZN, Sawicki DR, Seestaller L, Wu L, Katz A, Sullivan D, Tio C, Zhang ZY (1999) PTP1B inhibition and antihyperglycemic activity in the ob/ob mouse model of novel 11-arylbenzo[b] naphtho[2,3-d]furans and 11-arylbenzo[b] naphtho [2,3-d] thiophenes. J Med Chem 42:3199–3202

Wu C, Sun M, Liu L, Zhou GW (2003) The function of the protein tyrosine phosphatase SHP-1 in cancer. Gene 306:1–12

Xie LP, Zhang YL, Zhang ZY (2002) Design and characterization of an improved protein tyrosine phosphatase substrate-trapping mutant. Biochemistry 41:4032–4039

Xin ZL, Oost TK, Abad-Zapatero C, Hajduk PJ, Pei ZH, Szczepankiewicz BG, Hutchins CW, Ballaron SJ, Stashko MA, Lubben T, Trevillyan JM, Jirousek MR, Liu G (2003) Potent, selective inhibitors of protein tyrosine phosphatase 1B. Bioorg Med Chem Lett 13:1887–1890

Yahiro K, Niidome T, Kimura M, Hatakeyama T, Aoyagi H, Kurazono H, Imagawa K, Wada A, Moss J, Hirayama T (1999) Activation of Helicobacter pylori VacA toxin by alkaline or acid conditions increases its binding to a 250-kDa receptor protein-tyrosine phosphatase beta. J Biol Chem 274:36693–36699

Yahiro K, Wada A, Nakayama M, Kimura T, Ogushi K, Niidome T, Aoyagi H, Yoshino K, Yonezawa K, Moss J, Hirayama T (2003) Protein-tyrosine phosphatase alpha, RPTP alpha, is a Helicobacter pylori VacA receptor. J Biol Chem 278:19183–19189

Yang J, Cheng ZL, Niu TQ, Liang XS, Zhao ZZJ, Zhou GW (2000) Structural basis for substrate specificity of protein-tyrosine phosphatase SHP-1. J Biol Chem 275:4066–4071

Ye B, Burke TR (1995) L-O-(2-malonyl)tyrosine (L-OMT) a new phosphotyrosyl mimic suitably protected for solid-phase synthesis of signal- transduction inhibitory peptides. Tetrahedron Lett 36:4733–4736

Ye B, Burke TR (1996) Synthesis of a difluorophosphonomethyl-containing phosphatase inhibitor designed from the X-ray structure of a ptp1b-bound ligand. Tetrahedron 52:9963–9970

Ye B, Akamatsu M, Shoelson SE, Wolf G, Giorgetti-Peraldi S, Yan X, Roller PP, Burke TR Jr (1995) L-*O*-(2-Malonyl)tyrosine: a new phosphotyrosyl mimetic for the preparation of Src homology 2 domain inhibitory peptides. J Med Chem 38:4270–4275

Yi TL, Pathak MK, Lindner DJ, Ketterer ME, Farver C, Borden EC (2002) Anticancer activity of sodium stibogluconate in synergy with IFNs. J Immunol 169:5978–5985

Zabolotny JM, Bence-Hanulec KK, Stricker-Krongrad A, Haj F, Wang Y, Minokoshi Y, Kim YB, Elmquist JK, Tartaglia LA, Kahn BB, Neel BG (2002) PTP1B regulates leptin signal transduction in vivo. Dev Cell 2:489–495

Zhang ZY, Lee SY (2003) PTP1B inhibitors as potential therapeutics in the treatment of type 2 diabetes and obesity. Expert Opin Investig Drugs 12:223–233

Zhang YL, Yao ZJ, Sarmiento M, Wu L, Burke TR, Zhang ZY (2000) Thermodynamic study of ligand binding to protein-tyrosine phosphatase 1B and its substrate-trapping mutants. J Biol Chem 275:34205–34212

Zhang Z-Y, MacLean D, McNamara DJ, Sawyer TK, Dixon JE (1994a) Protein tyrosine phosphatase specificity: size and phosphotyrosine positioning requirements in peptide substrates. Biochemistry 33:2285–2290

Zhang Z-Y, Thieme-Sefler AM, MacLean D, McNamara DJ, Dobrusin EM, Sawyer TK, Dixon JE (1993) Substrate specificity of the protein tyrosine phosphatases. Proc Natl Acad Sci USA 90:4446–4450

Zhang Z-Y, Wang YA, Dixon JE (1994b) Dissecting the catalytic mechanism of protein-tyrosine phosphatases. Proc Natl Acad Sci USA 91:1624–1627

Zinker BA, Rondinone CM, Trevillyan JM, Gum RJ, Clampit JE, Waring JF, Xie N, Wilcox D, Jacobson P, Frost L, Kroeger PE, Reilly RM, Koterski S, Opgenorth TJ, Ulrich RG, Crosby S, Butler M, Murray SF, McKay RA, Bhanot S, Monia BP, Jirousek MR (2002) PTP1B antisense oligonucleotide lowers PTP1B protein, normalizes blood glucose, and improves insulin sensitivity in diabetic mice. Proc Natl Acad Sci USA 99:11357–11362

HEP (2005) 167:263–293

Biological Validation of the CD45 Tyrosine Phosphatase as a Pharmaceutical Target

D. R. Alexander

Laboratory of Lymphocyte Signalling and Development, The Babraham Institute, Babraham, Cambridge, CB2 4AT, UK
denis.alexander@bbsrc.ac.uk

Abstract The CD45 phosphotyrosine phosphatase is expressed on all nucleated haematopoietic cells and plays an important role in regulating immune receptor signalling thresholds. CD45 substrates include Src tyrosine kinase family members, and in T cells both $p56^{lck}$ and $p59^{fyn}$ are substrates. Src kinases such as $p56^{lck}$ have negative regulatory C-terminus Tyr phosphorylation sites that are phosphorylated by the c-Src kinase and dephosphorylated by CD45, thereby switching $p56^{lck}$ into a fully functional mode. Active $p56^{lck}$, and to a lesser extent $p59^{fyn}$, are involved in coupling the T cell antigen receptor to the intracellular signalling pathways that lead to T cell development and activation. In $CD45^{-/-}$ mice, the threshold for receptor signalling is high and there are significant defects in thymic development resulting in a greater than 90% reduction in the repertoire of mature peripheral T cells. Those $CD45^{-/-}$ T cells that do exit to the periphery are markedly non-responsive to mitogens. The $p56^{lck}$ kinase also has an activating autophosphorylation site that can be dephosphorylated by CD45 under some circumstances. However, the overall regulatory actions of CD45 on p56^{lck} function in the context of T cell antigen receptor coupling are positive, and this is confirmed by restoration of the CD45$^{-/-}$ phenotype with the *lck*^{Y505F} transgene. Up to eight CD45 isoforms are generated by alternative splicing of which at least five are expressed on lymphocytes at significant levels. Differential CD45 isoform expression is tightly controlled during lymphocyte development and activation, but putative differences in the molecular actions of the different isoforms remain poorly understood. CD45 is an attractive therapeutic target as a means to suppress T cell activation, of relevance in autoimmunity, protection against organ graft rejection and inflammation. CD45 may also be of use in cancer therapies. Current therapeutic strategies utilise CD45 monoclonal antibodies or phosphatase inhibitors. Increasing knowledge of CD45 structure and function will facilitate a more systematic and rational approach to drug design.

Keywords CD45 · Tyrosine phosphatase · Inhibitor · CD45 isoform · Monoclonal antibody

1 Introduction

The CD45 phosphotyrosine phosphatase (previously known as the leucocyte common antigen, LCA) is expressed on all nucleated haematopoietic cells and plays an important role in regulating receptor signalling thresholds in several types of immune cell. The molecule comprises a large heavily glycosylated ectodomain (391–552 amino acids) and an extensive cytoplasmic tail (700 amino acids) containing homologous domains 1 and 2 (Fig. 1). Domain 1 contains the protein tyrosine phosphatase (PTPase) activity, whereas the role of domain 2 appears to be largely regulatory. Alternative splicing generates eight or more isoforms that differ markedly in their ectodomain structures and glycosylation profiles.

An extensive range of reviews on CD45 is available (Thomas 1989; Trowbridge and Thomas 1994; Alexander 1997; Ashwell and Doro 1999; Thomas and Brown 1999; Alexander 2000; Justement 2001; Alexander 2003; Hermiston et al. 2003). This chapter will focus on the biological validation of CD45 as a pharmaceutical target and on the various approaches that have been used to inhibit CD45 activity and function.

2 CD45 Regulates Receptor Thresholds

2.1 CD45 and Lymphocyte Development

The first indication that CD45 has a positive role in regulating signals mediated by antigen receptors came from the investigation of T cell lines and T cell clones that lack CD45 expression. In these contexts it was found that

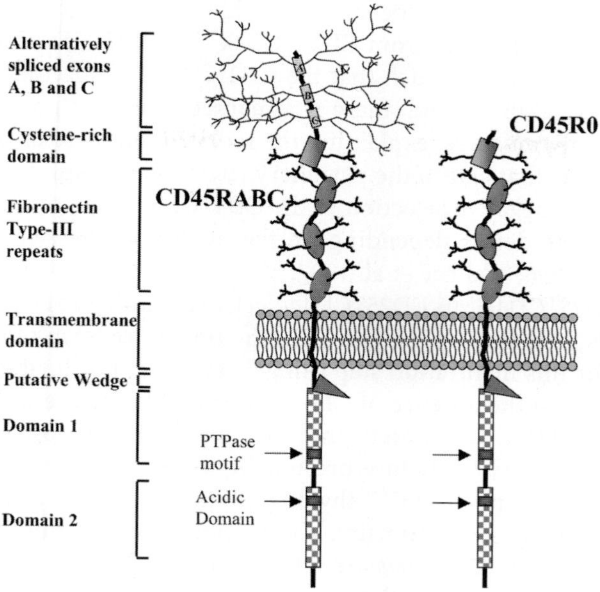

Fig. 1 Domain structure of the CD45 molecule. The extensive CD45 ectodomain is characterised by three fibronectin type III (FN-III) repeats, a cysteine-rich domain and the three alternatively spliced exons A, B and C at the N-terminus. The ectodomain is heavily glycosylated, mainly N-linked in the FN-III and cysteine-rich regions and *O*-linked in the A, B and C exon-encoded regions. The CD45R0 isoform lacks the A, B and C exon-encoded regions. The protein tyrosine phosphatase (*PTPase*) signature motif VHCSAGVGRTG is located in the C-terminal portion of *domain 1*. Domain 2 contains a characteristic 24 amino acid acidic sub-domain and a partial PTPase signature motif, but is not thought to display PTPase activity

stimulation of the T cell antigen receptor (TCR) no longer induced intracellular activating signals, demonstrating that the signal transduction coupling threshold of the receptor was greatly increased in the absence of CD45 (Pingel and Thomas 1989; Koretzky et al. 1990). Later, these findings were extended and confirmed by the generation of three CD45-targeted mouse-lines in which CD45 exons 6, 9 or 12 were deleted to generate mice in which nearly all the CD45 was absent (exon 6) (Kishihara et al. 1993) or was completely absent (exons 9 and 12) (Byth et al. 1996; Mee et al. 1999). The low levels of CD45 that remain expressed on the surface of peripheral T cells in the exon 6-targeted mice (Kong et al. 1995b) may in fact have a marked effect in regulating TCR signalling thresholds: low levels of CD45 (as little as 6%–8% of wild-type levels) are sufficient to restore T cell development and functions (Ogilvy et al. 2003). In mice completely lacking CD45 expression there are striking defects in thymic development so that only about 5% of the normal numbers of mature T cells exit to the periphery (Byth et al.

1996). Three distinct defects occur during development: first, there is a partial defect in the transition from $CD25^+CD44^-$ to $CD25^-CD44^-$ cells lacking CD4 and CD8 expression, such that the $CD25^+CD44^-$ subset accumulates in the absence of CD45; second, there is a marked failure of positive selection of $CD4^+CD8^+$ thymocytes, explaining the reduced numbers of mature $CD4^+$ and $CD8^+$ T cells that exit to the periphery (Byth et al. 1996); third, there is a partial defect in negative selection at the $CD4^+CD8^+$ stage of differentiation, the extent of the defect depending on the avidity of the selecting antigen (Conroy et al. 1996; Wallace et al. 1997; Mee et al. 1999). The reduced transition from $CD25^+CD44^-$ to $CD25^-CD44^-$ cells is readily explained by defects in the signals mediated by the pre-TCR, the immature form of the TCR that is required for this maturation step (Pingel et al. 1999). A further thymic defect that occurs in the absence of CD45 is a marked increase in the basal apoptosis of the $CD4^+CD8^+$ subset: since this population comprises the bulk of the thymus, this survival failure presumably explains much of the 50% reduction in size of the $CD45^{-/-}$ thymus (Byth et al. 1996). Stimulation of $CD45^{-/-}$ thymocytes in vitro using a CD3 monoclonal antibody (mAb) has shown that intracellular signals are typically reduced by 50%–80% (Stone et al. 1997). This contrasts with the virtual ablation of TCR signal transduction observed in most CD45-deficient T cell lines. In fact, optimal TCR stimulation can induce calcium signals in $CD45^{-/-}$ thymocytes to levels comparable with wild-type cells, although the twofold increase in TCR expression on $CD45^{-/-}$ $CD4^+CD8^+$ thymocytes (Stone et al. 1997) may compensate for defects in signalling to some extent. Taken together, these findings suggest that only a very potent CD45 inhibitor, with efficacy higher than 90%, would be likely to have any effect on murine thymic differentiation.

B cell development is less affected in the absence of CD45 than T cell development. Whereas the early stages of B cell differentiation appear to be normal, the maturation from IgM^{hi} IgD^{hi} (immunoglobulin-M^{hi}immunoglobulin-D^{lo}; T2) cells into the IgM^{lo} IgD^{hi} phenotype typical of follicular B cells is impaired (Byth et al. 1996). The thresholds for B cell selection events are altered in $CD45^{-/-}$ mice in a manner analogous to the changes observed in the T lineage. In $CD45^{-/-}$ mice back-crossed to mice carrying immunoglobulin genes specific for hen egg lysozyme (HEL), the circulating HEL autoantigen which mediates negative selection in wild-type mice instead positively selects HEL-binding B cells, leading to their accumulation as long-lived IgD^{hi} cells (Cyster et al. 1996).

The few patients who have been described to date lacking CD45 expression all display a severe combined immunodeficiency (SCID) (Kung et al. 2000; Tchilian et al. 2001) similar to that noted in the $CD45^{-/-}$ mice. Overall, therefore, observations from both mouse and human are consistent with the idea that CD45 plays a dominantly positive role during lymphocyte development by increasing the threshold for antigen receptor signal transduction.

2.2
CD45 and Lymphocyte Function

The B cell antigen receptor (BCR) is almost completely uncoupled from proliferative signals in CD45$^{-/-}$ B cells (Benatar et al. 1996; Byth et al. 1996), correlating with defects in calcium signalling and in activation of the Erk-2/pp90-Rsk pathways (Benatar et al. 1996; Cyster et al. 1996). The transition from IgM^{hi} IgD^{hi} cells into the IgM^{lo} IgD^{hi} phenotype is known to require a range of BCR-mediated intracellular signals, including Btk and Vav 1/2 regulation (Doody et al. 2001; Meade et al. 2002), so this maturation defect is most likely explained by the high threshold for BCR signalling in the absence of CD45 at this developmental stage.

Nevertheless, CD45-deficient mice appear to mount normal immune responses to T cell-independent antigens (Kong et al. 1995a), whereas T cell-dependent responses are severely defective (Kong et al. 1995a; Ogilvy et al. 2003). Adoptive transfer studies have also shown that B cells from exon 6-targeted mice (Kong et al. 1995a), as well as from exon 9-targeted mice (N. Holmes, unpublished), are capable of isotype switching in response to T-dependent antigens, providing T cells are present from CD45$^{+/+}$ mice. Therefore the defect in antigenic responses in CD45-deficient mice is localised to the T cell compartment.

As a result of the shifts in the thresholds of selection events during T cell differentiation in the CD45$^{-/-}$ thymus, self major histocompatibility complex peptides (MHC-peptides) that would normally have caused deletion of self-reactive TCRs now result instead in positive selection, leading to a high proportion of T cells expressing autoreactive TCRs (Trop et al. 2000). However, the development of autoimmunity in CD45$^{-/-}$ mice is not as aggressive as this finding might suggest, presumably because the few T cells that exit to the periphery are markedly non-responsive to antigenic stimulation. TCR stimulation in CD45$^{-/-}$ purified mature peripheral T cells results in virtually no proliferation (Stone et al. 1997) and the production of cytokines such as interleukin-2, interleukin-4 and interleukin-10 (IL-2, IL-4 and IL-10) is also much reduced (L. Perry and D.R. Alexander, unpublished). Therefore the results so far indicate that CD45-deficient mature T cells are remarkably non-responsive to stimulation, although the generation of a normal mature T cell repertoire by conditional silencing of the CD45 gene will be important in order to distinguish clearly between the consequences of aberrant development and defects caused directly by the absence of the CD45 molecule.

2.3
CD45 and Macrophages

CD45$^{-/-}$ macrophages display abnormally high integrin receptor-mediated adherence compared with wild-type controls, correlating with the maturation of fewer bone marrow-derived macrophages when differentiated in vitro (Roach et al. 1997). Therefore in contrast to the situation with antigen receptors, CD45 appears to exert a predominantly negative effect on integrin signalling. Consistent with this observation, in a CD45-deficient T cell line, enhanced adhesion to fibronectin via the $\alpha_5\beta_1$ (VLA-5) integrin but not via $\alpha_4\beta_1$ (VLA-4) has been noted (Shenoi et al. 1999).

2.4
CD45 and Mast Cells

Investigation of mast cell function in CD45 exon 6 targeted mice has suggested that CD45 is essential for degranulation triggered via the high-affinity immunoglobulin E receptor (Fc-ϵR1) (Berger et al. 1994). Similar results have been obtained using CD45-deficient cell lines (Zhang and Siraganian 1999; Murakami et al. 2000). On the other hand, stimulation of the Fc-ϵR1 receptor in mast cells from either exon 9-targeted (N. Holmes, unpublished results) or exon 12-targeted (V. Tybulewicz, unpublished results) mice has not revealed any obvious defect in primary mast cell degranulation when CD45 is completely absent. Therefore the precise role of CD45 in Fc-ϵR1 signal transduction remains to be clearly resolved.

2.5
CD45 and Natural Killer Cells

A marked increase in the numbers of natural killer (NK) cells has been noted in the spleen of both CD45 exon 6 and exon 9-targeted mice. Nevertheless, the NK cells appeared to have normal cytotoxic activities and could also differentiate normally into lymphokine-activated killer cells upon culture with IL-2 (Yamada et al. 1996; Martin et al. 2001). In addition, using the exon 9-targeted mice lacking CD45 expression, some subtle defects have been noted in the development and function of NK cells and of NK-T cells (Martin et al. 2001). For example, the cytotoxic NK cells were functionally unable to secrete interferon (IFN)-γ. In addition to NK cells there is a subset of lymphocytes that share receptor structures common to both T and NK cell lineages, the NK-T cells. These can be divided into two distinct subsets, those that are $CD4^+$ or $CD4^-CD8^-$ and that develop in a thymus-dependent manner, and a $CD8^+$ population that are thymus-independent in their development. In exon 9-targeted $CD45^{-/-}$ mice, the NK-T cell population was maintained in the intestinal intraepithelial lymphoid compartment but not in the spleen and was found to comprise the thymus-independent $CD8^+$ subset. Functionally these cells were unable to secrete IL-4 in response to TCR ligation. Therefore CD45 is required for the development of thymus-dependent NK-T cells, and for normal cytokine secretion in both NK cells and in the $CD8^+$ NK-T cell subset.

3
CD45 Substrates

3.1
The Src Tyrosine Kinases

The only molecules that have to date been unambiguously identified as substrates for CD45 are members of the Src family of tyrosine kinases. The Src member that has received most attention is $p56^{lck}$, a kinase mainly restricted in expression to the T-lineage. In fact, the regulation of $p56^{lck}$ by CD45 is sufficient to explain most if not all the results obtained using CD45-deficient cell lines and knockout mice. The $p56^{lck}$ kinase, as with other members of the Src kinase family, is regulated by a wide range of factors. These include: localisation of the kinase in reference to the plasma membrane; binding of proteins containing Pro-rich motifs to the $p56^{lck}$ SH3 domain; engagement of its SH2 domain by pTyr residue-containing proteins; autophosphorylation of the activatory Tyr-394 residue; and phosphorylation by the C-terminal Src kinase (Csk) of the inhibitory Tyr-505 residue. In the absence of CD45 in membranes in vitro (Mustelin et al. 1989; Mustelin and Altman 1990), in T cell lines (Ostergaard et al. 1989; McFarland et al. 1993; Sieh et al. 1993) or primary T cells (Stone et al. 1997), $p56^{lck}$ becomes hyper-phosphorylated at Tyr-505. This causes the kinase to adopt a 'closed conformation' in which the pTyr-505 residue forms an intramolecular association with its SH2 domain (Sieh et al. 1993; Stone et al. 1997). This version of the kinase lacks optimal activity and, perhaps more importantly, could render the $p56^{lck}$ SH2 and SH3 domains less available to engage exogenous proteins. One candidate protein for such interactions is pTyr-319 in the linker region of ZAP-70 which has been proposed to engage with the $p56^{lck}$ SH2 domain (Pelosi et al. 1999). Upon dephosphorylation of pTyr-505 by CD45, $p56^{lck}$ then adopts an 'open conformation', with a modest increase in kinase activity, and with its SH2 and SH3 domains now fully available for exogenous liaisons. It should be noted that dephosphorylation of pTyr-505 is not the only way in which such an open conformation is promoted. For example, a proline motif-containing peptide in the CD28 cytoplasmic tail can bind to the $p56^{lck}$ SH3 domain (Holdorf et al. 1999) and the *Herpes saimiri* viral Tip protein can disrupt the relatively weak interaction between the $p56^{lck}$ SH2 domain and pTyr-505 (Hartley et al. 1999), in both cases leading to increased $p56^{lck}$ functionality. The idea that dephosphorylation of $p56^{lck}$ pTyr-505 by CD45 is a physiologically relevant action of this PTPase is supported by the finding that in $CD45^{-/-}$ mice back-crossed to mice expressing a mutant lck^{Y505F} transgene, there is significant restoration of T cell development and reversal of the increased apoptosis that characterises $CD45^{-/-}$ $CD4^{+}CD8^{+}$ thymocytes (Pingel et al. 1999; Seavitt et al. 1999).

Mutational analysis of p56^{lck} has shown that autophosphorylation of the Tyr-394 residue plays a stronger positive role in promoting the enzyme activity of the kinase in comparison with the relatively weak inhibitory effect of Tyr-505 phosphorylation (Doro et al. 1996). In some CD45-deficient transformed cell lines (Doro et al. 1996) as well as murine CD45$^{-/-}$ thymocytes (Baker et al. 2000), increased phosphorylation at Tyr-394 has been observed, suggesting that CD45 also has the capability to dephosphorylate this residue. Indeed, the overall p56^{lck} kinase activity in the CD45$^{-/-}$ thymus is higher than in the wild-type (Doro and Ashwell 1999), consistent with the idea that it is the pTyr-394 site that is most potent in regulating activity. Dramatic confirmation that CD45 could dephosphorylate p56^{lck} pTyr-394 in vivo came from the observation that aggressive T cell lymphomas develop in CD45$^{-/-}$p56$^{lck-Y505F}$ mice, caused by the conversion of the mutant p56$^{lck-Y505F}$ into an oncogene by increased Tyr-394 phosphorylation in the absence of CD45 (Baker et al. 2000). It therefore appears that in the CD45-deficient T cell, pools of p56^{lck} may exist that are either hyper-phosphorylated at Tyr-505, or at Tyr-394, and perhaps at both sites simultaneously.

Recent analysis of the 'immune synapse' that is formed when MHC-peptides engage the TCR has given some clues as to how CD45 might be involved in regulating the two different regulatory phosphorylation sites of p56^{lck}. The engagement of antigen receptors by ligand results in the formation of a highly structured ensemble of molecules at the receptor contact point known as 'the immune synapse', 'immunological synapse' or 'supramolecular activation cluster' (SMAC). All these terms refer to the same entity. It is thought that the immune synapse is a consequence of initial signalling events and provides a mechanism to facilitate a prolonged and carefully orchestrated transmission of intracellular signals during the period of time required for full lymphocyte activation. As Fig. 2 illustrates, selective repertoires of molecules characterise the central and peripheral regions of the immune synapse (cSMAC and pSMAC, respectively) (Monks et al. 1998). The immune synapse is a dynamic system in which molecules rapidly traffic between its various regions.

The important question as to the precise relationship between CD45 localisation and the immune synapse has not yet been fully resolved, partly because the results obtained have varied somewhat depending on the model system utilised. A critical question is how CD45 localises in relation to its p56^{lck} kinase substrate. Initially in T cells p56^{lck} appears to co-cluster in the cSMAC but then moves to the periphery within a few minutes of receptor stimulation (Monks et al. 1998; Ehrlich et al. 2002; Holdorf et al. 2002). At the same time, the immune synapse appears to be replenished with more p56^{lck} from intracellular stores (Ehrlich et al. 2002). The question, then, is how CD45 relates to this moving target. Some imaging studies using either T cells (Leupin et al. 2000) or B cells (Batista et al. 2001) have suggested that CD45 is excluded from the immune synapse. However,

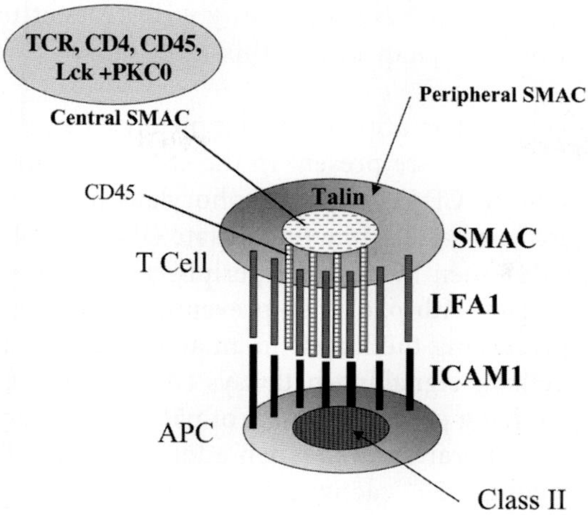

Fig. 2 The location of CD45 in a T cell "supramolecular activation cluster". The T cell antigen receptor (*TCR*) expressed on a T cell engages class II MHC-peptides presented on an antigen-presenting cell (*APC*). At 45 s following engagement the SMAC begins to form, Talin is localised in the central portion of the SMAC (*cSMAC*) and LFA1 is activated and binds to intercellular adhesion molecule (*ICAM*)-1 on the APC. At 3 min the TCR, CD45, CD4, Lck and PKCθ are localised in the cSMAC followed by activation of the $p56^{lck}$ kinase. By 7 min active ZAP-70 tyrosine kinase is found in the cSMAC and increased protein tyrosine phosphorylation in the cSMAC and peripheral SMAC (*pSMAC*), and CD45 has moved out to a region beyond the pSMAC. The model and kinetic data are based on the findings of Freiberg et al. (2002). It is possible that different CD45 isoforms are localised differently and with distinctive kinetics within the various SMAC regions

in a careful kinetic study in which three-dimensional immunofluorescence microscopy was utilised to study the interaction between primary T cells and cognate peptide presented on an antigen presenting cell, both CD45 and $p56^{lck}$ were initially identified in the cSMAC (Freiberg et al. 2002). Then, following 7 min of receptor stimulation, CD45 moved out of the cSMAC to a region peripheral to the pSMAC. Even in the absence of antigen-presenting cells, using a system in which the MHC-peptide ligand was presented to T cells on beads, CD45 was still initially found in the cSMAC in close association with the TCR, showing that recruitment of CD45 to the immune synapse was not caused by an exogenous ligand (Freiberg et al. 2002). In a different study in which planar lipid bilayers containing MHC-peptide and the adhesion molecule intercellular adhesion molecule (ICAM)-1 were used for antigen presentation, CD45 was at first excluded from the cSMAC, but within 10 min was then recruited back to the centre of the contact area (Johnson et al. 2000). The discrepancies between these results may be due to the different experimental systems utilised, in particular the use of lipid bilayers for antigen presentation in contrast to antigen presenting cells. A further intriguing possibility is that different CD45 isoforms (see below) might behave differently with respect to their localisation within the immune synapse, and this question was not addressed in the cited studies.

Overall, although the data are not yet completely clear, a likely scenario is that both CD45 and $p56^{lck}$ are present in the cSMAC at the earliest stage of its formation, enabling CD45 to dephosphorylate $p56^{lck}$ at pTyr-505 and maintain the kinase in a basally functional state (Fig. 2). Following $p56^{lck}$ kinase activation, CD45 then moves to a peripheral region where it may not have continued contact with $p56^{lck}$, so preventing rapid dephosphorylation of pTyr-394 and preserving the kinase in an activated state to facilitate TCR coupling to intracellular signalling pathways (Alexander 2000). In this context, it is of interest that a potent inhibitor of $p56^{lck}$ kinase activity completely inhibited T cell proliferation even when added 1 h after TCR stimulation, suggesting that ongoing $p56^{lck}$ activity is important for the T cell activation process (Ehrlich et al. 2002).

The pharmaceutical relevance of this potentially dual action of CD45 on $p56^{lck}$ is that CD45 inhibitors could, in principle, exert either an activatory or inhibitory effect on the kinase depending on which of the two phosphorylation sites was dominant. Since $p56^{lck}$ Tyr-394 phosphorylation is amplified only upon activation of the kinase, and activation is hindered by hyperphosphorylation at Tyr-505, it seems reasonable to conclude based on the CD45-deficient cell studies that the dominant effect of CD45 inhibition would be a concomitant inhibition of $p56^{lck}$ due to increased Tyr-505 phosphorylation, so preventing the generation of pTyr-394 as a 'second substrate' for CD45. Nevertheless, it cannot yet be excluded that partial inhibition of CD45 might change the ratio between the phosphorylation status of the two sites in subtle ways, and it could eventually emerge that the regulation of this ratio is the key to the development of CD45 as a successful pharmaceutical target.

In addition to $p56^{lck}$, the $p59^{fyn}$ tyrosine kinase has also been shown to be regulated by CD45 in vivo in both T cell lines (Shiroo et al. 1992; McFarland et al. 1993) and in primary thymocytes (Stone et al. 1997). The adapter protein SKAP-55 may play a role in binding to CD45 and mediating its effects on $p59^{fyn}$ (Wu et al. 2002). The precise function of CD45-regulated $p59^{fyn}$ in coupling the TCR or other receptors to specific signalling pathways has not as yet been completely defined.

It has proved much more difficult to establish unambiguous CD45 substrates in B cells as compared to T cells. Indeed, BCR-stimulated tyrosine phosphorylation events appear normal in $CD45^{-/-}$ B cells. The reason for this may be the greater degree of redundancy in the utilisation of tyrosine kinases by the BCR in comparison with the TCR. Furthermore $p59^{lyn}$, a further member of the Src family of tyrosine kinases, is involved not only in coupling the BCR to intracellular signals, but also in mediating negative signals via the CD22 co-receptor, so there is scope for compensation between different receptors expressed on the same B cell. In fact, recruitment of the Syk tyrosine kinase to the BCR proceeds normally in a CD45-deficient cell-line, even though $p59^{lyn}$ is hyper-phosphorylated at its C-terminus inhibitory Tyr-508 regulatory site and is no longer itself recruited to the receptor (Pao 1997).

Whether $p59^{lyn}$ is the key B cell substrate for CD45 under physiological conditions, explaining the defects observed in BCR signalling, remains controversial. In CD45-deficient B cell lines there is evidence that the kinase is hyper-phosphorylated at both its autophosphorylation and C-terminus inhibitory regulatory Tyr residues, correlating with reduced activity of the kinase (Yanagi et al. 1996). But in a different CD45-deficient B cell line, basal $p59^{lyn}$ kinase activity is normal despite hyper-phosphorylation of $p59^{lyn}$ (Pao and Cambier 1997), whereas in a CD45-deficient sub-clone of the WEHI-231 B cell line, overall $p59^{lyn}$ activity is higher with increased phosphorylation at both regulatory Tyr residues (Katagiri et al. 1999). In contrast to these cell-line studies, dysfunctional regulation of $p59^{lyn}$ in primary $CD45^{-/-}$ B cells has not yet been reported. One possible reason for these conflicting results may be that different pools of Src family kinases are differentially regulated by CD45 and by other tyrosine phosphatases depending on their subcellular localisation (Biffen et al. 1994). Measurements of the 'average' activities and phosphorylation states of kinases by using enzyme immunoprecipitates from whole cell lysates may not sufficiently discriminate between such pools. Therefore in B cells, physiological CD45 substrates have not yet been unambiguously established.

In macrophages from the CD45 exon 6-targeted mice, the $p56/p59^{hck}$ and $p59^{lyn}$ tyrosine kinase members of the Src kinase family are both hyper-active, indicating that these are the likely physiologically relevant substrates for CD45 in this lineage (Roach et al. 1997).

3.2
Other Possible CD45 Substrates

In addition to members of the Src kinase family, several other CD45 substrates have been proposed. For example, CD45 may negatively regulate cytokine receptor coupling to intracellular signals by dephosphorylating the Janus kinases (JAKs) (Irie-Sasaki 2001; Yamada et al. 2002). The JAKs positively regulate cytokine receptor signalling by phosphorylating transcription factors known as the signal transducers and activators of transcription (STATs) which, upon phosphorylation, translocate to the nucleus where they regulate genes involved in the cytokine response. Hyper-phosphorylation of Jak-2 following IL-3 stimulation was noted in bone-marrow-derived mast cells derived from either the exon 6- or exon 9-targeted mice, correlating with increased phosphorylation of STAT-3 and STAT-5 (Irie-Sasaki 2001). Mice lacking CD45 also displayed increased protection against the picornavirus coxsackievirus B3 (CVB3) (Irie-Sasaki 2001), although a similar protection has been noted in *lck*$^{-/-}$ mice (Liu et al. 2000), so it is possible that increased protection in the absence of CD45 is an indirect consequence of its well-established regulation of p56^{lck}, rather than a reflection of JAK activation.

Other substrates that have been suggested for CD45 include ZAP-70 (Mustelin et al. 1995) and TCR-ζ (Furukawa et al. 1994; Hegedus et al. 1999). It has been suggested that the CD45 D2 domain may be involved in the recruitment of TCR-ζ as a substrate (Kashio et al. 1998). A complication in the assessment of TCR-ζ as a potential CD45 substrate in vivo is that the polypeptide is phosphorylated by CD45-activated p56^{lck}, so in CD45$^{-/-}$ thymocytes, for example, there is a marked reduction in TCR-ζ phosphorylation (Stone et al. 1997). This means that in the absence of CD45, its putative TCR-ζ substrate is not generated normally, so even if it were a substrate it would not be expected to be hyper-phosphorylated. The expression of mutant hyper-active lck^{Y505F} in murine T lymphoma cell lines lacking CD45 expression (Baker et al. 2000) potentially overcomes this problem, but in these cells there is no evidence for TCR-ζ hyper-phosphorylation (D. Higgins and D.R.Alexander, unpublished). A caveat to these findings is that the TCR-ζ polypeptide expression is very low in these cells, and therefore its hyper-phosphorylation might be difficult to detect. Overall, therefore, the possibility that CD45 dephosphorylates one or more of the six potential pTyr sites in TCR-ζ cannot yet be excluded.

4
CD45 Isoforms

CD45 is expressed as multiple isoforms resulting from alternative RNA splicing of exons 4, 5 and 6 (also denoted A, B and C, respectively) (Trowbridge and Thomas 1994; Alexander 1997). The exons 4–6 encode only about 50–60 amino acids, each located at the ectodomain N-terminus, but the effects of splicing out these alternative exons is amplified by the loss of their multiple *O*-linked glycosylation sites (Fig. 1). The cytoplasmic tail is identical in all CD45 isoforms. In theory alternative splicing of exons 4–6 generates up to eight different isoforms, but in practice only five of these isoforms have been reported as proteins expressed at significant levels in lymphocytes: CD45RABC, CD45RAB, CD45RBC, CD45RB and CD45R0, varying in molecular weight from 180 to 240 kDa (Rogers et al. 1992; Fukuhara et al. 2002). Alternative splicing (by mechanisms reviewed in Hermiston et al. 2003) has been most studied in the T lineage, where it is under tight regulatory control during thymic development and in the activation of mature T cells. For example, CD45R0 is up-regulated on CD4^{+}CD8^{+} thymocytes, but then declines following positive selection with up-regulation of higher molecular weight isoforms (such as CD45RB in the mouse) in $CD4^+$ and $CD8^+$ thymocytes (Fukuhara et al. 2002). Human cord blood T cells that have not previously been exposed to antigen express low CD45R0 levels relative to higher molecular weight isoforms containing the A-exon product. With increasing age the proportion of peripheral T cells expressing CD45R0 gradually increases until it typically reaches 40%–60% of the total repertoire in the adult (Hayward et al. 1989). Indeed, when $CD45RA^+$ T cells are activated in vitro they up-regulate CD45R0 and down-regulate the $CD45RA^+$ isoforms over a period of several days (Akbar et al. 1988). However, this conversion is never complete, and all T cells express more than one CD45 isoform. It is not, therefore, possible to purify primary T cell subsets from wild-type mouse or human and assess the properties of single CD45 isoforms in isolation. The up-regulation of CD45R0 on antigen-experienced T cells, and upon T cells activated in vitro, has led to the idea that $CD45R0^+$ T cells comprise, or contain a population, of 'memory/effector' cells. However, this suggestion remains controversial and the only clear conclusion at present is that in the mature T cell repertoire CD45R0 is a marker for previously activated T cells. There is also evidence suggesting that conversion to a $CD45R0^{hi}$ phenotype is a reversible process, so in vivo it seems probable that CD45R0 is not only a marker for previously activated T cells, but also for T cells stimulated relatively recently.

T cells that accumulate at sites of inflammation generally express high levels of CD45R0. For example, many of the T cells found in the inflamed synovium in rheumatoid arthritis (Matthews et al. 1993) and in inflammatory dermatoses (Markey et al. 1990) are in a pseudo-activated state and express high levels of CD45R0, HLA-DR and other activation markers. Interestingly, several therapeutic reagents have now been shown to selectively deplete $CD45R0^+$ T cells in patients. For example, alefacept is a fusion protein consisting of the first extracellular domain of lymphocyte function-associated antigen 3 (LFA-3, CD58), fused to the human IgG_1 hinge, C_H2 and C_H3 domains, that binds to CD2 expressed on T cells. The fusion protein prolongs cardiac allograft survival in primates (Kaplon et al. 1996) and has recently been licensed following phase II and phase III clinical trials for the treatment of chronic plaque psoriasis (Ellis and Krueger 2001), a disease characterised by infiltration of memory/effector type $CD45R0^+$ lymphocytes. Alefacept has been shown to reduce the number of $CD45RO^+$ cells in psoriasis patients, a finding that correlated with improvement of the psoriatic lesions (Ellis and Krueger 2001); and selective killing of $CD45R0^+$ rather than $CD45RA^+$ T cells by autologous NK cells in the presence of alefacept has also been demonstrated in vitro (Cooper et al. 2003). Therefore the selective depletion of activated/memory type T cells appears to be a promising avenue for anti-inflammatory therapeutic intervention.

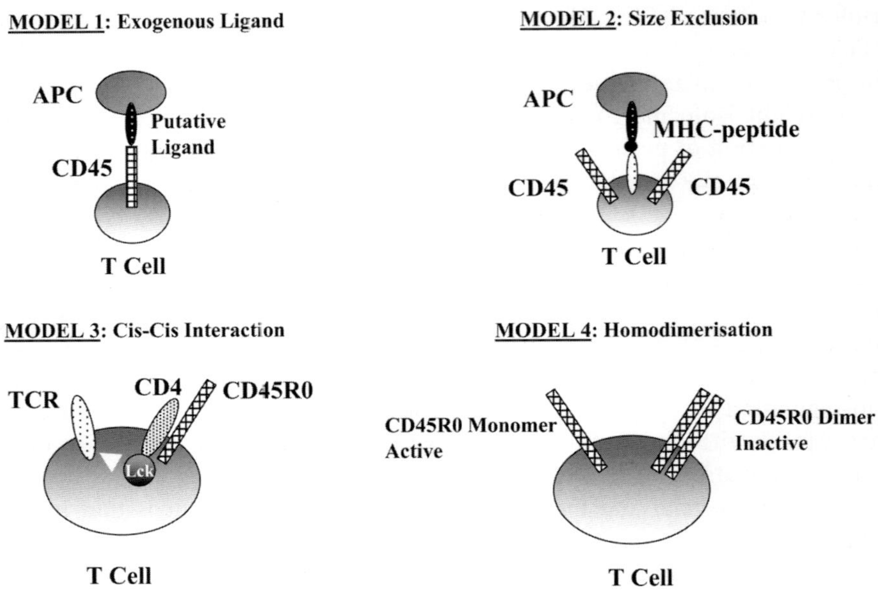

Fig. 3 Four possible models to explain the molecular actions of CD45 isoforms

As Fig. 3 illustrates, four models have been suggested to explain the different molecular actions of CD45 isoforms, and these models will be briefly reviewed. None of the models are mutually exclusive.

4.1 The Exogenous Ligand Model

It is a reasonable assumption that CD45 might have exogenous ligands, either in soluble form or expressed on other cells such as antigen presenting cells, and that such ligands could vary between different CD45 isoforms. However, until now, no physiologically relevant CD45 ligands have been described. Although CD45 binds effectively to lectins, not surprisingly in light of its abundant oligosaccharide branches, such interactions have not as yet been demonstrated to play a role in vivo in modulating the actions of CD45.

4.2 The Size Exclusion Model

An equally reasonable assumption is that the larger CD45 isoform ectodomain might sterically hinder the presentation of MHC-peptides to the TCR, whereas the relatively small CD45R0 ectodomain would exert little or no hindrance (Davis and van der Merwe 1996). This possibility is closely related to the question as to how and when CD45 localises within the 'immune synapse' as discussed in Sect. 3.1. An intriguing possibility is that CD45 isoforms differentially localise within the immune synapse, thereby modulating the speed and/or intensity of T cell responses. For example, in a variant of the size-exclusion model, CD45R0 could be present at the earliest formation of the cSMAC, promoting the activation of $p56^{lck}$, whereas CD45 isoforms with larger ectodomains might be excluded from the cSMAC, thereby reducing the speed of response in the initiation of TCR signalling. However, the mere size of the CD45 ectodomain per se does not seem to be the main arbiter of CD45 function. Thus, in one study three chimaeric proteins, each containing the CD45 cytoplasmic tail but having small (Thy-1), intermediate (CD2) or large (CD43) ectodomains, were expressed in a CD45-deficient T cell line (Irles et al. 2003). The expectation in this investigation was that the large ectodomain would prevent superantigen-mediated TCR stimulation by preventing the close apposition of the ligand. Unexpectedly, however, the CD43–CD45 chimaera was found to be most efficient at restoring TCR signalling, whereas the chimaeras with small ectodomains were poor in this respect. This correlated with the localisation of the CD43–CD45 chimaera in lipid rafts, whereas chimaeras with smaller ectodomains were excluded from rafts. This study therefore provides no support for the size-exclusion model.

It is important to resolve the issue of CD45, and more particularly of CD45 isoform, sub-cellular localisation in relation to the micro-architecture of the immune synapse, because disruption of the correct location of a specific CD45 isoform might prove to be a potent method for disrupting CD45 function. This possibility will be assessed further below.

4.3 The *Cis–Cis* Interaction Model

There is an extensive literature describing the association of CD45 with other proteins in *cis–cis* interactions at the cell surface (the earlier literature is reviewed in Alexander 1997). Reconstitution of a CD45-deficient murine cell line with CD45 isoforms suggested that the CD45R0 isoform promoted greater IL-2 secretion upon engagement of the TCR with the cognate MHC-peptide as compared to other isoforms (Novak et al. 1994). Co-capping experiments in these cells revealed preferential CD4–CD45R0 association (Leitenberg et al. 1996). However, more detailed capping and co-immunoprecipitation studies indicated a basal association of CD45R0 with the TCR independent of CD4 expression and suggested that co-capping of CD4 with CD45R0 was mediated by this prior CD45R0–TCR association (Leitenberg et al. 1999). Nevertheless, CD4–CD45 association has also been described in primary $CD4^+$ T cells (Mittler et al. 1991; Bonnard et al. 1997). In a further study in which fluorescence resonance energy transfer (FRET) analysis was used to investigate *cis–cis* interactions, different CD45 isoforms were transfected into a CD45-deficient T cell line expressing the TCR, CD4 and CD8. The results suggested that CD45R0 preferentially associated with CD4 and CD8 relative to the CD45RBC and CD45RABC isoforms (Dornan et al. 2002). The CD45R0–CD4 association correlated with up-regulated protein tyrosine phosphorylation events under both basal and TCR-stimulated conditions. These studies suggest a model in which the juxtaposition of CD45 PTPase activity in relation to its CD4- or CD8-associated $p56^{lck}$ kinase substrate promotes the action of the kinase, thereby up-regulating TCR-stimulated intracellular phosphorylation events.

Attractive as such a model may be, one problem with such cell line studies is that the glycosylation status of CD45 isoforms and their associating glycoproteins may not be the same as in primary cells, resulting in associations that do not accurately reflect those found under more physiological conditions. To address this question, $CD45^{-/-}$ mice have been reconstituted with specific CD45 isoforms. In one study it was shown that either CD45R0 or CD45RABC transgenes, driven by a proximal *lck* promoter, restored T cell numbers to near normal in lymph nodes, while no restoration of T cell populations in the spleen was found (Kozieradzki et al. 1997). In contrast, the Vav promoter has more recently been utilised to generate several lines of transgenic mice expressing either CD45R0 or CD45RB on the $CD45^{-/-}$ background in all haematopoietic lineages (Ogilvy et al. 2003). When expressed at levels comparable with the total CD45 expression found in hemizygous $CD45^{+/-}$ mice, thymic development was restored to apparently normal levels and reconstitution of mature T cells in both the lymph nodes and spleen was observed. In fact expression of CD45R0 at a level only 6%–8% of the total wild-type CD45 expression level was sufficient to restore thymic development to levels equivalent to wild-type. Mice expressing either the CD45R0 or CD45RB isoforms at comparable levels were equally efficient in their ability to mount T-dependent antigenic responses. Interestingly, however, neither isoform at this level of expression was able to restore effective B cell maturation, nor BCR-stimulated proliferation, showing that CD45 isoforms play unique roles which differ between the T and B lineages.

Overall, therefore, there is considerable support, based largely on cell line studies, for the *cis–cis* interaction model, but the model remains to be confirmed as being relevant to the function of CD45 isoforms in the whole animal context.

4.4 The Homodimerisation Model

The possibility that homodimerisation of transmembrane PTPases leads to the inhibition of phosphatase activity has received recent attention. An indication that the actions of CD45 might be regulated in this manner was suggested by studies using a chimaeric receptor with an epidermal growth factor receptor (EGFR) ectodomain and a CD45 cytoplasmic tail. This chimaera successfully restored TCR signal transduction in a CD45-deficient cell line, but TCR signalling was largely abrogated upon subsequently dimerising the artificial receptor by the addition of EGF (Desai et al. 1993). Mutation of a putative wedge domain (Fig. 1) within the CD45 tail portion of the chimaera significantly blunted the ability of EGF to inhibit TCR-mediated signals, suggesting that the wedge domain might be critical in promoting homodimerisation (Majeti et al. 1998). Introduction of a point mutation at the same site in CD45 in a mouse model in situ resulted in a severe lymphoproliferative and lupus-like syndrome with autoantibody production, consistent also with de-inhibition of CD45 PTPase activity (Majeti et al. 2000). However, since the point mutation was introduced into the germ-line, CD45 in all haematopoietic lineages presumably carries the same mutation, so the question of which cell-type is responsible for the observed abnormalities is important.

CD45 has been shown to dimerise in several different studies. For example, CD45 was found to dimerise to a small extent after chemical cross-linking of a T cell line (Takeda et al. 1992) and recombinant fragments of the rat extracellular domain can exist as dimers as well as monomers (Symons et al. 1999). Is it possible that CD45 isoforms might differentially homodimerise, thereby inhibiting specific pools of CD45 PTPase activity? Interestingly, in a study using FRET, it was found that CD45R0 preferentially homodimerises on the surface of a T cell line when compared with CD45RBC or CDRABC isoforms (Dornan et al. 2002). Similar findings were obtained using chemical cross-linking and a cysteine dimer-trapping method in which it was also shown that CD45R0 preferentially homodimerises in a manner hindered by sialylation and *O*-glycosylation (Xu and Weiss 2002).

As with the *cis–cis* interaction model, the homodimerisation model is also an attractive hypothesis for explaining the differential actions of CD45 isoforms. However, significant questions remain. For example, it is important to show by direct biochemical assay that CD45 homodimerisation causes inhibition of its PTPase activity. Furthermore, in the FRET study cited above, both CD45R0 homodimers and CD4/CD8–CD45R0 heterodimers were detected on the surface of the same cell, yet the net effect on TCR signal transduction of CD45R0 expression appeared to be positive (Dornan et al. 2002). In addition, in a series of transgenic lines expressing increasing amounts of CD45R0 at the T cell surface, in which comparable numbers of peripheral T cells were observed in the spleen and lymph nodes, a quantitative effect was noted in which T-dependent antigenic responses correlated positively with the CD45R0 expression level (Ogilvy et al. 2003). This result is difficult to explain if the main role of CD45R0 is to exert a negative effect on T cell responses. Therefore further work will be required to determine whether the homodimerisation model adequately explains the putative differential actions of CD45 isoforms in vivo.

Overall, our understanding of the molecular actions of specific CD45 isoforms remains significantly incomplete. Achieving a thorough understanding of the biological reasons for the existence and tight regulation of CD45 isoform expression in immune cells remains one of the outstanding challenges in the CD45 research field.

5
CD45 as a Therapeutic Target

CD45 is an attractive therapeutic target as a means to suppress T cell activation, of relevance in autoimmunity, protection against organ graft rejection, inflammation and in cancer therapies. Numerous attempts have been made by pharmaceutical companies to target $p56^{lck}$ selectively, and to some extent $p59^{fyn}$, in order to induce immunosuppression, but inhibition of CD45 would presumably inhibit the actions of both kinases simultaneously, thereby achieving the same goal more effectively. The putative dual action of a CD45 inhibitor in down-regulating the functions of both kinases is important because there is considerable evidence for redundancy between the two enzymes (Seddon et al. 2000; Seddon and Zamoyska 2002) Thus a selective $p56^{lck}$ inhibitor might not be as potent in suppressing T cell activation as expected, since $p59^{fyn}$ appears able to substitute for the actions of $p56^{lck}$ to a considerable extent. A CD45 inhibitor would overcome this potential problem.

An important question to be addressed in considering CD45 as a target is the suggested dual role for the phosphatase as both an activator and inhibitor of $p56^{lck}$. As discussed in Sect. 3.1, only when $p56^{lck}$ pTyr-505 becomes dephosphorylated does the kinase become fully functional, thereby leading to increased phosphorylation at Tyr-394. In a sense, therefore, the enzyme has its own internal 'security system' with respect to a CD45 inhibitor, since hyper-phosphorylation at Tyr-505 caused by CD45 inhibition would tend to reduce Tyr-394 phosphorylation. Nevertheless, in $CD45^{-/-}$ thymocytes at least, there is a modest increase in $p56^{lck}$ Tyr-394 phosphorylation (Baker et al. 2000), so the possibility cannot be excluded that at some critical level of CD45 inhibition a specific intracellular pool of $p56^{lck}$ might be activated rather than inhibited. This possibility will require careful assessment during any attempt to target CD45 therapeutically.

The biological studies described above suggest that the dominant effect of a CD45 inhibitor would be on the T lineage, since the phenotypic effects of CD45 deficiency in other lineages are relatively mild, at least in the murine context. Based on the mouse models, T-independent antigenic responses would remain intact even in the presence of the most potent CD45 inhibitor, and it is striking that quite low levels of CD45 expression are sufficient to restore immune responses to T-dependent antigens (Ogilvy et al. 2003).

Nevertheless, possible side effects of CD45 therapy on cell types such as macrophages and NK cells will require careful assessment.

Two main approaches are being utilised to target CD45: the use of specific antibodies and direct inhibition of its PTPase activity.

5.1
The Use of CD45 Monoclonal Antibodies

There is a very extensive literature concerning the actions of CD45 mAbs on T cells, and earlier publications have been reviewed elsewhere (Alexander 1997). It should first be noted that there is an important difference in the potential mechanism of action of CD45 mAbs, depending whether or not secondary cross-linking antibody is utilised in the experimental system. During the late 1980s and early 1990s many publications appeared claiming that the dominant action of CD45 was negative with respect to TCR signal transduction coupling (reviewed in Alexander 1997). These results were based on experiments in which CD3 mAb against the relatively rare TCR was cross-linked with the very abundant CD45 molecule. Since in many of the cell systems utilised CD3 ligation was required to induce intracellular signals, extensive cross-linking with abundant CD45 thereby produced a 'dilution effect' whereby CD3 ligation became less effective and, not surprisingly, the intracellular signals were inhibited. However, it was later shown using chemically engineered divalent antibodies consisting of F(ab′) fragments against both CD3 and CD45, that when this dilution effect is prevented by fixing the CD3/CD45 ratio, then there is no inhibition (Alexander et al. 1992; Shivnan et al. 1992). In fact, under these conditions the enforced juxtaposition of CD45 with the TCR amplifies T cell activation responses, consistent with the dominantly positive effect of CD45 on TCR signal transduction coupling. Therefore results based on cross-linking the abundant CD45 molecule with other receptors using secondary antibody should be treated with caution, particularly in the absence of relevant controls.

By contrast, there are many instances in which specific CD45 mAbs have striking effects on T cells under conditions in which cross-linking is not an issue. In animal models, one of the main uses of CD45 mAbs has been to induce tolerance to tissue transplants. The most extensive studies have been carried out using a CD45RB mAb called MB23G2 that has been shown to induce long-term engraftment of islets tissue into MHC-disparate diabetic mice (Auersvald et al. 1997; Basadonna et al. 1998), to prevent renal allograft rejection (Lazarovits et al. 1996; Zhong and Lazarovits 1998) and to be useful in the treatment of preclinical models of autoimmunity (Zhong and Lazarovits 1998). Tolerance could be adoptively transferred by transfusion of tolerant mouse $CD4^+$ splenic lymphocytes into naïve allografted animals (Gao et al. 1999). The induction of tolerance was associated with a partial depletion of peripheral blood lymphocytes and with a shift in CD45 isoform expression on T cells from higher molecular weight isoforms to a proportionally greater increase in CD45R0 (Basadonna et al. 1998). In further studies to investigate the mechanism of action of MB23G2 in tolerance induction, it was found that mAb treatment of mice was followed by a rapid up-regulation on T cells of CTLA-4, a receptor that mediates negative signals, inhibiting T cell activation (Fecteau et al. 2001). Administration of a blocking CTLA-4 mAb at the time of transplantation prevented the anti-CD45RB therapy from prolonging the survival of islet allografts, suggesting that CTLA-4 up-regulation was playing a role in tolerance induction. In addition, treatment with cyclosporin A blocked the MB23G2-induced CTLA-4 expression and promoted acute rejection. How the CD45RB mAb treatment causes up-regulation of CTLA-4 on T cells remains an intriguing question.

Rat models have also been developed to investigate the actions of CD45 mAbs in vivo. The rat anti-rat RT7 mAb has been extensively used. In the rat, two allomorphic forms of the RT7 antigen exist, known as $RT7^a$ and $RT7^b$ (previously known as ART-1 and Ly-1) (Wonigeit 1979a,b). In animals expressing the $RT7^a$ allotype, the $RT7^a$ mAb binds to all $CD45^+$ cells. Treatment of rats with the $RT7^a$ mAb causes a massive depletion of peripheral leucocytes as well as bone-marrow precursor cells (Dahlke et al. 2002), and this is associated with tolerance induction to fully MHC-mismatched grafts (Ko et al. 2001). Interestingly, mature B cells, although well coated with the mAb, are protected from depletion. Leucocyte depletion showed an identical pattern in complement-deficient as in normal rats, suggesting that complement lysis is probably not important for the depleting effect (Dahlke et al. 2002). However, $RT7^a$ mAbs (IgG2b) of other isotypes were much less effective at depletion, indicating that Fc-receptor-mediated interactions are important. Besides the actions of such mAbs in tolerance induction, depletion of stem cells has potential in the therapy of haematopoietic malignancies and also in the conditioning of bone-marrow for other indications.

The mechanism of action of the $RT7^a$ mAb in depleting leucocytes remains unknown, but CD45 ligation using certain mAbs has been shown to directly induce apoptosis in either murine or human T and B cells (Klaus et al. 1996; Lesage et al. 1997). The ligation of CD45 is associated with its localisation to the detergent-insoluble cell fraction. Results based on expression of CD45 mutants in the CD45-deficient BW5147 thymoma T cell line have suggested that CD45 PTPase activity and in fact most of the cytoplasmic tail are not required for the apoptosis induced by CD45 ligation (Fortin et al. 2002). The role of CD45 in regulating apoptosis has also been suggested by the finding that in $CD45^{-/-}$ $CD4^+CD8^+$ thymocytes there is a marked increase in basal apoptosis (Byth et al. 1996) that is reversed upon expression of the active lck^{Y505F} transgene (Baker et al. 2000), implicating CD45-regulated $p56^{lck}$ in the induction of survival signals. It is, therefore, possible that perturbation of CD45 using specific mAbs might interfere with the ability of CD45-regulated $p56^{lck}$ to maintain survival signals. However, this does not appear to be the mechanism in the BW5147 experimental system, since the CD45 PTPase activity appears to be dispensable (Fortin et al. 2002).

CD45 mAbs have also been widely used with some success in pre-clinical radiotherapy animal model systems to target $CD45^+$ cancer cells with various isotopes (Matthews et al. 1992, 1999; Ruffner et al. 2001; Nemecek and Matthews 2002; Sandmaier et al. 2002; Vallera et al. 2003). Isotopes used in these studies include ^{125}I, ^{131}I, ^{213}Bi and ^{90}Y. The potential for CD45 mAbs in therapy for haematological malignancies has also been highlighted by animal studies in which the CD45 mAb inhibited the proliferation of cancer cells (Nemecek and Matthews 2002). For example, a CD45 mAb was effective in inhibiting growth of systemically disseminated human non-Hodgkin's lymphoma B cells in SCID mice (Dekroon et al. 1996).

Increasing understanding of the differential molecular actions of the different CD45 isoforms will influence future strategies used for developing CD45 mAbs as therapeutic reagents. For example, if the heterodimerisation model of CD45 isoform actions developed using cell line model systems (Dornan et al. 2002) proves to be relevant to primary T cells, then potentially mAbs could be developed that blocked, for example, the proposed interaction between CD4 and CD45R0, thereby down-regulating T cell activation.

5.2
The Use of Chemical Inhibitors

Until now much of the published data on CD45 PTPase inhibitors has been reported as an adjunct to results presented on the inhibition of other PTPases (Lee and Burke 2003). The non-availability of CD45 crystal structures illustrating PTPase active site interactions with inhibitors has also hindered rational drug design. Nevertheless, certain classes of compounds have been shown to be potent inhibitors of CD45, and their actions in cell-based systems, at least in the T lineage, are consistent with the dominantly positive role of CD45 in regulating receptor signalling.

A variety of reagents, which may be divided into metal-containing or non-metal-containing, exert inhibitory effects on a broad range of PTPases, including CD45, but their lack of specificity render them of less interest in the therapeutic context (Lee and Burke 2003). For example, suramin is a potent inhibitor of CD45, with complete inhibition within 10 min at low micromolar concentrations, but it also inhibits a wide range of other PTPases (Ghosh and Miller 1993). Small molecules such as peroxynitrite (Takakura et al. 1999) and sulphotyrosyl peptides (Desmarais et al. 1998) are also nonspecific CD45 inhibitors

Various classes of phosphorus-containing analogues have been shown to be effective CD45 inhibitors, such as the phosphonate-containing class of small molecule inhibitors. These include nitroarylhydroxymethylphosphonic acid derivatives which demonstrate low micromolar affinity (IC_{50} values ranging from 2 to 12 μM) against CD45 together with some selectivity for CD45 when compared to PTP1B (Beers et al. 1997). The arylmethylphosphonic moieties in such compounds act as surrogates of phenylphosphate functionality. In contrast, a variety of compounds have been identified through natural product screens that do not contain phosphorus. For example, the aporphine alkaloid nornuciferine from *Rollinia ulei* extracts shows an IC_{50} of 5.3 μM towards CD45 (Miski et al. 1995). Screening of *Streptomyces* extracts led to the discovery of the hydroquinone dephostatin that inhibits CD45 with an IC_{50} of 7.7 μM (Imoto et al. 1993; Watanabe et al. 1995). An unsaturated lactam called pulchellalactam was isolated from the marine fungus *Corollospora pulchella* and displayed selectivity in inhibiting CD45 as compared to PTP1B (Alvi et al. 1998).

Small molecule screens have generated some non-phosphorus-containing compounds that show some promise as selective CD45 inhibitors. The benzimidazole derivative TU-572 inhibits CD45 with an IC_{50} of 0.28 μM (Hamaguchi et al. 2000) and shows considerable specificity in comparison with a range of other phosphatases. The compound was also shown to suppress IgE-mediated anaphylaxis and murine contact hypersensitivity reactions (Hamaguchi et al. 2001). Derivatives of phenanthrenediones have also been found to be potent and reversible CD45 inhibitors at low micromolar concentrations, inhibiting T cell proliferation in biological assays (Urbanek et al. 2001).

Although the achievements in the field of CD45 inhibition have been somewhat modest relative to other PTPases, it is expected that the availability of crystal structures will accelerate the search for biologically relevant and selective inhibitors. A focused effort in this direction may well prove rewarding.

5.3
Other Possible Approaches to Perturbing CD45

Even without a CD45 crystal structure, it is already clear that the cytoplasmic D2 domain plays an important role in regulating the actions of CD45. Thus, mutation of various conserved residues surrounding the Cys^{1144} in the pseudo-active site of domain 2 caused a 50% reduction in the PTPase activity of domain 1 (Johnson et al. 1992), whereas mutation of Glu^{1180} to Gly in domain 2 abrogated PTPase activity completely (Ng et al. 1995). Evidence using recombinant polypeptides in vitro suggests that domain 2 stabilises domain 1 and increases its PTPase activity: the destabilising Glu^{1180} to Gly point mutation affected this stabilisation (Felberg and Johnson 1998, 2000). Furthermore, the spacer region between the two tandem repeats appears to interact with domain 2 (Hayami-Noumi et al. 2000). In functional experiments in which TCR signalling was examined following reconstitution of a CD45-deficient cell line with mutant forms of CD45, substitution of domain 2 with that from the LAR PTPase abrogated the production of IL-2 (Kashio et al. 1998). This defect could not be explained by ablation of the PTPase activity, suggesting a specific role for domain 2.

Taken together, these findings suggest that the targeting of the D2 domain might be an alternative strategy for perturbing CD45 function. Disruption of the normal interaction(s) expected between the D2 and D1 domains might be dynamically equivalent to the actions of a PTPase inhibitor, or even directly cause PTPase inhibition. Although speculative, this approach is worth considering.

6 Conclusions

Considering that the CD45 gene was cloned and its alternatively spliced forms were already recognised in the mid-1980s, the precise functions of the molecule in vivo have proved remarkably challenging to unravel. Nevertheless, the main outline of how CD45 mediates its effects is now clear. The precise molecular actions of the different CD45 isoforms remain poorly understood, and elucidation of their functions may facilitate novel rationales for therapeutic intervention. Without doubt, CD45 remains an attractive pharmaceutical target in order to achieve immunosuppression, and its targeting might prove to have certain advantages when compared with the alternative strategy of inhibiting the $p56^{lck}$ tyrosine kinase.

Acknowledgements The literature on CD45 is vast and I apologise to those whose work has not been cited due only to restrictions on space. This is a selective review and I have not attempted to cover every aspect of the field. I would like to thank the Biotechnology and Biological Sciences Research Council for financial support and my many colleagues, listed as co-authors on our publications, who have worked with me over the years on this fascinating topic.

References

Akbar AN, Terry L, Timms A, Beverley PCL, Janossy G (1988) Loss of CD45R and gain of UCHL1 reactivity is a feature of primed T-cells. J Immunol 140:2171–2178

Alexander D, Shiroo M, Robinson A, Biffen M, Shivnan E (1992) The role of CD45 in T-cell activation—resolving the paradoxes. Immunol Today 13:477–481

Alexander DR (1997) The role of the CD45 phosphatase in lymphocyte signalling. In: Harnett MM, Rigley KP (eds) Lymphocyte signalling: mechanisms, subversion and manipulation. John Wiley and Sons, Sussex, pp 107–140

Alexander DR (2000) The CD45 tyrosine phosphatase: a positive and negative regulator of immune cell function. Semin Immunol 12:349–359

Alexander DR (2003) The CD45 Phosphotyrosine Phosphatase. In: Arino J, Alexander DR (eds) Signalling through protein phosphatases. Springer, Heidelberg, pp 231–252

Alvi KA, Casey A, Nair BG (1998) Pulchellalactam: a CD45 protein tyrosine phosphatase inhibitor from the marine fungus Corollospora pulchella. J Antibiot (Tokyo) 51:515–517

Ashwell JD, Doro U (1999) CD45 and Src-family kinases: and now for something completely different. Immunol Today 20:412–416

Auersvald LA, Rothstein DM, Oliveira SC, Khuong CQ, Onodera H, Lazarovits AI, Basadonna GP (1997) Indefinite islet allograft survival in mice after a short course of treatment with anti-CD45 monoclonal antibodies. Transplantation 63:1355–1358

Baker M, Gamble J, Tooze R, Higgins D, Yang FT, O'Brien PCM, Coleman N, Pingel S, Turner M, Alexander DR (2000) Development of T-leukaemias in CD45 tyrosine phosphatase-deficient mutant lck mice. EMBO J 19:4644–4654

Basadonna GP, Auersvald L, Khuong CQ, Zheng XX, Kashio N, Zekzer D, Minozzo M, Qian HY, Visser L, Diepstra A, Lazarovits AI, Poppema S, Strom TB, Rothstein DM (1998) Antibody-mediated targeting of CD45 isoforms: a novel immunotherapeutic strategy. Proc Natl Acad Sci USA 95:3821–3826

Batista FD, Iber D, Neuberger MS (2001) B cells acquire antigen from target cells after synapse formation. Nature 411:489–494

Beers SA, Malloy EA, Wu W, Wachter MP, Gunnia U, Cavender D, Harris C, Davis J, Brosius R, Pellegrino-Gensey JL, Siekierka J (1997) Nitroarylhydroxymethylphosphonic acids as inhibitors of CD45. Bioorg Med Chem 5:2203–2211

Benatar T, Carsetti R, Furlonger C, Kamalia N, Mak T, Paige CJ (1996) Immunoglobulin-mediated signal-transduction in B-cells from CD45-deficient mice. J Exp Med 183:329-334

Berger SA, Mak TW, Paige CJ (1994) Leukocyte common antigen (CD45) is required for immunoglobulin E-mediated degranulation of mast cells. J Exp Med 180:471–476

Biffen M, McMichael-Phillips D, Larson T, Venkitaraman A, Alexander D (1994) The CD45 tyrosine phosphatase regulates specific pools of antigen receptor-associated P59(Fyn) and CD4-associated P56(Lck) tyrosine kinases in human T-cells. EMBO J 13:1920–1929

Bonnard M, Maroun CR, Julius M (1997) Physical association of CD4 and CD45 in primary, resting CD4(+) T cells. Cell Immunol 175:1-11

Byth KF, Conroy LA, Howlett S, Smith AJH, May J, Alexander DR, Holmes N (1996) CD45-null transgenic mice reveal a positive regulatory role for CD45 in early thymocyte development, in the selection of CD4(+)CD8(+) thymocytes, and in B-cell maturation. J Exp Med 183:1707–1718

Conroy LA, Byth KF, Howlett S, Holmes N, Alexander DR (1996) Defective depletion of CD45-null thymocytes by the Staphylococcus aureus enterotoxin B superantigen. Immunol Lett 54:119–122

Cooper JC, Morgan G, Harding S, Subramanyam M, Majeau GR, Moulder K, Alexander DR (2003) Alefacept selectively promotes NK cell-mediated deletion of CD45R0+ human T cells. Eur J Immunol 33:666–675

Cyster JG, Healy JI, Kishihara K, Mak TW, Thomas ML, Goodnow CC (1996) Regulation of B-lymphocyte negative and positive selection by tyrosine phosphatase CD45. Nature 381:325–328

Dahlke MH, Lauth OS, Jager MD, Roeseler T, Timrott K, Jackobs S, Neipp M, Wonigeit K, Schlitt HJ (2002) In vivo depletion of hematopoietic stem cells in the rat by an anti-CD45 (RT7) antibody. Blood 99:3566–3572

Davis SJ, van der Merwe PA (1996) The structure and ligand interactions of CD2: implications for T-cell function. Immunol Today 17:177–187

DeKroon J, Depaus RA, Kluinnelemans HC, Kluin PM, Vanbergen CAM, Munro AJ, Hale G, Willemze R, Falkenburg JHF (1996) Anti-CD45 and Anti-Cd52 (Campath) monoclonal-antibodies effectively eliminate systemically disseminated human non-Hodgkins-lymphoma B-cells in Scid mice. Exp Hematol 24:919–926

Desai DM, Sap J, Schlessinger J, Weiss A (1993) Ligand-mediated negative regulation of a chimeric transmembrane receptor tyrosine phosphatase. Cell 73:541–554

Desmarais S, Jia ZC, Ramachandran C (1998) Inhibition of protein tyrosine phosphatases PTP1B and CD45 by sulfotyrosyl peptides. Arch Biochem Biophys 354:225–231

Doody GM, Bell S, Vigorito E, Clayton E, McAdam S, Tooze R, Fernandez C, Lee IJ, Turner M (2001) Vav-2 plays a role in the generation of the humoral immune response and collaborates with Vav-1 in signalling for B cell maturation. Nat Immunol 2:542–547

Dornan S, Sebestyen Z, Gamble J, Nagy P, Bodnar A, Alldridge L, Doe S, Holmes N, Goff LK, Beverley P, Szollosi J, Alexander DR (2002) Differential association of CD45 isoforms with CD4 and CD8 regulates the actions of specific pools of p56lck tyrosine kinase in T cell antigen receptor signal transduction. J Biol Chem 277:1912–1918

Doro U, Ashwell JD (1999) Cutting edge: the CD45 tyrosine phosphatase is an inhibitor of Lck activity in thymocytes. J Immunol 162:1879–1883

Doro U, Sakaguchi K, Appella E, Ashwell JD (1996) Mutational analysis of Lck in CD45-negative T-cells—dominant role of tyrosine-394 phosphorylation in kinase-activity. Mol Cell Biol 16:4996–5003

Ehrlich LI, Ebert PJ, Krummel MF, Weiss A, Davis MM (2002) Dynamics of p56lck translocation to the T cell immunological synapse following agonist and antagonist stimulation. Immunity 17:809–822

Ellis CN, Krueger GG (2001) Treatment of chronic plaque psoriasis by selective targeting of memory effector T lymphocytes. N Engl J Med 345:248–255

Fecteau S, Basadonna GP, Freitas A, Ariyan C, Sayegh MH, Rothstein DM (2001) CTLA-4 up-regulation plays a role in tolerance mediated by CD45. Nat Immunol 2:58–63

Felberg J, Johnson P (1998) Characterization of recombinant CD45 cytoplasmic domain proteins—evidence for intramolecular and intermolecular interactions. J Biol Chem 273:17839–17845

Felberg J, Johnson P (2000) Stable interdomain interaction within the cytoplasmic domain of CD45 increases enzyme stability. Biochem Biophys Res Commun 271:292–298

Fortin M, Steff AM, Felberg J, Ding I, Schraven B, Johnson P, Hugo P (2002) Apoptosis mediated through CD45 is independent of its phosphatase activity and association with leukocyte phosphatase-associated phosphoprotein. J Immunol 168:6084–6089

Freiberg BA, Kupfer H, Maslanik W, Delli J, Kappler J, Zaller DM, Kupfer A (2002) Staging and resetting T cell activation in SMACs. Nat Immunol 3:911–917

Fukuhara K, Okumura M, Shiono H, Inoue M, Kadota Y, Miyoshi S, Matsuda H (2002) A study on CD45 isoform expression during T-cell development and selection events in the human thymus. Hum Immunol 63:394–404

Furukawa T, Itoh M, Krueger NX, Streuli M, Saito H (1994) Specific interaction of the CD45 protein-tyrosine-phosphatase with tyrosine-phosphorylated CD3 zeta-chain. Proc Natl Acad Sci USA 91:10928–10932

Gao ZH, Zhong R, Jiang JF, Garcia B, Xing JJ, White MJ, Lazarovits AI (1999) Adoptively transferable tolerance induced by CD45RB monoclonal antibody. J Am Soc Nephrol 10:374–381

Ghosh J, Miller RA (1993) Suramin, an experimental chemotherapeutic drug, irreversibly blocks T-cell CD45-protein tyrosine phosphatase in-vitro. Biochem Biophys Res Commun 194:36–44

Hamaguchi T, Takahashi A, Kagamizono T, Manaka A, Sato M, Osada H (2000) Synthesis and characterization of a potent and selective protein tyrosine phosphatase inhibitor, 2. Bioorg Med Chem Lett 10:2657–2660

Hamaguchi T, Takahashi A, Manaka A, Sato M, Osada H (2001) TU-572, a potent and selective CD45 inhibitor, suppresses IgE-mediated anaphylaxis and murine contact hypersensitivity reactions. Int Arch Allergy Immunol 126:318–324

Hartley DK, Hurley TR, Hardwick JS, Lund TC, Medveczky PG, Sefton BM (1999) Activation of the Lck tyrosine-protein kinase by the binding of the tip protein of herpesvirus Saimiri in the absence of regulatory tyrosine phosphorylation. J Biol Chem 274:20056–20059

Hayami-Noumi K, Tsuchiya T, Moriyama Y, Noumi T (2000) Intra- and intermolecular interactions of the catalytic domains of human CD45 protein tyrosine phosphatase. FEBS Lett 468:68–72

Hayward AR, Lee J, Beverley PCL (1989) Ontogeny of expression of Uchl1 antigen on TCR-1+ (CD4/8) and TCR-delta+ T-cells. Eur J Immunol 19:771–773

Hegedus Z, Chitu V, Toth GK, Finta C, Varadi G, Ando I, Monostori E (1999) Contribution of kinases and the CD45 phosphatase to the generation of tyrosine phosphorylation patterns in the T-cell receptor complex zeta chain. Immunol Lett 67:31–39

Hermiston ML, Xu Z, Weiss A (2003) CD45: a critical regulator of signaling thresholds in Immune Cells. Annu Rev Immunol 21:107–137

Holdorf AD, Green JM, Levin SD, Denny MF, Straus DB, Link V, Changelian PS, Allen PM, Shaw AD (1999) Proline residues in CD28 and the Src homology (SH)3 domain of Lck are required for T cell costimulation. J Exp Med 190:375–384

Holdorf AD, Lee KH, Burack WR, Allen PM, Shaw AS (2002) Regulation of Lck activity by CD4 and CD28 in the immunological synapse. Nat Immunol 4:4

Imoto M, Kakeya H, Sawa T, Hayashi C, Hamada M, Takeuchi T, Umezawa K (1993) Dephostatin, a novel protein-tyrosine-phosphatase inhibitor produced by streptomyces .1. Taxonomy isolation and characterization. J Antibiot (Tokyo) 46:1342–1346

Irie-Sasaki Jea (2001) CD45 is a JAK phosphatase and negatively regulates cytokine receptor signalling. Nature 409:349–354

Irles C, Symons A, Michel F, Bakker TR, van der Merwe PA, Acuto O (2003) CD45 ectodomain controls interaction with GEMs and Lck activity for optimal TCR signaling. Nat Immunol 4:189–197

Johnson KG, Bromley SK, Dustin ML, Thomas ML (2000) A supramolecular basis for CD45 tyrosine phosphatase regulation in sustained T cell activation. Proc Natl Acad Sci U S A 97:10138–10143

Johnson P, Ostergaard HL, Wasden C, Trowbridge IS (1992) Mutational analysis of CD45—a leukocyte-specific protein tyrosine phosphatase. J Biol Chem 267:8035–8041

Justement LB (2001) The role of the protein tyrosine phosphatase CD45 in regulation of B lymphocyte activation. Int Rev Immunol 20:713–738

Kaplon RJ, Hochman PS, Michler RE, Kwiatkowski PA, Edwards NM, Berger CL, Xu H, Meier W, Wallner BP, Chisholm P, Marboe CC (1996) Short course single agent therapy with an LFA-3-IgG1 fusion protein prolongs primate cardiac allograft survival. Transplantation 61:356–363

Kashio N, Matsumoto W, Parker S, Rothstein DM (1998) The second domain of the CD45 protein tyrosine phosphatase is critical for interleukin-2 secretion and substrate recruitment of TCR-zeta in vivo. J Biol Chem 273:33856–33863

Katagiri T, Ogimoto M, Hasegawa K, Arimura Y, Mitomo K, Okada M, Clark MR, Mizuno K, Yakura H (1999) CD45 negatively regulates Lyn activity by dephosphorylating both positive and negative regulatory tyrosine residues in immature B cells. J Immunol 163:1321–1326

Kishihara K, Penninger J, Wallace VA, Kundig TM, Kawai K, Wakeham A, Timms E, Pfeffer K, Ohashi PS, Thomas ML, Furlonger C, Paige CJ, Mak TW (1993) Normal B-lymphocyte development but impaired T-cell maturation in CD45-exon 6 protein-tyrosine-phosphatase deficient mice. Cell 74:143–156

Klaus SJ, Sidorenko SP, Clark EA (1996) CD45 ligation induces programmed cell-death in T-lymphocyte and B-lymphocyte. J Immunol 156:2743–2753

Ko S, Jager MD, Tsui TY, Deiwick A, Dinkel A, Rohde F, Dahlke MH, Lauth O, Wonigeit K, Schlitt HJ (2001) Long-term allograft acceptance induced by single dose anti-leukocyte common antigen (RT7) antibody in the rat. Transplantation 71:1124–1131

Kong YY, Kishihara K, Sumichika H, Nakamura T, Kaneko M, Nomoto K (1995a) Differential requirements of CD45 for lymphocyte development and function. Eur J Immunol 25:3431–3436

Kong YY, Kishihara K, Yoshida H, Mak TW, Nomoto K (1995b) Generation of T-cells with differential responses to alloantigens in CD45 exon 6-deficient mice. J Immunol 154:5725–5735

Koretzky GA, Picus J, Thomas ML, Weiss A (1990) Tyrosine phosphatase CD45 is essential for coupling T-cell antigen receptor to the phosphatidyl inositol pathway. Nature 346:66–68

Kozieradzki I, Kundig T, Kishihara K, Ong CJ, Chiu D, Wallace VA, Kawai K, Timms E, Ionescu J, Ohashi P, Marth JD, Mak TW, Penninger JM (1997) T cell development in mice expressing splice variants of the protein tyrosine phosphatase CD45. J Immunol 158:3130–3139

Kung C, Pingel JT, Heikinheimo M, Klemola T, Varkila K, Yoo LI, Vuopal K, Poyhonen M, Uhari M, Rogers M, Speck SH, Chatila T, Thomas ML (2000) Mutations in the tyrosine phosphatase CD45 gene in a child with severe combined immunodeficiency disease. Nat Med 6:343–345

Lazarovits AI, Poppema S, Zhang Z, Khandaker M, Lefeuvre SK, Garcia BM, Ogasa N, Jevnikar AM, White MJ, Singh G, Stiller CR, Zhong RZ (1996) Prevention and reversal of renal allograft rejection by antibody against CD45RB. Nature 380:717–720

Lee K, Burke TR Jr (2003) CD45 protein-tyrosine phosphatase inhibitor development. Curr Top Med Chem 3:797–807

Leitenberg D, Novak TJ, Farber D, Smith BR, Bottomly K (1996) The extracellular domain of CD45 controls association with the CD4-T cell-receptor complex and the response to antigen-specific stimulation. J Exp Med 183:249–259

Leitenberg D, Boutin Y, Lu DD, Bottomly K (1999) Biochemical association of CD45 with the T cell receptor complex: regulation by CD45 isoform and during T cell activation. Immunity 10:701–711

Lesage S, Steff AM, Philippoussis F, Page M, Trop S, Mateo V, Hugo P (1997) CD4(+)CD8(+) thymocytes are preferentially induced to die following CD45 cross-linking, through a novel apoptotic pathway. J Immunol 159:4762–4771

Leupin O, Zaru R, Laroche T, Muller S, Valitutti S (2000) Exclusion of CD45 from the T-cell receptor signaling area in antigen-stimulated T lymphocytes. Curr Biol 10:277–280

Liu P, Aitken K, Kong YY, Opavsky MA, Martino T, Dawood F, Wen WH, Kozieradzki I, Bachmaier K, Straus D, Mak TW, Penninger JM (2000) The tyrosine kinase p56lck is essential in coxsackievirus B3-mediated heart disease. Nat Med 6:429–434
Majeti R, Bilwes AM, Noel JP, Hunter T, Weiss A (1998) Dimerization-induced inhibition of receptor protein tyrosine phosphatase function through an inhibitory wedge. Science 279:88–91
Majeti R, Xu Z, Parslow TG, Olson JL, Daikh DI, Killeen N, Weiss A (2000) An inactivating point mutation in the inhibitory wedge of CD45 causes lymphoproliferation and autoimmunity. Cell 103:1059–1070
Markey AC, Allen MH, Pitzalis C, Macdonald DM (1990) T-cell inducer populations in cutaneous inflammation—a predominance of T-helper-inducer lymphocytes (Thi) in the infiltrate of inflammatory dermatoses. Br J Dermatol 122:325–332
Martin SM, Mehta IK, Yokoyama WM, Thomas ML, Lorenz RG (2001) Development of intestinal intraepithelial lymphocytes, NK cells, and NK 1.1(+) T cells in CD45-deficient mice. J Immunol 166:6066–6073
Matthews DC, Badger CC, Fisher DR, Hui TE, Nourigat C, Appelbaum FR, Martin PJ, Bernstein ID (1992) Selective radiation of hematolymphoid tissue delivered by anti-CD45 antibody. Cancer Res 52:1228–1234
Matthews DC, Appelbaum FR, Eary JF, Fisher DR, Durack LD, Hui TE, Martin PJ Mitchell D, Press OW, Storb,R, Bernstein ID (1999) Phase I study of I-131-anti-CD45 antibody plus cyclophosphamide and total body irradiation for advanced acute leukemia and myelodysplastic syndrome. Blood 94:1237–1247
Matthews N, Emery P, Pilling D, Akbar A, Salmon M (1993) Subpopulations of primed-T helper-cells in rheumatoid-arthritis. Arthritis Rheum 36:603–607
McFarland EDC, Hurley TR, Pingel JT, Sefton BM, Shaw A, Thomas ML (1993) Correlation between Src family member regulation by the protein-tyrosine-phosphatase CD45 and transmembrane signaling through the T-cell receptor. Proc Natl Acad Sci USA 90:1402–1406
Meade J, Fernandez C, Turner M (2002) The tyrosine kinase Lyn is required for B cell development beyond the T1 stage in the spleen: rescue by over-expression of Bcl-2. Eur J Immunol 32:1029–1034
Mee PJ, Turner M, Basson AM, Costello PS, Zamoyska R, Tybulewicz VLJ (1999) Greatly reduced efficiency of both positive and negative selection of thymocytes in CD45 tyrosine phosphatase-deficient mice. Eur J Immunol 29:2923–2933
Miski M, Shen X, Cooper R, Gillum AM, Fisher DK, Miller RW, Higgins TJ (1995) Aporphine alkaloids, CD45 protein-tyrosine-phosphatase inhibitors, from Rollinia-ulei. Bioorg Med Chem Lett 5:1519–1522
Mittler RS, Rankin BM, Kiener PA (1991) Physical associations between CD45 and CD4 or CD8 occur as late activation events in antigen receptor-stimulated human T-cells. J Immunol 147:3434–3440
Monks CRF, Freiberg BA, Kupfer H, Sciaky N, Kupfer A (1998) Three-dimensional segregation of supramolecular activation clusters in T cells. Nature 395:82–86
Murakami K, Sato S, Nagasawa S, Yamashita (2000) T Regulation of mast cell signaling through high-affinity IgE receptor by CD45 protein tyrosine phosphatase. Int Immunol 12:169–176
Mustelin T, Altman A (1990) Dephosphorylation and activation of the T-cell tyrosine kinase p56lck by the leukocyte common antigen (CD45). Oncogene 5:809–813
Mustelin T, Coggeshall KM, Altman A (1989) Rapid activation of the T-cell tyrosine kinase $pp56^{lck}$ by the CD45 phosphotyrosine phosphatase. Proc Natl Acad Sci USA 86:6302–6306

Mustelin T, Williams S, Tailor P, Couture C, Zenner G, Burn P, Ashwell JD, Altman A (1995) Regulation of the P70(Zap) tyrosine protein-kinase in T-cells by the CD45 phosphotyrosine phosphatase. Eur J Immunol 25:942–946

Nemecek ER, Matthews DC (2002) Antibody-based therapy of human leukemia. Curr Opin Hematol 9:316–321

Ng DHW, Maiti A, Johnson P (1995) Point mutation in the 2nd phosphatase domain of CD45 abrogates tyrosine phosphatase-activity. Biochem Biophys Res Commun 206:302–309

Novak TJ, Farber D, Leitenberg D, Hong SC, Johnson P, Bottomly K (1994) Isoforms of the transmembrane tyrosine phosphatase CD45 differentially affect T-cell recognition. Immunity 1:109–119

Ogilvy S, Louis-Dit-Sully C, Cooper J, Cassady RL, Alexander DR, Holmes N (2003) Either of the CD45RB and CD45RO isoforms are effective in restoring T cell, but not B cell, development and function in CD45-null mice. J Immunol 171:1792–1800

Ostergaard HL, Shackelford DA, Hurley TR, Johnson P, Hyman R, Sefton BM, Trowbridge IS (1989) Expression Of CD45 alters phosphorylation of the Lck-encoded tyrosine protein-kinase in murine lymphoma T-cell lines. Proc Natl Acad Sci USA 86:8959–8963

Pao LI, Cambier JC (1997) Syk, but not Lyn, recruitment to B cell antigen receptor and activation following stimulation of CD45(-) B cells. J Immunol 158:2663–2669

Pelosi M, DiBartolo V, Mounier V, Mege D, Pascussi JM, Dufour E, Blondel A, Acuto O (1999) Tyrosine 319 in the interdomain B of ZAP-70 is a binding site for the Src homology 2 domain of Lck. J Biol Chem 274:14229–14237

Pingel JT, Thomas ML (1989) Evidence that the leukocyte-common antigen is required for antigen-induced lymphocyte-T proliferation. Cell 58:1055–1065

Pingel S, Baker M, Turner M, Holmes N, Alexander DR (1999) The CD45 tyrosine phosphatase regulates CD3-induced signal transduction and T cell development in recombinase-deficient mice: restoration of pre-TCR function by active p56(lck). Eur J Immunol 29:2376–2384

Roach T, Slater S, Koval M, White L, McFarland EC, Okumura M, Thomas M, Brown E (1997) CD45 regulates Src family member kinase activity associated with macrophage integrin-mediated adhesion. Curr Biol 7:408–417

Rogers PR, Pilapil S, Hayakawa K, Romain PL, Parker DC (1992) CD45 alternative exon expression in murine and human CD4+ T-cell subsets. J Immunol 148:4054–4065

Ruffner KL, Martin PJ, Hussell S, Nourigat C, Fisher DR, Bernstein ID, Matthews DC (2001) Immunosuppressive effects of $^{(131)}$I-anti-CD45 antibody in unsensitised and donor antigen-presensitised H2-matched, minor antigen-mismatched murine transplant models. Cancer Res 61:5126–5131

Sandmaier BM, Bethge WA, Wilbur DS, Hamlin DK, Santos EB, Brechbiel MW, Fisher DR, Storb R (2002) Bismuth 213-labeled anti-CD45 radioimmunoconjugate to condition dogs for nonmyeloablative allogeneic marrow grafts. Blood 100:318–326

Seavitt JR, White LS, Murphy KM, Loh DY, Perlmutter RM, Thomas ML (1999) Expression of the p56(lck) Y505F mutation in CD45-deficient mice rescues thymocyte development. Mol Cell Biol 19:4200–4208

Seddon B, Zamoyska R (2002) TCR signals mediated by Src family kinases are essential for the survival of naive T cells. J Immunol 169:2997–3005

Seddon B, Legname G, Tomlinson P, Zamoyska R (2000) Long-term survival but impaired homeostatic proliferation of naive T cells in the absence of p56lck. Science 290:127–131

Shenoi H, Seavitt J, Zheleznyak A, Thomas ML, Brown EJ (1999) Regulation of integrin-mediated T cell adhesion by the transmembrane protein tyrosine phosphatase CD45. J Immunol 162:7120–7127
Shiroo M, Goff L, Biffen M, Shivnan E, Alexander D (1992) CD45-tyrosine phosphatase-activated p59fyn couples the T-cell antigen receptor to pathways of diacylglycerol production, protein-kinase-C activation and calcium influx. EMBO J 11:4887-4897
Shivnan E, Biffen M, Shiroo M, Pratt E, Glennie M, Alexander D (1992) Does coaggregation of the CD45 and CD3 antigens inhibit T-cell antigen receptor complex-mediated activation of phospholipase-C and protein-kinase-C. Eur J Immunol 22:1055–1062
Sieh M, Bolen JB, Weiss A (1993) CD45 specifically modulates binding of Lck to a phosphopeptide encompassing the negative regulatory tyrosine Of Lck. EMBO J 12:315–321
Stone JD, Conroy LA, Byth KF, Hederer RA, Howlett S, Takemoto Y, Holmes N, Alexander DR (1997) Aberrant TCR-mediated signalling in CD45-null thymocytes involves dysfunctional regulation of Lck, Fyn, TCR-ζ and ZAP-70. J Immunol 158:5773–5782
Symons A, Willis AC, Barclay AN (1999) Domain organization of the extracellular region of CD45. Protein Eng 12:885–892
Takakura K, Beckman JS, MacMillanCrow LA, Crow JP (1999) Rapid and irreversible inactivation of protein tyrosine phosphatases PTP1B, CD45, and LAR by peroxynitrite. Arch Biochem Biophys 369:197–207
Takeda A, Wu JJ, Maizel AL (1992) Evidence for monomeric and dimeric forms of CD45 associated with a 30-kDa phosphorylated protein. J Biol Chem 267:16651–16659
Tchilian EZ, Wallace DL, Wells RS, Flower DR, Morgan G, Beverley PC (2001) A deletion in the gene encoding the CD45 antigen in a patient with SCID. J Immunol 166:1308–1313
Thomas ML (1989) The leukocyte common antigen family. Annu Rev Immunol 7:339–369
Thomas ML, Brown EJ (1999) Positive and negative regulation of Src-family membrane kinases by CD45. Immunol Today 20:406–411
Trop S, Charron J, Arguin C, Hugo P (2000) Thymic selection generates T cells expressing self-reactive TCRs in the absence of CD45. J Immunol 165:3073–3079
Trowbridge IS, Thomas ML (1994) CD45— an emerging role as a protein-tyrosine-phosphatase required for lymphocyte-activation and development. Annu Rev Immunol 12:85–116
Urbanek RA, Suchard SJ, Steelman GB, Knappenberger KS, Sygowski LA, Veale CA, Chapdelaine MJ (2001) Potent reversible inhibitors of the protein tyrosine phosphatase CD45. J Med Chem 44:1777–1793
Vallera DA, Elson M, Brechbiel MW, Dusenbery KE, Burns LJ, Skubitz KM, Jaszcz WB, Ramsay NK, Panoskaltsis-Mortari A, Kuroki DW, Wagner JE, Kersey JH (2003) Preclinical studies targeting normal and leukemic hematopoietic cells with Yttrium-90-labeled anti-CD45 antibody in vitro and in vivo in nude mice. Cancer Biother Radiopharm 18:133–145
Wallace VA, Penninger JM, Kishihara K, Timms E, Shahinian A, Pircher H, Kundig TM, Ohashi PS, Mak TW (1997) Alterations in the level of CD45 surface expression affect the outcome of thymic selection. J Immunol 158:3205–3214
Watanabe T, Takeuchi T, Otsuka M, Tanaka S, Umezawa K (1995) Synthesis and protein tyrosine phosphatase inhibitory activity of dephostatin analogs. J Antibiot (Tokyo) 48:1460–1466
Wonigeit K (1979a) Characterization of the RT-Ly-1 and RT-Ly-2 alloantigenic systems by congenic rat strains. Transplant Proc 11:1631–1635

Wonigeit K (1979b) Definition of lymphocyte antigens in rats: RT-Ly-1, RT-Ly-2, and a new MHC-linked antigen system. Transplant Proc 11:1334–1336

Wu L, Fu J, Shen SH (2002) SKAP55 coupled with CD45 positively regulates T-cell receptor-mediated gene transcription. Mol Cell Biol 22:2673–2686

Xu Z, Weiss A (2002) Negative regulation of CD45 by differential homodimerization of the alternatively spliced isoforms. Nat Immunol 3:764–771

Yamada H, Kishihara K, Kong YY, Nomoto K (1996) Enhanced generation of NK cells with intact cytotoxic function in CD45 exon 6-deficient mice. J Immunol 157:1523–1528

Yamada T, Zhu D, Saxon A, Zhang K (2002) CD45 controls interleukin-4-mediated IgE class switch recombination in human B cells through its function as a Janus kinase phosphatase. J Biol Chem 277:28830–28835

Yanagi S, Sugawara H, Kurosaki M, Sabe H, Yamamura H, Kurosaki T (1996) CD45 modulates phosphorylation of both autophosphorylation and negative regulatory tyrosines of Lyn in B-cells. J Biol Chem 271:30487–30492

Zhang J, Siraganian RP (1999) CD45 is essential for Fc epsilon RI signaling by ZAP70, but not Syk, in Syk-negative mast cells. J Immunol 163:2508–2516

Zhong RZ, Lazarovits AI (1998) Monoclonal antibody against CD45RB for the therapy of rejection and autoimmune diseases. J Mol Med 76:572–580

HEP (2005) 167:295–317

Serine/Threonine Protein Phosphatase Inhibitors with Antitumor Activity

R. E. Honkanen

Department of Biochemistry and Molecular Biology, University of South Alabama, MSB 2362, College of Medicine, Mobile, AL 36688, USA
honkanen@sungcg.usouthal.edu

Abstract Recent studies with fostriecin and derivatives of cantharidin suggest that the development of specific, or highly selective, inhibitors of serine/threonine protein phosphatases, notably PP2A, PP4, and PP5, may prove useful for the medical management of human cancer. This chapter will review the discovery and development of natural compounds that were originally shown to have marked antitumor activity and subsequently found to act as potent inhibitors of certain PPP-family phosphatases. The review will focus on two compounds, cantharidin and fostriecin, addressing discovery, molecular mechanisms of action, affects on cultured cell, clinical use, toxicity, plasma pharmacokinetics, and a brief review of data from a phase I human clinical trial.

Keywords Fostriecin · Cantharidin · Phosphatase · Inhibitor · Tumor · Human · Serine

1 Introduction

In eukaryotic organisms, reversible phosphorylation influences the biological activity of many proteins. Phosphorylation occurs commonly on serine, threonine, and tyrosine residues and represents a fundamental mechanism for controlling intracellular events as diverse as metabolism, contractility, membrane transport, gene transcription, cell motility, and protein synthesis. Protein phosphorylation is a dynamic process. Therefore, at any point in time the phosphorylation status of a given protein reflects the combined actions of both the protein kinases and the protein phosphatases that recognize a particular protein as a substrate. Since reversible phosphorylation has been implicated in the control of many critical aspects of cell growth and differentiation, it seems logical that the development of agents to modify the actions of specific protein kinases or phosphatases should prove useful for the treatment of human cancers. Indeed, as discussed in other chapters of this volume, a considerable effort has been devoted to the development of pharmacological agents which regulate the actions of protein kinases. In contrast, until recently the serine/threonine protein phosphatases have been all but ignored as clinically relevant targets for drug development.

One of the reasons serine/threonine phosphatases have been overlooked as targets for drug development is that they were viewed as simple housekeeping enzymes, functioning to "mop up" after the more important "regulatory" kinases. This concept, however, is simply not true, as there is substantial evidence that protein phosphatases, like their kinase counterparts, are highly regulated and dynamic enzymes. Another complicating factor is that, in the human genome, roughly 383 genes encode kinases that act to catalyze the phosphorylation of serine/threonine residues on proteins (Manning et al. 2002). In contrast, as few as 32 genes encode phosphatases that act on serine/threonine phosphoesters. Thus, the serine/threonine phosphatases are outnumbered more than ten to one by their kinase counterparts. This suggests that a compound which inhibits the catalytic activity of a given phosphatase may have a broad range of biological activity, making it difficult to predict possible side effects. Finally, there are concerns that some inhibitors (i.e., okadaic acid and microcystin-LR) may act as tumor-promoting agents.

In spite of these perceived difficulties, it seems that nature has produced a number of compounds that act as potent inhibitors of serine/threonine phosphatases, and some demonstrate substantial antitumor activity. In this chapter, I will review studies leading to the development of phosphatase inhibitors into drugs that have antitumor activity, focusing on two compounds (cantharidin and fostriecin) that have been tested in humans.

1.1 Target Phosphatases for Drug Development

For "rational drug development," one of the first steps is the identification of suitable cellular targets, and to date most targets are proteins. In the development of antitumor agents, many protein kinases have been designated as developmental drug targets based on the roles they play in the regulation of signaling pathways known to affect cellular proliferation. However, for the serine/threonine phosphatases the process has been quite the opposite. That is, compounds with antitumor activity were identified first via conventional methods (i.e., the screening of natural product extracts). The realization that these antitumor drugs acted on protein phosphatases came much later, when investigations into the molecular mechanisms leading to the suppression of tumor progression revealed that the antitumor drugs acted as potent inhibitors of protein phosphatases.

To understand how phosphatase inhibitors with antitumor activity were discovered and developed, it will be helpful to first briefly review the enzymes upon which they act. Traditionally, serine/threonine phosphatases have been placed into four major groups (PP1, PP2A, PP2B, and PP2C) based on their biochemical properties. These enzymes have also been divided into two major gene families [protein phosphatase P (PPP) and protein phosphatase M (PPM)] based on the similarity of their primary amino acid sequence (Cohen 1997). The PPP gene family consists of PP1, PP2A, PP2B, PP4, PP5, PP6, and PP7. It should also be noted that in humans there are actually three genes encoding four isoforms of PP1, two gene encoding isoforms of PP2A, two genes encoding isoforms of PP7, and three genes encoding at least six isoforms of PP2B, with the additional isoforms produced by alternative splicing of mRNA (Honkanen and Golden 2002).

The catalytic subunits of all PPP-family members are structurally similar (Fig. 1). Nonetheless, they can be further classified by their sensitivity to a number of natural compounds that inhibit catalytic activity [i.e., okadaic acid, calyculin A, fostriecin, microcystin, cantharidin, and tautomycin (for review see Honkanen and Golden 2002; Lewy et al. 2002). PP1–PP6 are sensitive to inhibition and contain a similar "toxin"-binding domain near the C-terminal region of the catalytic subunit. In contrast, PP2B and PP7 have regions within the inhibitor-binding domains that are not conserved, and these "inserts" render them less sensitive, or insensitive, to the above listed inhibitors. The PPM family of enzymes, which is not affected by the above-mentioned inhibitors, consists of the Mg^{2+}/Mn^{2+}-dependent phosphatases (biochemically classified as PP2C) and the pyruvate dehydrogenase phosphatases (Cohen 1997).

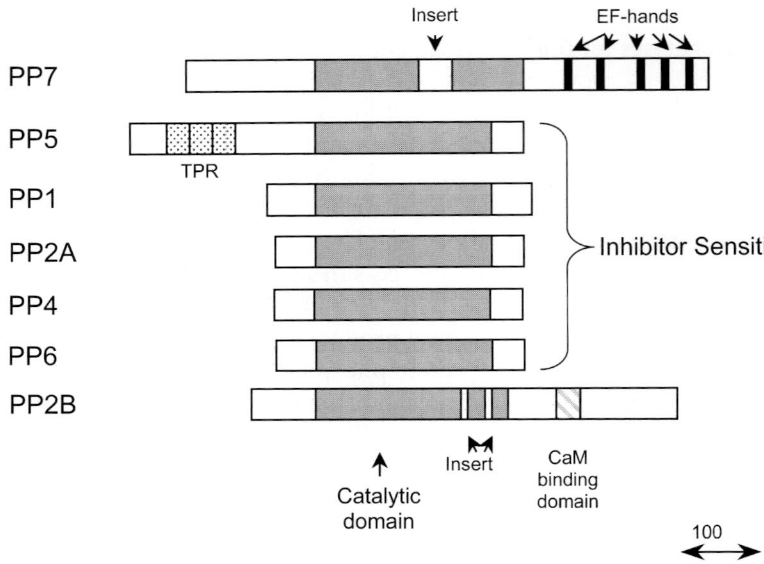

Fig. 1 Homology of serine/threonine protein phosphatases. A schematic representation depicting the amino acid similarity of human PPP-family serine/threonine protein phosphatases. PP1–PP7 contain a common catalytic core domain that is highly conserved. PP1, PP2A, PP4, and PP6 are highly homologous enzymes, differing primarily in their C- and N-terminal regions. PP2B differs in that it contains a Ca^{2+}-calmodulin (*CaM*)-binding domain in its C-terminal region and two small divergent regions (indicated by *arrows* and *open boxes*) in the catalytic domain near the okadaic acid/microcystin binding site. The amino-terminal region of PP5 contains three tetratricopeptide (*TPR*) domains. PP7 differs from all of the other PPase families in that it contains EF-hand motifs in the C-terminal region (indicated by *filled squares*) and a larger (44 amino acid) insert in the catalytic core domain (indicated by an *open box*). The inhibitor-insensitive enzymes contain divergent regions (*inserts*) in the inhibitor binding domain, which have been designated as the β12–β13 loop based on the crystal structure of PP1

2 Cantharidin

Although the mode of action was unknown at the time, an inhibitor of PP1–PP6 actually represent one of the oldest treatments for cancer in recorded history. Writings dating back over 2,000 years describe the use of a concoction, "Mylabris", that is produced from the dried body of the Chinese blister beetle (*Mylabris phalerata* or *Mylabris cichorii*) for the treatment of both cancer and warts (Wang et al. 1989). The active constituent of Mylabris is exo, exo-2,3-dimethyl-7-oxabicyclo[2.2.1]heptane-2,3-dicarboxylic acid anhydride, which is commonly referred to as cantharidin (Fig. 2). Cantharidin is a natural vesicant produced by as many as 1,500 different species of beetles belonging to the order Coleoptera, which produce it as a mechanism for defense.

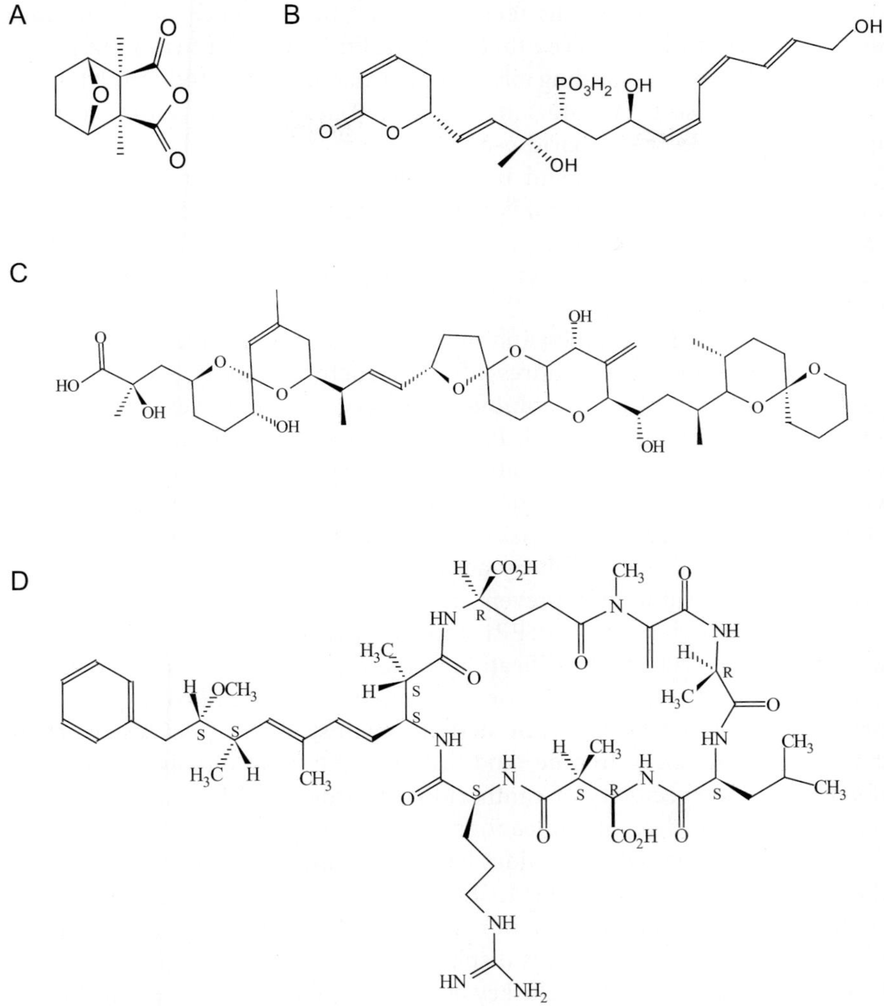

Fig. 2A–D Structures of natural products with inhibitory activity against PP1, PP2A, PP4, PP5, and PP6. **A** Cantharidin (exo, exo-2,3-dimethyl-7-oxabicyclo[2.2.1]heptane-2,3-dicarboxylic acid anhydride). **B** Fostriecin {2*H*-pyran-2-one, 5, 6-dihydro-6-[3,6,13-trihydroxy-3-methyl-4-(phosphonooxy)-1,7,9,11-tridecatetraenyl]}. **C** Okadaic acid. **D** Microcystin-LR

2.1
Molecular Mechanism of Action

Although cantharidin was identified as the active constituent of Mylabris in the early 1800s, the first stereospecific synthesis was not reported until the 1950s (Stork 1999), and the understanding of the molecular mechanism underlying its biological actions remained elusive for another 40 years. Then, in a key study it was observed that cantharidin binds with high affinity to a specific and saturable binding site in a cytosolic fraction produced from homogenized mouse liver (Graziano et al. 1997, 1998). Purification revealed that the high affinity cantharidin-binding site was protein phosphatase type 2A (Li and Casida 1992), and further characterization demonstrated that cantharidin acts as a strong inhibitor of PP1 and PP2A and a weaker inhibitor of PP2B (Honkanen 1993). Today we know that cantharidin also affects PP4 and PP5 (Hastie and Cohen 1998; Borthwick et al. 2001; Honkanen and Golden 2002).

Cantharidin is the simplest inhibitor of PP1 and PP2A identified to date, and several studies have addressed the structure–activity relationship of cantharidin by testing the inhibitory effects of derivatives against PP1, PP2A, and PP2B (Sodeoka et al. 1997; McCluskey et al. 2000a,b, 2001; Essers etal 2001). Details of specific modifications have been discussed in recent reviews (McCluskey and Sakoff 2001; Honkanen and Golden 2002; McCluskey et al. 2002b), so here the discussion will be brief. The consensus is that ring opening is needed for inhibitory activity, as attempts to modify the anhydride of cantharidin that prevent ring opening suppress (or eliminate) the inhibitory activity against PP1 and PP2A (McCluskey and Sakoff 2001; McCluskey et al. 2002b). Modification of the 7-O bridgehead is not tolerated, and bulky substitutions at C5, or even modest substitutions at the C1/C4 bridgeheads, suppress inhibitor activity against PP2A (McCluskey et al. 2002b). Unfortunately, to date modifications that substantially improve the potency or the specificity of cantharidin towards PP1/PP2A have not been reported. Nonetheless, modifications of the anhydride moiety on norcantharidins to produce cantharimides have been shown to produce compounds that retain inhibitory activity (McCluskey et al. 2001). This suggests that the synthesis of additional analogs of cantharidin that retain biological activity should be possible, and analogs displaying selectivity (although modest) for PP1 have been reported (McCluskey et al. 2002). The synthesis of fluorinated cantharidin analogs have also been reported (Essers etal 2001). Unfortunately, the effects of fluorination on inhibitory activity were not reported.

2.2 Effects of Cantharidin on Cells

Cantharidin and structurally related compounds have been shown to produce cytotoxic effects in a number of human cell lines, including bone, leukemia, neuroblastoma, ovarian, and colon cancer cells. Cantharidin also has cytotoxic activity against a number of primary tumor cells, with 5–10 μM cantharidin sufficient to induce death in 24–120 h (Walter 1989; Wang et al. 1990; McCluskey et al. 2000a,b, 2003; McCluskey and Sakoff 2001). In most cells cantharidin can elicit an apoptotic response (McCluskey et al. 2003).

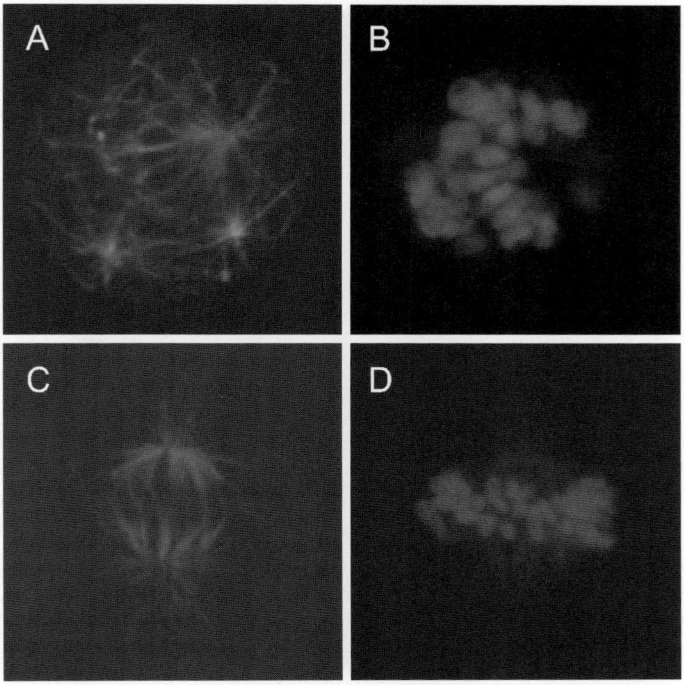

Fig. 3A–D Abnormal spindle formation and chromosome condensation in human tumor cells treated with cantharidin. A549 lung carcinoma cells were treated with 4 μM cantharidin (**A**,**B**) or solvent alone (**C**,**D**) were fixed 18 h after treatment, and tubulin was visualized by immunofluorescence following treatment with anti-α-tubulin (primary) and fluorescein isothiocyanate (FITC)-labeled (secondary) antibodies (**A**, **C**). DNA was visualized by staining with propidium iodine (**B**, **D**)

Still, to date we know little about the molecular mechanisms by which the inhibition of phosphatase activity produces a cytotoxic/antitumor effect.

Studies in CHO cells have revealed that cantharidin treatment induces G2/M-phase growth arrest that is characterized by the formation of aberrant mitotic spindles and occurs prior to induction of apoptosis (Cheng et al. 1998). Similar results have been seen in human lung adenocarcinoma (A549) cells (Fig. 3). G2/M-phase growth arrest has been also noted in glioblastoma cell lines following treatment with norcantharidin, and post-G2/M induction of apoptosis was shown to be dependent on the presence of the p53 gene (Hong et al. 2000). In Drosophila, genetic studies have revealed that the depletion of either PP2A or PP4 results in mitotic failure. The deficiency of PP2A is associated with the uncoupling of nuclear and centrosome cycles and elongated microtubules (Snaith et al. 1996), while depletion of PP4 in embryos results in the absence of microtubules emanating from centrosomes or aberrant microtubules that are unconnected to the centrosomes

(Helps et al. 1998). In *Caenorhabditis elegans*, the suppression of PPH-4.1 (one of two PP4 homologs expressed in *C. elegans*) results in similar aberrant microtubule organization, suggesting that PP4 is needed for the activation of microtubule nucleation at the centrosome (Sumiyoshi et al. 2002). Therefore, in lower eukaryotic organisms the antiproliferative effects of cantharidin may result from the suppression of PP4. Still, until a specific inhibitor for PP2A or PP4 is developed, it is not possible to predict if the mitotic aberrations produced by cantharidin in human cells result for the suppression of PP2A, PP4, or both.

2.3 Clinical Use of Cantharidin

Cantharidin has a long history of use by dermatologists as a treatment for molluscum contagiosum and warts, which continues to this date (Nickolls and Tear 1954; Stoughton and Bagatell 1959; Bagatell et al. 1969; Graziano et al. 1988; Nicholls et al. 1990; Moed et al. 2001). In the United States, the Food and Drug Administration (FDA) approved cantharidin for this purpose prior to 1962. Subsequently, the Food Drug and Cosmetic Act was amended to require drug efficacy data. The data were not supplied by the manufacturers, and cantharidin was removed from the U.S. market (Moed et al. 2001).

As an antitumor agent, cantharidin has been used as a traditional medicine in China for over 2,000 years. It was also used briefly as an antitumor drug in Europe during the 1800s, but by the early 1900s it was generally considered by physicians as too toxic for internal use (Oaks et al. 1960). More recently, the clinical use of cantharidin was found effective against primary hepatoma, but its usefulness was limited by severe toxicity in mucous membranes (Sakoff et al. 1999). Interestingly, in contrast to many types of conventional chemotherapy, cantharidin has been shown to stimulate the production of white blood cells by the bone marrow in a limited number of patients (McCluskey and Sakoff 2001), but renal toxicity has hindered its development for use as an antitumor drug (McCluskey and Sakoff 2001; McCluskey et al. 2002b).

2.4 Toxicity

The clinical testing of cantharidin as an antitumor drug revealed marked kidney toxicity, which has limited further evaluation and suggests that cantharidin is simply too toxic for use in mainstream oncology (McCluskey and Sakoff 2001). Therefore, the amount of human toxicity data from formal clinical trials is limited. However, the erroneous concept that extracts of cantharidin-producing beetles (i.e., “Spanish fly”) can be used as an aphrodisiac has resulted in numerous poisonings, and the medical records from patients suffering from the illicit use of cantharidin provide considerable insight into the toxic effects of cantharidin in humans. If injected, a lethal dose of cantharidin is 10–65 mg, with death usually ensuing in less than 24 h. Ingestion of cantharidin produces painful urogenital tract irritation that can produce priapism in men and pelvic engorgement in women. This likely underlies the myth that cantharidin acts as an aphrodisiac. However, cantharidin poisoning is more commonly characterized by nausea, severe abdominal pain, dysphasia, lumbar pain, urinary tract urgency, shock, convulsions, coma, and death (Wang et al. 1989; Sakoff et al. 1999; McCluskey and Sakoff 2001; McCluskey et al. 2002b).

3 Fostriecin

Fostriecin, also referred to as CI-920, NSC 339638, or PD 110,161, was developed as an antitumor drug by Park Davis, and it entered human phase I clinical trials before it was shown to act as an inhibitor of protein phosphatases. Fostriecin was discovered in the course of a screening program designed to identify new antitumor agents contained in the fermentation broth of an actinomycete. The actinomycete that produces fostriecin was originally isolated from a Brazilian soil sample and subsequently characterized as *Streptomyces pulveraceus* (subspecies *fostreus*). Fostriecin, and two structurally related compounds (PD113,270 and PD113,271), were identified as water-soluble components of an extract that was observed to inhibit the growth of murine L1210 lymphoid and P388 lymphocytic leukemia cells in tissue culture without having significant antimicrobial activity (Stampwala et al. 1983; Tunac et al. 1983). Further characterization revealed that all three compounds were phosphate esters containing an unsaturated lactone and a conjugated triene system. Chemical and spectral techniques revealed the structure of fostriecin as depicted in Fig. 2 {2*H*-pyran-2-one,5,6-dihydro-6-[3,6,13-trihydroxy-3-methyl-4-(phosphonooxy)-1,7,9,11-tridecatetraenyl]} (Stampwala et al. 1983; Hokanson and French 1985). Because fostriecin is unstable above pH 8 and very labile in dilute acid, it can only be purified with isolation steps performed within the pH range of 5.5–7.5 (Tunac et al. 1983; Jackson et al. 1985). Accordingly, fostriecin is purified as a sodium salt. For clinical studies it was formulated with sodium ascorbate to improve stability against oxidation.

3.1 Molecular Mechanism of Action

Initial observations with fostriecin revealed that it inhibited the proliferation of several types of tumor cells both in vitro and in vivo (Stampwala et al.

1983; Leopold et al 1984; Jackson et al. 1985). Therefore, early studies were directed toward understanding how fostriecin's structure influenced its activity. Investigations revealed that fostriecin has cytotoxic activity against a number of tumor cell lines in vitro and marked antileukemic activity in mice (Leopold et al 1984). Tissue culture studies on the structure–activity relationship of fostriecin revealed that the removal of the primary alcohol moiety (PD113,270) had little effect on cytotoxicity against L1210 and HCT-8 cells in vitro. Hydroxylation of the lactone ring (PD 113,271) caused a moderate reduction in activity (Jackson et al. 1985), and removal of the phosphate ester (PD114,631) or opening of the lactone ring (PD 113,027) resulted in a considerable loss of cytotoxic activity (Jackson et al. 1985). Together, these studies suggest that both the phosphate ester and the lactone ring contribute to the biological activity of fostriecin.

Initial biochemical studies revealed that fostriecin produced a marked inhibition of macromolecular synthesis. Treatment of L1210 murine leukemia cells with 10 μM fostriecin resulted in a decrease in the rate of DNA, RNA, and protein synthesis within 45 min, with maximal inhibition occurring within 60 min (Fry et al. 1984a). Measurement of ribonucleotide and deoxyribonucleotide pools in fostriecin-treated cells indicated that the ATP and 2′-deoxyribo-ATP (dATP) pools did not differ significantly from the control values, and the levels of the other ribonucleoside and deoxyribonucleoside trisphosphates were either elevated or unchanged relative to control cells (Fry et al. 1984a; Jackson et al. 1985). These observations suggested the inhibition of nucleic acid synthesis was not due to precursor depletion. However, no effects on DNA polymerase, RNA polymerase, or enzymes within the purine or pyrimidine biosynthetic pathways were noted, and the mechanism of nucleic acid synthesis inhibition remained elusive (Fry et al. 1984a; Jackson et al. 1985; Scheithauer et al. 1986).

3.2 Inhibition of Cell Cycle Progression

To gain further insight into the mechanism by which fostriecin inhibits tumor cell proliferation, studies designed to determine the phase of the cell cycle at which fostriecin induced growth arrest were conducted (Jackson et al. 1985; Baguley et al. 1989). Treatment of L1210 cells with a cytostatic concentration of fostriecin (1.5 μM) for 24 h followed by flow cytometric analysis of propidium iodide-stained DNA revealed that fostriecin produced a marked increase in accumulation of cells in the G2/M phase of the cell cycle (Boritzki et al. 1988). In HL-60 and MOLT-4 cells (human promyelocytic and lymphocytic leukemic cells, respectively) 1 μM fostriecin also resulted in the suppression of progression through the G2-phase of the cell cycle. Treatment with 15 μM fostriecin, which is cytotoxic, also produced S-phase growth arrest (Hotz et al. 1992a,b). Similar results were observed in CHO cells, where fostriecin induced G2/M-phase growth arrest and, like cantharidin, caused the appearance of multiple aberrant mitotic spindles (Cheng et al. 1998). Effects of fostriecin at higher concentrations (25–500 μM) also affected cell cycle progression in HL-60 cells, and at these higher concentrations fostriecin triggered endonucleolytic DNA degradation resulting in apoptotic cell death (Hotz et al. 1992a; Graziano et al. 1997). The ability of fostriecin to induce apoptotic cell death at high concentrations (>20 μM) is addressed in more detail in a recent review of preclinical data obtained with fostriecin (de Jong et al. 1997).

3.3 Inhibition of Topoisomerase II Activity

Topoisomerase II is a nuclear enzyme that binds covalently with DNA, cleaves both DNA strands, passes another part of double-stranded DNA through the break, and then reseals the DNA. Because of its critical role in DNA replication, topoisomerase II is the target for many chemotherapeutic drugs, and the inhibition of topoisomerase II activity arrests growth with a cell cycle distribution similar to that observed following treatment with fostriecin. Early reports indicated that fostriecin inhibited type II DNA topoisomerase (Boritzki et al. 1988). At a concentration of 100 μM, fostriecin completely inhibited the relaxation of supercoiled DNA typically affected by type II topoisomerase (IC_{50} 40 μM). In contrast to other type II topoisomerase inhibitors, however, fostriecin did not induce DNA strand breaks, suggesting that it did not stabilize a cleavable complex (Boritzki et al. 1988). Rather, it was felt that fostriecin probably inhibited the catalytic activity of sensitive topoisomerases directly. Correlative studies in three small cell lung carcinoma cell lines showing topoisomerase II-related drug resistance compared the concentration of fostriecin that inhibits tumor cell growth with the relative amount of topoisomerase II in the cancerous cells. There was a lack of cross-resistance to fostriecin and a relationship between topoisomerase II activity and fostriecin sensitivity (de Jong etal. 1991). Nonetheless, despite these reports, fostriecin was not found to have an inhibitory effect on topoisomerase II when an in vitro excision-repair system was employed to study the effects of topoisomerase poisoning (Forsina and Rossi 1992). Other investigators conducting studies in CME or K562 leukemia cell lines with topoisomerase inhibitors that do not stabilize DNA–topoisomerase II complexes also failed to observe an inhibitory effect of fostriecin on topoisomerase II (Chen and Beck 1993; Fattman et al. 1996).

3.4
Inhibition of Protein Phosphatase Activity

More recent studies suggest an alternative mechanism of action of fostriecin. In a variety of rodent, simian, and human cell lines, fostriecin inhibits a mitotic entry checkpoint and induces chromosome condensation in interphase cells in a manner comparable to okadaic acid, a known inhibitor of several PPP-family serine/threonine protein (PP1, PP2A, PP4, PP5, and PP6) (Roberge et al. 1994; Cohen 1997; Honkanen and Golden 2002). Further investigations revealed that fostriecin inhibits the activity of both PP1 and PP2A (Roberge et al. 1994; Walsh et al. 1997; Cheng et al. 1998), suggesting that the antitumor activity of fostriecin could also originate from its ability to interfere with the reversible phosphorylation of proteins that are critical for progression through the cell cycle (Roberge et al. 1994; Guo et al. 1995; Ho and Roberge 1996; Walsh et al. 1997; Cheng et al. 1998). Fostriecin-induced chromosome condensation correlates with an increase in histone H2A and H3 phosphorylation in mouse mammary tumor cells, and fostriecin-induced hyperphosphorylation of vimentin correlates with the reorganization of intermediate filaments in hamster kidney cells (Ho and Roberge 1996). However, as observed with the effects on topoisomerase II activity, the amount of fostriecin that was associated with enhanced phosphorylation was higher than that associated with antitumor activity: $\geq$25 μM fostriecin was needed to demonstrate histone hyperphosphorylation and $\geq$50 μM for vimentin hyperphosphorylation (Ho and Roberge 1996). The higher concentrations may reflect the short time course of the studies (generally less than 4 h), and the intracellular concentration of fostriecin was not determined.

Detailed studies conducted with the purified catalytic subunits of mammalian serine/threonine phosphatases as well as the endogenous enzymes contained in diluted whole cell extracts have confirmed the inhibitory activity of fostriecin against certain eukaryotic serine/threonine phosphatases. When the purified catalytic subunits of PP1 and PP2A from rabbit muscle or bovine brain were used in these inhibition studies, fostriecin displayed potent inhibitory activity against PP2A (IC_{50}=1.5–3.2 nM) and weak inhibitory activity against PP1 (IC_{50}=131 μM) (Walsh et al. 1997; Cheng et al. 1998; Hastie and Cohen 1998). Fostriecin also potently inhibits the activity of PP4 ($IC_{50}\cong$3.0 nM) (Hastie and Cohen 1998) and weakly affects the activity of PP5 ($IC_{50}\cong$70 μM) (Honkanen and Golden 2002). Fostriecin also inhibits endogenous, divalent cation-insensitive phosphatase activity of diluted whole cell extracts of RINm5F insulinoma (Walsh et al. 1997) and CHO (Cheng et al. 1998) cells, rat and pig myocyte homogenates (Armstrong et al. 1997; Weinbrenner et al. 1997), and homogenates of rabbit ventricular biopsies (Weinbrenner et al. 1997). The divalent, cation-independent phosphatase activity contained in these homogenates is derived primarily from

PP1, PP2A, PP4, PP5, and possibly PP6 (Weinbrenner et al. 1997), and the inhibition kinetics obtained were similar to predicted values for a homogenate composed of these enzymes (Walsh et al. 1997; Weinbrenner et al. 1997; Cheng et al. 1998). The kinetics of fostriecin-induced inhibition of PP2A and PP4 correlate well with the ability of fostriecin to inhibit tumor cell proliferation both in vivo and in vitro, suggesting that additional studies into the relationship of these phosphatases to cell cycle progression is warranted. In addition, the effects of fostriecin related to G2 growth arrest [e.g., the formation of aberrant mitotic spindles (Cheng et al. 1998) and the induction of apoptosis (Gorczyca et al. 1993a,b,c; Hotz et al. 1992a,b)] can be mimicked by other phosphatase inhibitors (i.e., okadaic acid and cantharidin) when applied at concentrations that inhibit activity to a comparable extent (Boe et al. 1991; Hotz et al. 1992a; Ishida et al. 1992; Kiguchi et al 1994; Walsh et al. 1997; McDermott et al. 1998; Cheng et al. 1998).

The relationship between fostriecin actions on topoisomerase II, serine/threonine phosphatase inhibition, and ultimate cytoxicity are not well understood. Both phosphatase and topoisomerase inhibitors induce G2-growth arrest and apoptosis (Jackson et al. 1985; Boe et al. 1991; Kiguchi et al 1994; Cheng et al. 1998; Gorczyca et al. 1993a,b,c). In addition, in many studies the concentrations of fostriecin needed to induce enhanced phosphorylation of nuclear proteins, inhibition of topoisomerase II, or induction of apoptosis were substantially higher (>20 μM) than those associated with antitumor activity. Cellular uptake may be limited by the transport capacity of the reduced folate transporter, which appears to be required for the cellular uptake of fostriecin (see below). Alternatively, only some of the fostriecin-sensitive phosphatases or topoisomerases may be associated with antitumor activity. At concentrations associated in vitro as well as in vivo with antitumor activity, fostriecin inhibits only half of the divalent cation-independent phosphatase activity contained in RINm5F insulinoma cells and CHO cells (Walsh et al. 1997; Cheng et al. 1998). The inhibition data obtained with the dilute cell extracts is similar to that predicted for a mixture of PP1, PP2A, and PP4; however, because of the lack of truly type-specific inhibitors, the contribution of individual phosphatases cannot be assessed experimentally at this time. Furthermore, although it is clear that fostriecin can induce an apoptotic response, it is still not clear if the response arises from the inhibition of one of the affected enzymes or if it is triggered as a consequence of prolonged G2/M-phase growth arrest.

3.5 Cellular Uptake of Fostriecin

To date, only a few studies have addressed the mechanism of fostriecin uptake. Fostriecin is water soluble, and the evidence available suggests that it enters the cell by a carrier-mediated mechanism (Fry et al. 1984 Jackson et al. 1985; Spinella et al. 1995). Reduced folates (leucovorin and 5-methyltetrahydrofolate) completely protect L1210 cells from the inhibitory growth effects of fostriecin, while folic acid, which is transported by a process distinct from that for reduced folates, does not provide protection (Fry et al. 1984). Therefore, fostriecin appears to enter L1210 leukemia cells via the reduced folate carrier system. Fostriecin also acts as a potent inhibitor of methotrexate influx with a K_i of 30 μM (slope) and K_i (intercept) of 58.8 μM (Fry et al. 1984). Cells that have been made resistant (~70-fold) to the cytotoxic effects of fostriecin by continuous exposure to increasing concentrations of the drug are also cross-resistant to methotrexate and collaterally sensitive to trimetrexate (a hydrophobic antifolate). This fostriecin-resistant cell line also has a severely impaired reduced folate carrier system, exhibiting a methotrexate influx rate of less than 1% of controls.

3.6 Effects of Fostriecin on Cells

Fostriecin has demonstrated marked antitumor activity against a wide spectrum of tumor cells in vitro and in vivo. In cultured tumor cells, fostriecin proved cytotoxic against a number of cell lines (i.e., L1210, HCT-8, P338), and structure–activity relationship studies comparing fostriecin analogs and cytotoxicity indicate that both the lactone ring and phosphate group are important for cytotoxicity of fostriecin in vitro (Lewy et al. 2002). Recently, the total synthesis of fostriecin has been reported (Boger et al. 2001), so analogs for further evaluation should be forthcoming (Lewy et al. 2002).

In mice, fostriecin exhibits potent cytotoxic activity P388 and L1210 leukemias when administered via i.p. injection. Fostriecin was also active against B16 melanomas. In vitro, fostriecin proved efficacious in L1210-bearing mice with an IC_{50} of 0.46 μM for continuous exposure and 4.4 μM for a 1-h exposure. Scheduling studies indicated that once-daily treatment for 5- or 9-day periods was more effective then two or three single doses every 4 days, and i.p. dosing at 6.25 mg/kg per day on days 1–9 proved to be curative in the L1210 mouse model (de Jong et al. 1997).

In a clonogenic human solid tumor screening assay, in which fostriecin (2.2 μM for 1 h) was tested on a number of tumor specimens derived from patients, fostriecin was found to be highly active and compared favorably to 17 clinically used anticancer drugs including etoposide and doxorubicin (de Jong et al. 1997). Fostriecin produced a 50% or greater decrease in tumor colony forming units in 42% of breast, 33% of the ovarian, and 38% of the non-small cell lung cancer samples (de Jong et al. 1997). In solid tumor mice models, fostriecin produced rapid necrosis in advanced implanted murine colon tumors (Baguley et al. 1989). In other studies, fostriecin proved inactive against a range of solid tumors; however, because the tumors were also insensitive to methotrexate this failure was attributed to the absence of the reduced-folate carrier (de Jong et al. 1997).

Another interesting development is that fostriecin was shown to provide protection to ischemic cardiac tissue comparable to that produced by ischemic preconditioning. Ischemic preconditioning is a phenomenon whereby the heart is protected from an ischemic insult by a previous brief episode of ischemia and reperfusion. Although the mechanism of the protection provided by ischemic preconditioning has remained elusive, several lines of evidence suggest that the activation of protein kinases, such as protein kinase C (Weinbrenner et al. 1998) and the p38 MAPK cascade (Ytrehus et al. 1994) may contribute to this protective response (for review see; Downey and Cohen 1997). To test the potential of fostriecin as an inhibitor of ischemic damage, studies were conducted in perfused, isolated rabbit hearts (Weinbrenner et al. 1997) and isolated ventricular cardiomyocytes from rabbit (Armstrong et al. 1997; Weinbrenner et al. 1997; Armstrong et al. 1998) and pig (Armstrong et al. 1997, 1998). In both pig and rabbit models 0.1–10 μM fostriecin mimicked the protection of preconditioning in both rabbit and pig cardiomyocytes (Armstrong et al. 1997, 1998; Weinbrenner et al. 1997). In isolated, perfused rabbit hearts fostriecin was administered starting either 15 min prior to or 10 min after the onset of a 30-min period of regional ischemia and continuing until the onset of reperfusion. In hearts pretreated with fostriecin, only 8% of the ischemic zone infarcted, which was significantly less than that in the untreated control hearts (33%). Fostriecin also provided significant protection in hearts treated only after the onset of ischemia (18% infarction; $p<0.05$ vs control). Together, these studies suggest that type-selective phosphatase inhibitors may also offer promise as infarct size-limiting drugs.

3.7 Human Clinical Trials and Plasma Pharmacokinetics

Because of its spectrum of activity and unique mechanism of action, the Clinical Trials Evaluation Program of the United States National Cancer Institute initiated phase I clinical trials. To determine the pharmacokinetics of fostriecin, a high-pressure liquid chromatographic method to measure fostriecin in plasma samples was developed (Pillon et al. 1994). Fostriecin is extracted from plasma samples with acetonitrile and then dichloromethane. It is then analyzed by HPLC with a mobile phase of 7.5% acetonitrile in 0.067 M phosphate buffer after separation on a reverse phase C_{18} column. The extraction efficiency is reported as 70% and the sensitivity limit 100 ng/ml.

3.7.1 Stability of Fostriecin

In whole blood, fostriecin was found to be stable for the first 2 h, and aqueous fostriecin remained stable for approximately 12 days. Fostriecin concentration in frozen (−20°C) plasma samples decreased after approximately 14 days. The decrease in fostriecin concentration was not affected by adding ascorbic acid to protect the samples from oxidation. At −70°C samples remained stable for approximately 49 days; stability decreased rapidly thereafter (Pillon et al. 1994).

3.7.2 Pharmacokinetics in Rabbits

The pharmacokinetic properties of fostriecin in rabbits were assessed after bolus intravenous injection of 12 mg/m^2 (Pillon et al. 1994). Disappearance from plasma was best described by a monoexponential equation representing a one-compartment model. The mean distribution space was determined as 4.4 l/m^2 (~8 times the plasma volume) and the plasma clearance was 302 ml/min/m^2 (75% of hepatic plasma flow). The plasma half-life of fostriecin was 12.0+/−8.6 min.

3.7.3 Pharmacokinetics in Humans

Only limited data on the pharmacokinetics of fostriecin in humans have been published. The available data are from a phase I oncology study that enrolled 20 patients whose tumors were unresponsive to established treatments (de Jong et al. 1997, 1999). Fostriecin was supplied by NCI as a lyophilized powder and diluted with 0.9% NaCl. It was administered daily as an intravenous infusion for 1 h on each of 5 days at 4-week intervals. The fostriecin doses used were 2, 4, 6.6, 10, 12.2, and 20 mg/m^2 per day). Three patients were entered into the study at each dose level, with patients receiving the next higher dose when no limiting toxicity was noted at the previous dose. Blood samples were obtained on day 1 prior to infusion, at 30 and 45 min during and at the end of the infusion, and at 10, 20, and 30 min and 1, 1.5, 2, 4, 7 and 17 h after the end of infusion. Urine was collected before the start of infusion and again at 0–2, 2–5, and 15–18 h after the start of the infusion.

A close linear association was observed between drug dose, maximum plasma concentration, and AUC (area under the curve), suggesting linear pharmacokinetics within the dose range investigated. Plasma pharmacokinetics was best described by a two-compartment model. Mean plasma half-life was 0.36 h ($t_{1/2\alpha}$) and 1.51 h ($t_{1/2\beta}$). Mean apparent total body clearance was 2.90 l/h/m^2 (=48.3 ml/min/m^2; 95% CI, 2.24–3.57 l/h/m^2). Mean residence time was 1.19 h (95% CI, 0.41–1.97 h). The mean volume of distribution was 5.64 l/m^2 (95% CI, 2.16–9.11 l/m^2). Only approximately 15% of the fostriecin was excreted in the urine. After approximately 25 min a metabolite, postulated to be dephosphorylated fostriecin, appeared in the plasma and urine of patients receiving more than 12.2 mg/m^2 fostriecin (de Jong et al. 1998, 1999).

3.8 Toxicity Studies

Preclinical toxicological evaluation of fostriecin was conducted primarily in mice and rats, and to date only a limited amount of toxicity data has been released from human clinical trials.

3.8.1 Toxicity in Rodents

Single-dose intravenous administration of fostriecin at dose levels of 8.8–48 mg/kg resulted in death at a dose of 35 mg/kg (60%) and 48 mg/kg (90%), with most deaths occurring on day 1 or 2 of the study (Susick et al. 1990). The 10% lethal dose (LD_{10}) in mice was 2 mg/m^2 per day. In most cases, animals exhibited labored breathing, tremors, hypoactivity, hypothermia, and loss of the righting reflex prior to death. Clinical signs were not restricted to animals that died. The majority of animals surviving the study exhibited labored breathing and hypoactivity immediately after dosing, which lasted for approximately 1 week. Major toxic effects were observed primarily at doses exceeding or equal to 17.5 mg/kg and consisted of bone marrow hypocellularity, leukopenia, neutropenia, thrombocytopenia, and diffuse necrosis of lymphoid tissues. The effects were reversible. One target organ was the kidney. Renal effects were observed primarily at doses of 20 mg/kg. Increases in serum BUN, creatinine, and 24-h glucose excretion were noted, but were reversible. After dosing at 10 and 20 mg/kg, 24-h Na^+ and K^+ excretion and urine osmolarity decreased. Renal lesions were most prevalent at the dose of 20 mg/kg, and consisted of vacuolization and necrosis of the proximal and distal tubular epithelium at the corticomedullary junction with extension to the medulla.

The effect of schedule and route of administration was also assessed. In mice, fostriecin was both inactive and nontoxic when given orally. Subcutaneous treatment was without antileukemic activity and may have even enhanced toxicity (Jackson et al. 1985). In rats, repeated daily intravenous administration of fostriecin for 5 days at dose levels of 2.5–26.5 mg/kg resulted in death at greater than or equal to 10 mg/kg with similar hematological, bone marrow, lymphoid, and renal changes observed following a single treatment (Susick et al. 1990). All rabbits receiving fostriecin at a dose of 12 mg/m^2 exhibited a 15-fold increase in serum alanine aminotransferase

(ALT) and a 60-fold increase in serum aspartate aminotransferase (AST). Maximal rises were observed within 4 h after treatment. There was an 11-fold increase in serum bilirubin 24 h after administration, but levels returned to normal within 48 h.

3.8.2 Toxicity in Humans

In the phase I trial, liver and renal toxicities were observed. In contrast to preclinical trials in rodents, almost no hematological toxicity was evident (Susick et al. 1990; de Jong et al. 1998, 1999). Abnormalities of liver function were not associated with symptoms, and often lessened despite continued administration of fostriecin.

To assess renal toxicity, serum concentrations of creatinine, urea, and electrolytes were measured immediately before the start of treatment, daily during the treatment, and twice weekly during treatment-free intervals. In most patients, significant elevations of serum creatinine were observed at the starting dose, and in all patients at doses exceeding or equal to 4 mg/m^2 per day. But at daily doses above 4 mg/m^2, a plateau in serum creatinine was reached, with no further increases observed as the dose rose. Serum creatinine levels generally rose after the first dose, reached their maximal level on day 3, stabilized despite continuing drug administration, and recovered in 1–2 weeks (median recovery 10–11 days, range 5–19 days) after discontinuation of the drug (de Jong et al. 1998, 1999). Renal hemodynamics was also measured with clearance studies employing ^{125}I-iothalamate and ^{131}I-hippuran in 8 patients taking doses exceeding or equal to 4 mg/m^2 per day. Measurements were made at baseline and on day 3 or 4 during and 3 weeks after the first course. The median change in effective renal plasma flow was −23%, and glomerular filtration rate fell by 36%. The filtration fraction decreased in all patients during the first course of treatment. Urinary β2-microglobulin concentrations increased dramatically (median 150-fold), which is compatible with impaired tubular reabsorption. It was concluded that fostriecin induces a considerable decrease in renal function compatible with renal tubular damage (de Jong et al. 1998, 1999). The rapid recovery and reversibility of renal hemodynamic changes suggest a predominantly functional disorder rather than extensive necrosis. There was no indication of cumulative toxicity (de Jong et al. 1998, 1999); however, the maximal tolerated dose was not determined.

4 Conclusions

Cantharidin appears to be too toxic for use as an antitumor drug in most clinical settings. Still, the in vitro antitumor activity of cantharidin is impressive, and the observation that it stimulates the production of white blood cells by bone marrow seems worthy of further investigation. In addition, the recent syntheses of derivatives that retain inhibitory activity suggest that more selective inhibitors can be developed.

Based on in vitro investigations with fostriecin and the limited data available from the phase I clinical trial, it is not yet clear if blood concentrations of fostriecin predicted to have antitumor activity and achievable at doses of 30–40 mg/m^2 can be reached in humans. Unfortunately, concerns regarding drug purity and storage stability of the naturally produced material lead to the discontinuation of the trial before dose-limiting toxicities or therapeutic plasma levels were reached. Therefore, further dose escalation is still necessary to define the maximum tolerated dose (MTD) of fostriecin. Nonetheless, the toxicities encountered over the dose ranges investigated to date, and in particular their limited progression with increasing doses, indicate that further dose escalation will be possible (de Jong et al. 1999). The possibility of developing fostriecin for the protection of cardiac tissue under ischemic conditions is also promising. Plasma concentrations (1.5–7.5 μM) of fostriecin achieved with doses of 6.6–20 mg/m^2 are above the 1 μM concentration that provided protection to isolated rabbit hearts, and the short half-life and reversibility of the observed toxic effects suggest that even higher doses may be employed clinically for a single treatment. If so, then fostriecin may be useful in limiting the damage to ischemic cardiac tissue. Clearly, additional studies with this interesting molecule will be necessary to provide additional insight into the molecular mechanisms underlying the actions for fostriecin.

Acknowledgements This work was supported in part by grants for the National Institutes of Health Grant (CA60750 and HL HL-59154).

References

Armstrong SC, Kao R, Gao W, Shivell LC, Downey JM, Honkanen RE, Ganote CE (1997) Comparison of in vitro preconditioning responses of isolated pig and rabbit cardiomyocytes: effects of a protein phosphatase inhibitor, fostriecin. J Mol Cell Cardiol 29:3009–24

Armstrong SC, Gao W, Lane JR, Ganote CE (1998) Protein phosphatase inhibitors calyculin A and fostriecin protect rabbit cardiomyocytes in late ischemia. J Mol Cell Cardiol 30:61–73

Bagatell FK, Dugan K, Wilgram GF (1969) Structural and biochemical changes in tissues isolated from the cantharidin-poisoned rat with special emphasis upon hepatic subcellular particles. Toxicol Appl Pharmacol 15:249–61

Baguley BC, Calveley SB, Crowe KK, Fray LM, O'Rourke SA, Smith GP (1989) Comparison of the effects of flavone acetic acid, fostriecin, homoharringtonine and tumour necrosis factor alpha on colon 38 tumours in mice. Eur J Cancer Clin Oncol 25:263–9

Boe R, Gjertsen BT, Vintermyr OK, Houge G, Lanotte M, Doskeland SO (1991) The protein phosphatase inhibitor okadaic acid induces morphological changes typical of apoptosis in mammalian cells. Exp Cell Res 195:237–46

Boger DL, Ichikawa S, Zhong W (2001) Total synthesis of fostriecin (CI-920). J Am Chem Soc 123:4161–7

Boritzki TJ, Wolfard TS, Besserer JA, Jackson RC, Fry DW (1988) Inhibition of type II topoisomerase by fostriecin. Biochem Pharmacol 37:4063–8

Borthwick EB, Zeke T, Prescott AR, Cohen PTW (2001) Nuclear localization of protein phosphatase 5 is dependent on the carboxy-terminal region. FEBS Lett 491:279–84

Chen M, Beck WT (1993) Teniposide-resistant CEM cells, which express mutant DNA topoisomerase II alpha, when treated with non-complex-stabilizing inhibitors of the enzyme, display no cross-resistance and reveal aberrant functions of the mutant enzyme. Cancer Res 53:5946–53

Cheng A, Balczon R, Zuo Z, Koons JS, Walsh AH, Honkanen RE (1998) Fostriecin-mediated G2/M-phase growth arrest correlates with abnormal centrosome replication, the formation of aberrant mitotic spindles, and the inhibition of serine/threonine protein phosphatase activity. Cancer Res 58:3611–9

Cohen PTW (1997) Novel protein serine/threonine phosphatases: variety is the spice of life. Trends Biochem Sci 22:245–51

de Jong S, Zijlstra JG, Mulder NH, de Vries EG (1991) Lack of cross-resistance to fostriecin in a human small-cell lung carcinoma cell line showing topoisomerase II-related drug resistance. Cancer Chemother Pharmacol 28:461–4

de Jong RS, de Vries EG, Mulder NH (1997) Fostriecin: a review of the preclinical data. Anticancer Drugs 8:413–8

de Jong RS, de Vries EG, Meijer S, de Jong PE, Mulder NH (1998) Renal toxicity of the anticancer drug fostriecin. Cancer Chemother Pharmacol 42:160–4

de Jong RS, Mulder NH, Uges DR, Sleijfer DT, Hoppener FJ, Groen HJ, Willemse PH, van der Graaf WT, deVries EG (1999) Phase I and pharmacokinetic study of the topoisomerase II catalytic inhibitor fostriecin. Br J Cancer 79:882–7

Downey JM, Cohen MV (1997) Signal transduction in ischemic preconditioning. Adv Exp Med Biol 430:39–55

Essers M, Wibbeling B, Haufe G (2001) Synthesis of the first fluorinated cantharidin analogues. Tetrahedron Lett 42:5429–33

Fattman CL, Allan WP, Hasinoff BB, Yalowich JC (1996) Collateral sensitivity to the bisdioxopiperazine dexrazoxane (ICRF-187) in etoposide (VP-16)-resistant human leukemia K562 cells. Biochem Pharmacol 52:635–42

Frosina G, Rossi O (1992) Effect of topoisomerase poisoning by antitumor drugs VM 26, fostriecin and camptothecin on DNA repair replication by mammalian cell extracts. Carcinogenesis 13:1371–7

Fry DW, Besserer JA, Boritzki TJ (1984) Transport of the antitumor antibiotic Cl-920 into L1210 leukemia cells by the reduced folate carrier system. Cancer Res 44:3366–70

Fry DW, Boritzki TJ, Jackson RC (1984a) Studies on the biochemical mechanism of the novel antitumor agent, CI-920. Cancer Chemother Pharmacol 13:171–5

Gorczyca W, Gong J, Ardelt B, Traganos F, Darzynkiewicz Z (1993a) The cell cycle related differences in susceptibility of HL-60 cells to apoptosis induced by various antitumor agents. Cancer Res 3:3186–92

Gorczyca W, Gong J, Darzynkiewicz Z (1993b) Detection of DNA strand breaks in individual apoptotic cells by the in situ terminal deoxynucleotidyl transferase and nick translation assays. Cancer Res 53:1945–51

Gorczyca W, Bigman K, Mittelman A, Ahmed T, Gong J, Melamed MR, Darzynkiewicz Z (1993c) Induction of DNA strand breaks associated with apoptosis during treatment of leukemias. Leukemia 7:659–70

Graziano MJ, Waterhouse AL, Casida JE (1987) Cantharidin poisoning associated with specific binding site in liver. Biochem Biophys Res Commun 149:79–85

Graziano MJ, Pessah IN, Matsuzawa M, Casida JE (1988) Partial characterization of specific cantharidin binding sites in mouse tissues. Mol Pharmacol 33:706–12

Guo XW, Th'ng JP, Swank RA, Anderson HJ, Tudan C, Bradbury EM, Roberge M (1995) Chromosome condensation induced by fostriecin does not require p34cdc2 kinase activity and histone H1 hyperphosphorylation, but is associated with enhanced histone H2A and H3 phosphorylation. EMBO J 14:976–85

Hastie CJ, Cohen PTW (1998) Purification of protein phosphatase 4 catalytic subunit: inhibition by the antitumour drug fostriecin and other tumour suppressors and promoters. FEBS Lett 431:357–61

Helps NR, Brewis ND, Lineruth K, Davis T, Kaiser K, Cohen PTW (1998) Protein phosphatase 4 is an essential enzyme required for organisation of microtubules at centrosomes in Drosophila embryos. J Cell Sci 111:1331–40

Ho DT, Roberge M (1996) The antitumor drug fostriecin induces vimentin hyperphosphorylation and intermediate filament reorganization. Carcinogenesis 17(5):967–72

Hokanson GC, French JC (1985) Novel antitumor agents CI-920, Pd 113271, PD113,271 III; Structure determination. J Org Chem 50:462–6

Hong CY, Huang SC, Lin SK, Lee JJ, Chueh LL, Lee CH, Lin JH, Hsiao M (2000) Norcantharidin-induced post-G(2)/M apoptosis is dependent on wild-type p53 gene. Biochem Biophys Res Commun 76:278–85

Honkanen RE (1993) Cantharidin, another natural toxin that inhibits the activity of serine/threonine protein phosphatases types 1 and 2A. FEBS Lett 330:283–6

Honkanen RE, Golden T (2002) Regulators of serine/threonine protein phosphatases at the dawn of a clinical era. Curr Med Chem 9:2055–75

Hotz MA, Traganos F, Darzynkiewicz Z (1992a) Changes in nuclear chromatin related to apoptosis or necrosis induced by the DNA topoisomerase II inhibitor fostriecin in MOLT-4 and HL-60 cells are revealed by altered DNA sensitivity to denaturation. Exp Cell Res 201:184–91

Hotz MA, Del Bino G, Lassota P, Traganos F, Darzynkiewicz Z (1992b) Cytostatic and cytotoxic effects of fostriecin on human promyelocytic HL-60 and lymphocytic MOLT-4 leukemic cells. Cancer Res 52:1530–5

Ishida Y, Furukawa Y, Decaprio JA, Saito M, Griffin JD (1992) Treatment of myeloid leukemic cells with the phosphatase inhibitor okadaic acid induces cell cycle arrest at either G1/S or G2/M depending on dose. J Cell Physiol 150:484–92

Jackson RC, Fry DW, Boritzki TJ, Roberts BJ, Hook KE, Leopold WR (1985) The biochemical pharmacology of CI-920, a structurally novel antibiotic with antileukemic activity. Adv Enzyme Regul 23:193–215

Kiguchi K, Glesne D, Chubb CH, Fujiki H, Huberman E (1994) Differential induction of apoptosis in human breast tumor cells by okadaic acid and related inhibitors of protein phosphatases 1 and 2A. Cell Growth Differ 5:995–1004

Leopold WR, Shillis JL, Mertus AE, Nelson JM, Roberts BJ, Jackson RC (1984) Anticancer activity of the structurally novel antibiotic Cl-920 and its analogues. Cancer Res 44:1928–32

Lewy DS, Gauss CM, Soenen DR, Boger DL (2002) Fostriecin: chemistry and biology. Curr Med Chem 9:2005–32

Li, Y-M, Casida JE (1992) Cantharidin-binding protein: identification as protein phosphatase 2A. Proc Nat Acad Sci USA 89:11867–70

Manning G, Whyte DB, Martinez R, Hunter T, Sudarsanam S (2002) The protein kinase complement of the human genome. Science 298:1912–34

McCluskey A, Sakoff JA (2001) Small molecule inhibitors of serine/threonine protein phosphatases. Mini Rev Med Chem 1:43–55

McCluskey A, Keane MA, Mudgee LM, Sim AT, Sakoff J, Quinn RJ (2000a) Anhydride modified cantharidin analogues. Is ring opening important in the inhibition of protein phosphatase 2A? Eur J Med Chem 35:957–64

McCluskey A, Bowyer, MC, Collins E, Sim ATR, Sakoff J, Baldwin ML (2000b) Anhydride modified cantharidin analogues: synthesis, inhibition of protein phosphatases 1 and 2A and anticancer activity. Bioorganic Med Chem Letts 10:1687–90

McCluskey A, Walkom C, Bowyer MC, Ackland SP, Gardiner E, Sakoff J (2001) Cantharimides: a new class of modified cantharidin analogues inhibiting protein phosphatases 1 and 2A. Bioorg Med Chem Letts 11:2941–46

McCluskey A, Keane MA, Walkom CC, Bowyer MC, Sim AT, Young DJ, Sakoff JA (2002a) The first two cantharidin analogues displaying PP1 selectivity. Bioorg Med Chem Lett 12:391–3

McCluskey A, Sim AT, Sakoff JA (2002b) Serine-threonine protein phosphatase inhibitors: development of potential therapeutic strategies. J Med Chem 45:1151–75

McCluskey A, Ackland SP, Bowyer MC, Baldwin ML, Garner J, Walkom CC, Sakoff JA (2003) Cantharidin analogues: synthesis and evaluation of growth inhibition in a panel of selected tumour cell lines. Bioorg Chem 31:68–79

McDermott CM, Nho CW, Howard W, Holton B (1998) The cyanobacterial toxin, microcystin-LR, can induce apoptosis in a variety of cell types. Toxicon 36:1981–96

Moed L, Shwayder TA, Chang MW (2001) Cantharidin revisited: a blistering defense of an ancient medicine. Arch Dermatol 137:1357–60

Nicholls DSH, Med D, Christmas TI, Greig DE (1990) Oedemerid Blister beetle dermatosis: a review. J Am Acad Dermatol 22:815–9

Nickolls LC, Tear D (1954) Poisoning by cantharidin. Br Med J 2:1384–86

Oaks WW, DiTunno JF, Magnani T, Levey HA, Mills, LC (1960) Cantharidin poisoning. Arch Intern Med 105:106–14

Pillon L, Moore MJ, Thiessen JJ (1994) Determination of fostriecin pharmacokinetics in plasma using high-pressure liquid chromatography assay. Ther Drug Monit 16:186–90

Roberge M, Tudan C, Hung SM, Harder KW, Jirik FR, Anderson H (1994) Antitumor drug fostriecin inhibits the mitotic entry checkpoint and protein phosphatases 1 and 2A. Cancer Res 54:6115–21

Sakoff JA, McCluskey A, Keane MA, Ackland SP (1999) Anticancer activity and protein phosphatase 1 and 2A inhibition of a new generation of cantharidin analogues. Proc Am Assoc Cancer Res 40:2610–10

Scheithauer W, Von Hoff DD, Clark GM, Shillis JL, Elslager EF (1986) In vitro activity of the novel antitumor antibiotic fostriecin (CI-920) in a human tumor cloning assay. Eur J Cancer Clin Oncol 22:921–6

Snaith HA, Armstrong CG, Guo Y, Kaiser K, Cohen PTW (1996) Deficiency of protein phosphatase 2A uncouples the nuclear and centrosome cycles and prevents attachment of microtubules to the kinetochore in Drosophila microtubule star (mts) embryos. J Cell Sci 109:3001–12

Sodeoka M, Baba Y, Kobayashi S Hirukawa N (1997) Structure-activity relationship of cantharidin derivatives to protein phosphatases 1, 2A1, and 2B. Bioorg Med Chem Lett 7:1833–36

Spinella MJ, Brigle KE, Sierra EE, Goldman ID (1995) Distinguishing between folate receptor-alpha-mediated transport and reduced folate carrier-mediated transport in L1210 leukemia cells. J Biol Chem 270:7842–9

Stampwala SS, Bunge RH, Hurley TR, Willmer NE, Brankiewicz AJ, Steinman CE, Smitka TA, French JC (1983) Novel antitumor agents CI-920, PD 113,270 and PD 113,271. II. Isolation and characterization. J Antibiot (Tokyo) 36:1601–5

Stork G (1999) Some contributions to regio and stereo control: from Cincholoipon and Cantharidin to the present. Med Res Rev 19:370–87

Stoughton RB, Bagatell F (1959) Cantharidin treatment of warts. J Invest Dermatol 33:287–92

Sumiyoshi E, Sugimoto A, Yamamoto M (2002) Protein phosphatase 4 is required for centrosome maturation in mitosis and sperm meiosis in C. elegans. J Cell Sci 115:1403–10

Susick RL Jr, Hawkins KL, Pegg DG (1990) Preclinical toxicological evaluation of fostriecin, a novel anticancer antibiotic, in rats. Fundam Appl Toxicol 15:258–69

Tunac JB, Graham BD, Dobson WE (1983) Novel antitumor agents CI-920, PD 113,270 and PD 113,271. I. Taxonomy, fermentation and biological properties. J Antibiot (Tokyo) 36:1595–6000

Walsh AH, Cheng A, Honkanen RE (1997) Fostriecin, an antitumor antibiotic with inhibitory activity against serine/threonine protein phosphatases types 1 (PP1) and 2A (PP2A), is highly selective for PP2A. FEBS Lett 416:230–4

Walter WG (1989) Antitumor imide derivatives fo 7-oxabicyclo[2.2.1]heptane-2,3-dimethyl-2,3-dicarboxylic acid. J Pharm Sci 78:66–7

Wang CC, Wu CH, Hsieh KJ, Yen KY, Yang LL (1990) Cytotoxic effects of cantharidin on the growth of normal and carcinoma cells. Toxicology 147:77–87

Wang G-S (1989) Medical use of mylabris in ancient China and recent studies. J Ethnopharmacol 26:147–62

Weinbrenner C, Liu GS, Cohen MV, Downey JM (1997) Phosphorylation of tyrosine 182 of p38 mitogen-activated protein kinase correlates with the protection of preconditioning in the rabbit heart. J Mol Cell Cardiol 29:2383–91

Weinbrenner C, Baines CP, Liu GS, Armstrong SC, Ganote CE, Walsh AH, Honkanen RE, Cohen MV, Downey JM (1998) Fostriecin, an inhibitor of protein phosphatase 2A, limits myocardial infarct size even when administered after onset of ischemia. Circulation 98:899–905

Ytrehus K, Liu Y, Downey JM (1994) Preconditioning protects ischemic rabbit heart by protein kinase C activation. Am J Physiol 266:H1145–52

Part IV
Inhibitors in Clinical Use or Advanced Clinical Trials

HEP (2005) 167:321–359

Clinical Immunosuppression using the Calcineurin-Inhibitors Ciclosporin and Tacrolimus

N. R. Banner (✉) · H. Lyster · M. H. Yacoub

Harefield Hospital, Royal Brompton and Harefield NHS Trust, Harefield, Middx, UB9 6JH, UK
n.banner@rbh.nthames.nhs.uk

Abstract T cells play a key role in orchestrating the immune response to an allograft. The discovery of a potent and immunologically specific inhibitor of T cell activation, ciclosporin, dramatically improved the results of renal transplantation and transformed other types of organ transplantation from experimental to standard therapy. The discovery of a second drug, tacrolimus, that was structurally unrelated to ciclosporin but which had an identical mechanism of action, facilitated research which clarified the mechanisms underlying T cell activation. Although these drugs are powerful immunosuppressants, their clinical use is limited by their nephrotoxicity. In transplantation, this has led to their use in lower doses in combination with other immunosuppressive drugs. However long-term nephrotoxicity remains a significant problem, and this has curtailed the use of calcineurin-inhibitors for indications outside the field of transplantation. Ciclosporin and tacrolimus are metabolised by cytochrome P450 3A and are substrates for the P-glycoprotein transporter system. This results in complex pharmacokinetics with large variations in bioavailability and metabolism between individuals as well as a great number of clinically significant drug interactions. Therapeutic drug monitoring has been used to address these issues. For the foreseeable future, these powerful immunosuppressive agents are likely to continue to play a role in organ transplantation. However, newer immunosuppressants that are not nephrotoxic may begin to replace calcineurin-inhibitors for long-term maintenance therapy after transplantation.

Keywords Ciclosporin · Cyclosporine · Tacrolimus · Calcineurin-inhibitor · Immunosuppression · Transplantation · Nephrotoxicity · Autoimmune disease

1 Introduction

Pharmacological immunosuppression is essential for all types of allogeneic organ transplantation (Banner and Lyster 2003). Immunosuppressive therapy is also used to treat a range of autoimmune diseases and will be essential for xenotransplantation if this becomes a clinical reality in the future (Azimzadeh et al. 2003). The efficacy of such immunosuppression depends on the mechanism of action of agents used and their capacity to specifically target those aspects of the immune response which play a key role in the alloimmune response. The discovery of cyclosporin A (hereafter ciclosporin) was a major advance in immunosuppressive therapy because of its specific effect on lymphocytes and their role in the cognate immune response while leaving the functions of the innate immune system and other aspects of the adaptive immune response intact (Borel et al. 1976). The introduction of ciclosporin into clinical transplantation was associated with improved results in the fields of kidney (The Canadian Multicentre Transplant Study Group 1986), heart (Oyer et al. 1983) and liver transplantation (Starz et al. 1981); in addition, lung transplantation became a successful procedure for the first time (Reitz et al. 1982; Toronto Lung Transplant Group 1986). Ciclosporin was also effective in the control of graft-versus-host disease (GVHD) after allogeneic bone marrow transplantation (Deeg et al. 1985) and was found to

Table 1 Introduction of immunosuppressive agents into clinical use for organ transplantation

Approximate date	Agent
1960	Azathioprine
	Corticosteroids
	Antithymocyte globulin
1970	Ciclosporin
1980	Muromonab-CD3
	Tacrolimus
1990	Mycophenolate
	Basiliximab/daclizumab
	Sirolimus
2000	Everolimus

have a role in the management of autoimmune disease (Ellis et al. 1986; Forre et al. 1987; Tejani et al. 1987). Subsequently, further immunosuppressive agents have been introduced into clinical transplantation (Table 1). One of these was tacrolimus (Kino et al. 1987); it was found to have a similar mechanism of action as ciclosporin but a completely different molecular structure (Sawada et al. 1987). The availability of ciclosporin and tacrolimus facilitated research to establish their mechanism of action (Schreiber and Crabtree 1992). Here, we review the clinical pharmacology of both drugs with particular emphasis on their role in organ transplantation.

2 The Alloimmune Response and Allograft Rejection

Allograft rejection is conventionally divided into three syndromes according to the time of its occurrence; each of these has a different pathogenesis. Acute rejection may involve cellular or humoral mechanisms, although the former usually predominate. Pharmacological immunosuppression based on the calcineurin inhibitors has been effective in the control of acute cellular rejection, which is one of the most common problems early after organ transplantation, but it has had less impact on the other forms of rejection.

Hyperacute rejection was first described in renal transplantation (Williams et al. 1968; Patel and Terasaki 1969; Terasaki et al. 1971) and it has subsequently been recognised to occur in other types of transplant (Smith et al. 1993; Choi et al. 1999; Scornik et al. 1999). Preformed antibodies against antigens of either the ABO blood group system or human leukocyte antigens (HLA) bind to the endothelium of the allograft causing endothelial activation. This causes complement binding and intravascular coagulation which leads to the rapid destruction of the graft (Wu et al. 2003). This rapid form of rejection can be prevented by ABO matching between the recipient and donor and by screening transplant candidates for anti-HLA antibodies; those who have such antibodies must also undergo a lymphocytotoxic cross match against the donor before a transplant can be safely performed (Smith et al. 1993). When hyperacute rejection does occur, it requires specific treatment aimed at both the removal of the preformed antibodies and preventing the synthesis of further antibody (Bittner et al. 2001; Pierson et al. 2002).

Acute rejection typically first occurs within the first 3 months of transplantation but may occur later. It is predominantly a cellular process (Hall et al. 1978; Rosenberg et al. 1987) and is initiated by helper T cells which recognise either foreign HLA on the surface of cells within the graft (direct recognition) or antigens from the allograft which have been processed by antigen-presenting cells (APCs) of the host (indirect recognition) (Hornick and Lechler 1997). Direct recognition appears to be the most important mechanism in acute rejection. Thus, the T cell plays a central role in orchestrating the immune response to the allograft (Fig. 1) (Rose and Hutchinson 2003).

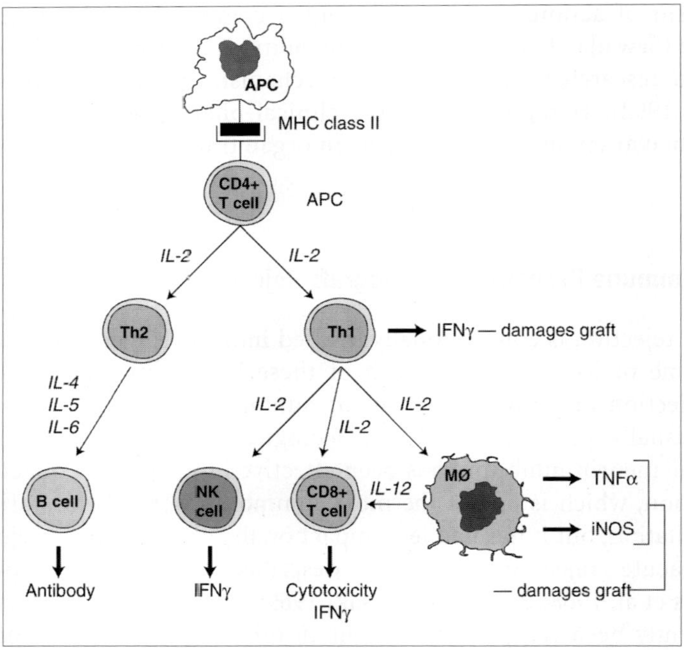

Fig. 1 Role of the helper T cell in orchestration the alloimmune response. Activation of $CD4^+$ T cells results in Th1 or Th2 cells, production of their characteristic cytokine profiles and maturation of effector mechanisms. *APC*, antigen-presenting cell; *MHC*, major histocompatibility complex; *IFN*, interferon; *TNF*, tumour necrosis factor; *iNOS* inducible nitric oxide synthase; *MØ*, macrophage; *IL*, interleukin. (Reproduced by permission from Rose et al. 2003)

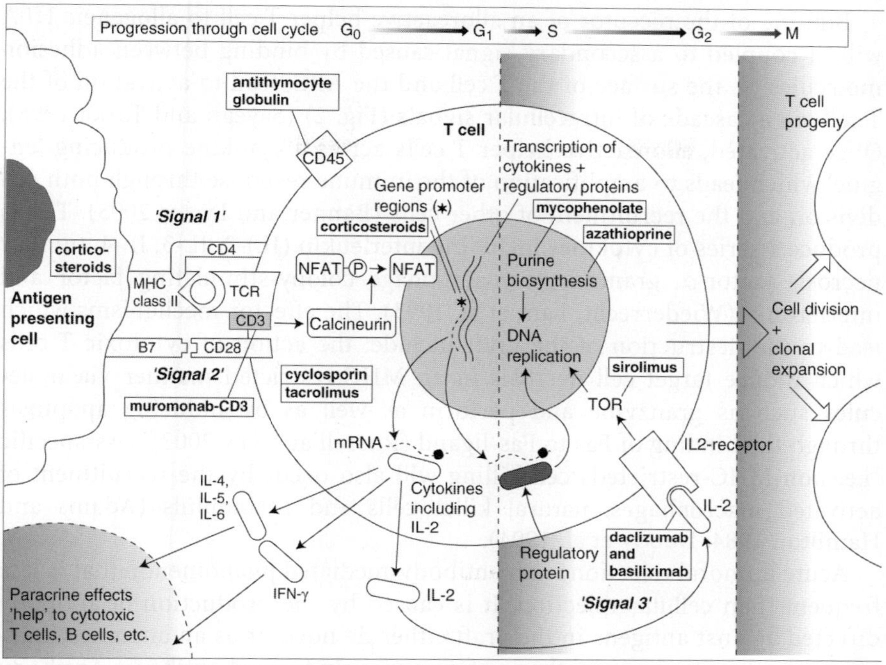

Fig. 2 Steps in the T cell activation cascade. Simplified model of the events which occur during T cell activation. The early, calcium-dependent, phase of activation begins when the T cell receptor (*TCR*) binds to a complementary MHC class II molecule with an associated peptide in its antigen-presentation grove *'Signal 1'*. Full activation also requires a second signal (*'Signal 2'*) which is caused by binding between complementary adhesion molecules on the surface of the antigen-presenting cell and the T cell. Signal transduction from the TCR occurs via the CD3 complex. Subsequent intracellular signalling involves the inositol triphosphate/diacylglycerol pathway and mobilisation of intracellular calcium. This leads to activation of the protein phosphatase calcineurin. Calcineurin dephosphorylates the nuclear factor of activated T cells (*NFAT*) allowing its active moiety to translocate to the nucleus and so bind to the promoter regions of various genes encoding cytokines such as interleukin-2 (*IL-2*), regulatory proteins and the IL-2 receptor. The pattern of cytokine expression depends on the nature of the T cell (Th1 or Th2) and can lead to either recruitment of cytotoxic T cells and other effector cells or to the provision of help to B cells for antibody production. The expression of IL-2 leads to autocrine stimulation of the T cell. Binding of IL-2 to its receptor initiates a second sequence of intracellular signals involving the mammalian target of rapamycin (*TOR*) which leads to DNA synthesis and replication and which culminates in cell division. The sites of action of various immunosuppressive agents are shown. Polyclonal antithymocyte globulin is shown as binding to the common leukocyte antigen (*CD45*) although, in reality, it contains antibodies which bind to many different T cell antigens. Abbreviations: *IL*, interleukin; *MHC*, major histocompatibility complex; *NFAT*, nuclear factor of activated T cells; *TCR*, T cell receptor; *TOR*, target of rapamycin; *IFN*, interferon. (Reproduced by permission from Banner and Lyster 2003)

Binding of the receptor of an alloreactive helper T cell to allogeneic HLA will, if coupled to a secondary signal caused by binding between adhesion molecules on the surface of the T cell and the APC, lead to activation of the T cell via a cascade of intracellular signals (Fig. 2) (Sayegh and Turka 1998). Once activated, alloreactive helper T cells act as a cytokine producing 'engine' which leads to amplification of the immune response through both cell division and the recruitment of other cells (Banner and Lyster 2003). T cells produce a series of cytokines including interleukin (IL)-2, IL-3, IL-4, tumour necrosis factor-α, granulocyte–macrophage colony-stimulating factor and interferon-γ (Wiederrecht, Lam et al. 1993). The effector mechanisms which lead to the destruction of the graft include: the action of cytotoxic T cells which induce target cell necrosis in an MHC-restricted manner via molecules such as granzyme and perforin as well as by inducing apoptosis through the binding of Fas to Fas-ligand (Russell and Ley 2002); less-specific (i.e. non-MHC-restricted) cell killing will also occur by the recruitment of activated macrophages, natural killer cells and eosinophils (Adams and Hamilton 1984; Doody et al. 1994).

Acute humoral rejection is an antibody-mediated phenomenon that is less frequent than cellular rejection. It is caused by the production of antibody directed against antigens in the graft either de novo or as an anamnestic response leading to the resynthesis of a previously formed antibody. Antibody binding to the graft leads to complement-mediated injury with prominent vascular features (acute 'vascular' rejection) (Cherry et al. 1992; Bohmig et al. 2001; Feucht 2003). In severe rejection, cellular and humoral mechanisms often co-exist (Abe, Sawada et al. 2003). Once established, this type of rejection cannot be controlled by conventional immunosuppression based on the calcineurin inhibitors and requires additional specific treatment to remove the antibody and inhibit its resynthesis (Grandtnerova et al. 1995; Hickstein et al. 1998; Garrett et al. 2002).

Chronic rejection is a multifactorial process which is driven by both immune and non-immune mechanisms. Episodes of acute cellular rejection and the formation of alloreactive antibody as well as autoimmune antibodies against non-polymorphic antigens all appear to play a role (Rose and Hutchinson 2003). Immunosuppression based on calcineurin inhibitors has an indirect influence on these processes by reducing the incidence of acute rejection and reducing T cell help to B cells for de novo antibody synthesis. However, it has not overcome the problem of chronic rejection, which remains one of the commonest long-term complications of organ transplantation.

3
Discovery of Ciclosporin and Tacrolimus

Prior to the discovery of ciclosporin, there were a limited number of agents available for clinical immunosuppression (Table 1). Acute rejection was a frequent problem that could lead to graft loss and the use of drugs such as corticosteroids in high doses for a prolonged period, which led to a high incidence of complications, particularly infection. Ciclosporin proved to be an important advance because of its selective and reversible effect on T cell activation (Kahan 1989).

Ciclosporin was discovered in the early 1970s by a team led by Borel working at Sandoz laboratories. The compound was identified from cultures containing the fungi *Tolypocladium inflatum* and *Cylindrocarpon lucidum* (Kay 1989). It was found to have immunosuppressive properties in murine models (Borel et al. 1976). Short-term experiments in small laboratory animals did not identify nephrotoxicity as a problem, and so it was a surprise that early clinical experience showed ciclosporin to be nephrotoxic in man (Calne et al. 1978). Subsequent experience and clinical trials confirmed that ciclosporin was an effective immunosuppressive agent and that its use was associated with improved graft survival (European multicentre trial group 1983); however, the issue of nephrotoxicity has remained as one of the main limitations of ciclosporin therapy. A number of metabolites and synthetic analogues of ciclosporin have been investigated but none has been found to be free of this problem; immunosuppressive effect and renal toxicity appear to change in parallel in this group of drugs (Siga et al. 1991).

Tacrolimus (formerly FK506) was also discovered through a process of screening fungal metabolites. It was isolated from cultures of the soil fungus *Streptomyces tsukubaensis* by researchers at the Fujisawa Pharmaceuticals in 1984. Subsequently, it was found to have similar immunosuppressive properties to ciclosporin but a much greater potency and a completely different molecular structure (Fig. 3) (Kino et al. 1987).

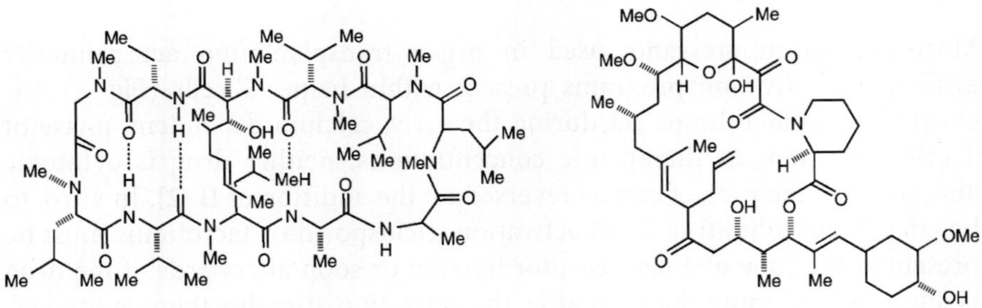

Ciclosporin Tacrolimus

Fig. 3 Molecular structures of ciclosporin and tacrolimus. Despite their common immunosuppressive action, the two drugs have no structural similarity

4
Structure and Binding to the Immunophilins

Ciclosporin is a hydrophobic cyclic undecapeptide (Fig. 3). In contrast, tacrolimus is a macrolide which has structural similarities to sirolimus (rapamycin) and everolimus but no features in common with ciclosporin. The structural dissimilarity of tacrolimus to ciclosporin and its structural connection with another immunosuppressive agent that has a different mechanism of action, sirolimus, was important in the search for the molecular targets of these agents.

Both ciclosporin and tacrolimus bind to intracellular proteins now known as immunophilins. These are ubiquitous and abundant small intracellular proteins which have been highly conserved during phylogeny (Wiederrecht, Lam et al. 1993). The major receptor for tacrolimus (FK506) is a 12-kDa protein designated FK binding protein 12 (FKBP12). The major receptor for ciclosporin is a 17-kDa protein designated cyclophilin-A (Handschumacher, Harding et al. 1984; Siekierka, Hung et al. 1989).

Despite their different structure, the immunophilins share an enzymatic activity catalysing the isomerisation of peptidyl–proline bonds; they are believed to play a role in protein folding (rotamase activity). Ciclosporin and tacrolimus are inhibitors of their cognate immunophilin's enzymatic activity, but they do not cross-inhibit the other family of immunophilins. The initial hypothesis that inhibition of the immunophilins isomerase activity played a key role in the action of these drugs was refuted by the discovery of congeners which inhibited that activity but that either differed in their mechanism of immunosuppression (sirolimus) or that lacked immunosuppressive activity altogether (Bierer et al. 1990; Dumont et al. 1990). Immunophilins play a role in the clinical pharmacokinetics of these drugs.

5
Mechanism of Action

Most immunosuppressants used in organ transplantation act primarily against the activation programs present within helper T cells (Fig. 2). Ciclosporin and tacrolimus act during the early, calcium-dependent, phase of T cell activation. At therapeutic concentrations, neither drug is cytotoxic and, in vitro, their effect can be reversed by the addition of IL-2). In vitro, to be effective in inhibiting T cell activation, ciclosporin or tacrolimus must be present at the time of T cell receptor ligation or soon afterwards; if the drug is administered more than 6 h after the activation stimulus there is little effect on T cell proliferation (Kay et al. 1983; Kumagai et al. 1988; Tocci et al. 1989).

Activation is initiated following the cognate interaction of an alloreactive T cell receptor with a MHC–peptide complex on an APC, coupled with a second signal involving the binding between costimulatory molecules such as B7–1 and 2 on the APC and CD28 on the T cell (Crabtree 1989; Sayegh and Turka 1998). This activates tyrosine kinases, which phosphorylate tyrosine residues of CD3 within the receptor complex (Fig. 4) (Shaw and Dustin 1997). Subsequent intracellular pathways are activated including the inositol triphosphate (IP_3) and diacylglycerol (DAG) pathway. IP_3 stimulates the release of calcium from the endoplasmic reticulum and opens a calcium channel in the membrane, producing an influx of calcium into the cell (Parekh et al. 1997; Shaw and Dustin 1997; Fierro et al. 2000).

Research using ciclosporin, tacrolimus and their analogues clarified the sequence of events that transduce this calcium signal into gene transcription within the T cell (Schreiber and Crabtree 1992; Liu 1993). Affinity matrices of FKBP and cyclophilin were used to identify ligands for complexes of FKBP–tacrolimus and cyclophilin–ciclosporin. Both were found to bind the same set of proteins in a calcium-dependent fashion (Liu et al. 1991). The target proteins were identified as the phosphatase calcineurin and the regulatory protein calmodulin (Klee et al. 1988; Liu 1993). Binding of each drug–immunophilin complex to calcineurin–calmodulin inhibited the phosphatase activity of calcineurin (Liu 1993). In vitro, calcineurin activity was completely abolished by doses of ciclosporin or tacrolimus (hereafter calcineurin inhibitors or CNIs) that inhibited transcription of IL-2 (Fruman, Klee et al. 1992). Calcineurin consists of a catalytic domain coupled to a control region, a calmodulin-binding region and an autoinhibitory domain. Phosphatase activity is activated by the binding of calcium and calmodulin (Kincaid et al. 1986; Hubbard and Klee 1989).

Calcineurin dephosphorylates a number of substrates that play a role in intracellular regulation. The steps linking calcineurin phosphatase activity to the regulation of IL-2 are now understood, but the mechanisms that link this calcium-dependent pathway to effects that do not involve transcription and to the many adverse effects of CNIs are far less clear (Schreiber and Crabtree 1992). However, the correlation of immunosuppressive potency and nephrotoxicity within CNIs and their analogues supports the view that inhibition of calcineurin underlies the toxicity of these compounds (Sigal et al. 1991; Wiederrecht et al. 1993).

Calcineurin dephosphorylates the nuclear factor for activated T cells (NFAT) family of transcription factors. NFAT plays a key role in gene transcription within the activated lymphocyte (Shaw et al. 1988; Luo et al. 1996). NFAT1 is present in the cytoplasm of resting T cells and translocates into the nucleus in response to the calcium signal that follows T cell activation (Figs. 2 and 4) (Shaw et al. 1995; Loh et al. 1996). The event that initiates the nuclear import of NFAT1 is its dephosphorylation by calcineurin (Shaw et al. 1995; Luo et al. 1996). By inhibiting the translocation of NFAT to the nu-

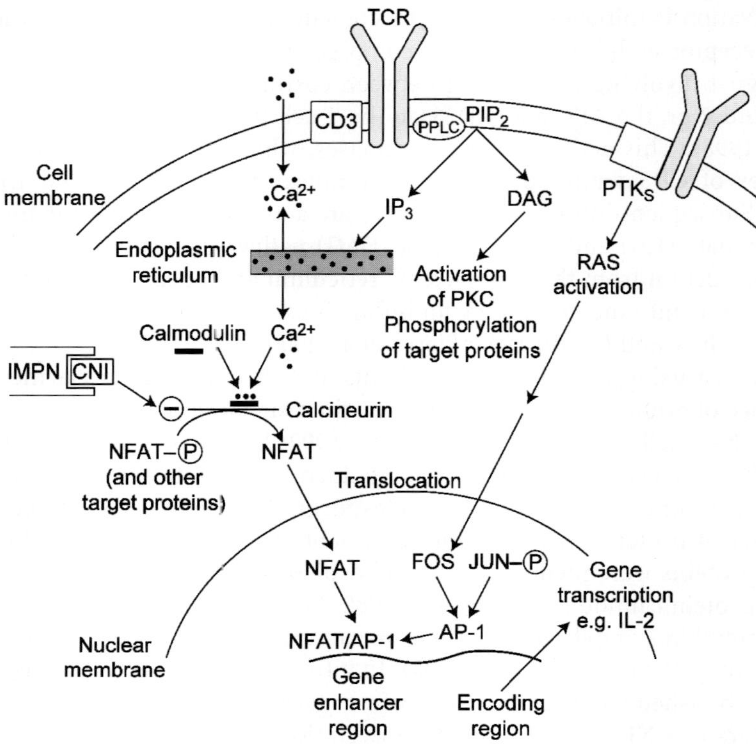

Fig. 4 Mechanism of action of the calcineurin inhibitors. Binding of an MHC–peptide complex to its cognate T cell receptor (*TCR*) initiates a cascade of signalling events which constitute the early, calcium-dependent, phase of T cell activation. TCR-associated protein tyrosine kinases (*PTKs*) become activated and lead to the phosphorylation of phosphatidylinositol phospholipase C (*PPLC*). PPLC then catalyses the breakdown of the membrane phospholipid phosphatidylinositol bisphosphate (PIP_2) to form inositol triphosphate (IP_3) and diacylglycerol (DAG). IP_3 induces the release of calcium (Ca^{2+}) from the endoplasmic reticulum (*ER*). The phosphatase calcineurin is then activated by the binding of calcium and the regulatory protein calmodulin. Calcineurin dephosphorylates regulatory proteins including the cytoplasmic form of the nuclear factor of activated T cells (*NFAT*). Dephosphorylated NFAT can then be imported into the nucleus where it binds to the enhancer region of genes such as that for IL-2. DAG, in combination with calcium, activates protein kinase C (*PKC*), which phosphorylates other regulatory proteins. Other PTKs, activated by cognate binding of the TCR, phosphorylate substrates that activate guanosine triphosphate-binding proteins such as Ras. The Ras pathway links to a mitogen-activated protein (*MAP*) cascade (not shown) that ultimately leads to the transcription of Fos and the activation of Jun by phosphorylation. Fos and Jun-P combine to form the transcription factor activator protein (*AP*)-1 which binds to the enhancer region of the IL-2 gene. A number of factors can bind to the enhancer region of the IL-2 gene, including NFAT, AP-1, nuclear factor (*NF*)-κB and Oct-1; once bound, they serve to co-operatively activate the transcription of the gene. NFAT plays a key role in gene activation and the calcineurin inhibitors (*CNIs*) interfere with T cell activation by preventing its translocation into the cell nucleus. Ciclosporin and tacrolimus act as prodrugs which bind to their corresponding immunophilins (*IMPN*) to form a CNI–IMPN

cleus, calcineurin inhibition prevents the co-operation of NFAT with other transcription factors in enabling the expression of IL-2 and other cytokines (Durand et al. 1988; Wiederrecht et al. 1991; Schreiber and Crabtree 1992).

Experimentally, alternative pathways of T cell activation can bypass calcium-dependent activation of calcineurin, but their relevance to clinical allograft rejection and clinical immunosuppression remains uncertain (June et al. 1987; Lin et al. 1991). The clinical practice of combining a CNI with other types of immunosuppressant may mitigate the effect of such pathways (Banner and Lyster 2003).

6 Clinical Use of the Calcineurin Inhibitors

6.1 Transplantation

6.1.1 Maintenance Immunosuppression

The introduction of the original Sandimmun (or Sandimmune) formulation of ciclosporin as a clinical immunosuppressant for renal transplantation was associated with a marked improvement in patient and graft survival (Canadian Multicenter Transplant Study Group 1983; European Multicentre Trial Group 1983). In the Canadian trial, ciclosporin and prednisone were compared to azathioprine and prednisone; in the European study, ciclosporin monotherapy was compared to azathioprine plus steroids. However, in the Canadian trial, serum creatinine levels were higher in the ciclosporin group, suggesting nephrotoxicity; and in the European study, 24 of 84 patients in the ciclosporin group who had functioning grafts were switched to conventional immunosuppression because of nephrotoxicity. These early studies established ciclosporin as a more effective immunosuppressive agent while illustrating the problem of nephrotoxicity.

The results of liver and heart transplantation were both improved following the introduction of ciclosporin, although once again renal function was found to be worse in the heart transplant patients who received ciclosporin (Starzl et al. 1981; Oyer et al. 1983; Emery et al. 1986). The availability of ciclosporin was one of the factors that enabled lung transplantation to be per-

complex that inhibits calcineurin. They thereby prevent the dephosphorylation of NFAT and hence the expression of IL-2 and other genes. It is believed that many of the toxic non-immunosuppressive effects of the ciclosporin and tacrolimus are related to the effect of calcineurin inhibition on the function of other regulatory proteins

formed successfully (Reitz et al. 1982; Toronto Lung Transplant Group 1986).

The use of ciclosporin gradually evolved with lower dose regimens being introduced in combination with other immunosuppressive agents and the development of dose adjustment according to the concentration of ciclosporin present in the patient's blood (therapeutic drug monitoring, TDM). The aim of combination therapy was to obtain synergistic immunosuppression by using drugs that act at different stages of the T cell activation cascade but which have non-overlapping toxicities (Fig. 2) (Banner and Lyster 2003).

The introduction of tacrolimus for organ transplantation made its greatest impact in the field of liver transplantation. Absorption of the Sandimmun formulation of ciclosporin is dependent on bile flow. Early after liver transplantation, when a T-tube biliary diversion is normally in place, Sandimmun was not absorbed effectively, necessitating intravenous therapy. In contrast, oral therapy with tacrolimus can be established early after liver transplantation. Clinical trials found that the use of tacrolimus, when compared with Sandimmun, was associated with lower acute rejection rates, including corticosteroid-resistant rejection, and similar graft and patient survival (European FK506 Multicentre Liver Study Group 1994; U.S. Multicenter FK506 Liver Study 1994). In renal transplantation, tacrolimus use was again associated with lower rates of rejection (Vincenti et al. 1996; Mayer et al. 1997; Jensik 1998; Knoll and Bell 1999). In heart transplantation, a tacrolimus-based immunosuppression regimen had a similar efficacy to one based on ciclosporin but with a different profile of side effects (Taylor et al. 1999).

Based on data indicating that pharmacokinetic variability associated with the Sandimmun formulation of ciclosporin was a factor limiting efficacy (Lindholm and Kahan 1993; Kahan et al. 1996), a new formulation of ciclosporin (Neoral) was introduced. Direct comparison of the two formulations in heart transplant recipients showed similar safety together with graft and patient survival rates, while there was a reduction in the incidence of steroid-resistant rejection (Eisen et al. 2001).

Due to the very different potency and pharmacokinetic profiles of ciclosporin and tacrolimus together with the need for TDM (which necessitates 'open label' clinical trials), it has not been possible to establish a clear advantage for one agent over the other except in specific circumstances. There are, however, differences in the side effects of the two CNIs.

6.1.2 Treatment of Acute Rejection

Although CNIs are effective in the prophylaxis of rejection, alone they are inadequate for the treatment of established acute rejection. This is because a range of effector mechanisms have been initiated which are not sensitive to calcineurin inhibition (Rose and Hutchinson 2003). Nevertheless, proper maintenance of immunosuppression, including a CNI, is an essential part of treatment because it will control the T cell-mediated cytokine release. Treatment of acute rejection normally includes the use of high-dose corticosteroids with or without antithymocyte globulin or muromonab-CD3 (Banner and Lyster 2003).

6.1.3 Rescue Therapy

Many studies have examined the role of transferring patients from ciclosporin to tacrolimus as 'rescue therapy' for acute rejection that is refractory to conventional therapy. Unfortunately, the nature of the study populations and the clinical situation has precluded the use of randomised studies. Therefore, the data from such studies have been anecdotal and uncontrolled. Nevertheless there are data to support the view that switching from ciclosporin to tacrolimus can be a beneficial part of the treatment for refractory rejection (Woodle et al. 1996; Mentzer et al. 1998).

6.1.4 Hyperacute and Chronic Rejection

Hyperacute rejection is caused by preformed antibodies and will not be influenced by the administration of a CNI. Acute rejection is a risk factor for chronic rejection, and so CNI-based immunosuppression may indirectly help to prevent chronic rejection; but there is little evidence that CNIs are efficacious in the treatment of established chronic rejection.

6.1.5 Current Practice

In recent years, regimens for maintenance immunosuppression after organ transplantation have usually consisted of a CNI combined with one or more other drugs. Corticosteroids are almost invariably used and are usually combined with a third agent such as azathioprine (Amenabar et al. 1998), mycophenolate (European Mycophenolate Mofetil Cooperative Study Group 1995), sirolimus (Kahan 2000) or everolimus (Eisen et al. 2003). Doses of ciclosporin and tacrolimus are normally adjusted in the light of blood concentrations, clinical response and evidence of nephrotoxicity. There are no laboratory investigations that can directly determine the appropriate degree of immunosuppression for an individual patient.

6.2 Allogeneic Bone Marrow Transplantation

Both ciclosporin and tacrolimus have a role increasing the rate of engraftment and in prophylaxis against, as well as treatment of, GVHD (Hows et al. 1982; Storb et al. 1986; Storb et al. 1988; Przepiorka et al. 1996; Arranz et al. 2002).

6.3 Indications Other than Organ Transplantation

From their mechanism of action, the CNIs might be expected to have a role in the management of autoimmune disease. However, their impact in this area has been limited. They act at the earliest stage of activation of the cognate immune system. In transplantation, where the timing of the antigenic stimulus from the allograft is known, they can be used prophylactically. However, in autoimmune disease, the initial stimulus to the immune system is obscure and the fault may lie in immune regulation rather than a response to an external trigger. By the time the disease is recognised clinically, multiple mechanisms may be involved, many of which are insensitive to the actions of CNIs. The adverse effects of the CNIs, including their nephrotoxicity, have been acceptable in the field of transplantation, where the objective is to maintain the function of a life-sustaining allograft and where there have been few alternatives. In autoimmune disease, however, the objective is usually to minimise morbidity rather than to avoid mortality, and so the acceptable level for toxicity is less. Nephrotoxicity may limit the long-term use of CNIs, and relapse of the disease is often a problem when the drug is discontinued. Furthermore, for many of autoimmune diseases there are often alternative treatments available. Generally, in the treatment of autoimmune disease the dose of CNI has been adjusted according to renal function rather than the drug concentration in blood, with the aim to emphasise the need of minimising toxicity rather than maximising efficacy. Currently, the CNIs are not first-line treatment for any autoimmune disease, but they may be of value in cases that have proved refractory to other treatment or where other therapy has caused unacceptable toxicity.

6.3.1 Nephrotic Syndrome

This clinical syndrome of oedema and hypoalbuminaemia coupled with heavy proteinuria and associated dyslipidaemia is caused by a number of renal pathologies including minimal change nephropathy, focal segmental glomerular sclerosis, membranous nephropathy and mesangial proliferative glomerulonephritis. Minimal change disease often responds well to corticosteroid with or without cyclophosphamide, but ciclosporin is also effective and can be used in cases where a remission can only be maintained with unacceptable levels of steroid treatment or where relapses are frequent (Niaudet 1994; Bargman 1999). Combination treatment using ciclosporin and corticosteroids can be of value in focal segmental glomerulonephritis (Cattran et al. 1999). There are few data on the role of ciclosporin in treating nephrotic syndrome of other causes (Muirhead 1999).

6.3.2 Rheumatoid Arthritis

Rheumatoid arthritis is a serious chronic systemic inflammatory disorder characterised by a deforming symmetrical erosive polyarthritis that may be associated with a number of extra-articular complications which include vasculitis, interstitial pneumonitis, mononeuritis multiplex and Sjögren's syndrome. Treatment involves the use of anti-inflammatory drugs plus disease-modifying agents and corticosteroids. Ciclosporin is effective but is regarded as a second-line agent because of the potential for renal toxicity (Berg et al. 1986; Dougados et al. 1988; Forre 1994; Panayi and Tugwell 1997). Tacrolimus also has a disease-modifying effect (Furst et al. 2002). In refractory cases, ciclosporin has been used in combination with other disease-modifying drugs (Tugwell et al. 1995; van den Borne et al. 1998).

6.3.3 Dermatological Disorders

CNIs are also effective in treating a number of dermatological disorders that are mediated by the cellular components of the adaptive immune system. Systemically administered ciclosporin has been used in the treatment of psoriasis (Ruzicka 1996) and atopic dermatitis (Sowden et al. 1991). However, long-term use is limited by nephrotoxicity. Systemically administered tacrolimus is effective in the treatment of psoriasis with a similar risk of nephrotoxicity (Jegasothy et al. 1992; The European FK 506 Multicentre Psoriasis Study Group 1996).

Tacrolimus and an analogue, pimecrolimus, penetrate the skin and are available as topical formulations (Marsland and Griffiths 2002; Reynolds and Al-Daraji 2002). Topical tacrolimus is effective in the treatment of atopic eczema (Nghiem et al. 2002), but is not effective in chronic plaque psoriasis (Zonneveld et al. 1998), possibly as a result of insufficient skin penetration. The systemic absorption of topically administered tacrolimus or pimecrolimus is low and the levels observed are considerably lower than those used in transplantation.

6.3.4 Other Conditions

Ciclosporin has been investigated as a treatment for a number of other autoimmune conditions where it has not been found to have a major role either because of limited efficacy or nephrotoxicity. Ciclosporin is active against uveitis (Nussenblatt et al. 1985) but because of problems with nephrotoxicity (Palestine et al. 1986; Austin et al. 1989) it is usually reserved for cases which are refractory to other therapy or severe bilateral sight-threatening uveitis (Walton et al. 1998).

Type 1 diabetes is an autoimmune disease. Ciclosporin has been found to increase the frequency and duration of early remission of disease but has not been found to alter the long-term outcome or need for insulin therapy (The Canadian-European Randomized Control Trial Group 1988).

Ciclosporin has been used in the treatment of acute severe ulcerative colitis that has failed to respond to high-dose corticosteroid therapy. However, these patients are usually referred for colectomy because remission may only be short term and because of the risk of nephrotoxicity (McCormack et al. 2002). Ciclosporin may have a role as a corticosteroid-sparing agent in patients with chronic ulcerative colitis (Actis et al. 1999).

7 Toxicity

7.1 General Effect of Immunosuppression

Pharmacological immunosuppression is not specific for the response to the transplanted organ or the disease under treatment. Therefore patients receiving immunosuppressive treatment are at increased risk of infection and of certain types of malignancy (Fishman and Rubin 1998; Penn 2000; Euvrard et al. 2003). Calcineurin-inhibitors principally affect the adaptive immune response of T cells and leave the innate immune system intact. Therefore conditions such as chronic viral infection that are particularly controlled by T cell responses would be expected to be increased in patients receiving CNIs (Cohen 2000; Banner 2003). However, because CNIs are used in combination with other immunosuppressive agents, their selective effect on the immune system is lost and a wide spectrum of infections may be encountered (Kahan 1989; Fishman and Rubin 1998).

7.2 Specific Toxicity

Although the calcineurin-inhibitors are potent immunosuppressive agents, their clinical use is limited by their toxicity. The commonest serious and dose-limiting problem is nephrotoxicity. A large number of other side effects can also occur. There are some differences between the toxicity of ciclosporin and tacrolimus (Table 2).

Table 2 Comparison of the toxicity of ciclosporin and tacrolimus

	Ciclosporin	Tacrolimus
Nephrotoxicity	++	++
Hypertension	++	+
Neurotoxicity	+	++
Glucose intolerance and diabetes mellitus	+	++
Hyperlipidaemia	++	+
Gingival hypertrophy	++	–
Hypertrichosis	+	–
Alopecia	–	+
Hyperuricaemia and gout	+	+
Hyperkalaemia and hypomagnesaemia	+	+
Liver dysfunction	+/–	+/–
Gastrointestinal symptoms	+	+
Pancreatitis	+	+
Haemolytic-uraemic syndrome/TTP	+	+
Gynaecomastia	+	+

Reproduced with permission from Banner and Lyster (2003).

7.3 Nephrotoxicity

The toxic effect of the CNIs on the kidney is well known, although the mechanisms underlying it are not completely understood (Wilkinson and Cohen 1999). It had been aptly described as the Achilles' heal of this form of therapy (Bennett et al. 1996). Data from kidney transplantation are difficult to interpret because the function of the renal allograft is influenced both by alloimmune injury and drug toxicity. Additionally, the renal allograft may be somewhat protected by virtue of the sympathetic denervation that accompanies transplantation. CNI nephrotoxicity has been clearly recognised after heart, liver and lung transplantation, as well as in patients being treated for autoimmune disease (Zaltzman et al. 1992; Falkenhain et al. 1996). Toxicity occurs in an acute, potentially reversible, and a chronic irreversible form. Less commonly, the kidney can be affected by the thrombotic microangiopathy. The mechanisms underlying the nephrotoxicity appear to be closely linked to the inhibition of calcineurin and are therefore similar for ciclosporin and tacrolimus.

7.3.1 Acute Toxicity

This syndrome is associated with renal vasoconstriction and functional changes that are potentially reversible. The mechanisms involved include alterations in endothelial function and in the regulation of vasomotor tone. Vasoconstriction leads to a reduction in glomerular filtration rate, salt and water retention and associated hypertension. Experimentally, endothelin appears to play a role in the vasoconstriction (Kon et al. 1995). Additionally, there is increased activity in the renin angiotensin system with increased numbers of granules in the juxtaglomerular apparatus and in hilar arterioles as well as increased expression of angiotensin type 1 receptors (Tufro-McReddie et al. 1993). Ciclosporin inhibits endothelial nitric oxide production (Andoh et al. 1997; Assis et al. 1997), endothelium-dependent vasodilation and the release of prostacyclin (Bossaller et al. 1989). Furthermore, it increases sympathetic-mediated vasoconstriction (Scherrer et al. 1990).

7.3.2 Chronic Toxicity

Chronic toxicity is associated with structural changes in the kidney. In native kidneys there is global and segmental glomerular sclerosis. Surviving glomeruli tend to be larger, indicating hyperfiltration, and proteinuria is common (Myers et al. 1988; Bertani et al. 1991). The changes are believed to be secondary to afferent arteriolar vasculopathy leading to glomerular ischaemia and tubular atrophy. The tubular atrophy and fibrosis follow a striped pattern which begins in the medullar and progresses into the medullary rays of the cortex (Palestine et al. 1986; Andoh and Bennett 1998) (Fig. 5). This anatomy means that the extent of fibrosis is often underestimated by a percutaneous core renal biopsy.

During the early phase of the disease, the correlation between the degree of structural damage and functional changes is poor (Myers et al. 1988; Ruggenenti et al. 1994; Hartmann et al. 1996). Renal function, measured by creatinine and creatinine clearance, may be stable, but structural changes may be occurring with progressive tubulointerstitial injury. This dissociation between functional and structural changes can also be demonstrated in animal models (Elzinga et al. 1993).

The renin angiotensin system appears to play a role in renal fibrosis (Kon et al. 1995; Shihab et al. 1996). Ciclosporin increases the expression of transforming growth factor-β and may thereby increase the fibrotic response to injury (Khanna et al. 1997). Tacrolimus may not have this effect (Mohamed

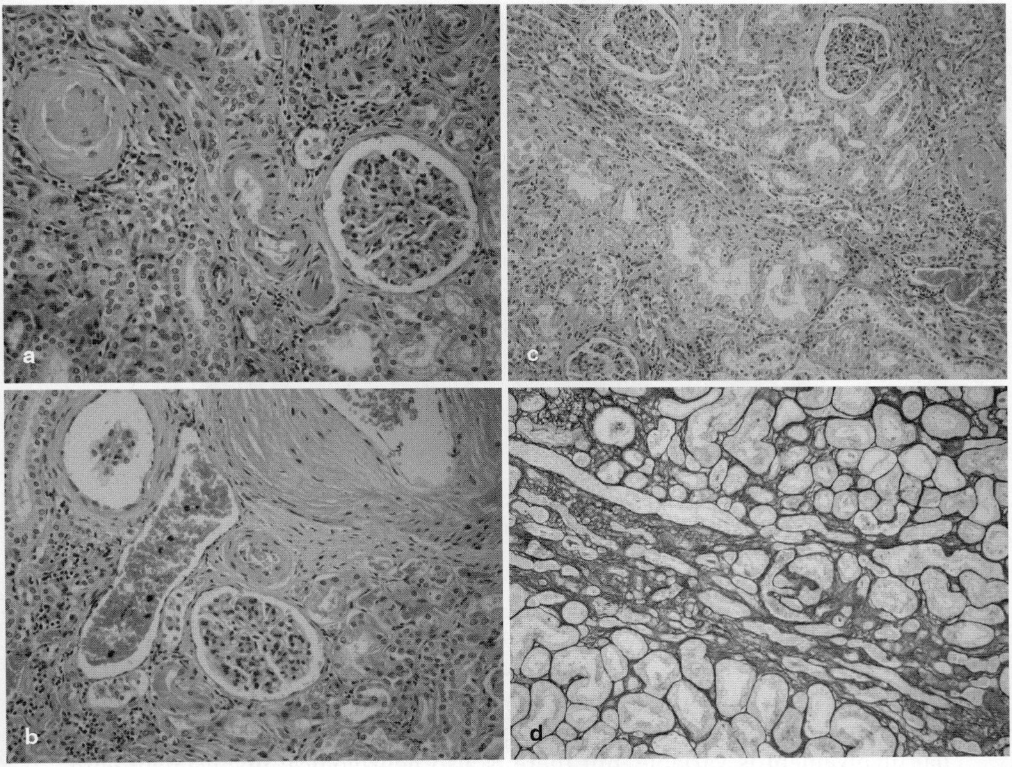

Fig. 5a–d Renal histopathological changes of chronic ciclosporin nephropathy. **a** Hyaline arteriolosclerosis, focal interstitial nephritis, glomerulosclerosis and focal tubular atrophy. **b** Intimal sclerosis of an artery, interstitial nephritis, hyaline arteriolosclerosis. **c** Focal tubular atrophy with striped fibrosis, glomerulosclerosis and hypertrophied tubules to either side of the zone of atrophy. **d** Striped fibrosis: atrophied tubules enmeshed in dense reticulin (corresponding to the zone of striped fibrosis in panel **c**). Staining: Grocott's silver methenamine. (Photomicrographs courtesy of Dr. Margaret Burke)

et al. 2000). It has therefore been argued that tacrolimus might be associated with less nephrotoxicity than ciclosporin; however, this has not been established in clinical studies, and another study failed to confirm this mechanistic difference between the two agents (Khanna et al. 1999).

7.3.3 Thrombotic Microangiopathy

The two uncommon related thrombotic microangiopathic (TMA) syndromes, haemolytic–uraemic syndrome (HUS) and thrombotic thrombocytopoenic purpura (TTP), are associated with infection, drug toxicity and pregnancy, and occur in familial and idiopathic forms. Both have been asso-

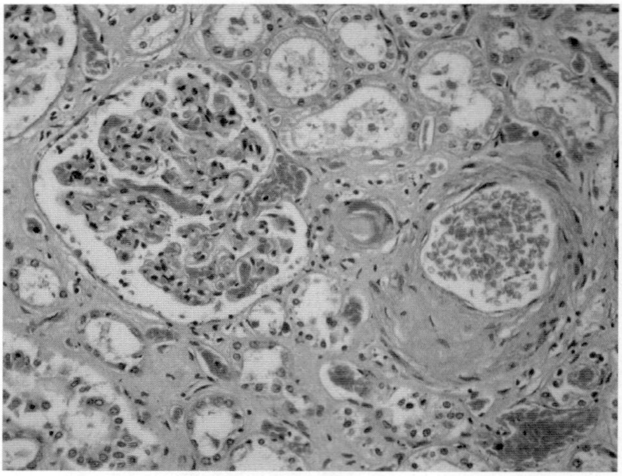

Fig. 6 Renal histopathological changes associated with the haemolytic–uraemic syndrome. Fibrinoid necrosis in an afferent arteriole and hyaline intimal thickening of an artery. (Photomicrograph courtesy of Dr. Margaret Burke)

ciated with the use of calcineurin inhibitors. The clinical features of HUS are a non-immune (Coombs' test-negative) microangiopathic haemolytic anaemia, acute renal failure and thrombocytopaenia associated with microvascular thrombosis (Fig. 6). TTP shares these features, although the degree of renal involvement is variable, but there is also neurological involvement with changing symptoms and signs. There may be a fever in either HUS or TTP. The pathophysiology of both conditions is believed to be injury to the endothelium and its consequent dysfunction (Kulzer and Wanner 1998).

CNI-associated TMA has mainly been observed in renal transplantation but has also occurred after other types of organ and bone-marrow transplantation (Ichihashi et al. 1992; Verburgh et al. 1996; Young et al. 1996). The risk may be increased by high levels of drug exposure and in some cases a cofactor such as infection can be demonstrated. An idiosyncratic susceptibility may be involved, but cases have been described where the CNI has been successfully used again once the TMA has resolved (Guella et al. 1998).

7.3.4 Management

Acute nephrotoxicity is dose-related and normally reversible by either dose reduction or, where possible, withdrawal of the CNI.

Chronic toxicity is more difficult to detect at an early stage because of the poor correlation between functional and structural changes. The use of lower doses of CNIs (combining them with other immunosuppressive drugs) and the use of dose adjustments based on the measurement of blood levels has led to some reduction in toxicity, but the effect has not been dramatic and the problem remains unsolved (Myers et al. 1988). This may be partly because of the limitations of therapeutic drug monitoring (see below), but is also because of the close link between the calcineurin inhibition that is necessary for immunosuppression and the nephrotoxicity. This means that there is no true 'therapeutic range' where efficacy can be achieved while simultaneously avoiding toxicity. Furthermore, it appears that patients vary in their susceptibility to nephrotoxicity, although the basis of this variation is currently unknown.

Tight control of blood pressure is important in slowing any progression, as is the treatment of proteinuria, usually by use of an angiotensin-converting enzyme inhibitor or a receptor blocker (Joint National Committee 1997; Mackenzie and Brenner 1998). CNI dose reduction, and when feasible, withdrawal may be of value. However, this increases the risk of allograft rejection. Additionally, some patients with established chronic nephrotoxicity may show a progressive fall in renal function despite withdrawal of the drug (Myers et al. 1988; Zietse et al. 1994). Those who develop end-stage renal failure need renal replacement therapy and will subsequently require renal transplantation (Kuo et al. 1995).

The treatment of CNI-associated thrombotic microangiopathy consists of withdrawing the drug, plasma exchange (Bell et al. 1991; Onundarson et al. 1992) and supportive therapy, including renal replacement therapy if necessary. The role of anticoagulation and antiplatelet agents is unproved. The prognosis of CNI-associated TMA is uncertain because information about this syndrome is based on case reports and no large case series has been published.

7.4 Hypertension

Hypertension is common after all forms of organ transplantation and this is related to the use of CNIs. The mechanisms linking the CNIs to hypertension are not fully understood but, as previously described, they interfere with vascular control mechanisms and increase activity of the sympathetic nervous system. In addition, the nephrotoxicity caused by these drugs may play a role in the development of hypertension (Andoh et al. 2001; Johnson et al. 2002). Interestingly, tacrolimus appears to be less potent in inducing hypertension than ciclosporin, although the reason for this remains unknown (Taylor et al. 1999).

7.5 Dyslipidaemia

Dyslipidaemia is common in organ transplant recipients. Its prevalence is partly due to the frequent use of corticosteroids, but the CNIs also play a role (Ballantyne et al. 1989; Kasiske et al. 1991). Once again, tacrolimus has a less adverse effect than ciclosporin (Taylor et al. 1999). Treatment of hypercholesterolemia must take into account the interaction between the CNIs and statins (Ballantyne 2000; Christians et al. 2002).

7.6 Diabetes Mellitus

Diabetes mellitus is another common complication of organ transplantation that is related to corticosteroid use. The CNIs are a further contributory factor (Roth et al. 1989). There is evidence that the risk is greater with tacrolimus (Pirsch et al. 1997), although this finding has not been confirmed in all studies (Taylor et al. 1999).

7.7 Neurotoxicity

Acute neurotoxicity is an infrequent but severe complication of CNI use. The syndrome consists of headache, visual impairment (including cortical blindness), generalised tonic–clonic seizures, encephalopathy and coma; less frequently dysphasia and cerebellar symptoms can occur. Paraesthesia and a burning sensation in hands and feet occasionally occur. Headache, visual disturbance and seizures are the most common manifestations. The syndrome occurs within days or weeks of starting CNI treatment. It is more common in children and adolescents than in adults and is also commoner after liver and bone marrow transplantation than after other types of organ transplant. Additional features that are sometimes present include hypertension, hypomagnesaemia and hypocholesterolaemia (de Groen et al. 1987; Jarosz et al. 1997; Derici et al. 2001). Hypocholesterolaemia and activity of the P-glycoprotein transport system may affect the concentration of the CNI present within the central nervous system (CNS) (de Groen et al. 1987; Sugawara et al. 1990; Schinkel et al. 1995). The differential diagnosis includes other CNS drug toxicity, opportunistic CNS infection (meningitis and encephalitis) and TTP. Typical findings on magnetic resonance imaging (MRI) are cerebral oedema within the cortex and juxtacortical white matter of the posterior cerebral hemispheres (Schwartz et al. 1995; Coley et al. 1999). The pathogenesis of the condition is not fully understood but seems to be related to CNI vascular toxicity. The MRI findings closely resemble those seen in hypertensive encephalopathy (Schwartz et al. 1995). The oedema appears to be vasogenic in nature rather than reflecting ischaemia (Coley et al. 1999). Treatment involves control of any hypertension, reduction in the dose and blood level of the CNI, together with supportive measures, including the use of analgesics and anticonvulsants as necessary. The clinical and MRI findings are usually completely reversible, although irreversible injury has been reported (Esterl et al. 1996). Recurrence of this acute syndrome during long-term therapy is unusual.

Chronic neurological side effects of the CNIs include headaches, which are often migrainous in nature, and tremor (Plosker and Foster 2000). The headaches can occasionally can be severe but usually respond to conventional therapy (Maghrabi and Bohlega 1998). Hand tremor can be troublesome in some patients but usually improves as the dose of CNI is reduced with increasing time after transplantation.

7.8 Other Side Effects

These are summarised in Table 2 and have been described in detail elsewhere (Kahan 1989; Plosker and Foster 2000). Cosmetic side effects of ciclosporin which can be troublesome for women (hirsutism) and children (hirsutism and coarsening of the facial features during growth) are absent with tacrolimus. In addition, the troublesome gingival hypertrophy which happens in some patients on ciclosporin does not occur with tacrolimus.

8 Pharmacokinetics and Drug Interactions

Both ciclosporin and tacrolimus are substrates for the cytochrome P450 (CP450) family of enzymes and P-glycoprotein (Pgp) transport system. This leads to a complex set of pharmacokinetic considerations that are important for the effective clinical use of the CNIs (Fig. 7). CP450 and Pgp underlie many of the drug interactions that occur between the CNIs and other therapeutic agents (Christians et al. 2002).

An orally administered CNI is subject to countertransport by P-glycoprotein and metabolism by CP450 3A within the wall of the small intestine (Lin et al. 1999). Variation in the activity of these two systems results in differences between individuals in the oral bioavailability of the CNIs (Ptachcinski et al. 1986; Shimada et al. 1994). Furthermore, the administration of drugs or other substances that alter Pgp and CP450 activity can radically change bioavailability of the CNIs (Christians et al. 2002). Following absorption, the CNI is subject to further 'first pass' metabolism by CP450 in the liver before reaching the systemic circulation (Karanam et al. 1994; Bekersky et al. 2001). The resulting metabolites are primarily excreted in the bile, although

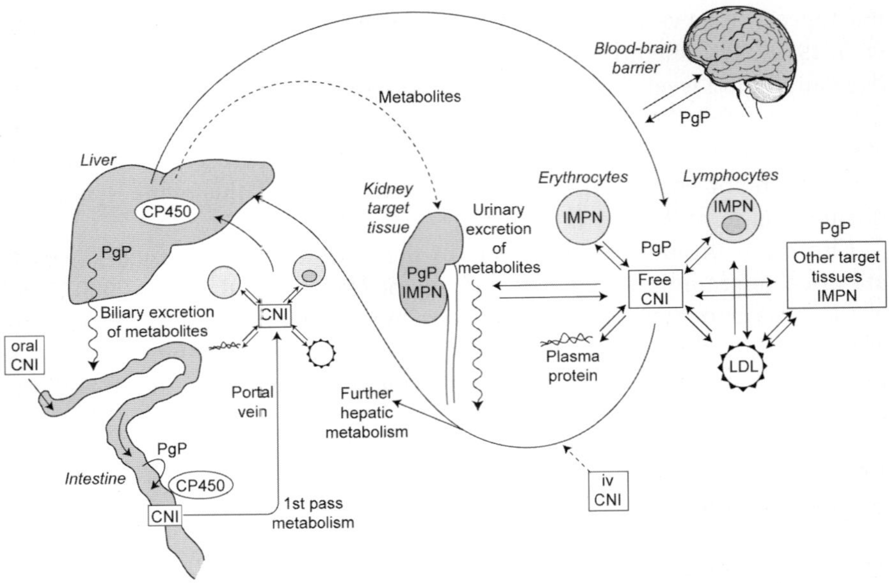

Fig. 7 Pharmacokinetics of the calcineurin inhibitors. When orally administered, the calcineurin inhibitors (*CNIs*) ciclosporin and tacrolimus are subject to countertransport by P-glycoprotein (*Pgp*) and metabolism by cytochrome P450 (*CP450*) 3A in the wall of the intestine. Absorbed drug passes via the portal circulation to the liver where further metabolism occurs. The majority of CNI metabolites are excreted via the bile. In health, only a small fraction of metabolites are excreted in the urine. Drug that has entered the systemic circulation is metabolised during recirculation through the liver. In the blood, only a small fraction of these drugs exist in the free state; most is bound to cells (both drugs) and plasma proteins (tacrolimus) or lipoproteins including low-density lipoprotein or LDL (ciclosporin). Free drug appears to enter cells via diffusion although, in the case of ciclosporin, entry may also be facilitated by lipoproteins. Intracellular drug is subject to countertransport by Pgp. The drug concentration measured during TDM is the total concentration in blood, which differs from the concentration at the intracellular site of action. Intravenously administered drug (*iv CNI*) bypasses 'first pass' metabolism in the intestine and liver so that the dose required intravenously will be lower than the oral dose

a small proportion will also enter the circulation. This proportion will increase in the face of hepatic dysfunction (Bekersky et al. 2001). Although the CNIs are metabolised in the liver, dose adjustment may be needed if a patient develops renal failure; this is probably because uraemia can interfere with hepatic metabolism by down-regulation of hepatic CP450 (Pichette and Leblond 2003).

When administered intravenously, the CNI will avoid 'first pass' metabolism in the intestine and liver and directly enter the systemic circulation. Consequently, the intravenous dose required to achieve any blood concentration is considerably lower than the oral dose (Banner and Lyster 2003). For the same reason, intersubject variation is reduced during intravenous administration. Drug elimination from the systemic circulation is principally via hepatic metabolism.

Only a very small proportion of CNI is unbound in the blood. The majority is associated with its binding proteins within red cells or bound to plasma proteins (in the case of tacrolimus) or lipoproteins (in the case of ciclosporin) (de Groen 1988; Nagase, Iwasaki et al. 1994). Therefore, the total concentration of CNI in blood that is measured during therapeutic drug monitoring (TDM) will be influenced by the haematocrit and the concentration of proteins and lipoproteins in the blood. Additionally, activity of the P-glycoprotein transporter will determine the relationship of the intra- to extracellular drug concentration (Chaudhary et al. 1992). Thus, there is no simple and predictable relationship between the measured concentration and that present at the drug's site of action (Sugawara et al. 1990; Sandborn et al. 1995; Schinkel et al. 1995). Further details of the pharmacokinetics of the CNIs are available elsewhere (Ptachcinski et al. 1985; Kahan 1989; Venkataramanan et al. 1995; Christians et al. 2002).

Most pharmacokinetic drug interactions involving the CNIs are based on either induction or inhibition of CP450 3A (Banner and Lyster 2003). However it is now becoming clear that alterations in Pgp activity contribute to these effects and, by altering the distribution of drug within compartments, Pgp can alter the drug's immunosuppressive and toxic effect independently from the total concentration measured in blood (Christians et al. 2002). Recognised interactions where other drugs alter the metabolism of the CNIs are summarised in Table 3; interactions where the CNIs make an important alteration to the metabolism of other drugs are listed in Table 4. Pharmacodynamic interactions also occur where the toxicity of other drugs are additive or synergistic with those of the CNIs. Since nephrotoxicity is a frequent problem during therapy with the CNIs, other drugs with a potential for nephrotoxicity are a particular problem, e.g. non-steroidal antiinflammatory agents (Sheiner et al. 1994), amphotericin (Kennedy et al. 1983) and foscarnet (Morales et al. 1995). Physicians prescribing for patients being treated with CNIs should be cognisant of such interactions and be able to anticipate their potential effect. Close observation and dose adjustment with the help of TDM is required to prevent an unnecessary loss of efficacy or toxicity (Banner and Lyster 2003). Pharmacodynamic interactions must be assessed by clinical observation and laboratory surveillance of the function of the relevant organ (e.g. serum creatinine and creatinine clearance in the case of nephrotoxicity).

Factors that influence the distribution of the drug will alter the relationship between the total concentration measured in the blood and the concentration at the site of action within the cell. Drugs that affect the P-glycoprotein transport system may influence this equilibrium and, thus, could alter the drug's concentration at its intracellular site of action, thereby modulating both immunosuppressive efficacy and toxicity (Sugawara et al. 1990;

Table 3 Some important pharmacokinetic interactions affecting the bioavailability of ciclosporin and/or tacrolimus

Drugs that increase CNI metabolism and reduce bioavailability	
Rifampicin (rifampin)	Furlan et al. 1995; Hebert et al. 1999
Anticonvulsants	
Phenytoin	Keown et al. 1984
Phenobarbitone	Carstensen et al. 1986
Carbamazepine	Cooney et al. 1995
Prednisolone	Undre and Schafer 1998
St John's Wort	Barone et al. 2000
Drugs that reduce CNI metabolism and increase bioavailability	
Imidazole antifungal agents	
Fluconazole	Assan et al. 1994; Manez et al. 1994
Itraconazole	Banerjee et al. 2001
Ketoconazole	Keogh et al. 1995; Floren et al. 1997
Clotrimazole	Mieles et al. 1991
Macrolide antibiotics	
Erythromycin	Ptachcinski et al. 1985; Furlan et al. 1995
Clarithromycin	Wolter et al. 1994; Sadaba et al. 1998
Sirolimus (effect on tacrolimus only)	Lampen et al. 1995; Lampen et al. 1998
Chloramphenicol	Schulman et al. 1998
Calcium channel blockers	
Verapamil	Robson et al. 1988
Diltiazem	Valantine et al. 1992; Hebert and Lam 1999
Methylprednisolone	Klintmalm and Sawe 1984
Theophylline	Boubenider et al. 2000
HIV protease inhibitors	Sheikh et al. 1999; Schvarcz et al. 2000
Danazol	Shapiro et al. 1993; Passfall et al. 1994
Grapefruit juice	Edwards et al. 1999

Table 4 Pharmacokinetic interactions where the CNIs make an important change to the metabolism of another drug

Reduced metabolism and increased drug effect	
HMG-CoA reductase inhibitors (statins)	
Lovastatin	Norman et al. 1988; Olbricht et al. 1997
Simvastatin	Weise and Possidente 2000
Atorvastatin	Jacobsen et al. 2000
TOR inhibitors	
Sirolimus	Christians and Sewing 1993; Kaplan et al. 1998; Lampen et al. 1998
Everolimus	Crowe et al. 1999; Jacobsen et al. 2001
Divergent effects	
Mycophenolate/mycophenolic acid	
Metabolism increased by ciclosporin	Smak Gregoor et al. 1999
Metabolism decreased/unchanged by tacrolimus	Zucker et al. 1997; Christians et al. 2002

Chaudhary et al. 1992; Schinkel et al. 1995). This may be one of the mechanisms underlying the increase in ciclosporin nephrotoxicity that has been observed when it has been used in combination with sirolimus or everolimus (Andoh et al. 1996; Kahan 2000; MacDonald 2001; Eisen et al. 2003). However, this explanation remains a hypothesis, and one study conducted in primates failed to demonstrate an altered distribution of ciclosporin when it was co-administered with everolimus (Serkova et al. 2000).

9
Therapeutic Drug Monitoring

Methods of monitoring therapy with CNIs have become an established part of clinical practice. The reasons for this include: the potential for serious toxicity with CNIs, the importance of maintaining immunosuppressive efficacy to protect life-sustaining organ transplants, the wide range of variation between individuals in bioavailability and metabolism together with the large number of drug interactions between CNIs and other agents (Banner and Lyster 2003). Guidelines have been developed for the monitoring of ciclosporin and tacrolimus (Jusko et al. 1995; Oellerich et al. 1995).

The concentrations measured are those in whole blood and are only indirectly related to those at the site of action (Holt et al. 1994; Oellerich et al. 1998). Consequently, the TDM results must be interpreted in the light of other information including efficacy (lack of acute rejection) and toxicity (particularly renal). A 'therapeutic range' derived for a population of patients is usually wide and individuals with drug levels within the range may still experience rejection, nephrotoxicity or opportunistic infection. The appropriate therapeutic range will be determined by a series of factors including the time after transplantation and the other immunosuppressive agents being used (Banner and Lyster 2003). The choice of a specific 'target range' for an individual patient remains a matter of clinical judgement which must be based on the patient's individual response.

'Trough levels' are usually measured just before the administration of the next dose. In the case of tacrolimus, such levels appear to be a good measure of systemic exposure to the drug (Jusko et al. 1995). However, the correlation of trough level to exposure is less good in the case of the Neoral formulation of ciclosporin, and alternatives, such as the blood concentration 2 h after an oral dose, appear to be better measures (Levy 2001).

10 Conclusion

The discovery of the CNIs was one of the most significant advances in clinical organ transplantation. Ciclosporin improved the results of renal transplantation and transformed other types of organ transplantation from experimental to standard therapy. Both the newer agent tacrolimus and the reformulation of ciclosporin, Neoral, have advantages over the original Sandimmun formulation. The problem of nephrotoxicity remains a factor that limits the use of these drugs outside the field of transplantation. Furthermore, chronic renal failure has become one of the long-term complications of organ transplantation. Attempts to ameliorate this problem through careful drug monitoring and by using reduced doses of these drugs in combination with other immunosuppressive agents have only been partially successful. New approaches to long-term immunosuppressive treatment are needed and alternative drugs are becoming available. The potent immunosuppressive effect of the CNIs means that they are likely to continue to play a role in the initial period after transplantation when the risk of rejection is greatest, but it seems likely that they may be replaced with other drugs in the long-term maintenance treatment of patients with allografts.

References

Abe M, Sawada T, et al (2003) C4d deposition in peritubular capillary and alloantibody in the allografted kidney suffering severe acute rejection. Clin Transplant 17 Suppl 10:14–9

Actis GC, Volpes R, et al (1999) Oral microemulsion cyclosporin to reduce steroids rapidly in chronic active ulcerative colitis. Eur J Gastroenterol Hepatol 11:905–8

Adams DO, Hamilton TA (1984) The cell biology of macrophage activation. Annu Rev Immunol 2:283–318

Amenabar JJ, Gomez-Ullate P, et al (1998) A randomized trial comparing cyclosporine and steroids with cyclosporine, azathioprine, and steroids in cadaveric renal transplantation. Transplantation 65:653–61

Andoh TF, Bennett WM (1998) Chronic cyclosporine nephrotoxicity. Curr Opin Nephrol Hypertens 7:265–70

Andoh TF, Lindsley J, et al (1996) Synergistic effects of cyclosporine and rapamycin in a chronic nephrotoxicity model. Transplantation 62:311–6

Andoh TF, Gardner MP, et al (1997) Protective effects of dietary L-arginine supplementation on chronic cyclosporine nephrotoxicity. Transplantation 64:1236–40

Andoh TF, Johnson RJ, et al (2001) Subclinical renal injury induced by transient cyclosporine exposure is associated with salt-sensitive hypertension. Am J Transplant 1:222–7

Arranz R, Conde E, et al (2002) CsA-based post-graft immunosuppression: the main factor for improving outcome of allografted patients with acquired aplastic anemia. A retrospective survey by the Spanish Group of Hematopoietic Transplantation. Bone Marrow Transplant 29:205–11

Assan R, Fredj G, et al (1994) FK 506/fluconazole interaction enhances FK 506 nephrotoxicity. Diabete Metab 20:49–52
Assis SM, Monteiro JL, et al (1997) L-Arginine and allopurinol protect against cyclosporine nephrotoxicity. Transplantation 63:1070–3
Austin HA, Palestine AG 3rd , et al (1989) Evolution of ciclosporin nephrotoxicity in patients treated for autoimmune uveitis. Am J Nephrol 9:392–402
Azimzadeh A, C Schroeder, et al (2003) Xenotransplantation. In: Banner NR, Polak JM, Yacoub MH (eds) Lung transplantation. Cambridge University Press, Cambridge, pp 374–385
Ballantyne CM (2000) Statins after cardiac transplantation: which statin, what dose, and how low should we go? J Heart Lung Transplant 19:515–7
Ballantyne CM, Podet EJ, et al (1989) Effects of cyclosporine therapy on plasma lipoprotein levels. Jama 262:53–6
Banerjee R, Leaver N, et al (2001) Coadministration of itraconazole and tacrolimus after thoracic organ transplantation. Transplant Proc 33:1600–2
Banner NR (2003) Cytomegalovirus infection. In: Banner NR, Polak JM, Yacoub MH (eds) Lung transplantation. Cambridge University Press, Cambridge, pp 261–273
Banner NR, Lyster H (2003) Pharmacological immunosuppression. In: Banner NR, Polak JM, Yacoub MH (eds) Lung transplantation. Cambridge University Press, Cambridge, pp 205–42
Bargman JM (1999) Management of minimal lesion glomerulonephritis: evidence-based recommendations. Kidney Int Suppl 70:S3–16
Barone GW, Gurley BJ, et al (2000) Drug interaction between St. John's wort and cyclosporine. Ann Pharmacother 34:1013–6
Bekersky I, Dressler D, et al (2001) Comparative tacrolimus pharmacokinetics: normal versus mildly hepatically impaired subjects. J Clin Pharmacol 41:628–35
Bell WR, Braine HG, et al (1991) Improved survival in thrombotic thrombocytopenic purpura-hemolytic uremic syndrome. Clinical experience in 108 patients. N Engl J Med 325:398–403
Bennett WM, DeMattos A, et al (1996) Chronic cyclosporine nephropathy: the Achilles' heel of immunosuppressive therapy. Kidney Int 50:1089–100
Berg KJ, Forre O, et al (1986) Side effects of cyclosporin A treatment in patients with rheumatoid arthritis. Kidney Int 29:1180–7
Bertani T, Ferrazzi P, et al (1991) Nature and extent of glomerular injury induced by cyclosporine in heart transplant patients. Kidney Int 40:243–50
Bierer BE, Mattila PS, et al (1990) Two distinct signal transmission pathways in T lymphocytes are inhibited by complexes formed between an immunophilin and either FK506 or rapamycin. Proc Natl Acad Sci U S A 87:9231–5
Bittner HB, Dunitz J, et al (2001) Hyperacute rejection in single lung transplantation—case report of successful management by means of plasmapheresis and antithymocyte globulin treatment. Transplantation 71:649–51
Bohmig GA, Regele H, et al (2001) C4d-positive acute humoral renal allograft rejection: effective treatment by immunoadsorption. J Am Soc Nephrol 12:2482–9
Borel JF, Feurer C, et al (1976) Biological effects of cyclosporin A: a new antilymphocytic agent. Agents Actions 6:468–75
Bossaller C, Forstermann U, et al (1989) Ciclosporin A inhibits endothelium-dependent vasodilatation and vascular prostacyclin production. Eur J Pharmacol 165:165–9
Boubenider S, Vincent I, et al (2000) Interaction between theophylline and tacrolimus in a renal transplant patient. Nephrol Dial Transplant 15:1066–8

Calne RY, White DJ, et al (1978) Cyclosporin A in patients receiving renal allografts from cadaver donors. Lancet 2:1323–7

Canadian-European Randomized Control Trial Group (1988) Cyclosporin-induced remission of IDDM after early intervention. Association of 1 yr of cyclosporin treatment with enhanced insulin secretion. The Canadian-European Randomized Control Trial Group. Diabetes 37:1574–82

Canadian Multicenter Transplant Study Group (1983) A randomized clinical trial of cyclosporine in cadaveric renal transplantation. N Engl J Med 309:809–15

Canadian Multicentre Transplant Study Group (1986) A randomized clinical trial of cyclosporine in cadaveric renal transplantation. Analysis at three years. N Engl J Med 314:1219–25

Carstensen H, Jacobsen N, et al (1986) Interaction between cyclosporin A and phenobarbitone. Br J Clin Pharmacol 21:550–1

Cattran DC, Appel GB, et al (1999) A randomized trial of cyclosporine in patients with steroid-resistant focal segmental glomerulosclerosis. North America Nephrotic Syndrome Study Group. Kidney Int 56:2220–6

Chaudhary PM, Mechetner EB, et al (1992) Expression and activity of the multidrug resistance P-glycoprotein in human peripheral blood lymphocytes. Blood 80:2735–9

Cherry R, Nielsen H, et al (1992) Vascular (humoral) rejection in human cardiac allograft biopsies: relation to circulating anti-HLA antibodies. J Heart Lung Transplant 11:24–9; discussion 30

Choi JK, Kearns J, et al (1999) Hyperacute rejection of a pulmonary allograft. Immediate clinical and pathologic findings. Am J Respir Crit Care Med 160:1015–8

Christians U, Sewing KF (1993) Cyclosporin metabolism in transplant patients. Pharmacol Ther 57:291–345

Christians U, Jacobsen W, et al (2002) Mechanisms of clinically relevant drug interactions associated with tacrolimus. Clin Pharmacokinet 41:813–51

Cohen JI (2000) Epstein-Barr virus infection. N Engl J Med 343:481–92

Coley SC, Porter DA, et al (1999) Quantitative MR diffusion mapping and cyclosporine-induced neurotoxicity. AJNR Am J Neuroradiol 20:1507–10

Cooney GF, Mochon M, et al (1995) Effects of carbamazepine on cyclosporine metabolism in pediatric renal transplant recipients. Pharmacotherapy 15:353–6

Crabtree GR (1989) Contingent genetic regulatory events in T lymphocyte activation. Science 243:355–61

Crowe A, Bruelisauer A, et al (1999) Absorption and intestinal metabolism of SDZ-RAD and rapamycin in rats. Drug Metab Dispos 27:627–32

de Groen PC (1988) Cyclosporine, low-density lipoprotein, and cholesterol. Mayo Clin Proc 63:1012–21

de Groen PC, Aksamit AJ, et al (1987) Central nervous system toxicity after liver transplantation. The role of cyclosporine and cholesterol. N Engl J Med 317:861–6

Deeg HJ, Storb R, et al (1985) Cyclosporine as prophylaxis for graft-versus-host disease: a randomized study in patients undergoing marrow transplantation for acute nonlymphoblastic leukemia. Blood 65:1325–34

Derici U, Arinsoy T, et al (2001) Cyclosporine-A induced neurotoxicity after renal transplantation. Acta Neurol Belg 101:124–7

Doody DP, Stenger KS, et al (1994) Immunologically nonspecific mechanisms of tissue destruction in the rejection of skin grafts. J Exp Med 179:1645–52

Dougados M, Awada H, et al (1988) Cyclosporin in rheumatoid arthritis: a double blind, placebo controlled study in 52 patients. Ann Rheum Dis 47:127–33

Dumont FJ, Staruch MJ, et al (1990) Distinct mechanisms of suppression of murine T cell activation by the related macrolides FK-506 and rapamycin. J Immunol 144:251–8

Durand DB, Shaw JP, et al (1988) Characterization of antigen receptor response elements within the interleukin-2 enhancer. Mol Cell Biol 8:1715–24

Edwards DJ, Fitzsimmons ME, et al (1999) 6',7'-Dihydroxybergamottin in grapefruit juice and Seville orange juice: effects on cyclosporine disposition, enterocyte CYP3A4, and P-glycoprotein. Clin Pharmacol Ther 65:237–44

Eisen HJ, Hobbs RE, et al (2001) Safety, tolerability, and efficacy of cyclosporine microemulsion in heart transplant recipients: a randomized, multicenter, double-blind comparison with the oil-based formulation of cyclosporine—results at 24 months after transplantation. Transplantation 71:70–8

Eisen HJ, Tuzcu EM, et al (2003) Everolimus for the prevention of allograft rejection and vasculopathy in cardiac-transplant recipients. N Engl J Med 349:847–58

Ellis CN, Gorsulowsky DC, et al (1986) Cyclosporine improves psoriasis in a double-blind study. Jama 256:3110–6

Elzinga LW, Rosen S, et al (1993) Dissociation of glomerular filtration rate from tubulointerstitial fibrosis in experimental chronic cyclosporine nephropathy: role of sodium intake. J Am Soc Nephrol 4:214–21

Emery RW, Cork R, et al (1986) Cardiac transplant patient at one year. Cyclosporine vs conventional immunosuppression. Chest 90:29–33

Esterl RM Jr, Gupta N, et al (1996) Permanent blindness after cyclosporine neurotoxicity in a kidney-pancreas transplant recipient. Clin Neuropharmacol 19:259–66

European FK506 Multicentre Liver Study Group (1994) Randomised trial comparing tacrolimus (FK506) and cyclosporin in prevention of liver allograft rejection. Lancet 344:423–8

European multicentre trial group (1983) Cyclosporin in cadaveric renal transplantation: one-year follow-up of a multicentre trial. Lancet 2:986–9

European Mycophenolate Mofetil Cooperative Study Group (1995) Placebo-controlled study of mycophenolate mofetil combined with cyclosporin and corticosteroids for prevention of acute rejection. European Mycophenolate Mofetil Cooperative Study Group. Lancet 345:1321–5

Euvrard S, Kanitakis J, et al (2003) Skin cancers after organ transplantation. N Engl J Med 348:1681–91

Falkenhain ME, Cosio FG, et al (1996) Progressive histologic injury in kidneys from heart and liver transplant recipients receiving cyclosporine. Transplantation 62:364–70

Feucht HE (2003) Complement C4d in graft capillaries—the missing link in the recognition of humoral alloreactivity. Am J Transplant 3:646–52

Fierro L, Lund PE, et al (2000) Comparison of the activation of the Ca2+ release-activated Ca2+ current ICRAC to InsP3 in Jurkat T-lymphocytes, pulmonary artery endothelia and RBL-1 cells. Pflugers Arch 440:580–7

Fishman JA, Rubin RH (1998) Infection in organ-transplant recipients. N Engl J Med 338:1741–51

Floren LC, Bekersky I, et al (1997) Tacrolimus oral bioavailability doubles with coadministration of ketoconazole. Clin Pharmacol Ther 62:41–9

Forre O (1994) Radiologic evidence of disease modification in rheumatoid arthritis patients treated with cyclosporine. Results of a 48-week multicenter study comparing low-dose cyclosporine with placebo. Norwegian Arthritis Study Group. Arthritis Rheum 37:1506–12

Forre O, Bjerkhoel F, et al (1987) An open, controlled, randomized comparison of cyclosporine and azathioprine in the treatment of rheumatoid arthritis: a preliminary report. Arthritis Rheum 30:88–92

Fruman DA, Klee CB, et al (1992) Calcineurin phosphatase activity in T lymphocytes is inhibited by FK 506 and cyclosporin A. Proc Natl Acad Sci U S A 89:3686–90

Furlan V, Perello L, et al (1995) Interactions between FK506 and rifampicin or erythromycin in pediatric liver recipients. Transplantation 59:1217–8

Furst DE, Saag K, et al (2002) Efficacy of tacrolimus in rheumatoid arthritis patients who have been treated unsuccessfully with methotrexate: a six-month, double-blind, randomized, dose-ranging study. Arthritis Rheum 46:2020–8

Garrett HE Jr, Groshart K, et al (2002) Treatment of humoral rejection with rituximab. Ann Thorac Surg 74:1240–2

Grandtnerova B, Javorsky P, et al (1995) Treatment of acute humoral rejection in kidney transplantation with plasmapheresis. Transplant Proc 27:934–5

Guella A, Daoud M, et al (1998) Uneventful re-treatment with cyclosporin in two cases of cyclosporin-induced haemolytic uraemic syndrome. Nephrol Dial Transplant 13:1864–5

Hall BM, Dorsch S, et al (1978) The cellular basis of allograft rejection in vivo. I. The cellular requirements for first-set rejection of heart grafts. J Exp Med 148:878–89

Handschumacher RE, Harding MW, et al (1984) Cyclophilin: a specific cytosolic binding protein for cyclosporin A. Science 226:544–7

Hartmann A, Andereassen AK, et al (1996) Five years' follow-up of renal glomerular and tubular functions in heart transplant recipients. J Heart Lung Transplant 15:972–9

Hebert MF, Lam AY (1999) Diltiazem increases tacrolimus concentrations. Ann Pharmacother 33:680–2

Hebert MF, Fisher RM, et al (1999) Effects of rifampin on tacrolimus pharmacokinetics in healthy volunteers. J Clin Pharmacol 39:91–6

Hickstein H, Korten G, et al (1998) Protein A immunoadsorption (i.a.) in renal transplantation patients with vascular rejection. Transfus Sci 19 Suppl:53–7

Holt DW, Johnston A, et al (1994) Methodological and clinical aspects of cyclosporin monitoring: report of the Association of Clinical Biochemists task force. Ann Clin Biochem 31:420–46

Hornick P, Lechler R (1997) Direct and indirect pathways of alloantigen recognition: relevance to acute and chronic allograft rejection. Nephrol Dial Transplant 12:1806–10

Hows JM, Palmer S, et al (1982) Use of cyclosporin A in allogeneic bone marrow transplantation for severe aplastic anemia. Transplantation 33:382–6

Hubbard MJ, Klee CB (1989) Functional domain structure of calcineurin A: mapping by limited proteolysis. Biochemistry 28:1868–74

Ichihashi T, Naoe T, et al (1992) Haemolytic uraemic syndrome during FK506 therapy. Lancet 340:60–1

Jacobsen W, Kuhn B, et al (2000) Lactonization is the critical first step in the disposition of the 3-hydroxy-3-methylglutaryl-CoA reductase inhibitor atorvastatin. Drug Metab Dispos 28:1369–78

Jacobsen W, Serkova N, et al (2001) Comparison of the in vitro metabolism of the macrolide immunosuppressants sirolimus and RAD. Transplant Proc 33:514–5

Jarosz JM, Howlett DC, et al (1997) Cyclosporine-related reversible posterior leukoencephalopathy: MRI. Neuroradiology 39:711–5

Jegasothy BV, Ackerman CD, et al (1992) Tacrolimus (FK 506)—a new therapeutic agent for severe recalcitrant psoriasis. Arch Dermatol 128:781–5

Jensik SC (1998) Tacrolimus (FK 506) in kidney transplantation: three-year survival results of the US multicenter, randomized, comparative trial. FK 506 Kidney Transplant Study Group. Transplant Proc 30:1216–8

Johnson RJ, Herrera J-Acosta, et al (2002) Subtle acquired renal injury as a mechanism of salt-sensitive hypertension. N Engl J Med 346:913–23

Joint National Committee (1997) The sixth report of the Joint National Committee on prevention, detection, evaluation, and treatment of high blood pressure. Arch Intern Med 157:2413–46

June CH, Ledbetter JA, et al (1987) T cell proliferation involving the CD28 pathway is associated with cyclosporine-resistant interleukin 2 gene expression. Mol Cell Biol 7:4472–81

Jusko WJ, Piekoszewski W, et al (1995) Pharmacokinetics of tacrolimus in liver transplant patients. Clin Pharmacol Ther 57:281–90

Jusko WJ, Thomson AW, et al (1995) Consensus document: therapeutic monitoring of tacrolimus (FK-506). Ther Drug Monit 17:606–14

Kahan BD (1989) Cyclosporine. N Engl J Med 321:1725–38

Kahan BD (2000) Efficacy of sirolimus compared with azathioprine for reduction of acute renal allograft rejection: a randomised multicentre study. The Rapamune US Study Group. Lancet 356:194–202

Kahan BD, Welsh M , et al (1996) Variable oral absorption of cyclosporine. A biopharmaceutical risk factor for chronic renal allograft rejection. Transplantation 62:599–606

Kaplan B, Meier-Kriesche HU , al et (1998) The effects of relative timing of sirolimus and cyclosporine microemulsion formulation coadministration on the pharmacokinetics of each agent. Clin Pharmacol Ther 63:48–53

Karanam BV, Vincent SH, et al (1994) FK 506 metabolism in human liver microsomes: investigation of the involvement of cytochrome P450 isozymes other than CYP3A4. Drug Metab Dispos 22:811–4

Kasiske BL, Tortorice KL, et al (1991) The adverse impact of cyclosporine on serum lipids in renal transplant recipients. Am J Kidney Dis 17:700–7

Kay JE (1989) Inhibitory effects of cyclosporin A on lymphocyte activation. In: Thomson AW (ed) Cyclosporin. Kluwer Academic, Dordrecht, pp 1–23

Kay JE, Benzie CR, et al (1983) Effect of cyclosporin A on lymphocyte activation by the calcium ionophore A23187. Immunology 50:441–6

Kennedy MS, Deeg HJ, et al (1983) Acute renal toxicity with combined use of amphotericin B and cyclosporine after marrow transplantation. Transplantation 35:211–5

Keogh A, Spratt P, et al (1995) Ketoconazole to reduce the need for cyclosporine after cardiac transplantation. N Engl J Med 333:628–33

Keown PA, Laupacis A, et al (1984) Interaction between phenytoin and cyclosporine following organ transplantation. Transplantation 38:304–6

Khanna A, Kapur S, et al (1997) In vivo hyperexpression of transforming growth factor-beta1 in mice: stimulation by cyclosporine. Transplantation 63:1037–9

Khanna A, Cairns V, et al (1999) Tacrolimus induces increased expression of transforming growth factor-beta1 in mammalian lymphoid as well as nonlymphoid cells. Transplantation 67:614–9

Kincaid RL, Martensen TM, et al (1986) Modulation of calcineurin phosphotyrosyl protein phosphatase activity by calmodulin and protease treatment. Biochem Biophys Res Commun 140:320–8

Kino T, Hatanaka H, et al (1987) FK-506, a novel immunosuppressant isolated from a Streptomyces. II. Immunosuppressive effect of FK-506 in vitro. J Antibiot (Tokyo) 40:1256–65

Klee CB, Draetta GF, et al (1988) Calcineurin. Adv Enzymol Relat Areas Mol Biol 61:149–200
Klintmalm G, Sawe J (1984) High dose methylprednisolone increases plasma cyclosporin levels in renal transplant recipients. Lancet 1:731
Knoll GA, Bell RC (1999) Tacrolimus versus cyclosporin for immunosuppression in renal transplantation: meta-analysis of randomised trials. Bmj 318:1104–7
Kon V, Hunley TE, et al (1995) Combined antagonism of endothelin A/B receptors links endothelin to vasoconstriction whereas angiotensin II effects fibrosis. Studies in chronic cyclosporine nephrotoxicity in rats. Transplantation 60:89–95
Kulzer P, Wanner C (1998) Thrombotic microangiopathy: a challenge with uncertain outcome. Nephrol Dial Transplant 13:2154–60
Kumagai N, Benedict SH, et al (1988) Cyclosporin A inhibits initiation but not progression of human T cell proliferation triggered by phorbol esters and calcium ionophores. J Immunol 141:3747–52
Kuo PC, Luikart H, et al (1995) Clinical outcome of interval cadaveric renal transplantation in cardiac allograft recipients. Clin Transplant 9:92–7
Lampen A, Christians U, et al (1995) Metabolism of the immunosuppressant tacrolimus in the small intestine: cytochrome P450, drug interactions, and interindividual variability. Drug Metab Dispos 23:1315–24
Lampen A, Zhang Y, et al (1998) Metabolism and transport of the macrolide immunosuppressant sirolimus in the small intestine. J Pharmacol Exp Ther 285:1104–12
Levy GA (2001) C2 monitoring strategy for optimising cyclosporin immunosuppression from the Neoral formulation. BioDrugs 15:279–90
Lin CS, Boltz RC, et al (1991) FK-506 and cyclosporin A inhibit highly similar signal transduction pathways in human T lymphocytes. Cell Immunol 133:269–84
Lin JH, Chiba M, et al (1999) Is the role of the small intestine in first-pass metabolism overemphasized? Pharmacol Rev 51:135–58
Lindholm A, Kahan BD (1993) Influence of cyclosporine pharmacokinetics, trough concentrations, and AUC monitoring on outcome after kidney transplantation. Clin Pharmacol Ther 54:205–18
Liu J (1993) FK506 and cyclosporin, molecular probes for studying intracellular signal transduction. Immunol Today 14:290–5
Liu J, Farmer Jr JD , et al (1991) Calcineurin is a common target of cyclophilin-cyclosporin A and FKBP-FK506 complexes. Cell 66:807–15
Loh C, Shaw KT, et al (1996) Calcineurin binds the transcription factor NFAT1 and reversibly regulates its activity. J Biol Chem 271:10884–91
Luo C, Shaw KT, et al (1996) Interaction of calcineurin with a domain of the transcription factor NFAT1 that controls nuclear import. Proc Natl Acad Sci U S A 93:8907–12
MacDonald AS (2001) A worldwide, phase III, randomized, controlled, safety and efficacy study of a sirolimus/cyclosporine regimen for prevention of acute rejection in recipients of primary mismatched renal allografts. Transplantation 71:271–80
Mackenzie HS, Brenner BM (1998) Current strategies for retarding progression of renal disease. Am J Kidney Dis 31:161–70
Maghrabi K, Bohlega S (1998) Cyclosporine-induced migraine with severe vomiting causing loss of renal graft. Clin Neurol Neurosurg 100:224–7
Manez R, Martin M, et al (1994) Fluconazole therapy in transplant recipients receiving FK506. Transplantation 57:1521–3
Marsland AM, Griffiths CE (2002) The macrolide immunosuppressants in dermatology: mechanisms of action. Eur J Dermatol 12:618–22

Mayer AD, Dmitrewski J, et al (1997) Multicenter randomized trial comparing tacrolimus (FK506) and cyclosporine in the prevention of renal allograft rejection: a report of the European Tacrolimus Multicenter Renal Study Group. Transplantation 64:436–43

McCormack G, McCormick PA, et al (2002) Cyclosporin therapy in severe ulcerative colitis: is it worth the effort? Dis Colon Rectum 45:1200–5

Mentzer RM Jr, Jahania MS, et al (1998) Tacrolimus as a rescue immunosuppressant after heart and lung transplantation. The U.S. Multicenter FK506 Study Group. Transplantation 65:109–13

Mieles L, Venkataramanan R, et al (1991) Interaction between FK506 and clotrimazole in a liver transplant recipient. Transplantation 52:1086–7

Mohamed MA, Robertson H, et al (2000) TGF-beta expression in renal transplant biopsies: a comparative study between cyclosporin-A and tacrolimus. Transplantation 69:1002–5

Morales JM, Munoz MA, et al (1995) Reversible acute renal failure caused by the combined use of foscarnet and cyclosporin in organ transplanted patients. Nephrol Dial Transplant 10:882–3

Muirhead N (1999) Management of idiopathic membranous nephropathy: evidence-based recommendations. Kidney Int Suppl 70:S47–55

Myers BD, Newton L, et al (1988) Chronic injury of human renal microvessels with low-dose cyclosporine therapy. Transplantation 46:694–703

Myers BD, Sibley R, et al (1988) The long-term course of cyclosporine-associated chronic nephropathy. Kidney Int 33:590–600

Nagase K, Iwasaki K, et al (1994) Distribution and protein binding of FK506, a potent immunosuppressive macrolide lactone, in human blood and its uptake by erythrocytes. J Pharm Pharmacol 46:113–7

Nghiem P, Pearson G, et al (2002) Tacrolimus and pimecrolimus: from clever prokaryotes to inhibiting calcineurin and treating atopic dermatitis. J Am Acad Dermatol 46:228–41

Niaudet P (1994) Treatment of childhood steroid-resistant idiopathic nephrosis with a combination of cyclosporine and prednisone. French Society of Pediatric Nephrology. J Pediatr 125:981–6

Norman DJ, Illingworth DR, et al (1988) Myolysis and acute renal failure in a heart-transplant recipient receiving lovastatin. N Engl J Med 318:46–7

Nussenblatt RB, Palestine AG, et al (1985) Cyclosporine therapy for uveitis: long-term followup. J Ocul Pharmacol 1:369–82

Oellerich M, Armstrong VW, et al (1995) Lake Louise Consensus Conference on cyclosporin monitoring in organ transplantation: report of the consensus panel. Ther Drug Monit 17:642–54

Oellerich M, Armstrong VW, et al (1998) Therapeutic drug monitoring of cyclosporine and tacrolimus. Update on Lake Louise Consensus Conference on cyclosporin and tacrolimus. Clin Biochem 31:309–16

Olbricht C, Wanner C, et al (1997) Accumulation of lovastatin, but not pravastatin, in the blood of cyclosporine-treated kidney graft patients after multiple doses. Clin Pharmacol Ther 62:311–21

Onundarson PT, Rowe JM, et al (1992) Response to plasma exchange and splenectomy in thrombotic thrombocytopenic purpura. A 10-year experience at a single institution. Arch Intern Med 152:791–6

Oyer PE, Stinson EB, et al (1983) Cyclosporine in cardiac transplantation: a 2 1/2 year follow up. Transplant Proc 15:2546–52

Palestine AG, Austin HA 3rd, et al (1986) Renal histopathologic alterations in patients treated with cyclosporine for uveitis. N Engl J Med 314:1293–8

Panayi GS, Tugwell P (1997) The use of cyclosporin A microemulsion in rheumatoid arthritis: conclusions of an international review. Br J Rheumatol 36:808–11

Parekh AB, Fleig A, et al (1997) The store-operated calcium current I(CRAC): nonlinear activation by InsP3 and dissociation from calcium release. Cell 89:973–80

Passfall J, Schuller I, et al (1994) Pharmacokinetics of cyclosporin during administration of danazol. Nephrol Dial Transplant 9:1807–8

Patel R, Terasaki PI (1969) Significance of the positive crossmatch test in kidney transplantation. N Engl J Med 280:735–9

Penn I (2000) Cancers in renal transplant recipients. Adv Ren Replace Ther 7:147–56

Pichette V, Leblond FA (2003) Drug metabolism in chronic renal failure. Curr Drug Metab 4:91–103

Pierson RN, Loyd JE 3rd , et al (2002) Successful management of an ABO-mismatched lung allograft using antigen-specific immunoadsorption, complement inhibition, and immunomodulatory therapy. Transplantation 74:79–84

Pirsch JD, Miller J, et al (1997) A comparison of tacrolimus (FK506) and cyclosporine for immunosuppression after cadaveric renal transplantation. FK506 Kidney Transplant Study Group. Transplantation 63:977–83

Plosker GL, Foster RH (2000) Tacrolimus: a further update of its pharmacology and therapeutic use in the management of organ transplantation. Drugs 59:323–89

Przepiorka D, Ippoliti C, et al (1996) Tacrolimus and minidose methotrexate for prevention of acute graft-versus-host disease after matched unrelated donor marrow transplantation. Blood 88:4383–9

Ptachcinski RJ, Carpenter BJ, et al (1985) Effect of erythromycin on cyclosporine levels. N Engl J Med 313:1416–7

Ptachcinski RJ, Venkataramanan R, et al (1985) Cyclosporine kinetics in renal transplantation. Clin Pharmacol Ther 38:296–300

Ptachcinski RJ, Venkataramanan R, et al (1986) Clinical pharmacokinetics of cyclosporin. Clin Pharmacokinet 11:107–32

Reitz BA, Wallwork JL, et al (1982) Heart-lung transplantation: successful therapy for patients with pulmonary vascular disease. N Engl J Med 306:557–64

Reynolds NJ, Al-Daraji WI (2002) Calcineurin inhibitors and sirolimus: mechanisms of action and applications in dermatology. Clin Exp Dermatol 27:555–61

Robson RA, Fraenkel M, et al (1988) Cyclosporin-verapamil interaction. Br J Clin Pharmacol 25:402–3

Rose ML, Hutchinson IV (2003) Immunological mechanisms of graft injury. In: Banner NR, Polak JM, Yacoub MH (eds) Lung transplantation. Cambridge University Press, Cambridge, pp 185–204

Rosenberg AS, Mizuochi T, et al (1987) Phenotype, specificity, and function of T cell subsets and T cell interactions involved in skin allograft rejection. J Exp Med 165:1296–315

Roth D, Milgrom M, et al (1989) Posttransplant hyperglycemia. Increased incidence in cyclosporine-treated renal allograft recipients. Transplantation 47:278–81

Ruggenenti P, Perico N, et al (1994) Following an initial decline, glomerular filtration rate stabilizes in heart transplant patients on chronic cyclosporine. Am J Kidney Dis 24:549–53

Russell JH, Ley TJ (2002) Lymphocyte-mediated cytotoxicity. Annu Rev Immunol 20:323–70

Ruzicka T (1996) Cyclosporin in less common immune-mediated skin diseases. Br J Dermatol 135:40–2
Sadaba B, Lopez de Ocariz A , et al (1998) Concurrent clarithromycin and cyclosporin A treatment. J Antimicrob Chemother 42:393–5
Sandborn WJ, Lawson GM, et al (1995) Early cellular rejection after orthotopic liver transplantation correlates with low concentrations of FK506 in hepatic tissue. Hepatology 21:70–6
Sawada S, Suzuki G, et al (1987) Novel immunosuppressive agent, FK506. In vitro effects on the cloned T cell activation. J Immunol 139:1797–803
Sayegh MH, Turka LA (1998) The role of T cell costimulatory activation pathways in transplant rejection. N Engl J Med 338:1813–21
Scherrer U, Vissing SF, et al (1990) Cyclosporine-induced sympathetic activation and hypertension after heart transplantation. N Engl J Med 323:693–9
Schinkel AH, Wagenaar E, et al (1995) Absence of the mdr1a P-Glycoprotein in mice affects tissue distribution and pharmacokinetics of dexamethasone, digoxin, and cyclosporin A. J Clin Invest 96:1698–705
Schreiber SL, Crabtree GR (1992) The mechanism of action of cyclosporin A and FK506. Immunol Today 13:136–42
Schulman SL, Shaw LM, et al (1998) Interaction between tacrolimus and chloramphenicol in a renal transplant recipient. Transplantation 65:1397–8
Schvarcz R, Rudbeck G, et al (2000) Interaction between nelfinavir and tacrolimus after orthoptic liver transplantation in a patient coinfected with HIV and hepatitis C virus (HCV). Transplantation 69:2194–5
Schwartz RB, Bravo SM, et al (1995) Cyclosporine neurotoxicity and its relationship to hypertensive encephalopathy: CT and MR findings in 16 cases. AJR Am J Roentgenol 165:627–31
Scornik JC, Zander DS, et al (1999) Susceptibility of lung transplants to preformed donor-specific HLA antibodies as detected by flow cytometry. Transplantation 68:1542–6
Serkova N, Hausen B, et al (2000) Tissue distribution and clinical monitoring of the novel macrolide immunosuppressant SDZ-RAD and its metabolites in monkey lung transplant recipients: interaction with cyclosporine. J Pharmacol Exp Ther 294:323–32
Shapiro R, Venkataramanan R, et al (1993) FK 506 interaction with danazol. Lancet 341:1344–5
Shaw AS, Dustin ML (1997) Making the T cell receptor go the distance: a topological view of T cell activation. Immunity 6:361–9
Shaw JP, Utz PJ, et al (1988) Identification of a putative regulator of early T cell activation genes. Science 241:202–5
Shaw KT, Ho AM, et al (1995) Immunosuppressive drugs prevent a rapid dephosphorylation of transcription factor NFAT1 in stimulated immune cells. Proc Natl Acad Sci U S A 92:11205–9
Sheikh AM, Wolf DC, et al (1999) Concomitant human immunodeficiency virus protease inhibitor therapy markedly reduces tacrolimus metabolism and increases blood levels. Transplantation 68:307–9
Sheiner PA, Mor E, et al (1994) Acute renal failure associated with the use of ibuprofen in two liver transplant recipients on FK506. Transplantation 57:1132–3
Shihab FS, Andoh TF, et al (1996) Role of transforming growth factor-beta 1 in experimental chronic cyclosporine nephropathy. Kidney Int 49:1141–51
Shimada T, Yamazaki H, et al (1994) Interindividual variations in human liver cytochrome P-450 enzymes involved in the oxidation of drugs, carcinogens and toxic

chemicals: studies with liver microsomes of 30 Japanese and 30 Caucasians. J Pharmacol Exp Ther 270:414–23
Siekierka JJ, Hung SH, et al (1989) A cytosolic binding protein for the immunosuppressant FK506 has peptidyl-prolyl isomerase activity but is distinct from cyclophilin. Nature 341:755–7
Sigal NH, Dumont F, et al (1991) Is cyclophilin involved in the immunosuppressive and nephrotoxic mechanism of action of cyclosporin A? J Exp Med 173:619–28
Smak Gregoor PJ, van Gelder T, et al (1999) Mycophenolic acid plasma concentrations in kidney allograft recipients with or without cyclosporin: a cross-sectional study. Nephrol Dial Transplant 14:706–8
Smith JD, Danskine AJ, et al (1993) The effect of panel reactive antibodies and the donor specific crossmatch on graft survival after heart and heart-lung transplantation. Transpl Immunol 1:60–5
Sowden JM, Berth J-Jones, et al (1991) Double-blind, controlled, crossover study of cyclosporin in adults with severe refractory atopic dermatitis. Lancet 338:137–40
Starzl TE, Klintmalm GB, et al (1981) Liver transplantation with use of cyclosporin A and prednisone. N Engl J Med 305:266–9
Storb R, Deeg HJ, et al (1986) Marrow transplantation for severe aplastic anemia: methotrexate alone compared with a combination of methotrexate and cyclosporine for prevention of acute graft-versus-host disease. Blood 68:119–25
Storb R, Deeg HJ, et al (1988) Cyclosporine v methotrexate for graft-v-host disease prevention in patients given marrow grafts for leukemia: long-term follow-up of three controlled trials. Blood 71:293–8
Sugawara I, Hamada H, et al (1990) Specialized localization of P-glycoprotein recognized by MRK 16 monoclonal antibody in endothelial cells of the brain and the spinal cord. Jpn J Cancer Res 81:727–30
Taylor DO, Barr ML, et al (1999) A randomized, multicenter comparison of tacrolimus and cyclosporine immunosuppressive regimens in cardiac transplantation: decreased hyperlipidemia and hypertension with tacrolimus. J Heart Lung Transplant 18:336–45
Tejani A, Butt K, et al (1987) Cyclosporine-induced remission of relapsing nephrotic syndrome in children. J Pediatr 111:1056–62
Terasaki PI, Kreisler M, et al (1971) Presensitization and kidney transplant failures. Postgrad Med J 47:89–100
The European FK 506 Multicentre Psoriasis Study Group (1996) Systemic tacrolimus (FK 506) is effective for the treatment of psoriasis in a double-blind, placebo-controlled study. The European FK 506 Multicentre Psoriasis Study Group. Arch Dermatol 132:419–23
Tocci MJ, Matkovich DA, et al (1989) The immunosuppressant FK506 selectively inhibits expression of early T cell activation genes. J Immunol 143:718–26
Toronto Lung Transplant Group (1986) Unilateral lung transplantation for pulmonary fibrosis. N Engl J Med 314:1140–5
Tufro-McReddie A, Gomez RA, et al (1993) Effect of CsA on the expression of renin and angiotensin type 1 receptor genes in the rat kidney. Kidney Int 43:615–22
Tugwell P, Pincus T, et al (1995) Combination therapy with cyclosporine and methotrexate in severe rheumatoid arthritis. The Methotrexate-Cyclosporine Combination Study Group. N Engl J Med 333:137–41
U.S. Multicenter FK506 Liver Study (1994) A comparison of tacrolimus (FK 506) and cyclosporine for immunosuppression in liver transplantation. The U.S. Multicenter FK506 Liver Study Group. N Engl J Med 331:1110–5

Undre NA, Schafer A (1998) Factors affecting the pharmacokinetics of tacrolimus in the first year after renal transplantation. European Tacrolimus Multicentre Renal Study Group. Transplant Proc 30:1261–3

Valantine H, Keogh A, et al (1992) Cost containment: coadministration of diltiazem with cyclosporine after heart transplantation. J Heart Lung Transplant 11:1–7; discussion 7–8

van den Borne BE, Landewe RB, et al (1998) Combination therapy in recent onset rheumatoid arthritis: a randomized double blind trial of the addition of low dose cyclosporine to patients treated with low dose chloroquine. J Rheumatol 25:1493–8

Venkataramanan R, Swaminathan A, et al (1995) Clinical pharmacokinetics of tacrolimus. Clin Pharmacokinet 29:404–30

Verburgh CA, Vermeij CG, et al (1996) Haemolytic uraemic syndrome following bone marrow transplantation. Case report and review of the literature. Nephrol Dial Transplant 11:1332–7

Vincenti F, Laskow DA, et al (1996) One-year follow-up of an open-label trial of FK506 for primary kidney transplantation. A report of the U.S. Multicenter FK506 Kidney Transplant Group. Transplantation 61:1576–81

Walton RC, Nussenblatt RB, et al (1998) Cyclosporine therapy for severe sight-threatening uveitis in children and adolescents. Ophthalmology 105:2028–34

Weise WJ, Possidente CJ (2000) Fatal rhabdomyolysis associated with simvastatin in a renal transplant patient. Am J Med 108:351–2

Wiederrecht G, Brizuela L, et al (1991) FKB1 encodes a nonessential FK 506-binding protein in Saccharomyces cerevisiae and contains regions suggesting homology to the cyclophilins. Proc Natl Acad Sci U S A 88:1029–33

Wiederrecht G, Lam E, et al (1993) The mechanism of action of FK-506 and cyclosporin A. Ann N Y Acad Sci 696:9–19

Wilkinson AH, Cohen DJ (1999) Renal failure in the recipients of nonrenal solid organ transplants. J Am Soc Nephrol 10:1136–44

Williams GM, Hume DM, et al (1968) Hyperacute renal-homograft rejection in man. N Engl J Med 279:611–8

Wolter K, Wagner K, et al (1994) Interaction between FK 506 and clarithromycin in a renal transplant patient. Eur J Clin Pharmacol 47:207–8

Woodle ES, Thistlethwaite JR, et al (1996) A multicenter trial of FK506 (tacrolimus) therapy in refractory acute renal allograft rejection. A report of the Tacrolimus Kidney Transplantation Rescue Study Group. Transplantation 62:594–9

Wu A, Buhler LH, et al (2003) ABO-incompatible organ and bone marrow transplantation: current status. Transpl Int 16:291–9

Young BA, Marsh CL, et al (1996) Cyclosporine-associated thrombotic microangiopathy/ hemolytic uremic syndrome following kidney and kidney-pancreas transplantation. Am J Kidney Dis 28:561–71

Zaltzman JS, Pei Y, et al (1992) Cyclosporine nephrotoxicity in lung transplant recipients. Transplantation 54:875–8

Zietse R, Balk AH, et al (1994) Time course of the decline in renal function in cyclosporine-treated heart transplant recipients. Am J Nephrol 14:1–5

Zonneveld IM, Rubins A, et al (1998) Topical tacrolimus is not effective in chronic plaque psoriasis. A pilot study. Arch Dermatol 134:1101–2

Zucker K, Rosen A, et al (1997) Augmentation of mycophenolate mofetil pharmacokinetics in renal transplant patients receiving Prograf and CellCept in combination therapy. Transplant Proc 29:334–6

HEP (2005) 167:361–389

Targeted Therapy with Imatinib: An Exception or a Rule?

D. Fabbro[1] (✉) · G. Fendrich[1] · V. Guez[1] · T. Meyer[1] · P. Furet[1] · J. Mestan[1] · J. D. Griffin[2] · P. W. Manley[1] · S. W. Cowan-Jacob[1]

[1] Department of Oncology, Novartis Pharma Inc., WKL-125.4.10, 4002 Basel, Switzerland
doriano.fabbro@pharma.novartis.com
[2] Dana-Farber Cancer Institute, Boston, MA 02115, USA

Abstract The discovery of STI571, a drug targeting the tyrosine kinase activity of Bcr-Abl, c-Kit, and platelet-derived growth factor receptor (PDGFR), has demonstrated the feasibility of ATP-competitive small-molecule kinase inhibitors for the chronic treatment of molecularly defined cancers. The presence of an activated form of protein kinases targeted by STI571 in various malignancies appears to be mandatory for a clinical response to this drug. This also indicates that a certain subset of molecularly defined tumors depends upon the overactivation of one or more signaling pathways, which can be attacked by targeted therapy. The finding that STI571 resistance is often associated with mutations in the kinase domain unambiguously demonstrates that the targets of STI571 in these tumors are Bcr-Abl, c-Kit, and/or PDGFR. Generation of resistance to STI571 is most likely due to the binding mode of STI571 that stabilizes the inactive conformation of the target kinases. Recent mutational analysis combined with structural biology has provided the basis for the understanding of the binding mode of STI571, and the resistance mechanisms as well as activation mechanisms of Bcr-Abl, c-Kit, and PDGFR. Although this binding mode is key for the exquisite selectivity and tolerability of STI571, it is also its "weakness", because it allows mutations to occur in the target kinase which appear not to affect the normal function of the kinase. Therefore, for an effective long-term cancer therapy with ATP-competitive small-molecule kinase inhibitors, it appears necessary to use more than one kinase inhibitor targeting different conformations of the same kinase, or each inhibitor needs to be aimed at a specific mutant and downstream signaling element.

Keywords Protein kinase inhibitors · STI571 · Gleevec · CML · Abl kinase · c-Kit · PDGFR

Abbreviations

ALL	Acute lymphoblastic leukemia
AML	Acute myelogenous leukemia
Bcr-Abl	Fusion protein arising from the breakpoint cluster region gene (BCR) fusing with the Abelson (ABL) gene
CML	Chronic myeloid leukemia
GIST	Gastrointestinal stromal tumor
CMML	Chronic myelomonocytic leukemia
DFSP	Dermatofibrosarcoma protuberans
HES	Hypereosinophilic syndrome
IC_{50}	Concentration causing 50% inhibition
Kit	Receptor of stem cell factor
PAP	Phenyl-aminopyrimidine
PDGF	Platelet-derived growth factor
PDGFR	Receptor of platelet-derived growth factor
PKC	Protein kinase C family of kinase subtypes involved in mitogenic signaling and metabolic pathways
PTK	Protein tyrosine kinase
RPTK	Receptor PTK

1 Introduction

The increased understanding of signal transduction pathways in normal and neoplastic cells has provided new strategies for therapeutic intervention in cancer (Hanahan and Weinberg 2000). Among the various signaling molecules, protein kinases have become an important group of drug targets, as these enzymes play a central role in diverse biological processes such as cell growth, differentiation, and apoptosis (Pawson and Nash 2000; Schlessinger 2000; Blume-Jensen and Hunter 2001; Manning et al. 2002). The recent development of specific kinase inhibitors blocking the activity of deregulated kinases appears to be sufficient to inhibit growth of tumors in vitro, in vivo, as well as in the clinic (Levitzki 1996; McMahon et al. 1998; Strawn and Shawver 1998; Matter 2001; Traxler et al. 2001).

The approach to design protein kinase inhibitors directed to the ATP binding site suffers from two major obstacles: access to the intracellular targets and selectivity. As there are more than 500 kinase in the human genome, the generation of inhibitors with an absolute specificity is unlikely to be achieved (Manning et al. 2002). The main emphasis, therefore, should be on inhibitors possessing a "reasonable" selectivity profile along with an "acceptable" side effect profile.

The recent discovery and development of STI571 (imatinib mesylate; Glivec; Gleevec; CGP57148), which was approved by the FDA on 10 May 2001 for the treatment of chronic myelogenous leukaemia (CML), shows that targeting the ATP binding of protein kinases for the treatment of various diseases is feasible.

Based upon its clear disease association in CML, the protein tyrosine kinase of Bcr-Abl, represents an ideal drug target to validate the clinical utility of protein kinase inhibitors as therapeutic agents (Daley et al. 1990; Gishizky et al. 1993; Gishizky 1996; Li et al. 1999). In fact, STI571 showed potent in vitro and in vivo antitumor activity in preclinical models that were selective not only for Bcr-Abl, but also for c-Kit and platelet-derived-growth factor receptor (PDGFR) kinases (Druker et al. 1996; Traxler et al 2001; Manley et al. 2002). Initially, clinical trials in CML and acute lymphoblastic leukaemia (ALL) demonstrated that STI571 is well tolerated and showed promising clinical responses (Druker et al. 2001; Kantarjian et al. 2002a,b; Sawyers et al. 2002; Talpaz et al. 2002; O'Brien et al. 2003). Later, clinical responses were reported for STI571 in diseases with deregulated PDGFR activity, like hypereosinophilic syndrome (HES) (Gleich et al. 2002; Cools et al. 2003a,b; Griffin et al. 2003), systemic mastocytosis (Pardanani et al. 2003), gastrointestinal stromal tumors (GIST) (Joensuu et al. 2001; Tuveson et al. 2001; VanOosterom et al. 2001; Heinrich et al. 2002, 2003a) and chronic myelogenous monocytic leukaemia (CMML) (Golub et al. 1994; Ross et al. 1998; Sjöblom et al. 1998; Magnusson et al. 2001; Schwaller et al. 2001; Steer and Cross 2002) or with deregulated c-Kit activity like GIST and/or in acute myelogenous leukaemia (AML) (Heinrich et al. 2002). Although STI571 showed impressive responses in chronic phase of CML, GIST, and HES, many advanced-stage patients develop drug resistance during treatment and subsequently relapse. Although the reasons for STI571 resistance in CML are multiple, mutations in the kinase domain appear to be the predominant mechanism (reviewed in Cowan-Jacob et al. 2004). Such resistance mechanisms might prove to be an issue for protein kinase inhibitors directed towards genetically unstable cells, and therefore a good understanding of this phenomenon is important for the development of new cancer therapies.

2
Development of STI571

Almost two decades ago, when protein kinases were only available as more or less well-characterized biochemical activities obtained following purification from various tissues, there were some ideas in the pharmaceutical industry that protein kinases could represent potential oncology targets. In 1985 at Ciba-Geigy (now Novartis), one medicinal chemistry project was focusing on protein kinase C (PKC). PKC was believed to be involved in tumor promotion and growth modulation, due to the fact that it represented at that time the major receptor for tumor-promoting phorbol esters (Asaoka et al. 1992; Dekker and Parker 1994). The first "lead compound" that was identified to effectively inhibit PKC was the natural compound staurosporine, which was believed, at that time, to be a PKC-specific inhibitor (Tamaoki et al. 1986). A medicinal chemistry program was subsequently initiated around the staurosporine scaffold, which yielded the more selective PKC inhibitor CGP41251 (PKC412; midostaurin) (Fabbro et al. 1999, 2000). Following several iterative rounds of derivatization and optimization on the staurosporines, it was decided to switch to a new scaffold directed towards the ATP-binding site of PKC. Soon a phenyl-amino pyrimidine (PAP) derivative was discovered which had very promising "lead-like" properties and a high potential for chemical derivatization. This PAP derivative, with a 3′-pyridyl group (Fig. 1, element 1), showed potent enzyme and cellular activity against PKC (Zimmermann et al. 1996a,b, 1997). The introduction of a "flag-methyl" group (Fig. 1, element 2) ortho to the anilino-amino group, then led to a so-called control PAP derivative devoid of PKC inhibitory activity. Most importantly, this "control PAP derivative" revealed protein tyrosine kinase activity against Abl, c-Kit, and PDGFR (Zimmermann et al. 1996a,b, 1997, 2001; Buchdunger 2000). It was rapidly recognized that the presence of an amide group on the phenyl ring provided potent inhibitory activity against these tyrosine kinases (Fig. 1, element 3). However, the first series of these Abl, c-Kit, and PDGFR inhibitors showed poor oral bioavailability and low solubility, which was improved by addition of a highly polar, *N*-methylpiper-

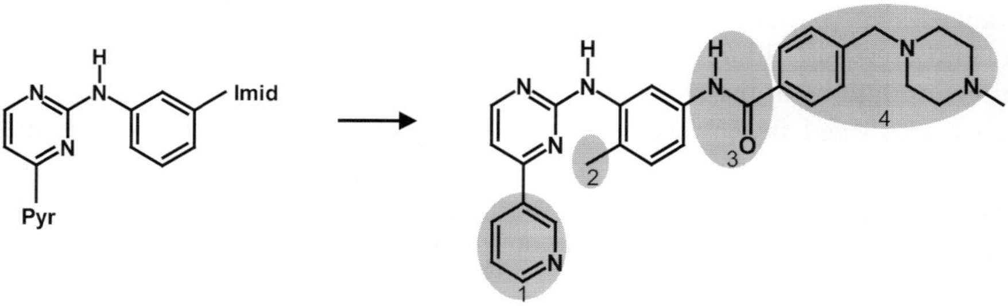

Fig. 1 Lead optimization: from PAP to STI571. An ATP-competitive lead from a smart screen (*left*) inhibited PKC, Abl, and PDGFR at IC_{50} of 1 μM, >10 μM, and >10 μM, respectively. Lead optimization led to STI571 (*right*), an ATP-competitive compound with the core structure of the lead compound, but enhanced cellular activity (*1*), switch of selectivity (loss of PKC inhibition) but inhibition of Abl, PDGFR, and Kit (*2*), potency against tyrosine protein kinases (*3*), and increased solubility and oral bioavailability (*4*)

azine side chain (Fig. 1, element 4). All of these PAP modifications resulted in the methyl piperazine derivative, originally coded CGP57148 and thereafter named STI571 (signal transduction inhibitor 571), imatinib mesylate, Glivec, or Gleevec (Zimmermann et al. 1996a,b, 1997, 2001; Buchdunger 2000).

3 Pharmacological Profile of STI571

3.1 Bcr-Abl (CML)

The hallmark of CML is the Philadelphia (Ph) chromosome, which is detected in virtually all cases of CML and in 20%–30% of cases of all adult ALL (Khouri et al. 1995; Cortes et al. 1996; Gishizky 1996; Warmuth et al. 1999). The majority of patients with CML and a significant fraction of Ph chromosome positive (Ph^+) ALL have one of the three different versions of this Bcr-Abl fusion protein (p185, p210, or p230 kDa), with additional rare cases of chromosomal translocation occurring where the Abl kinase (or Arg, a related Abl gene) (Okuda et al. 2001) comes under the control of yet other proteins (Khouri et al. 1995; Cortes et al. 1996; Gishizky 1996; Warmuth et al. 1999).

In vitro studies using purified enzymes showed that STI571 is an ATP-competitive inhibitor of Abl, Arg, c-Kit, and PDGFR, but is devoid of significant activity against most other kinases (Druker et al. 1996; Traxler et al. 2001; Zimmermann et al. 2001; Fabbro et al. 2002; Manley et al. 2002; Cowan-Jacob et al. 2004). This selectivity profile was also observed in cellular systems, where STI571 showed potent inhibition of autophosphorylation of p210Bcr-Abl (Druker et al. 1996; Carroll et al. 1997), p185Bcr-Abl, and Tel-Abl (Carroll et al.1997), as well as activated c-Kit or PDGFR, with these activities correlating with the inhibition of cell proliferation (Buchdunger et al. 1996, 2000; Carroll et al.1997; Gambacorti-Passerini et al. 1997; Beran et al. 1998; Dan et al. 1998; le Coutre et al. 1999; Heinrich et al. 2000; Fabbro et al. 2002). Bcr-Abl activates multiple signaling pathways, including the Ras-Raf-ERK, JAK-STAT, PI3 K, JNK/SAPK, NF-κB, and c-myc, which are inhibited by STI571 (Sillaber et al. 2000; Sattler and Griffin 2003). STI571 selectively induced apoptosis that is dependent on Stat5-induced up-regulation of Bcl-xL in Bcr-Abl-positive cell lines and primary leukemia cells from Ph^+ CML as well as ALL without affecting Ph chromosome-negative (Ph^-) cells (Horita et al. 2000). In addition, STI571 inhibited the colony formation from peripheral blood and bone marrow from Ph^+ CML patients, with a 92%–98% decrease in Bcr-Abl-positive colonies with little effect on normal hematopoiesis (Carroll et al. 1997; Deininger et al. 1997; Gambacorti-

Passerini et al. 1997; Beran et al. 1998; Dan et al. 1998; Kasper et al. 1999; le Coutre et al. 1999). STI571 also prevented down-regulation of p27 levels in Bcr-Abl expressing cells as this oncogene has been shown to promote cell cycle progression by activating cyclin-dependent kinases (cdk) and down-regulating the cdk inhibitor p27 (Gesbert et al. 2000; Jonuleit et al. 2000).

The finding that expression of Bcr-Abl in mice induces a disease resembling CML provided strong evidence that the Bcr-Abl oncoprotein was one of the major driving factors in the pathophysiology of CML (Daley et al. 1990; Gishizky et al. 1993; Li et al. 1999). The in vitro antiproliferative activity of STI571 was confirmed in animal models using Bcr-Abl-transformed 32D cells in syngeneic mice, while it showed no antitumor activity against tumors derived from v-src transformed 32D cells, compatible with the selectivity profile of the compound (Druker et al. 1996). The in vivo activity of STI571 against Bcr-Abl-driven tumors was confirmed and extended to models employing cells derived from CML patients in blast crisis (Druker et al. 1996; Deininger et al. 1997; Kasper et al. 1999). Oral treatment with STI571 led to the inhibition of p210Bcr-Abl tyrosine phosphorylation correlating with tumor-free survival of the animals, suggesting that a continuous exposure of STI571 was required for optimal anti-leukemic effects (Buchdunger et al. 1996; Druker et al. 1996). STI571 has also been shown to have good oral activity in a murine bone marrow transplantation model using retroviral p210bcr-abl transduction (Wolff and Ilaria 2001).

CML has a triphasic clinical course: a chronic phase, an accelerated phase, and a terminal blast crisis resembling acute leukemia in which myeloid or lymphoblast precursors fail to differentiate. The chronic phase of CML more closely resembles a myeloproliferative disorder rather than a leukemia, as during this phase of the disease the terminal differentiation of cells is normal (Tenen 2003). The defined pathogenic events and the chronic phase of CML, which represents an almost unique "hyperproliferative disease that depends solely on the Bcr-Abl oncoprotein" was key for the impressive clinical responses induced by STI571 in this limited set of cancer patients.

Since the initial phase I dose-escalation study with STI571 in June 1998 with patients that failed therapy with interferon (IFN)-α, the responses in chronic-phase CML to STI571 have been quite durable, although most patients with blast-phase CML or Ph^{+}ALL have developed resistance to STI571 and have relapsed (Druker et al. 2001; Kantarjian et al. 2002a,b; Sawyers et al. 2002; Talpaz et al. 2002; O'Brien et al. 2003). The reasons for this resistance and/or relapse appear to be multiple, but data from recent clinical trials show that half of the relapsed patients carry point mutations in the kinase domain of Bcr-Abl. More than 30 mutations have been identified so far in the Abl kinase domain that renders this enzyme less sensitive to STI571 (reviewed in Cowan-Jacob et al. 2004).

3.2 PDGFR

In addition to inhibiting Bcr-Abl, Abl, Arg, and c-Kit, STI571 also inhibits the PTK of the PDGFR. PDGF has important roles in the regulation of growth and differentiation of various mesenchymal cell types during embryonal development. In the adult, PDGF stimulates wound healing and also regulates the homeostasis of the connective tissue compartment (Heldin et al. 2002). Overactivation of PDGF signaling has been implicated in several disorders, including tumors, atherosclerosis, and fibrotic conditions.

3.2.1 Chronic Myelomonocytic Leukemia

As a consequence of a reciprocal t(5;12) chromosomal translocation, the trans-membrane and the intracellular domains of the PDGFRβ gene are fused to various partners like TEL (ETV6) (Golub et al. 1994), H4/D10S170 (Schwaller et al. 2001), HIP1(Ross et al. 1998) and RAB5 (Magnusson et al. 2001) all of which encode putative oligomerization domains. The resulting constitutive activation of the PDGFRβ kinase generates a myeloproliferative disorder which is characterized by eosinophilic leukemia or CMML (Steer and Cross 2002), a subtype of the myelodysplastic syndrome which may progress to an acute leukemia. STI571 not only inhibited the in vitro proliferation of cells transformed by these oncoproteins (Beran et al. 1998; Sjöblom et al. 1998) but has also displayed antitumor activity in vivo in a bone marrow transplantation model driven by TEL-PDGFRβ (Tomasson et al. 1999). STI571 treatment led to a normalization of eosinophils and peripheral blood cells in CMML patients involving PDGFRβ translocations (Apperley et al. 2002; Magnusson et al. 2002).

3.2.2 Hypereosinophilic Syndrome

HES is characterized by persistent eosinophilia that can result in damage to various organs (Weller and Bubley 1994). Clinical studies with STI571 have reported responses in HES patients that were associated with normalization of eosinophil counts (Gleich et al. 2002, 2003). About 50% of the HES patients with durable responses to STI571 were found to have a FIP1L1-PDGFRα fusion oncogene which harbors a constitutively activated PTK activity (Cools et al. 2003a; Griffin et al. 2003). This oncogenic FIP1L1-PDGFRα was also found in patients with systemic mastocytosis that have been found to respond to the STI571 treatment (Pardanani et al. 2003). Other genetic abnormalities resulting in the activation of a "putative STI571 sensitive protein kinase" are likely to be responsible for the responses observed in FIP1L1-PDGFRα-negative HES patients that have been treated with STI571. Interestingly, one HES patient with FIP1L1-PDGFRα which relapsed

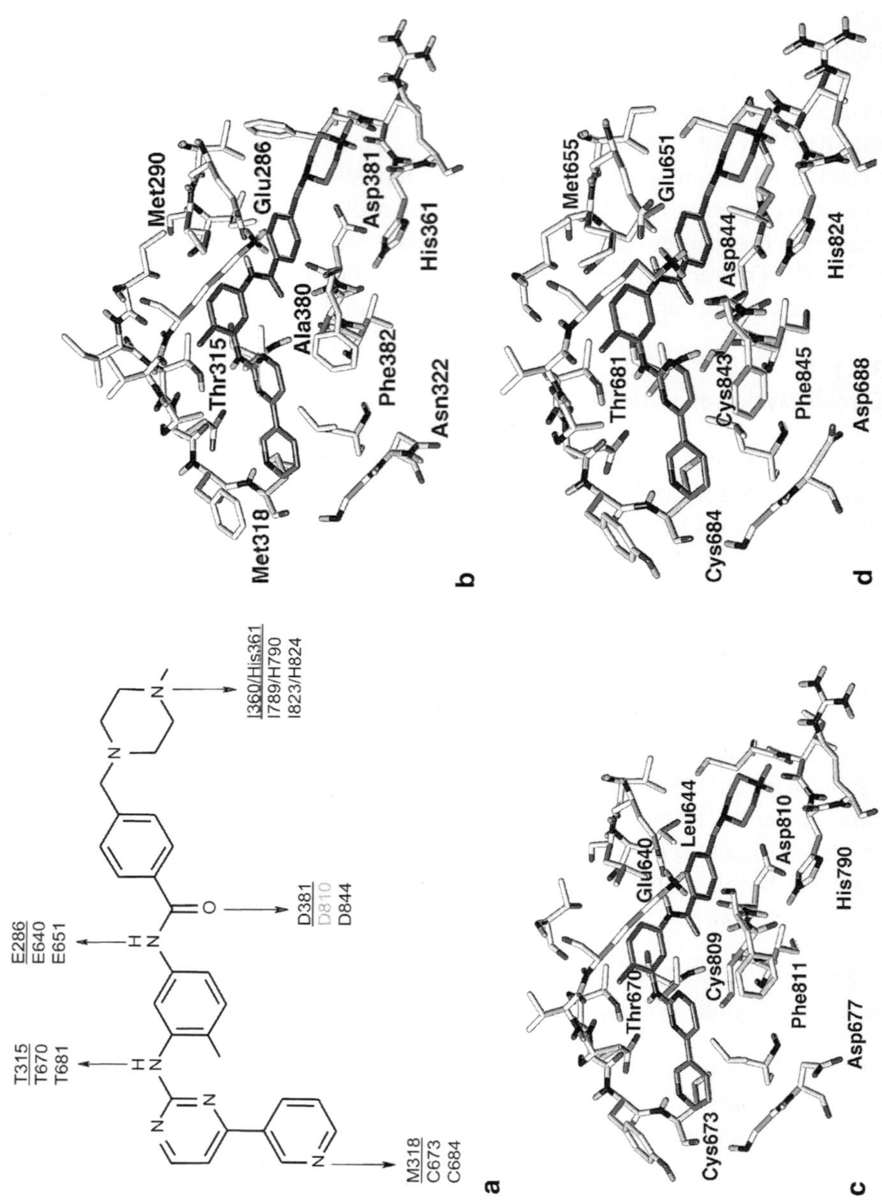

Fig. 2a–d STI571 binding to Abl, Kit, and PDGFRβ. **a** Hydrogen bonds between STI571 and Abl, Kit, or PDGFRβ. Hydrogen bonds between STI571 and the key residues in Abl, Kit, and PDGFRβ involve: anilino-NH of STI571 with *T315* of Abl, T670 of Kit, or T681 of PDGFRβ; amide-NH of STI571 with *E286* of Abl, E640 of Kit, or E651 in PDGFRβ; amide-carbonyl of STI571 with *D381* of Abl, not to D810 of Kit, but possibly to D844 of PDGFRβ (D of the DFG motif N-terminal A-loop); pyridine N of STI571 with to *M318* of Abl, C673 of Kit, or C684 in PDGFRβ; *N*-methylpiperazine of STI571 with *I360/H361* of Abl, I789/H790 of Kit, or I823/H824 in PDGFRβ. **b** STI571 binding to Abl. Details of the

under STI571 treatment was found to contain a T674I point mutation in the kinase domain of the PDGFRα, which corresponded to a STI571-resistant mutation (T315I) found in Bcr-Abl (Cools et al. 2003b; Fig. 2). The STI571-resistant FIP1L1-PDGFRα-T674I mutant was sensitive to another PDGFR inhibitor, PKC412, which targets a different conformation of the PDGFRα kinase domain compared to STI571 (Cools et al. 2003b).

3.2.3
Dermatofibrosarcoma Protuberans

Dermatofibrosarcoma protuberans (DFSP) is a locally invasive soft tissue tumor of the dermis which is characterized by translocations involving chromosomes 17 and 22 resulting in the fusion of the collagen type I α1 chain gene (Col) with PDGF-B chain (Mandahl et al. 1990; Craver et al. 1995; Naeem et al. 1995; Pedeutour et al. 1996; Simon et al. 1997). Expression of Col-PDGF-B in fibroblasts induced PDGFRβ autophosphorylation, morphological transformation, and in vivo tumor growth. Tumor growth of primary DFSP was strongly reduced by STI571 treatment, and the increase in PDGFRβ tyrosine phosphorylation, due to expression of Col-PDGF-B in primary cultures of human DFSP, was decreased by treatment with STI571 (Sjöblom et al. 2001). STI571 had a significant impact with respect to tumor growth and metastatic spread in patients with DFSP (Maki et al. 2002; Rubin et al. 2002).

In summary, these early clinical trials obtained with patients suffering from DFSP, CMML, and HES show the utility of STI571 in tumors that are driven by overactivation of PDGF signaling.

3.2.4
Glioblastomas and Sarcomas

Several observations provide a rationale for clinical studies with STI571 in the treatment of glioblastomas and sarcomas:

1. PDGFRα and PDGF-A chain are co-expressed in tumor cells with increasing frequency in high-grade, as compared to low-grade, tumors (Hermanson et al. 1996).

binding of STI571 (*dark*) to Abl kinase domain (*light*). Hydrogen bonds to (*from left to right*) M318, T315, E286, D381, I360, and H361. The inhibitor has packing interactions with Phe317, Phe382, Val256, Tyr253, Ile313, Lys271, Met290, Val299, Ala380, and Val289. **c** STI571 binding to Kit. Details of the binding of STI571 (*dark*) to Kit kinase domain (*light*). Hydrogen bonds to (*from left to right*) C673, T670, E640, I789, and H790. **d** STI571 binding to PDGFRβ. Details of the binding of STI571 (*dark*) to PDGFRβ kinase domain (*light*). Potential hydrogen bonds to (*from left to right*) C684, T681, E651, D844, I823, and H824

2. Amplified and oncogenic forms of the PDGFRα gene have been found in glioblastomas (Fleming et al. 1992; Kumabe et al. 1992; Clarke and Dirks 2003).
3. Expression of PDGF-B and PDGFRβ are frequently observed in various soft tissue tumors and sarcomas (Smits et al. 1992), while in Ewing family sarcomas the expression of PDGF-C is strongly up regulated (Zwerner and May 2001).
4. Experimental glioblastoma can be inhibited in in vivo animal models by STI571 (Shamah et al. 1993; Strawn et al. 1994; Kilic et al. 2000), while dominant-negative PDGF-C, as well as AG1296, a PDGFR kinase antagonist, inhibited growth of Ewing sarcoma cells in vitro (Zwerner and May 2002).

As mutations causing constitutive activation of PDGFRα have recently been found in a subset of GISTs that were responsive to STI571 (Heinrich et al. 2003a,b), it cannot be excluded that the PDGFR may be mutated more frequently in tumors, including glioblastoma and sarcomas. The utility of PDGF signaling inhibitors like STI571 for the treatment of sarcoma and glioblastoma will only be revealed in carefully controlled clinical trials.

3.2.5 PDGF Signaling in Non-oncological Indications

The rationale for PDGF signaling antagonists in non-oncological indications, such as vasculoproliferative disease, is linked to the upregulation of PDGF signaling in smooth muscle cells derived from atherosclerotic vessels, as well as from neointima lesions (Ross et al. 1990; Tanizawa et al. 1996; Ueda et al. 1996; Rubin et al. 1998). In animal models of restenosis, significant efficacy has been obtained either with neutralizing antibodies to PDGF or with different types of inhibitory approaches (Ferns et al. 1991; Myllarniemi et al. 1997; Sirois et al. 1997; Banai et al. 1998; Bilder et al. 1999; Giese et al. 1999; Hart et al. 1999; Yamasaki et al. 2001; Bilder et al. 2003). Although these studies are encouraging and have indicated that PDGF antagonists might be useful clinically for the treatment of vasculoproliferative diseases, there are some concerns as to whether inhibition of PDGF signaling alone will be sufficiently efficacious for the treatment atherosclerotic lesions that usually involve multiple pathways and cells (Sihvola et al. 1999; Kozaki et al. 2002; Sihvola 2003).

Reduced cell proliferation, collagen synthesis, and deposition have been observed in bleomycin-induced fibrosis with PDGFR antagonists like AG1296 or by expressing a soluble form of the PDGFRβ (Rice et al. 1999; Yoshida et al. 1999). Treatment of glomerulonephritis with either STI571 or PDGF aptamers led to a significant reduction in mesangial cell proliferation and collagen deposition preventing renal scarring, suggesting a therapeutic potential of PDGF antagonists in fibrotic conditions (Floege and Ostendorf 2001).

Last but not least, stimulation of PDGF signaling was found to contribute to increased interstitial fluid pressure (IFP) in experimental tumors (Pietras et al. 2001, 2002, 2003). Therefore, inhibition of PDGF signaling, with STI571 or other antagonists, may be useful in lowering the intra-tumoral fluid pressure, facilitating an increased uptake of cytotoxic drugs in tumors that result in an improved therapeutic efficacy.

3.3 c-Kit

3.3.1 STI571 in GIST

Deregulation of c-Kit has been implicated in the etiology of a number of cancers, including AML, small cell lung cancers, gliomas, testicular cancer, and GIST. The majority of the GIST patients carry mutations in c-Kit that result in constitutively enhanced ligand-independent PTK activity, which appears to play a key role in the pathogenesis of these tumors (Hirota et al. 1998; Lux et al. 2000; Demetri et al. 2002; Heinrich et al. 2002; Joensuu et al. 2002). Since these Kit mutations lead to uncontrolled cell proliferation via permanent stimulation of downstream signaling pathways, it was thought that GIST should prove sensitive to STI571. Although the activity of STI571 against c-Kit was initially of concern, due to the important role that this receptor appears to play in hematopoiesis, the c-Kit-activating mutations associated with GIST supported the use of STI571 in the treatment of this tumor, which is refractory to chemotherapy and radiation. The remarkable clinical activity of STI571 led to its approval in February 2002 for the treatment of advanced GISTs.

Clinical responses in GIST patients following treatment with STI571 appear to be closely associated with the presence of activating c-Kit mutations, as patients expressing wild-type Kit had a significantly lower response (Heinrich et al. 2003a,b). In the subset of patients that expressed wild-type c-Kit and responded to STI571 treatment, activating mutations in the PDGFRα have been found. These clinical trials demonstrated for the first time the presence of naturally occurring mutated forms of PDGFRα. The mutational status of PDGFRα could explain response and sensitivity to imatinib in GISTs lacking c-Kit mutations, because mutations in c-Kit and in PDGFRα appear to be mutually exclusive.

Although STI571 is an effective therapy in GIST with an impressive response rate of 62% after 15 months of treatment (Demetri et al. 2002; Joensuu et al. 2002), relapses have been observed in up to 20% of patients. It seems very likely that one of the underlying mechanisms for this STI571 resistance will be the emergence of clones carrying point-mutations in the kinase domain of c-Kit, in close analogy to the resistance induced in Bcr-Abl by STI571 in CML.

3.3.2 STI571 Binding to c-Kit and PDGFR

An understanding of the molecular interactions at the atomic level between STI571 and Abl was key to understand the binding mode between STI571 and the inactive conformation of c-Kit (Manley et al. 2002). Six hydrogen-bonding interactions between STI571 and c-Kit, which are found in the STI571-Abl structure, were suggested by homology modeling, and five of these were recently confirmed by analysis of the crystal structure of a complex between c-Kit and STI571 (Jacob et al. unpublished) (Fig. 2). The predicted amide-C=O interaction with D810 of the DFG motif does not occur due to a very slight twist of STI571 in binding to c-Kit compared to Abl. Assuming a similar auto-inhibitory conformation as in Abl and c-Kit, these H-bonds are also believed to be important interactions between STI571 and PDGFRβ (in PDGFRα the residues interacting with STI571 are identical) (Fig. 2).

The interactions comprise:

1. Anilino-NH with T670 (T315 in Abl and T681 in PDGFRβ).
2. Amide-NH with E640 (E286 in Abl and E651 in PDGFRβ).
3. Amide-C=O with D810 of the DFG motif does not occur in c-Kit (occurs in Abl with D381, and possibly in PDGFRβ with D844).
4. Pyridine-N with C673 (M318 in Abl and C684 in PDGFRβ).
5. *N*-methylpiperazine with I360 and H361 (I789/H790in Abl and I823/H824 in PDGFRβ).

Interestingly, STI571 is inactive against the activating mutations found in systemic mastocytosis, seminoma, and AML that affect position D816 (Heinrich et al. 2002). Mutations in D816, which lies four amino acids beyond the DFG motif in the A-loop, appear to disfavor the auto-inhibitory conformation of the A-loop such that STI571 does not bind.

4 Resistance to STI571

4.1 Kinase Domain Mutations

STI571 resistance may be caused by up-regulation of the Bcr-Abl, by STI571 efflux mechanisms, and/or plasma binding to α-1 acidic glycoprotein

(Gambacorti-Passerini et al. 2000, 2002, 2003; Mahon et al. 2000; Weisberg and Griffin 2000; Hughes et al. 2002; Jørgensen et al. 2002; le Coutre et al. 2003). However, the predominant mechanism of resistance appears to be due to mutations in the kinase domain of Bcr-Abl, which renders the kinase less sensitive to STI571 inhibition. More than 30 single missense mutations have been found in relapsed CML patients (Kuwazuru et al. 1990; Griffin 2000; Mahon et al. 2000; Gambacorti-Passerini et al. 2000, 2002, 2003; Weisberg and Griffin 2000; Barthe et al. 2001; Gorre et al. 2001a,b; Hochhaus et al. 2001, 2002, 2003; Al-Ali et al. 2002; Branford et al. 2002, 2003; Hofmann et al. 2002a; Hughes et al. 2002; Kreil et al. 2002; le Coutre et al. 2002; Leguay et al. 2002; Roche-Lestienne et al. 2002; von Bubnoff et al. 2002; Hochhaus 2003), some patients possess multiple cell populations with different Bcr-Abl mutations, and at least one patient has been observed to have two mutations in the same Bcr-Abl molecule (Shah et al. 2002).

Structural studies have provided evidence for the binding mode of STI571 to Abl and have revealed how point mutations identified in relapsed patients can lead to resistance (Schindler et al. 2000; Hantschel et al. 2003; Nagar et al. 2002, 2003; Cowan-Jacob et al. 2004). The structure of the catalytic domain of Abl complexed to STI571 (or a close analog thereof) showed that the Abl-kinase adopts a so-called auto-inhibited or inactive conformation (Xu et al.1999; Schindler et al. 2000; Manley et al. 2002; Nagar et al. 2002, 2003; Hantschel et al. 2003). The main feature of this binding mode is that the A-loop, which controls the catalytic activity of kinases, adopts a self-inhibitory conformation by imitating the bound substrate. This binding mode probably accounts for the relatively high selectivity of STI571, but at the same time allows mutations to occur which lower the affinity to STI571 without affecting the kinase activity or ATP-binding affinities (Shah et al. 2002; Cowan-Jacob et al. 2004).

Although various mutations display varying degrees of STI571 resistance, the affinities for ATP for the various mutant forms of recombinant Abl were similar to the wt-Abl kinase (Shah et al. 2002; Cowan-Jacob et al. 2004). The most common mutants in Ph^+ leukemias are E255K/V, T315I, and M351T, with G250E, Q252H/R, Y253H/F, F317L, and E355G being less frequent, while mutants most resistant to STI571 are T315I, G250E, E255K and Y253H. The mutations appear to pre-exist and may not to occur due to drug exposure (Shah et al. 2002; Branford et al. 2003). While most of the mutations that lead to STI571 resistance result in the destabilization of the auto-inhibited conformation of the Abl kinase domain, the Y253F/H, T315I, F317L, F359V, and F382L mutations directly affect the binding to STI571 (Shah et al. 2002; Cowan-Jacob et al. 2004). The mutations cluster in the following regions of the Abl kinase (Fig. 3):

- *The hinge region.* It connects the N-terminal with the C-terminal lobe and harbors the T315I mutant, which is one of the most resistant to STI571. This

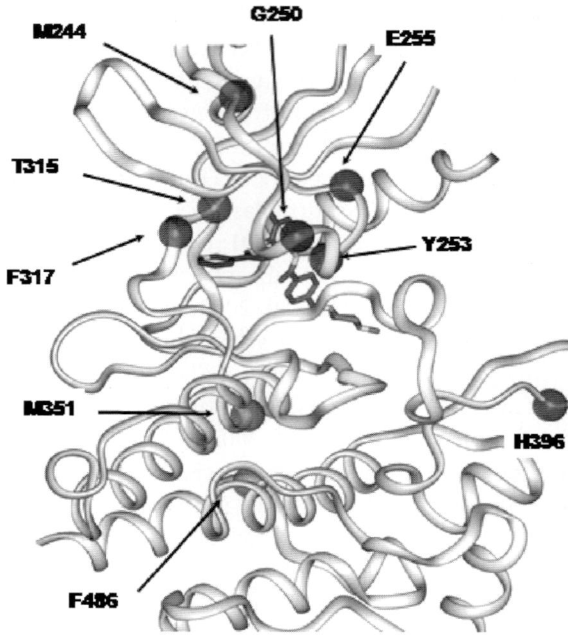

Fig. 3 STI571-resistant mutations in the Abl kinase domain. Locations of the main STI571-resistant mutations on the structure of Abl kinase in complex with STI571s. The IC_{50} (*in parentheses*) concentrations were determined in vitro with the recombinant versions of the Abl kinase that was used for crystallization: wtAbl (0.18 uM); single mutations in the ATP binding (T315I: >10 uM; F317L: 0.40 uM); G-loop (E255K: >10 uM; Y253H: >10 uM; G250E: 1.6 uM; E258G: 1.3 uM); A-loop (H369P: 0.90 uM); Distant Muts (M244 V: 0.68 μM; M351T: 0.30 μM; F486S: 0.87 μM; M244V: 0.68 μM)

change leads to a steric clash between the isoleucine side chain and STI571, together with the loss of an H-bond to the drug. A mutation of the analogous T674I gatekeeper residue has also been identified in the PDGFRα kinase of an HES patient who relapsed under STI571 treatment (Cools et al. 2003b), and is also likely to occur in c-Kit driven malignancies (T670I) (Fig. 2). In contrast to T315I, the other hinge region mutation in Abl, the F317L, causes a relatively minor disturbance in the STI571 binding (Shah et al. 2002; Cowan-Jacob et al. 2004).

- *The G-loop* (P-loop). It usually adopts a β-sheet conformation in the active Abl kinases; whereas when STI571 is bound to the inactive form, the G-loop forms a cage around the pyridine-pyrimidine rings of STI571, stabilized by numerous interactions to other parts of the kinase. Any mutations disrupting one of these interactions, or favoring other G-loop conformations will result in STI571 resistance. It should be pointed out that mutations within the G-loop may also lead to an enhanced activation of the kinase (increased oncogenicity) that prevents STI571 to "freeze" the inactive conformation of Abl.

- *A-loop.* Mutations in the activation segment, such as H396P or H396R, show weak resistance to STI571 (Hochhaus et al. 2002; Shah et al. 2002; von Bubnoff et al. 2002) resulting from the loss of an H-bond interaction between P396 and N414 (Cowan-Jacob et al. 2004). In contrast, the reasons for the loosening of STI571 binding of mutations clustered on the N-terminal part of the A-loop (V379I, F382L and L387M) can be quite diverse and have been discussed recently (Shah et al. 2002; Cowan-Jacob et al. 2004).
- *N-terminal lobe.* The M244 V and F311I mutations are located in the N-terminal lobe, which is a region that seems capable of adapting to the binding of different inhibitors (Al-Ali et al. 2002; Hochhaus et al. 2002; Kreil et al. 2002; Roche-Lestienne et al. 2002; Shah et al. 2002). Exactly how these mutations cause resistance is still poorly understood (Cowan-Jacob et al. 2004).
- *C-terminal lobe.* Another group of mutations is located in the C-terminal lobe, close to the piperazinyl group of STI571. Except for F359V, none of the other mutations (E355G, M351T, S417Y, E459 K, F486S) are in direct contact with STI571. The most frequently occurring mutant M351T displays only a moderate resistance to STI571 (Al-Ali et al. 2002; Branford et al. 2002; Hochhaus et al. 2002; Kreil et al. 2002; Roche-Lestienne et al. 2002; Shah et al. 2002). The mutation E459K at the bottom of the C-terminal lobe is very remote from the STI571 binding site but in close proximity to the myristoyl binding site of Abl (Hantschel et al. 2003; Nagar et al. 2003). It is conceivable that this mutation has a direct effect on destabilizing the assembled inactive state of Abl, therefore indirectly favoring an activated conformation of the kinase domain to which STI571 has a lower affinity. The inactive state of the "full-length" Abl has a similar arrangement of the SH3, SH2, and kinase domains as in Src, although the manner by which Src and Abl are kept in a catalytically inactive state differ, particularly with respect to helix C (Hantschel et al. 2003; Nagar et al. 2003; Xu et al. 1997, 1999).

Additional mutants outside of the kinase domain of Bcr-Abl will probably be identified in patients relapsing following STI571 treatment. As shown by an elegant in vitro random mutagenesis study, about 90 mutations were found in Bcr-Abl that imparted resistance to STI571, without affecting the transforming ability of Bcr-Abl (Azam et al. 2003). One third of all of these mutants were outside of the kinase domain and probably cause an allosteric destabilization of the auto-inhibited conformation by involving residues that participate in interactions between the kinase domain and the regulatory N-terminal cap, SH3 and SH2 domains (Azam et al. 2003).

4.2 Overcoming STI571 Resistance

While the kinase domain mutations that still retain some STI571 sensitivity (IC50<3 uM) may be overcome with more potent inhibitors that interact with the STI571 binding conformation, the resistance caused by mutants in the G-loop or the T315I mutant may require inhibitors that bind to Abl in an alternative mode or target the same conformation without engaging in an H-bond with the gatekeeper residue T315. Targeting the active, ATP-binding conformation of Abl has the advantage that the likelihood of emergence of resistant mutants is reduced. Prototype compounds in this regard are the pyrido[2,3-d]pyrimidine derivatives, one of which has been shown to bind to the catalytically active conformation of the Abl kinases, although the DFG motif is in a conformation that is unsuitable for optimal binding of ATP (Nagar et al. 2002). In addition, this pyrido[2,3-d]pyrimidine derivative has been reported to inhibit various mutants of the G-loop, the M351T mutant, as well as the A-loop mutant H396P, but not T315I (Dorsey et al. 2000; La Rosée et al. 2002; Cowan-Jacob et al. 2004). However, because the conformation of activated protein kinases is highly conserved, a major disadvantage of these types of inhibitors is the lack of selectivity against other kinases which might limit their tolerability (Kraker et al. 2000).

In contrast to the highly conserved conformations of activated protein kinases, the inactive states of protein kinases often adopt conformations in which there are large variations in size and shape of the ATP-binding pocket (Huse and Kuriyan 2002). Although targeting the inactive conformation of kinases may result in a better selectivity profile, the caveat is that these inhibitors will interact with many residues not involved in binding ATP, allowing mutations to arise which will prevent binding of the inhibitor without affecting the kinase activity.

Treatment strategies geared towards improving the STI571 therapy and/or circumventing STI571 resistance are multiple and may include:

1. Inhibition of other kinases acting downstream of Bcr-Abl, such as the Src family members Lyn and Hck (Danhauser-Riedel et al. 1996; Donato et al. 2003; Warmuth et al. 2003) or Btk (Hofmann et al. 2002b)
2. Inhibitors targeting other signaling molecules like Mek/Erk (Yu et al. 2002), PI3 K (Klejman et al. 2002), farnesyltransferase inhibitors (Topaly et al. 2002; Daley 2003; Hoover et al. 2002), protein degradation (Gatto et al. 2001), or Hsp90 (Gorre et al. 2002), all of which have shown to enhance the antiproliferative effects of cells expressing STI571 resistant Bcr-Abl

The most likely treatment of malignancies targeted by STI571 will be a cocktail of drugs designed to inhibit a particular class of STI571-resistant mutations or a mechanism of resistance reminiscent to the treatment of

HIV. Similar treatment strategies are likely to be applied in diseases other than CML where the drug targets the PTK of c-Kit and PDGFR (i.e., CMML, GIST, HES).

5
Conclusion and Perspectives

Although the clinical efficacy of STI571 has clearly demonstrated the utility and the potential of kinase inhibitors, the defined etiologies of diseases associated with expression of mutated PDGFR, c-Kit and Abl may make the success of this kinase inhibitor as single agent unique for a limited set of cancers. On the other hand, STI571 has taught us several lessons:

1. Protein kinase inhibitors with a "reasonable selectivity" are feasible and can be used for the chronic treatment of cancer patients with an acceptable tolerability and efficacy profile where the pathophysiology of the kinase target in the tumor is molecularly defined.
2. In almost all clinical studies with STI571, the clinical responses to drug treatment correlate with the presence of an activated form of the target kinase in the tumor. These findings indicate that at least some (subsets) of tumors may ultimately depend on the over-activation of one pathway which can be attacked using targeted therapy. To maximize the chances of success in targeted therapy it will be mandatory to stratify patients according to the relevance of the molecular target in the particular malignancy.
3. Although relapses under STI571 treatment may be due to various reasons, the finding that it is often associated with mutations in the kinase domain of the target enzyme unambiguously demonstrates that the target for STI571, thus far, can only be Bcr-Abl, c-Kit, and/or PDGFR.
4. The exquisite selectivity of STI571, which is achieved by targeting and/or inducing the "inactive conformation of the target kinase," is presumably key for the excellent tolerability to the drug but is at the same time also its "Achilles heel." The binding mode of STI571 to the target kinase allows mutations in residues that are not involved in ATP binding and consequently not deleterious to the normal function of the targeted kinase. Mutations leading to resistance are either less likely to occur, or will generate a different set of mutations if the compound targets the active rather than the inactive conformation. To optimize treatment, it appears obvious to use more than one kinase inhibitor targeting the same kinase, but different conformations.
5. A key to the discovery of new anti-cancer therapeutics is the selection of epidemiologically relevant, drugable protein kinase targets coupled to efficient lead optimization for potency, selectivity, efficacy, and biopharmaceutical properties. Mutational analysis combined with structural biology has

provided the understanding on the activation mechanisms of Bcr-Abl, Kit, and PDGFR as well as to its resistance to STI571.

Protein kinase inhibitors have and will continue to offer new therapies in the coming years and have started to add novel treatment modalities for cancer. Consequently, an effective long-term management of cancer is still likely to require cocktails of drugs, each aimed at a specific mutant and pathway.

References

Al-Ali HK, Lange T, Krahl R, Mueller C, Patzer G, Niederwieser D, Deininger MWN (2002) BCR-ABL kinase domain mutations in patients with secondary but not primary resistance to imatinib. Blood 100 (Suppl):368a

Apperley JF, Gardembas M, Melo JV, Russell-Jones R, Bain BJ, Baxter EJ, Chase A, Chessells JM, Colombat M, Dearden CE, Dimitrijevic S, Mahon FX, Marin D, Nikolova Z, Olavarria E, Silberman S, Schultheis B, Cross NC, Goldman JM (2002) Response to imatinib mesylate in patients with chronic myeloproliferative diseases with rearrangements of the platelet-derived growth factor receptor β. N Engl J Med 347:481–487

Asaoka Y, Nakamura S, Yoshida K, Nishizuka Y (1992) Protein kinase C, calcium and phospho-lipid degradation. TIBS 17:414-418

Azam M, Latek RR, Daley GQ (2003) Mechanisms of autoinhibition and STI-571/imatinib resistance revealed by mutagenesis of BCR-ABL. Cell 112:831–843

Banai S, Wolf Y, Golomb G, Pearle A, Waltenberger J, Fishbein I, Schneider A, Gazit A, Perez L, Huber R, Lazarovichi G, Rabinovich L, Levitzki A, Gertz SD (1998) PDGF-receptor tyrosine kinase blocker AG1295 selectively attenuates smooth muscle cell growth in vitro and reduces neointimal formation after balloon angioplasty in swine. Circulation 97:1960–1969

Barthe C, Cony-Makhoul P, Melo JV, Reiffers J, Mahon, F-X (2001) Roots of clinical resistance to STI-571 cancer therapy. Science 293:2163

Beran M, Cao X, Estrov Z, Jeha S, Jin G, O'Brien S, Talpaz M, Arlinghaus RB, Lydon NB, Kantarjian H (1998) Selective inhibition of cell proliferation and BCR-ABL phosphorylation in Acute Lymphoblastic Leukemia cells expressing Mr 190,000 BCR-ABL protein by a tyrosine kinase inhibitor (CGP 57148). Clin Cancer Res 4:1661–1672

Bilder G, Wentz T, Leadley R, Amin D, Byan L, O'Conner B, Needle S, Galczenski H, Bostwick J, Kasiewski C, Myers M, Spada A, Merkel L, Ly C, Persons P, Page K, Perrone M, Dunwiddie C (1999) Restenosis following angioplasty in the swine coronary artery is inhibited by an orally active PDGF-receptor tyrosine kinase inhibitor, RPR101511A. Circulation 99:3292–3299

Bilder G, Amin D, Morgan L, McVey M, Needle S, Galczenski H, Leadley R, He W, Myers M, Spada A, Luo Y, Natajaran C, Perrone M (2003) Stent-induced restenosis in the swine coronary artery is inhibited by a platelet-derived growth factor receptor tyrosine kinase inhibitor, TKI963. J Cardiovasc Pharmacol 41:817–829

Blume-Jensen P, Hunter T (2001) Oncogenic kinase signalling. Nature 41:355–365

Branford S, Rudzki Z, Walsh S, Grigg A, Arthur Ch, Taylor K, Herrmann R, Lynch KP, Hughes TP (2002) High frequency of point mutations clustered within the adenosine triphosphate-binding region of Bcr/Abl in patients with chronic leukemia or Ph-positive acute lymphoblastic leukemia who develop imatinib (STI571) resistance. Blood 99:3472–3475

Branford S, Rudzki Z, Walsh S, Parkinson I, Grigg A, Szer J, Taylor K, Herrmann R, Seymour JF, Arthur C, Joske D, Lynch K, Hughes T (2003) Detection of BCR-ABL mutations in patients with CML treated with imatinib is virtually always accompanied by clinical resistance, and mutations in the ATP phosphate-binding loop (P-loop) are associated with a poor prognosis. Blood 102:276–283

Buchdunger E, Zimmermann J, Mett H, Meyer T, Mueller M, Druker BJ, Lydon NB (1996) Effects of a selective inhibitor of the Abl tyrosine-kinase in vitro and in vivo by a 2-phenylaminopyrimidine derivative. Cancer Res 56:100–104

Buchdunger E, Cioffi CL, Law N, Stover D, Ohno-Jones S, Druker BJ, Lydon NB (2000) Abl protein-tyrosine kinase inhibitor STI571 inhibits in vitro signal transduction mediated by c-Kit and platelet-derived growth factor receptors. J Pharmacol Exp Ther 295:139–145

Carroll M, Ohno-Jones S, Tamura S, Buchdunger E, Zimmermann J, Lydon NB, Gilliland DG, Druker BJ (1997) CGP 57148, a tyrosine kinase inhibitor, inhibits the growth of cells expressing BCR-ABL, TEL-ABL, and TEL-PDGFR fusion proteins. Blood 90:4947–4952

Clarke ID, Dirks PB (2003) A human brain tumor-derived PDGFR-α deletion mutant is transforming. Oncogene 22:722–733

Cools J, DeAngelo DJ, Gotlib J, Stover EH, Legare RD, Cortes J, Kutok J, Clark J, Galinsky I, Griffin JD, Cross NC, Tefferi A, Malone J, Alam R, Schrier SL, Schmid J, Rose M, Vandenberghe P, Verhoef G, Boogaerts M, Wlodarska I, Kantarjian H, Marynen P, Coutre SE, Stone R, Gilliland DG (2003a) A tyrosine kinase created by fusion of the PDGFRA and FIP1L1 genes as a therapeutic target of imatinib in idiopathic hypereosinophilic syndrome. N Engl J Med 348:1201–1214

Cools J, Stover EH, Boulton CL, Gotlib J, Legare RD, Amaral SM, Duclos N, Rowan R, Curley DP, Kutok JL, Lee BH, Williams IR, Coutre SE, Stone SM, DeAngelo DJ, Marynen P, Meyer T, Fabbro D, Neuberg D, Weisberg E, Griffin JD, Gilliland DG (2003b) PKC412 overcomes resistance to imatinib in a murine model of FIP1L1-PDGFRα-induced myeloproliferative disease. Cancer Cell 3:459–469

Cortes JE, Talpaz M, Kantarjian H (1996) Chronic myelogenous leukemia: a review. Am J Med 100:555–570

Cowan-Jacob SW, Guez V, Fendrich G, Fabbro D, Furet P, Liebetanz J, Mestan J, Paul W, Manley (2004) Imatinib (STI571) Resistance in chronic myelogenous leukemia: molecular basis of the underlying mechanisms and potential strategies for treatment. Minireview Med Chem (in press)

Craver RD, Correa H, Kao YS, Van Brunt T, Golladay ES (1995) Aggressive giant cell fibroblastoma with a balanced t(17;22) translocation. Cancer Genet Cytogenet 80:20–22

Daley GQ (2003) Towards combination targeted-directed chemotherapy for chronic myeloid leukemia: Role of farnesyltransferase inhibitors. Semin Oncol 40 Suppl 2:11–15

Daley GQ, Van Etten RA, Baltimore D (1990) Induction of chronic myelogenous leukemia in mice by the P210bcr/abl gene of the Philadelphia chromosome. Science 247:824–830

Dan S, Naito M, Tsuruo T (1998) Selective induction of apoptosis in Philadelphia chromosome-positive chronic myelogenous leukemia cells by an inhibitor of BCR-ABL tyrosine kinase, CGP 57148B. Cell Death Differ 5:710–715

Danhauser-Riedel S, Warmuth M, Druker BJ, Emmerich B, Hallek M (1996) Activation of Src kinases p53/p56lyn and p59hck by p210bcr/abl in myeloid cells. Cancer Res 56:3589–3596

Deininger M, Goldman J, Lydon N, Melo JV (1997) The tyrosine kinase inhibitor CGP57148B selectively inhibits the growth of BCR-ABL-positive cells. Blood 90:3691–3698

Dekker LV, Parker PJ (1994) Protein kinase C a question of specificity. TIBS 19:73-77

Demetri GD, vonMehren M, Blanke CD, Van den Abbeele AD, Eisenberg, B, Roberts PJ, Heinrich MC, Tuveson DA, Singer S, Janicek M, Fletcher JA, Silverman SG, Silberman SL, Capdeville R, Kiese B, Peng B, Dimitrijevic S, Druker BJ, Corless C, Fletcher CDM, Joensuu H (2002) Efficacy and safety of imatinib mesylate in advanced gastrointestinal stromal tumors. N Engl J Med 347:472–480

Donato NJ, Wu JY, Stapley J, Gallick G, Lin H, Arlinghaus R, Talpaz M (2003) BCR-ABL independence and LYN kinase overexpression in chronic myelogenous leukemia cells selected for resistance to STI571. Blood 101:690–698

Dorsey JF, Jove R, Kraker AJ, Wu J (2000) The pyrido[2,3-d]pyrimidine derivative PD180970 inhibits p210Bcr-Abl tyrosine kinase and induces apoptosis of K562 leukemic cells. Cancer Res 60:3127–3131

Druker BJ, Tamura S, Buchdunger E, Ohno S, Segal GM, Fanning S, Zimmermann J, Lydon NB (1996) Effects of a selective inhibitor of the Abl tyrosine kinase on the growth of Bcr-Abl positive cells. Nat Med 2:561–566

Druker BJ, Sawyers CL, Kantarjian H, Resta DJ, Reese SF, Ford JM, Capdeville R, Talpaz M (2001) Activity of a specific inhibitor of the BCR-ABL tyrosine kinase in the blast crisis of chronic myeloid leukemia and acute lymphoblastic leukemia with the Philadelphia chromosome. N Engl J Med 344:1038–1042

Fabbro D, Buchdunger E, Wood J, Mestan J, Hofmann F, Ferrari S, Mett H, O'Reilly T, Meyer T (1999) CGP 41251 a protein kinase inhibitor with potential as an anticancer agent. Pharmacol Ther 82:293–301

Fabbro D, Ruetz S, Bodis S, Pruschy M, Csermak K, Man A, Campochiaro P, Wood J, O'Reilly T, Meyer T (2000) CGP 41251 a Protein Kinase Inhibitor with Potential as an Anticancer Agent. PKC412 a protein kinase inhibitor with a broad therapeutic potential. Anticancer Drug Des 15:17–28

Fabbro D, Ruetz S, Buchdunger E, Cowan-Jacob SW, Fendrich G, Liebetanz J, Mestan J, O'Reilly T, Traxler P, Chaudhuri B, Fretz H, Zimmermann J, Meyer T, Giorgio C, Furet P, Manley PW (2002) Protein kinases as targets for anti-cancer agents: from inhibitors to useful drugs. Pharmacol Ther 93:79–98

Ferns GA, Raines EW, Sprugel KH, Motani AS, Reidy MA, Ross R (1991) Inhibition of neointimal smooth muscle accumulation after angioplasty by an antibody to PDGF. Science 253:1129–1132

Fleming TP, Matsui T, Heidaran MA, Molloy CJ, Artrip J, Aaronson SA (1992) Demonstration of an activated platelet-derived growth factor autocrine pathway and its role in human tumor cell proliferation in vitro. Oncogene 7:1355–1359

Floege J, Ostendorf T (2001) Platelet-derived growth factor: a new clinical target on the horizon. Kidney Int 59:1592–1593

Gambacorti-Passerini C, Le Coutre P, Mologni L, Fanelli M, Bertazzoli C, Marchesi E, Di Nicola M, Biondi A, Corneo G M, Belotti D, Pogliani E, Lydon NB (1997) Inhibition of the ABL kinase activity blocks the proliferation of BCR/ABL+ leukemic cells and induces apoptosis. Blood Cells Mol Dis 23:380–394

Gambacorti-Passerini C, Barni R, le Coutre P, Zucchetti M, Cabrita G, Cleris L, Rossi F, Gianazza E, Brueggen J, Cozens R, Pioltelli P, Pogliani E, Corneo G, Formelli F,

D'Incalci M (2000) Role of alpha1 acid glycoprotein in the in vivo resistance of human BCR-ABL(+) leukemic cells to the abl inhibitor STI571. J Natl Cancer Inst 92:1641–1650

Gambacorti-Passerini C, le Coutre P, Zucchetti M, D'Incalci M (2002) Binding of imatinib by α1-acid glycoprotein. Blood 100:367–368

Gambacorti-Passerini C, Zucchetti M, Russo D, Frapolli R, Verga M, Bungaro S, Tornagi L, Rossi F, Pioltelli P, Pogliani E, Alberti D, Corneo G, D'Incalci M (2003) a1-Acid glycoprotein binds to imatinib (STI571) and substantially alters its pharmacokinetics in chronic myeloid leukemia patients. Clin Cancer Res 9:625–632

Gatto SR, Scappini B, Verstovsek S, Milella M, Onida F, Ball G, Kantarjian HM, Keating MJ, Cortes JE, Beran M (2001) In Vitro Effects of PS-341 Alone and in Combination with STI571 in BCR-ABL Positive Cell Lines Both Sensitive and Resistant to STI571. Blood 98 (Suppl):101a

Gesbert F, Sellers WR, Signoretti S, Loda M, Griffin JD (2000) BCR/ABL regulates expression of the cyclin-dependent kinase inhibitor p27Kip1 through the phosphatidylinositol 3-Kinase/AKT pathway. J Biol Chem 275:39223–39230

Giese NA, Marijianowski MMH, McCook O, Hancock A, Ramakrishnan V, Fretto LJ, Chen C, Kelly AB, Koziol JA, Wilcox JN, Hanson SR (1999) The role of α and β platelet-derived growth factor receptor in the vascular response to injury in nonhuman primates. Arterioscler Thromb Vasc Biol 19:900–909

Gilbert RE, Kelly DJ, McKay T, Chadban S, Hill PA, Cooper ME, Atkins RC, Nikolic-Paterson DJ (2001) PDGF signal transduction inhibition ameliorates experimental mesangial proliferative glomerulonephritis. Kidney Int 59:1324–1332

Gishizky ML (1996) Molecular mechanisms of Bcr-Abl-induced oncogenesis. Cytokines Mol Ther 2:251–261

Gishizky ML, Johnson-White J, Witte ON (1993) Efficient transplantation of BCR-ABL-induced chronic myelogenous leukemia-like syndrome in mice. *Proc Natl Acad Sci U S A* 90:3755–3759

Gleich GJ, Leiferman KM, Pardanani A, Tefferi A, Butterfield JH (2002) Treatment of hypereosinophilic syndrome with imatinib mesylate. Lancet 359:1577–1578

Golub TR, Barker GF, Lovett M, Gilliland DG (1994) Fusion of PDGF receptor β to a novel *ets*-like gene, *tel*, in chronic myelomonocytic leukemia with t(5;12) chromosomal translocation. Cell 77:307–316

Gorre ME, Mohammed M, Ellwood K, Hsu N, Paquette R, Rao PN, Sawyers CL (2001a) Clinical resistance to STI-571 cancer therapy caused by BCR-ABL gene mutation or amplification. Science 293:876–880

Gorre M, Shah N, Ellwood K, Nicoll J, Sawyer CL (2001b) Roots of clinical resistance to STI-571 cancer therapy. Science 293:2163a

Gorre M, Ellwood-Yen K, Chiosis Gl, Rosen N, Sawyers CL (2002) BCR-ABL point mutants isolated from patients with imatinib mesylate-resistant chronic myeloid leukemia remain sensitive to inhibitors of the BCR-ABL chaperone heat shock protein 90. Blood 100:3041–3044

Griffin JH, Leung J, Bruner RJ, Caligiuri MA, Briesewitz R (2003) Discovery of a fusion kinase in EOL-1 cells and idiopathic hypereosinophilic syndrome. Proc Natl Acad Sci USA 100:7830–7835

Hanahan D, Weinberg RA (2000) The hallmarks of cancer. Cell 100:57–70

Hart CE, Kraiss LW, Vergel S, Gilbertson D, Kenagy R, Kirkman T, Crandall DL, Tickle S, Finney H, Yarranton G, Clowes AW (1999) PDGFβ receptor blockade inhibits intimal hyperplasia in the baboon. Circulation 99:564–569

Hantschel O, Nagar B, Guettler S, Kretzschmar J, Dorey K, Kuriyan J, Superti-Furga G (2003) A myristoyl/phosphotyrosine switch regulates c-Abl. Cell 112:845–857

Heinrich MC, Griffith DJ, Druker BJ, Wait CL, Ott KA, Ziegler AJ (2000) Inhibition of c-kit receptor tyrosine kinase activity by STI 571, a selective tyrosine kinase inhibitor. Blood 96:925–932

Heinrich MC, Blanke CD, Druker BJ, Corless CL (2002) Inhibition of KIT tyrosine kinase activity. A novel molecular approach to the treatment of KIT-positive malignancies. J Clin Oncol 20:1692–1703

Heinrich MC, Corless CL, Demetri GD, Blanke CD, von Mehren M, Joensuu H, McGreevey LS, Chen C-J, Van den Abbeele AD, Druker BJ, Kiese B, Eisenberg B, Roberts PJ, Singer S, Fletcher CDM, Silberman S, Dimitrijevic S, Fletcher JD (2003a) Kinase mutations and imatinib response in patients with metastatic gastrointestinal stromal tumor. JCO 21:4342–4349

Heinrich MC, Corless CL, Duensing A, McGreevey L, Chen CJ, Joseph N, Singer S, Griffith DJ, Haley A, Town A, Demetri GD, Fletcher CD, Fletcher JA (2003b) PDGFRA activating mutations in gastrointestinal stromal tumors. Science 299:708–710

Heldin C-H, Eriksson U, Östman A (2002) New members of the platelet-derived growth factor family of mitogens. Arch Biochem Biophys 398:284–290

Hermanson M, Funa K, Koopmann J, Maintz D, Waha A, Westermark B, Heldin C-H, Wiestler OD, Louis DN, von Deimling A, Nistér M (1996) Association of loss of heterozygosity on chromosome 17p with high platelet-derived growth factor α receptor expression in human malignant gliomas. Cancer Res 56:164–171

Hirota S, Isozaki K, Moriyama Y, Taniguchi M, Nakamura J, Okazaki T, Kitamura Y (1998) Gain-of-function mutations of c-kit in human gastrointestinal stromal tumors. Science 279:577–580

Hochhaus A (2003) Cytogenetic and molecular mechanisms of resistance to imatinib. Semin Oncol 40 Suppl 2:69–79

Hochhaus A, Kreil S, La Rosee P, Lahaye T, Berger U, Cross NCP, Linkesch W, Druker BJ, Hehlmann R (2001) Roots of clinical resistance to STI-571 cancer therapy. Science 293:2163a

Hochhaus A, Kreil S, Corbin AS, La Rosée P, Müller MC, Lahaye T, Schoch C, Cross NCP, Berger U, Gschaidmeier H, Druker BJ, Hehlmann R (2002) Molecular and chromosomal mechanisms of resistance to imatinib (STI571) therapy. Leukemia 16:2190–2196

Hofmann W-K, Jones LC, Lemp NA, de Vos S, Gschaidmeier H, Hoelzer D, Ottmann OG, Koeffler HP (2002a) Ph+ acute lymphoblastic leukemia resistant to the tyrosine kinase inhibitor STI571 has a unique BCR-ABL gene mutation. Blood 95:1860–1862

Hofmann W-K, de Vos S, Elashoff D, Gschaidmeier H, Hoelzer D, Koeffler HP, Ottmann OG (2002b) Relation between resistance of Philadelphia-chromosome-positive acute lymphoblastic leukaemia to the tyrosine kinase inhibitor STI571 and gene-expression profiles: a gene-expression study. Lancet 359:481–486

Hoover R, Mahon F X, Melo JV, Daley GQ (2002) Overcoming STI571 resistance with the farnesyl transferase inhibitor SCH66336. Blood 100:1068–1071

Horita M, Andreu EJ, Benito A, Arbona C, Sanz C, Benet I, Prosper F, Fernandez-Luna JL (2000) Blockade of the Bcr-Abl kinase activity induces apoptosis of chronic myelogenousleukemia cells by suppressing signal transducer and activator of transcription 5-dependent expression of Bcl-xL. J Exp Med 191:977–984

Hughes TP, Kaeda J, Branford S, Rudzki Z, Hochhaus A, Hensley ML, Ganthmann I, Bolton AE, Van Hoomissen IC, Goldman JM, Radich JP (2002) Molecular responses to imatinib (STI571) or interferon + Ara-C as initial therapy for CML; results in the IRIS study. Blood 100 (Suppl):96a

Huse M, Kuriyan J (2002) The conformational plasticity of protein kinases. Cell 109:275–282

Joensuu H, Roberts PJ, Sarlomo-Rikala M, Andersson LC, Tervahartiala P, Tuveson D, Silberman SL, Capdeville R, Dimitrijevic S, Druker B, Demetri GD (2001) Effect of the tyrosine kinase inhibitor STI571 in a patient with a metastatic gastrointestinal stromal tumor. N Engl J Med 1052:1052–1056

Joensuu H, Fletcher C, Dimitrijevic S, Silberman S, Roberts P, Demetri G (2002) Management of malignant gastrointestinal stromal tumours. Lancet Oncol 3:655–664

Jonuleit T, van der Kuip H, Miething C, Michels H, Hallek M, Duyster J, Aulitzky WE (2000) Bcr-Abl kinase down-regulates cyclin-dependent kinase inhibitor p27 in human and murine cell lines. Blood 96:1933–1939

Jørgensen HG, Elliott MA, Allan EK, Carr CE, Holyoake TL, Smith KD (2002) a1-Acid glycoprotein expressed in the plasma of chronic myeloid leukemia patients does not mediate significant in vitro resistance to STI571. Blood 99:713–715

Kantarjian HM, Cortes J, O'Brien S, Giles FJ, Albitar M, Rios MB, Shan J, Faderl S, Garcia-Manero G, Thomas DA, Resta D, Talpaz M (2002a) Imatinib mesylate (STI571) therapy for Philadelphia chromosome-positive chronic myelogenous leukemia in blast phase. Blood 99:3547–3553

Kantarjian H, Sawyers C, Hochhaus A, Guilhot F, Schiffer C, Gambacorti-Passerini C, Niederwieser D, Resta D, Capdeville R, Zoellner U, Talpaz M, Druker B, the International STI571 CML Study Group (2002b) Hematologic and cytogenetic responses to imatinib mesylate in chronic myelogenous leukemia. N Engl J Med 346:645–652

Kasper B, Fruehauf S, Schiedlmeier B, Buchdunger E, Ho AD, Zeller WJ (1999) Favourable therapeutic index of a $p210^{BCR\text{-}ABL}$-specific tyrosine kinase inhibitor activity on lineage-committed and primitive chronic myelogenous leukemia progenitors. Cancer Chemother Pharmacol 44:433–438

Khouri I, Kantarijan H, Talpaz M, Andreeff M, Lee M-S, Champlin R, Deisseroth AB (1995) Chronic myeloid leukemia. In: MD Abeloff, Armitage JO, Lichter AS, Niederhuber JE (ed) Clinical Oncology. Churchill Livingstone, New York, pp 2035–2052

Kilic T, Alberta JA, Zdunek PR, Acar M, Iannarelli P, O'Reilly T, Buchdunger E, Black PM, Stiles CD (2000) Intracranial inhibition of platelet-derived growth factor-mediated glioblastoma cell growth by an orally active kinase inhibitor of the 2-phenylaminopyrimidine class. Cancer Res 60:5143–5150

Klejman A, Rushen L, Morrione A, Slupianek A, Skorski T (2002) Phosphatidylinositol-3 kinase inhibitors enhance the anti-leukemia effect of STI571. Oncogene 21:5868–5876

Kraker A J, Hartl BG, Amar AM, Barvian MR, Showalter HDD, Moore CW (2000) Biochemical and cellular effects of c-Src kinase-selective pyrido[2, 3-d]pyrimidine tyrosine kinase inhibitors. Biochem Pharmacol 60:885–898

Kreil S, Müller MC, Hanfstein B, La Rosée P, Corbin AS, Lahaye T, Schoch C, Berger U, Gschaidmeier H, Hehlmann R, Hochhaus A (2002) Roots and management of imatinib resistance in BCR-ABL positive leukemias. Blood 100 (Suppl):368a

Kumabe T, Sohma Y, Kayama T, Yoshimoto T, Yamamoto T (1992) Amplification of α-platelet-derived growth factor receptor gene lacking an exon coding for a portion of the extracellular region in a primary brain tumor of glial origin. Oncogene 7:627–633

Kuwazuru Y,Yoshimura A, Hanada S, Utsunomiya A, Makino T, Ishibashi, K, Kodama M, Iwahashi M, Arima T, Akiyama S (1990) Expression of the multidrug transporter, P-glycoprotein, in acute leukemia cells and correlation to clinical drug resistance. Cancer 66:868–73

La Rosée P, Corbin AS, Stoffregen EP, Deininger MW, Druker BJ (2002) Activity of the Bcr-Abl kinase inhibitor PD180970 against clinically relevant Bcr-Abl isoforms that cause resistance to imatinib mesylate (Gleevec, STI571). Cancer Res 62:7149–7153

le Coutre P, Mologni L, Cleris L, Marchesi E, Buchdunger E, Giardini R, Formelli F, Gambacorti-Passerini C (1999) In vivo eradication of human BCR/ABL-positive leukemia cells with an ABL kinase inhibitor. J Natl Cancer Inst 91:163–168

le Coutre P, Kreuzer K-A, Na I-K, Lupberger J, Holdhoff M, Appelt C, Schwarz M, Muller C, Gambacorti-Passerini C, Platzbecker U, Bonnet R, Ehninger G, Schmidt CA (2002) Determination of alpha-1 acid glycoprotein in patients with Ph+ chronic myeloid leukemia during the first 13 weeks of therapy with STI571. Blood Cells Mol Dis 28:75–85

Leguay T, Desplat V, Barthe C, Rousselot P, Reiffers J, Marit G, Mahon F-X (2002) Study of mutations in the ATP binding domain and the SH2/SH3 domain of BCR-ABL in 43 chronic myeloid leukemia patients treated by imatinib mesylate (STI571). Blood 100 (Suppl):369a

Levitzki A (1996) Targeting signal transduction for disease therapy. Curr Opin Cell Biol 8:239–244

Li S, Ilaria RL Jr, Million RP, Daley GQ, Van Etten RA (1999) The P190, P210, and P230 forms of the BCR/ABL oncogene induce a similar chronic myeloid leukemia-like syndrome in mice but have different lymphoid leukemogenic activity. *J Exp Med* 189:1399–1412

Lux ML, Rubin BP, Biase TL, Chen CJ, Maclure T, Demetri G, Xiao S, Singer S, Fletcher CD, Fletcher JA (2000) KIT extracellular and kinase domain mutations in gastrointestinal stromal tumors. Am J Pathol 156:791–5

Magnusson MK, Meade KE, Brown KE, Arthur DC, Krueger LA, Barrett AJ, Dunbar CE (2001) Rabaptin-5 is a novel fusion partner to platelet-derived growth factor β receptor in chronic myelomonocytic leukemia. Blood 98:2518–2525

Magnusson MK, Meade KE, Nakamura R, Barrett J, Dunbar CE (2002) Activity of STI571 in chronic myelomonocytic leukemia with a platelet-derived growth factor β receptor fusion oncogene. Blood 100:1088–1091

Mahon F-X, Deininger MW, Schultheis B, Chabrol J, Reiffers J, Goldman JM, Melo JV (2000) Selection and characterization of BCR-ABL positive cell lines with differential sensitivity to the tyrosine kinase inhibitor STI571: diverse mechanisms of resistance. Blood 96:1070–9

Maki RG, Awan RA, Dixon RH, Jhanwar S, Antonescu CR (2002) Differential sensitivity to imatinib of 2 patients with metastatic sarcoma arising from dermatofibrosarcoma protuberans. Int J Cancer 100:623–626

Mandahl N, Heim S, Willen H, Rydholm A, Mitelman F (1990) Supernumerary ring chromosome as the sole cytogenetic abnormality in a dermatofibrosarcoma protuberans. Cancer Genet Cytogenet 49:273–275

Manley PW, Bold G, Buchdunger E, Cowan-Jacob SW, Fabbro D, Fendrich G, Furet P, Meyer T, Wood J, Zimmermann J (2002) Structure and molecular design of tyrosine kinase inhibitors. 'Imatinib: a selective tyrosine kinase inhibitor. Eur J Cancer 38 Suppl 5 S19–27

Manning G, Whyte DB, Martinez IR, Hunter T, Sudarsanam S (2002) The protein kinase complement of the human genome. Science 298:1912–1934

Matter A (2001) Tumor angiogenesis as a therapeutic Target. Drug Discov Today 6:1005–1023

McMahon G, Sun L, Liang C, Tang C (1998) Protein kinase inhibitors: structural determinants for target specificity. Curr Opin Drug Discov Devel 1:131–146

Myllarniemi M, Calderon L, Lemström K, Buchdunger E, Hayry P (1997) Inhibition of platelet-derived growth factor receptor tyrosine kinase inhibits vascular smooth muscle cell migration and proliferation. FASEB J 11:1119–1126

Naeem R, Lux ML, Huang SF, Naber SP, Corson JM, Fletcher JA (1995) Ring chromosomes in dermatofibrosarcoma protuberans are composed of interspersed sequences from chromosomes 17 and 22. Am J Pathol 147:1553–1558

Nagar B, Bornmann WG, Pellicena P, Schindler T, Veach DR, Miller WT, Clarkson B, Kuriyan J (2002) Crystal structures of the kinase domain of c-Abl in complex with the small molecule inhibitors PD173955 and imatinib (STI-571). Cancer Res 62:4236–4243

Nagar B, Hantschel O, Young MA, Scheffzek K, Veach D, Bornmann W, Clarkson B, Superti-Furga G, Kuriyan J (2003) Structural basis for the autoinhibition of c-Abl tyrosine kinase. Cell 112:859–871

O'Brien SG, Guilhot F, Larson RA, Gathmann I, Baccarani M, Cervantes F, Cornelissen JJ, Fischer T, Hochhaus A, Hughes T, Lechner K, Nielsen JL, Rousselot P, Reiffers J, Saglio G, Shepherd J, Simonsson B, Gratwohl A, Goldman JM, Kantarjian H, Tayloer K, Verhoef G, Bolton AE, Capdeville R, Druker BJ, O'Brien SG, Guilhot F, Larson RA, et al (2003) The IRIS study: international randomized study of interferon and low-dose Ara-C versus STI571 (imatinib) in patients with newly diagnosed chronic phase chronic myeloid leukemia. N Engl J Med 348:994–1004

Okuda K, Weisberg E, Gilliland DG, Griffin JD (2001) ARG tyrosine kinase activity is inhibited by STI571. Blood 97:2440–2448

Pardanani A, Ketterling RP, Brockman SR, Flynn HC, Paternoster SF, Shearer BM, Reeder TL, Li CY, Cross NC, Cools J, Gilliland DG, Dewald GW, Tefferi A (2003) CHIC2 deletion, a surrogate for FIP1L1-PDGFRA fusion, occurs in systemic mastocytosis associated with eosinophilia and predicts response to imatinib therapy. Blood 102:3093–3096

Pawson T, Nash P (2000) Protein-protein interactions define specificity in signal transduction. Genes Dev 14:1027–1047

Pedeutour F, Simon MP, Minoletti F, Barcelo G, Terrier-Lacombe MJ, Combemale P, Sozzi G, Ayraud N, Turc-Carel C (1996) Translocation, t(17;22)(q22;q13), in dermatofibrosarcoma protuberans: a new tumor-associated chromosome rearrangement. Cytogenet Cell Genet 72:171–174

Pietras K, Östman A, Sjöquist M, Buchdunger E, Reed RK, Heldin C-H, Rubin K (2001) Inhibition of platelet-derived growth factor receptors reduces interstitial hypertension and increases transcapillary transport in tumors. Cancer Res 61:2929–2934

Pietras K, Rubin K, Sjöblom T, Buchdunger E, Sjöquist M, Heldin C-H, Östman A (2002) Inhibition of PDGF receptor signaling in tumor stroma enhances anti-tumor effect of chemotherapy. Cancer Res 62:5476–5484

Pietras K, Hubert M, Buchdunger E, Rubin K, Heldin C-H, Wartmann M, Östman A (2003) STI571 enhances the therapeutic index of Epothilone B by a tumor-selective increase of drug uptake. Clin Cancer Res 9:33–45

Rice PL, Porter SE, Koski KM, Ramakrishna G, Chen A, Schrump D, Kazlauskas A, Malkinson AM (1999) Reduced receptor expression for platelet-derived growth factor and epidermal growth factor in dividing mouse lung epithelial cells. Mol Carcinog 25:285–294

Roche-Lestienne C, Soenen-Cornu V, Grardel-Duflos N, Lai JL, Philippe N, Facon T, Fenaux P, Preudhomme C (2002) Several types of mutations of the Abl gene can be found in chronic myeloid leukemia patients resistant to STI571, and they can pre-exist to the onset of treatment. Blood 100:1014–1018

Ross R, Masuda J, Raines EW, Gown AM, Katsuda S, Sasahara M, Malden LT, Masuko H, Sato H (1990) Localization of PDGF-B protein in macrophages in all phases of atherogenesis. Science 248:1009–1012

Ross TS, Bernard OA, Berger R, Gilliland DG (1998) Fusion of Huntingtin interacting protein 1 to platelet-derived growth factor β receptor (PDGFβR) in chronic myelomonocytic leukemia with t(5;7)(q33;q11.2). Blood 91:4419–4426

Rubin K, Tingström A, Hansson GK, Larsson E, Rönnstrand L, Klareskog L, Claesson-Welsh L, Heldin C-H, Fellström B, Terracio L (1988) Induction of B-type receptors for platelet-derived growth factor in vascular inflammation: possible implications for development of vascular proliferative lesions. Lancet 1:1353–1356

Rubin BP, Schuetze SM, Eary JF, Norwood TH, Mirza S, Conrad EU, Bruckner JD (2002) Molecular targeting of platelet-derived growth factor B by imatinib mesylate in a patient with metastatic dermatofibrosarcoma protuberans. J Clin Oncol 20:3586–3591

Sattler M, Griffin JD (2003) Molecular mechanisms of transformation by Bcr-Abl. Semin Oncol 40 Suppl 2:4–11

Sawyers CL, Hochhaus A, Feldman E, Goldman JM, Miller CB, Ottmann OG, Schiffer CA, Talpaz M, Guilhot F, Deininger MWN, Fischer T, O'Brien, SG, Stone RM, Gambacorti-Passerini CB, Russell NH, Reiffers JJ, Shea TC, Chapuis B, Coutre S, Tura S, Morra E, Larson RA, Saven A, Peschel C, Gratwohl A, Mandelli F, Ben-Am M, Gathmann I, Capdeville R, Paquette RL, Druker BJ (2002) Imatinib induces hematologic and cytogenetic responses in patients with chronic myeloid leukemia in myeloid blast crisis: results of a phase II study. Blood 99:3530–3539

Schindler T, Bornmann W, Pellicena P, Miller WT, Clarkson B, Kuriyan, J (2000) Structural mechanism for STI-571 inhibition of Abelson tyrosine kinase. Science 289:1938–1942

Schlessinger J (2000) Cell signaling by receptor tyrosine kinases. Cell 103:211–225

Schwaller J, Anastasiadou E, Cain D, Kutok J, Wojiski S, Williams IR, LaStarza R, Crescenzi B, Sternberg DW, Andreasson P, Schiavo R, Siena S, Mecucci C, Gilliland DG (2001) H4(D10S170), a gene frequently rearranged in papillary thyroid carcinoma, is fused to the platelet-derived growth factor receptor β gene in atypical chronic myeloid leukemia with t(5;10)(q33;q22). Blood 97:3910–3918

Shah NP, Nicoll JM, Nagar B, Gorre ME, Paquette RL, Kuriyan J, Sawyers CL (2002) Multiple BCR-ABL kinase domain mutations confer polyclonal resistance to the tyrosine kinase inhibitor imatinib (STI571) in chronic phase and blast crisis chronic myeloid leukemia. Cancer Cell 2:117–125

Shamah SM, Stiles CD, Guha A (1993) Dominant-negative mutants of platelet-derived growth factor revert the transformed phenotype of human astrocytoma cells. Mol Cell Biol 13:7203–7212

Sillaber C, Gesbert F, Frank DA, Sattler M, Griffin JD (2000) STAT5 activation contributes to growth and viability in Bcr/Abl-transformed cells. Blood 95:2118–2125

Simon M-P, Pedeutour F, Sirvent N, Grosgeorge J, Minoletti F, Coindre J-M, Terrier-Lacombe M-J, Mandahl N, Craver RD, Blin N, Sozzi G, Turc-Carel C, O'Brien KP, Kedra D, Fransson I, Guilbaud C, Dumanski JP (1997) Deregulation of the platelet-derived growth factor B-chain gene via fusion with collagen gene COL1A1 in dermatofibrosarcoma protuberans and giant-cell fibroblastoma. Nat Genet 15:95–98

Sihvola R, Koskinen P, Myllärniemi M, Loubtchenkov M, Häyry P, Buchdunger E, Lemström K (1999) Prevention of cardiac allograft arteriosclerosis by protein tyrosine kinase inhibitor selective for platelet-derived growth factor receptor. Circulation 99:2295–2301

Sihvola RK, Tikkanen JM, Krebs R, Aaltola EM, Buchdunger E, Laitinen O, Koskinen PK, Lemstrom KB (2003) Platelet-derived growth factor receptor inhibition reduces allograft arteriosclerosis of heart and aorta in cholesterol-fed rabbits. Transplantation 75:334–339

Sirois MG, Simons M, Edelman ER (1997) Antisense oligonucleotide inhibition of PDGFR-β receptor subunit expression directs suppression of intimal thickening. Circulation 95:669–676

Sjöblom T, Boureux A, Rönnstrand L, Heldin C-H, Ghysdael J, Östman A (1998) Characterization of the chronic myelomonocytic leukemia associated TEL-PDGFβR fusion protein. Oncogene 18:7055–7062

Sjöblom T, Shimizu A, O'Brien KP, Pietras K, Dal Cin P, Buchdunger E, Dumanski JP, Östman A, Heldin C-H (2001) Growth inhibition of dermatofibrosarcoma protuberans tumors by the platelet-derived growth factor receptor antagonist STI571 through induction of apoptosis. Cancer Res 61:5778–5783

Smits A, Funa K, Vassbotn FS, Beausang-Linder M, af Ekenstam F, Heldin C-H, Westermark B, Nistér M (1992) Expression of platelet-derived growth factor and its receptors in proliferative disorders of fibroblastic origin. Am J Pathol 140:639–648

Steer EJ, Cross NC (2002) Myeloproliferative disorders with translocations of chromosome 5q31–35: role of the platelet-derived growth factor receptor β. Acta Haematol 107:113–122

Strawn LM, Shawver LK (1998) Tyrosine kinases in disease: overview of kinase inhibitors as therapeutic agents and current drugs in clinical trials. Expert Opin Investig Drugs 7:553–573

Strawn LM, Mann E, Elliger SS, Chu LM, Germain LL, Niederfellner G, Ullrich A, Shawver LK (1994) Inhibition of glioma cell growth by a truncated platelet-derived growth factor-β receptor. J Biol Chem 1994;269:21215–21222

Talpaz M, Silver RT, Druker BJ, Goldman JM, Gambacorti-Passerini C, Guilhot F, Schiffer CA, Fischer T, Deininger MWN, Lennard AL, Hochhaus A, Ottmann OG, Gratwohl A, Baccarani M, Stone R, Tura S, Mahon F-X, Fernandes-Reese S, Gathmann I, Capdeville R, Kantarjian HG, Sawyers CL (2002) Imatinib induces durable hematologic and cytogenetic responses in patients with accelerated phase chronic myeloid leukemia: results of a phase 2 study. Blood 99:1928–1937

Tamaoki T, Nomoto H, Takahashi I, Kato Y, Morimoto M, Tomita F (1986) Staurosporine, a potent inhibitor of phospholipid/calcium-dependent protein kinase. Biochem Biophys Res Commun 135:397–402

Tanizawa S, Ueda M, Van der Loos CM, Van der Wal AC, Becker AE (1996) Expression of platelet derived growth factor B chain and β receptor in human coronary arteries after percutaneous transluminal coronary angioplasty: An immunohistochemical study. Br Heart J 75:549–556

Tenen DG (2003) Disruption of differentiation in human cancer: AML shows the way. Nat Rev Cancer 3:89–101

Tomasson MH, Williams IR, Hasserjian R, Udomsakdi C, McGrath SM, Schwaller J, Druker B, Gilliland DG (1999) TEL/PDGFβR induces hematologic malignancies in mice that respond to a specific tyrosine kinase inhibitor. Blood 93:1707–1714

Topaly J, Zeller WJ, Fruehauf S (2002) Combination therapy with imatinib mesylate (STI571): Synopsis of in in vitro studies. Br J Haematol 119:3–14

Traxler P, Bold G, Buchdunger E, Caravatti G, Furet P, Manley P, O'Reilly T, Wood J, Zimmermann J (2001) Tyrosine kinase inhibitors: from rational design to clinical trials. Med Res Rev 21:499–512

Tuveson DA, Willis NA, Jacks T, Griffin JD, Singer S, Fletcher CDM, Fletcher JA, Demetri GD (2001) STI571 inactivation of the gastrointestinal stromal tumor c-KIT oncoprotein: biological and clinical implications. Oncogene 20:5054–5058

Ueda M, Becker AE, Kasayuki N, Kojima A, Morita Y, Tanaka S (1996) *In situ* detection of platelet-derived growth factor-A and -B chain mRNA in human coronary arteries after percutaneous transluminal coronary angioplasty. Am J Pathol 149:831–843

VanOosterom AT, Judson I, Verweij J, Stroobants S, DonatodiPaola E, Dimitrijevic S, Martens M, Webb A, Sciot R, Van Glabbeke M, Silberman S, Nielsen OS (2001) Safety and efficacy of imatinib (STI571) in metastatic gastrointestinal stromal tumours: a phase I study. Lancet 358:1421–1423

von Bubnoff N, Schneller F, Peschel C, Duyster J (2002) BCR-ABL gene mutations in relation to clinical resistance of Philadelphia-chromosome-positive leukaemia to STI571: a prospective study. Lancet 359:487–491

Warmuth M, Danhauser-Riedl S, Hallek M (1999) Molecular pathogenesis of chronic myeloid leukemia: implications for new therapeutic strategies. Ann Hematol 78:49–64

Warmuth M, Simon N, Mitina O, Mathes R, Fabbro D, Manley PW, Buchdunger E, Forster K, Moarefi I, Hallek M (2003) Dual-specific Src and Abl kinase inhibitors, PP1 and CGP76030, inhibit growth and survival of cells expressing imatinib mesylate-resistant Bcr-Abl kinases. Blood 101:664–672

Weisberg E, Griffin JD (2000) Mechanism of resistance of the ABL tyrosine kinase inhibitor STI571 in BCR/ABL-transformed hematopoietic cell lines. Blood 95:3498–505

Weller PF, Bubley GJ (1994) The idiopathic hypereosinophilic syndrome. Blood 83:2759–2779

Wolff NC, Ilaria RL (2001) Establishment of a murine model for therapy-treated chronic myelogenous leukemia using the tyrosine kinase inhibitor STI571. Blood 98:2808–2816

Xu W, Harrison SC, Eck MJ (1997) Three-dimensional structure of the tyrosine kinase c-Src. Nature 385:595–602

Xu W, Doshi A, Lei M, Eck MJ, Harrison SC (1999) Crystal structures of c-Src reveal features of its autoinhibitory mechanism. Mol Cell 3:629–638

Yamasaki Y, Miyoshi K, Oda N, Watanabe M, Miyake H, Chan J, Wang X, Sun L, Tang C, McMahon G, Lipson KE (2001) Weekly dosing with the platelet-derived growth factor receptor tyrosine kinase inhibitor SU9518 significantly inhibits arterial stenosis. Circ Res 88:630–636

Yoshida M, Sakuma-Mochizuki J, Abe Ky, Arai T, Mori M, Goya S, Matsuoka H, Hayashi S, Kaneda Y, Kishimoto T (1999) In vivo gene transfer of an extracellular domain of platelet-derived growth factor β receptor by the HVJ-liposome method ameliorates bleomycin-induced pulmonary fibrosis. Biochem Biophys Res Commun 265:503–508

Yu C, Krystal G, Varticovski L, McKinstry R, Rahmani M, Dent P, Grant S (2002) Pharmacologic Mitogen-activated protein/extracellular signal-regulated kinase/mitogen-activated protein kinase inhibitors interact synergistically with STI571 to induce apoptosis in Bcr/Abl-expressing human leukemia cell. Cancer Res 62:188–199

Zimmermann J, Caravatti G, Mett H, Meyer T, Müller M, Lydon NB, Fabbro D (1996a) Phenylamino-pyrimidines: A new class of potent and selective inhibitors of protein kinase C (PKC). Arch Pharm Pharm Med Chem 329:371–376

Zimmermann J, Buchdunger E, Mett H, Meyer T, Lydon NB,Traxler P (1996b) (Phenylamino) pyrimidine (PAP) derivatives: a new class of potent and highly selective PDGF-receptor autophosphorylation inhibitors. Bioorg Med Chem Lett 6:1221–1226

Zimmermann J, Buchdunger E, Mett H, Meyer T, Lydon NB (1997) Potent and selective inhibitors of the ABL-kinase: phenylamino-pyrimidine (PAP) derivatives. Bioorg Med Chem Lett 7:187–192

Zimmermann J, Furet P, Buchdunger E (2001) STI571—a new treatment modality for CML? In: Anticancer agents: frontiers in cancer chemotherapy. In: Ojima I, Vite G, Altmann K (eds) ACS Symposium Series 796. American Chemical Society, Washington, pp 245–259

Zwerner JP, May WA (2001) PDGF-C is an EWS/FLI induced transforming growth factor in Ewing family tumors. Oncogene 20:626–633

Zwerner JP, May WA (2002) Dominant negative PDGF-C inhibits growth of Ewing family tumor cell lines. Oncogene 21:3847–3854

HEP (2005) 167:391–410

Clinical Aspects of Imatinib Therapy

B. J. Druker

Howard Hughes Medical Institute, Oregon Health and Science University Cancer Institute, L592, 3181 SW Sam Jackson Park Road, Portland, OR 97239, USA
druker@ohsu.edu

Abstract Imatinib is an inhibitor of the ABL, platelet-derived growth factor receptors, and KIT tyrosine kinases. Given the pathogenetic role of the BCR-ABL tyrosine kinase in chronic myeloid leukemia, this was the first disease selected for clinical trials with imatinib. In the clinical trials, patients in all phases of the disease responded to imatinib and experienced minimal toxicity. Responses in patients with chronic phase disease have been durable, thus far. Clinical trials with imatinib were expanded and there are now examples of malignancies driven by each of the targets of imatinib where remarkable results have been seen. The rationale for the use of imatinib in these various diseases and the clinical trial results will be reviewed.

Keywords CML · BCR-ABL · Imatinib

1 Introduction

Imatinib mesylate (Gleevec, Glivec, formerly STI571) is an inhibitor of the ABL, platelet-derived growth factor receptor (PDGFR), and KIT tyrosine kinases. Preclinical data with this compound demonstrated specific killing of cells expressing the constitutively activated BCR-ABL tyrosine kinase. As *BCR-ABL* is the causative molecular abnormality of chronic myeloid leukemia (CML), this was the first disease selected for clinical trials with imatinib. In these clinical trials, rapid responses to imatinib were observed with durable responses in patients with CML in the chronic phase. A randomized study comparing imatinib to standard therapy with interferon-α for newly diagnosed patients with CML in the chronic phase demonstrated significantly improved outcomes for patients randomized to imatinib as initial therapy. Thus, imatinib has rapidly become the standard therapy for patients with newly diagnosed CML.

Other disease indications for which imatinib has shown clinical activity are based on the KIT and PDGFR inhibitory activities of this drug. Specifically, the majority of gastrointestinal stromal tumors (GISTs) have activating KIT mutations that drive the growth of these tumors, and imatinib has shown remarkable single agent activity in this disease. Interestingly, a subset of patients with GIST and wild-type KIT expression have activating mutations of the PDGFRA that are imatinib-sensitive, and patients with these tumors also respond to imatinib. Similarly, the subset of patients with chronic myelomonocytic leukemia (CMML) with EVT6-PDGFRB rearrangements have responded well to imatinib, as have patients with dermatofibrosarcoma protuberans (DFSP), due to the activation of the PDGFRB by constitutive production of the ligand for this receptor. Lastly, patients with hypereosinophilic syndrome (HES) have recently been shown to have an intrachromosomal deletion that results in the production of an activated PDGFRA, and these patients respond extremely well to imatinib. Whether additional uses for imatinib will be found is less clear, but at a minimum, the concept of effective and selective therapies arising by targeting pathogenetic events in tumors has been validated.

2
Clinical Features of CML

CML is a clonal hematopoietic stem cell disorder. It accounts for 15%–20% of all cases of leukemia with an annual incidence of 1 to 2 cases per 100,000 per year. The median age at diagnosis is between 50 and 60 years of age. Clinically, the disease progresses through distinct phases referred to as chronic or stable, accelerated, and blast. The chronic or stable phase of the disease is characterized by excess numbers of myeloid cells that differentiate normally. After an average of 4–6 years, the disease transforms through an "accelerated phase" to an invariably fatal acute leukemia, also known as blast crisis. Disease progression is likely due to the accumulation of molecular abnormalities that lead to a progressive loss of the capacity for terminal differentiation of the leukemic clone (Faderl et al. 1999; Sawyers 1999).

Treatment choices for patients with CML prior to the introduction of imatinib included stem cell transplantation, hydroxyurea, or interferon-α-based regimens, with allogeneic stem cell transplantation being the only proven curative therapy. As the average age of onset of CML is greater than 50 years of age, this factor, plus the inability to identify a suitably matched donor limits this option to a minority of patients. Thus, fewer than 20% of CML patients were cured with these treatment options (Faderl et al. 1999; Sawyers 1999).

3 BCR-ABL as a Therapeutic Target

Virtually all patients with CML express the BCR-ABL protein. This chimeric protein is generated as a result of a reciprocal (9;22) chromosomal translocation that produces a shortened chromosome 22, the so-called Philadelphia chromosome (Ph) (Nowell and Hungerford 1960; Rowley 1973; de Klein et al. 1982; Shtivelman et al. 1985; Ben-Neriah et al. 1986). In CML patients, the BCR-ABL fusion protein has a relative molecular mass of 210 kDa. This same fusion protein is present in approximately half of adult patients with Ph-positive acute lymphoblastic leukemia (ALL). The remainder of the Ph-positive adult ALL patients and the 3% of pediatric ALL patients that are Ph positive express a smaller BCR-ABL fusion protein termed p185 or p190BCR-ABL (Chan et al. 1987; Hermans et al. 1987; Clark et al. 1988). *BCR-ABL* has been conclusively established as a leukemic oncogene in a variety of animal models (Daley et al. 1990; Heisterkamp et al. 1990; Kelliher et al. 1990; Huettner et al. 2000) and the transforming function of the BCR-ABL protein is dependent on the tyrosine kinase activity of the ABL portion of this protein (Lugo et al. 1990). Thus, an inhibitor of the ABL protein tyrosine kinase would be predicted to be an effective and selective therapeutic agent for these leukemias.

Imatinib is a relatively specific inhibitor of the BCR-ABL tyrosine kinase (Druker and Lydon 2000; Buchdunger et al. 2001). Pre-clinical data showed significant specific activity against *BCR-ABL*-expressing cell lines in vitro and in vivo (Druker et al. 1996). In addition, imatinib could select for the growth of *BCR-ABL*-negative hematopoietic cells from CML patient samples in colony-forming assays and long-term marrow cultures (Druker et al. 1996; Deininger et al. 1997; Kasper et al. 1999). Based on the favorable pre-clinical data, imatinib was advanced to clinical trials.

4 Clinical Trials in CML

4.1 Phase I and Pharmacokinetic Studies

A standard dose-escalation phase I study of imatinib began in June 1998 at three centers in the United States. The initial study was a dose escalation trial designed to establish the maximum tolerated dose with a secondary endpoint of clinical efficacy (Druker et al. 2001b). Patients with Ph-positive CML were eligible if they had failed therapy with interferon-α and were in the chronic phase of the disease, defined as less than 15% blasts in the peripheral blood and bone marrow. Patients had to be off all anti-leukemia therapy for at least 1 week prior to starting imatinib and were required to have a white blood count (WBC) of at least 20×10^9/l. Imatinib was administered as once daily oral therapy and no other cytoreductive agents were allowed. Patients were treated continuously at their initial dose unless severe toxicity or disease progression developed.

This study enrolled 83 patients at 14 dose levels ranging from 25 to 1,000 mg. The median duration of disease at study entry was 3.8 years, and one-third of patients had signs of early progression to accelerated phase, with increased blasts or basophils in peripheral blood or marrow (Druker et al. 2001b). Imatinib was well tolerated with minimal side effects and a maximally tolerated dose could not be defined.

Pharmacokinetic studies showed that imatinib is rapidly absorbed after oral administration with a mean T_{max} of 2–4 h. The increase in mean plasma AUC was proportional to the administered dose for the dose range of 25 to 1,000 mg, although there was large interpatient variability (Peng et al. 2001). Normalizing the dose to either body weight or body surface area did not reduce interpatient variability in AUC. The mean plasma trough concentration was 0.57 μg/ml (about 1 μM) 24 h after the administration of 350 mg of imatinib at steady state, which exceeds the concentration required to inhibit proliferation of *BCR-ABL*-positive leukemic cells. The half-life of the drug is approximately 18 h (Peng et al. 2001).

Hematologic responses, defined as a 50% decrease in the WBC from baseline, maintained for at least 2 weeks, were achieved in all patients treated with 140 mg or greater of imatinib. Once doses of 300 mg or greater were reached, 53/54 patients (98%) achieved a complete hematological response (CHR), defined as a normal WBC and platelet count with no circulating immature myeloid cells, maintained for at least 4 weeks (Druker et al. 2001b). Lowering of the WBC was typically seen within the first 2–3 weeks of therapy with achievement of normal WBCs in 3–6 weeks. Normal WBCs were maintained in 51 of 53 patients with a median duration of follow-up of 310 days. At doses of imatinib of exceeding or equal to 300 mg, cytogenetic responses were seen within 5 months in 17/31 (53%) patients with 31% of patients achieving a major cytogenetic response (<35% Ph-positive) and 10% achieving a complete cytogenetic response (Druker et al. 2001b).

Given the effectiveness of imatinib in chronic-phase patients who had failed interferon, the phase I studies were expanded to include patients with CML in myeloid and lymphoid blast crisis and patients with relapsed or refractory Ph-positive ALL (Druker et al. 2001a). Patients were treated with daily doses of 300–1,000 mg of imatinib. In patients with myeloid blast crisis, 21/38 (55%) had a response to therapy, as defined by a decrease in percentage of marrow blasts to less than 15%. Seventeen of 38 (45%) cleared their marrows of blasts (<5%), with 4 of these patients (11%) meeting criteria for complete remission with full recovery of peripheral blood counts. Seven patients with myeloid blast crisis (18%) had responses lasting beyond 1 year (Druker et al. 2001a).

In patients with Ph-positive ALL or lymphoid blast crisis of CML, 14/20 (70%) responded to imatinib. Eleven of 20 (55%) completely cleared their marrow of blasts, with 4 patients (20%) meeting criteria for a complete hematologic response. All but one of the lymphoid phenotype patients relapsed between days 45 and 117 (Druker et al. 2001a).

4.2 Phase II Studies

Based on the unprecedented results in phase I studies, single agent imatinib was tested further in interferon-refractory and interferon-intolerant patients as well as in patients with accelerated phase disease and patients with CML in myeloid blast crisis and Ph-positive ALL. These studies accrued over 1,000 patients, at 30 centers in 6 countries, in 6 to 9 months. Results from these studies with 18 months of follow-up have been published (Kantarjian et al. 2002; Ottmann et al. 2002; Sawyers et al. 2002; Talpaz et al. 2002), and results updated to 30 months of follow-up are summarized in Table 1.

Table 1 Phase II results with imatinib

	Chronic phase (IFN failure)	Accelerated phase	Blast crisis
	Kantarjian et al. 2002	Talpaz et al. 2002	Sawyers et al. 2002
CHR	96%	40%	9%
MCR	64%	28%	16%
CCR	48%	20%	7%
Disease progression	13%	50%	90%

CCR, complete cytogenetic response; CHR, complete hematologic response; IFN, interferon; MCR, major cytogenetic response (Philadelphia chromosome-positive metaphases $\leq$35%).

Chronic phase patients who were refractory to or intolerant of interferon-α were treated with 400 mg per day of imatinib; 454 of the 532 enrolled patients had a confirmed diagnosis of chronic-phase disease and were evaluable for response. Eligibility criteria in this study allowed inclusion of patients with up to 15% blasts and 15% basophils in the marrow or peripheral blood. Median duration of disease was 34 months and median duration of previous interferon-α therapy was 14 months. With a median follow-up of 29 months, 96% of patients achieved a CHR, with the median time to CHR being less than 1 month. Imatinib induced major cytogenetic responses in 64% of patients, with a complete cytogenetic response rate of 48%. The estimated progression-free survival at 24 months was 87% (Kantarjian et al. 2002).

Cytogenetic responses have been durable and correlate with improved progression-free and overall survival. Thus, once a patient achieves a major cytogenetic response, it is estimated that 24 months later, 91% of these patients will not have progressed. Achievement of a major cytogenetic response at 3, 6, or within 12 months was associated with a statistically significant improvement in overall survival. For example, if patients achieve a major cytogenetic response within 12 months, the estimated survival at 24 months is 99% as compared to 86% for patients with less than a major cytogenetic response ($p<0.001$). Baseline features that independently predicted a high rate of major cytogenetic responses were the absence of blasts in the peripheral blood, a hemoglobin exceeding 12 g/dl, less than 5% blasts in the marrow, CML disease duration of less than 1 year, and a prior cytogenetic response to interferon-α (Kantarjian et al. 2002).

Results of the phase II study in patients with accelerated-phase disease were equally impressive (Talpaz et al. 2002). Accelerated phase was defined as 15%–30% blasts or more than 30% blasts plus promyelocytes in the peripheral blood or marrow, greater than 20% peripheral basophils, or a platelet count less than $100x10^9/l$, unrelated to therapy. In this study, 235 patients were enrolled. Of these, 181 had a confirmed diagnosis of accelerated phase and were analyzed for response. With follow-up of up to three years, 83% of patients showed some form of hematologic response, with 40% of patients achieving a CHR; 28% of patients achieved a major cytogenetic response, with 20% complete responses (Talpaz et al. 2002).

In this phase II study, 62 patients with a confirmed diagnosis of accelerated phase were treated with 400 mg per day of imatinib, while 119 additional patients were treated with 600 mg per day. A retrospective analysis showed that prognostic features, such as age, sex, performance status, spleen size, and hematological parameters including WBC, percentage of marrow blasts, peripheral basophils, and hemoglobin were well matched between these two groups. A significantly improved outcome for responses and survival were observed for patients treated with 600 mg per day as compared to patients treated with 400 mg. For example, using 400 mg per day, 31% of patients obtained a CHR as compared to 45% of patients treated with 600 mg per day. The rate of complete cytogenetic responses was 24% with 600 mg per day versus 13% with 400 mg per day. The estimated survival at 24 months was 44% for patients treated with 400 mg per day versus 66% for patients treated with 600 mg per day (p=0.009). Patients who obtained a CHR, maintained for at least 4 weeks, and patients with a major cytogenetic response at 3 months also had significantly improved survival. Based on these data, 600 mg per day of imatinib is the preferred dose of therapy for patients with advanced phase disease.

Results of the phase II study treating 229 patients with a confirmed diagnosis of myeloid blast crisis showed an overall response rate of 52%, with sustained hematologic responses lasting at least 4 weeks in 31% of patients. Nine percent of patients achieved a complete remission (CR=<5% blasts) with peripheral blood recovery and another 4% of patients cleared their marrows to less than 5% blasts but did not meet the criteria for CR because of persistent cytopenias. Finally, 18% of patients either returned to chronic phase or had partial responses. Major cytogenetic responses were seen in 16% of patients, with 7% having complete responses (Sawyers et al. 2002). Median survival was 6.9 months with an estimated survival of 17% at 24 months.

Baseline features predictive of prolonged survival were (1) a platelet count greater than or equal to 100×10^9/l, (2) peripheral blood blasts less than 50%, and (3) a hemoglobin at or greater than 10 gm/dl. For patients with all three of these features, the median survival was 21 months. However, if patients had none of these features, their median survival was only 4 months. Patients with a CHR or marrow blasts less than 5% at 2 months had a median survival of over 24 months and their survival was significantly longer than patients who were either returned to chronic phase or had no response. These results with single agent imatinib compare favorably with historical controls treated with chemotherapy for myeloid blast crisis in which the median survival is approximately 3 months. However, the high relapse rates suggest that imatinib should be viewed as either a bridge to allogeneic stem cell transplantation or that patients should be enrolled in clinical trials combining imatinib with other agents.

In patients with Ph-positive ALL, 29/48 (60%) responded to single agent imatinib. Unfortunately, the duration of response was relatively short, with a median estimated time to disease progression of only 2.2 months (Ottmann et al. 2002).

4.3
Phase III Comparison of Imatinib to Interferon in Newly Diagnosed Chronic Phase Patients

A phase III randomized study, comparing imatinib at 400 mg per day with interferon-α plus cytarabine (Ara-C) in newly diagnosed patients with chronic phase CML enrolled 1,106 patients from June 2000 to January 2001. Baseline characteristics of the 553 patients randomized to each treatment were well balanced for all features evaluated, including age, WBC, Sokal and Euro scores, and time from diagnosis. With a median follow-up of 19 months, patients randomized to imatinib had statistically significant better results than patients treated with interferon-α plus Ara-C in all parameters measured (Table 2), including rates of CHR, major and complete cytogenetic responses, tolerance of therapy, and freedom from disease progression (O'Brien et al. 2003). Despite the fact that 76% of patients randomized to imatinib achieved a complete cytogenetic response, the majority of these patients had detectable leukemia using *BCR-ABL* transcripts as analyzed by reverse transcriptase-polymerase chain reaction (RT-PCR) (Hughes et al. 2002). When analyzed by log reduction in *BCR-ABL* transcript levels, 39% of patients achieved at least a 3-log reduction in *BCR-ABL* levels, but only 13% and 3% achieved a 4- and 5-log reduction, respectively.

Table 2 Phase III results of imatinib versus interferon plus cytarabine for newly diagnosed chronic phase CML patients (O'Brien et al. 2003)

	Imatinib 400 mg	Interferon+Ara-C
CHR	97%	69%
MCR	87%	35%
CCR	76%	14%
Intolerance	3%	31%
Progressive disease	3%	8.5%

CCR, complete cytogenetic response; CHR, complete hematologic response; MCR, major cytogenetic response (Philadelphia chromosome-positive metaphases<35%).
Intolerance leading to discontinuation of first-line therapy. Progressive disease to accelerated phase or blast crisis. All of these differences are highly statistically significant with $p<0.001$.

5
Mechanisms of Relapse/Resistance to Imatinib

Response rates to imatinib in chronic phase patients are quite high and thus far, responses have been durable. Response rates are also quite high in pa-

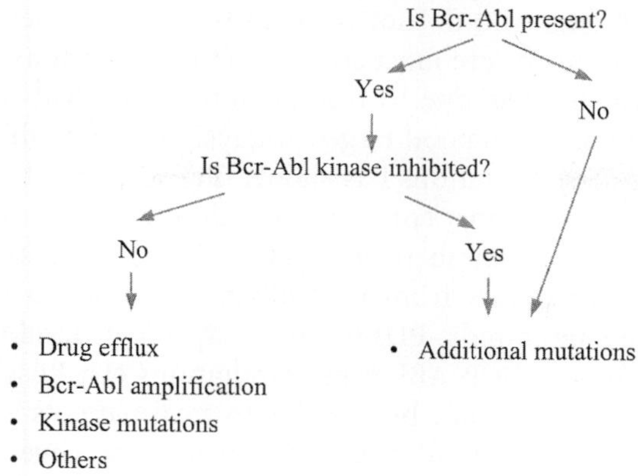

Fig. 1. Scheme for analyzing potential mechanisms of relapse

tients with advanced-phase disease, but relapses, despite continued therapy with imatinib, have been common. In all patients who have relapsed, the BCR-ABL protein remains present. A particularly useful categorization of relapsed/resistant CML patients has been to determine whether or not there is persistent inhibition of the BCR-ABL kinase (Fig. 1). Patients with persistent inhibition of the BCR-ABL kinase would be predicted to have additional molecular abnormalities besides BCR-ABL driving the growth and survival of the malignant clone. In contrast, patients with reactivation of the kinase would be postulated to have resistance mechanisms that either prevent imatinib from reaching the target or render the target insensitive to BCR-ABL. In the former category are mechanisms such as drug efflux or protein binding of imatinib. In the latter category would be mutations of the BCR-ABL kinase that render BCR-ABL insensitive to imatinib and amplification of the BCR-ABL protein.

In the largest studies of resistance or relapse, several consistent themes have emerged. In the majority of patients who respond to imatinib and then relapse while remaining on therapy, the BCR-ABL kinase has been reactivated (Gorre et al. 2001). BCR-ABL kinase activity was analyzed by assessing tyrosine phosphorylation of CRKL, a direct substrate of the BCR-ABL kinase, and the major tyrosine phosphorylated protein in CML patient samples (Oda et al. 1994; Druker et al. 2001b). In these studies, greater than 50% and perhaps as many as 90% of patients with hematologic relapse have BCR-ABL point mutations in at least 13 different amino acids scattered throughout the ABL kinase domain (Hofmann et al. 2001; Branford et al. 2002; Hochhaus et al. 2002; Roche-Lestienne et al. 2002; Shah et al. 2002; von Bubnoff et al. 2002). Some other patients have amplification of BCR-ABL at the genomic or transcript level. In contrast, in patients with primary resistance, that is, patients who do not respond to imatinib therapy, BCR-ABL-independent mechanisms are most common (Hochhaus et al. 2002).

In patients who relapse due to reactivation of the BCR-ABL kinase, the BCR-ABL kinase remains a good target. Analysis of the inhibitory activity of imatinib against these mutations has shown that some might be sensitive to dose escalation, but the most common mutation at amino acid 315 is completely insensitive to imatinib (Corbin et al. 2002). ABL kinase inhibitors with specificity that differs from imatinib have already been synthesized, and one of these compounds, PD180970, is capable of inhibiting some, but not all of the common BCR-ABL kinase mutations (La Rosee et al. 2002a). These data suggest that it may be possible to treat patients with several different ABL kinase inhibitors to circumvent resistance. Given that BCR-ABL kinase activity has been reactivated in relapsed patients, it might also be useful to target signaling pathways activated by BCR-ABL, such as RAF/MEK/ERK, PI-3 kinase, AKT, or RAS. For example, two groups recently reported in vitro sensitivity of imatinib-resistant BCR-ABL-positive cell lines to a farnesyl transferase inhibitor (Topaly et al. 2001; Hoover et al. 2002). Moreover, Hoover et al., observed that this compound sensitized cells to imatinib, even imatinib resistant cell lines (Hoover et al. 2002). Alternatively, strategies to decrease BCR-ABL protein expression using agents such as geldanamycin, 17-AAG, or arsenic trioxide might be useful (Topaly et al. 2001; Gorre et al. 2002; La Rosee et al. 2002b).

6
Safety and Tolerability

Imatinib has generally been well tolerated, with grade 3 or 4 nonhematologic toxicities being uncommon. The most common grade 1 or 2 toxicities include fluid retention, nausea, muscle cramps, skin rashes, fatigue, and diarrhea. Myelosuppression is more common in advanced phase patients than in chronic phase patients, and imatinib induced prolonged aplasia in 1% of blast crisis patients (Sawyers et al. 2002). In contrast, patients with GIST treated with 400 or 600 mg per day of imatinib had rates of grade 3/4 neutropenia and thrombocytopenia of 5% and less than 1%, respectively, demonstrating the specificity of this side effect to leukemia patients (Demetri et al. 2002). Thus, myelosuppression is more likely to be due to suppression of the BCR-ABL-positive clone as opposed to inhibition of normal hematopoiesis. For this reason, it is not clear how much is accomplished by dose reduction for myelosuppression.

7 Gastrointestinal Stromal Tumors and KIT

GISTs are mesenchymal neoplasms that can arise from any organ in the gastrointestinal tract or from the mesentery or omentum. Although GISTs morphologically resemble leiomyosarcomas and nerve sheath tumors, they are a distinct entity (Fletcher et al. 2002). More than 90% of GISTs express KIT (Hirota et al. 1998), and biochemical evidence of KIT activation can be found in almost all GISTs (Rubin et al. 2001). In approximately 90% of cases, this activation is linked to somatic mutations of KIT, usually involving exons 9 or 11 (Rubin et al. 2001). Several lines of evidence indicate that KIT mutations are an early pathogenetic event in GISTs: (1) a similar frequency and spectrum of mutations is seen in histologically benign vs malignant tumors and early/localized vs late/metastatic tumors; (2) familial syndromes of GIST are associated with germline mutations of KIT; (3) molecular studies suggest that KIT mutations are acquired before the development of cytogenetic abnormalities (Rubin et al. 2001; Corless et al. 2002; Heinrich et al. 2002c).

The standard treatment for localized GISTs is complete resection (Blanke et al. 2001). Recurrence after complete resection is common, occurring in up to 90% of patients with larger tumors (Ng et al. 1992), and survival following recurrence is short. Patients with advanced GIST have historically done poorly, with a 30% 6-month progression-free survival following initial chemotherapy. The chemosensitivity of GISTs has been difficult to define because most published series have not adequately distinguished GISTs from leiomyosarcomas and neurogenic tumors. However, the published data suggest that the response rate of GISTs to single- or multi-agent chemotherapy is less than 5%.

The concept that patients with GISTs might benefit from treatment with imatinib was based on the above data and two additional experimental observations: (1) treatment of GIST cell lines with imatinib inhibited proliferation and induced apoptosis; (2) several GIST-associated mutant KIT isoforms were potently inhibited by imatinib in vitro at concentrations similar to wild-type KIT (Heinrich et al. 2000; Tuveson et al. 2001). Based on the identification of mutated KIT as a therapeutic target in GIST and the lack of an effective conventional medical therapy, a patient with chemotherapy-resistant gastric GIST metastatic to omentum and liver was started on imatinib at 400 mg po daily in March 2000. The tumor in this patient expressed an exon 11 mutant KIT isoform and the patient responded dramatically to imatinib therapy (Joensuu et al. 2001).

The strong pre-clinical rationale, coupled with the clinical success in this solitary case, led to the development of two proof-of-principle GIST trials utilizing imatinib. An European Organization for Research and Treatment of Cancer (EORTC), dose-escalation study of imatinib included 40 patients, 36 of whom had advanced GIST. The imatinib dosage ranged from 400 mg daily to 500 mg twice daily. At the highest dose, 5 of 8 patients had grade 3 toxicity (nausea/vomiting in 3, edema in 1, and dyspnea in 1) and 400 mg twice daily was considered the maximally tolerated dose. Of the patients, 19 (53%) had objective partial responses, while 13 (36%) had stable disease and only 4 (11%) experienced frank progression (van Oosterom et al. 2001). Two patients who progressed on 400 mg subsequently responded to 800 mg. With a minimum follow-up of 11 months, 29/36 remained on treatment. None of the four patients in the trial with a non-GIST sarcoma responded to imatinib.

The GIST Working Group (a consortium of the Oregon Health and Science University Cancer Institute, the Fox Chase Cancer Center, the University of Turku, the University of Helsinki, and the Dana-Farber Cancer Institute) performed a phase II randomized trial of 400 mg daily vs 600 mg (Demetri et al. 2002): 147 patients with incurable GIST (51% pre-treated with systemic therapy) were accrued, with a median age of 54 and median performance status of 1. Of the patients, 94% had undergone previous surgery, often involving the stomach or other areas in the GI tract; therefore, drug absorption was a concern in this trial. Nevertheless, pharmacokinetic assessments showed that drug levels were actually higher than those seen in leukemia patients given imatinib. The half-life of the drug was 20 h.

Imatinib was highly effective in this advanced disease population: 62% of patients on 400 mg daily and 65% on 600 mg achieved a partial response (Demetri et al. 2002). Stable disease was seen in 19% and 20%, respectively, and 16% and 8% had primary resistance, manifested as initial disease progression. Of the patients that failed the lower dose, 28% responded when crossed over to the higher dose. With a median follow-up of 15 months, 73% of patients remained on study drug, with an overall median time-to-treatment failure of 72 weeks.

KIT mutation analysis was performed on pre-treatment tumor samples from 121 of the 147 patients in the GIST Working Group trial (Heinrich et al. 2002b). Using a combination of PCR amplification of tumor DNA, denaturing HPLC, and direct DNA sequencing, exons 9, 11, 13, and 17 of the *KIT* gene were examined for mutations. Activating mutations were found in 86% of cases, most commonly in exon 11. Despite the fact that previous studies had suggested KIT mutations in GIST were associated with a worse prognosis (Hirota et al. 1998), patients with an exon 11 mutation had a significantly higher partial response rate (72%) than those with no detectable mutations (9%), and time-to-treatment failure was statistically significantly longer as well. Patients whose tumor harbored an exon 9 mutation did less well than those with exon 11 mutation (partial rate of 32%), but responded better and had a longer time-to-treatment failure than those with no detectable mutation. Because the numbers of patients in the exon 9 mutation group and the no mutation group were relatively small, these findings need to be confirmed. It is currently recommended that imatinib be offered to all GIST patients who are candidates for systemic therapy. KIT mutation status may be helpful in assessing the risk-benefit ratio for adjuvant therapy, and might help identify patients with advanced disease who are likely to do poorly, so that alternative agents or combination therapies can be planned.

Several additional studies of imatinib in the treatment of GIST are ongoing. The EORTC enrolled a phase II trial treating GIST patients with 400 mg BID. Phase III trials of lower vs higher dose imatinib (400 vs 800 mg daily) were enrolled by a North American Intergroup and by a European Consortium (made up of the EORTC, ISG, and AGITG), and both trials accrued rapidly.

Given the high recurrence rate for GISTs, even following complete resection, and the sensitivity of the disease to imatinib, it is reasonable to test drug administration before or following surgery in higher-risk patients. At least three trials are assessing the neoadjuvant/adjuvant use of imatinib in GIST. As there is substantial evidence that KIT mutations are pathogenetic or at least occur before other molecular abnormalities, it is predicted that imatinib would be even more active in the early disease setting and may enhance surgical results by eliminating minimal residual disease (Heinrich et al. 2002c).

Besides GIST, a number of other human cancers are associated with *KIT* mutations, including mastocytosis, seminoma, and acute myeloid leukemia (AML). Although *KIT* mutations are found in almost all cases of mastocytosis, they are found in less than 10% of cases of seminoma and are rare in adult AML (Heinrich et al. 2002a). Unfortunately, the *KIT* mutation found in mastocytosis is biochemically resistant to imatinib (Ma et al. 2002), while the sensitivity of the mutations found in AML and seminoma have not been reported. Thus, it will be necessary to develop other KIT inhibitors with activity against the *KIT* mutation found in mastocytosis.

8
PDGFR as a Therapeutic Target

Translocations involving the *PDGFRB* gene have been identified in several myeloproliferative and myelodysplastic syndromes. The most common of these translocations, (5;12)(q33;p13), is seen in a subset of patients with CMML and results in fusion of the *EVT6* (*TEL*) and *PDGFRB* genes (Golub et al. 1994). *EVT6* is a member of the ETS family of transcription factors and contains an amino terminal domain that mediates homotypic oligomerization. When fused to the membrane-spanning region of PDGFRB, this domain leads to dimerization of PDGFRB and constitutive activation of its kinase activity (Carroll et al. 1996).

Both wild-type PDGFRB and EVT6-PDGFRB are inhibited by imatinib (Carroll et al. 1997); thus, EVT6-PDGFRB represents an attractive therapeutic target. In preliminary reports, several patients with CMML containing the (5;12)(q33;p13) translocation were treated with imatinib and all achieved complete hematologic remissions (Apperley et al. 2002; Magnusson et al. 2002). This encouraging result indicates that imatinib may be used to treat tumors that are dependent on PDGFR activation. There are additional chromosomal translocations that partner the *PDGFRB* gene with *H4, HIP1, CEV14*, or *Rab5*. Affected patients are described as having a myeloproliferative disorder with eosinophilia, eosinophilic leukemia, or CMML (Schwaller et al. 2001). Though rare, all of these PDGFRB-driven myeloid proliferations are potentially treatable with imatinib.

The PDGFRB pathway is also a target in DFSP, a low-grade sarcoma of the dermis that often recurs after surgical excision. These tumors are characterized by a (17;22) translocation involving the *COL1A1* and *PDGF-B* genes, which results in over-production of fusion COL1A1-PDGF-BB ligand and consequent hyperactivation of PDGFRB (Simon et al. 1997). It has been shown that imatinib inhibits the growth of DFSP cells both in culture and in immunodeficient mice (Sjoblom et al. 2001), and preliminary results in patients look promising (Maki et al. 2002; Rubin et al. 2002).

In the GIST clinical trials, it was observed that a small subset of patients with wild-type KIT expression responded well to imatinib. Careful examination of patients with wild-type KIT-expressing tumors showed that one third of these tumors had activating mutations of the PDGFRA (Heinrich et al. 2003). These mutations occurred in two different exons. One set of mutations was imatinib-sensitive and this accounted for responses observed in patients whose tumors expressed wild-type KIT (Heinrich et al. 2003).

Another disease in which imatinib has shown remarkable clinical benefits is HES. Imatinib had initially been used empirically in this disease and the dramatic results prompted investigations of the molecular basis for imatinib's activity in this disease. Two groups independently arrived at the conclusion that an intrachromosomal deletion on chromosome 4 resulted in a fusion between a gene of unknown function, FIP1L1, and a truncated PDGFRA in a large percentage of patients with this disorder (Cools et al. 2003; Griffin et al. 2003). The resulting FIP1L1-PRGFRA fusion protein is a constitutively activated tyrosine kinase that is imatinib sensitive, thus accounting for the responsiveness of this disease to imatinib.

Both KIT and the PDGF receptors are expressed in many common tumors and have been reported to be activated by both autocrine and paracrine mechanisms. In most of these tumors, it is unclear whether monotherapy with imatinib would be useful. Most likely, KIT and PDGFR activation have a supportive rather than a pathogenetic role in these tumors. Although imatinib may have a role in the treatment of such cancers, meaningful conclusions will only be derived from carefully designed clinical trials that incorporate proteomic and genomic assessment of target activation status.

9 Conclusions

The last few years have been filled with tremendous excitement as the dramatic activity of imatinib has been demonstrated in clinical trials. The clinical development of imatinib has shown that a combination of the right drug with the appropriate target disease and patient population can reveal the true potential of such targeted agents.

Acknowledgements Dr. Druker's laboratory is supported by the Howard Hughes Medical Institute and grants from the National Cancer Institute, The Leukemia and Lymphoma Society, the Burroughs Wellcome Fund, the T.J. Martell Foundation, and the Doris Duke Charitable Foundation.

References

Apperley JF, Gardembas M, Melo JV, Russell-Jones R, Bain BJ, Baxter EJ, Chase A, Chessells JM, Colombat M, Dearden CE, Dimitrijevic S, Mahon FX, Marin D, Nikolova Z, Olavarria E, Silberman S, Schultheis B, Cross NC, Goldman JM (2002) Response to imatinib mesylate in patients with chronic myeloproliferative diseases with rearrangements of the platelet-derived growth factor receptor beta. N Engl J Med 347:481–7

Ben-Neriah Y, Daley GQ, Mes-Masson A-M, Witte ON, Baltimore D (1986) The chronic myelogenous leukemia-specific P210 protein is the product of the bcr/abl hybrid gene. Science 233:212–214

Blanke CD, Eisenberg BL, Heinrich MC (2001) Gastrointestinal stromal tumors. Curr Treat Options Oncol 2:485–91

Branford S, Rudzki Z, Walsh S, Grigg A, Arthur C, Taylor K, Herrmann R, Lynch KP, Hughes TP (2002) High frequency of point mutations clustered within the adenosine triphosphate-binding region of BCR/ABL in patients with chronic myeloid leukemia or Ph-positive acute lymphoblastic leukemia who develop imatinib (STI571) resistance. Blood 99:3472–3475

Buchdunger E, Matter A, Druker BJ (2001) Bcr-Abl inhibition as a modality of CML therapeutics. Biochim Biophys Acta 1551:M11–18

Carroll M, Tomasson MH, Barker GF, Golub TR, Gilliland DG (1996) The Tel platelet-derived growth factor beta receptor (PDGF-beta-R) fusion in chronic myelomonocytic leukemia is a transforming protein that self-associates and activates PDGF-beta-R kinase-dependent signaling pathways. Proc Natl Acad Sci USA 93:14845–14850

Carroll M, Ohno-Jones S, Tamura S, Buchdunger E, Zimmermann J, Lydon NB, Gilliland DG, Druker BJ (1997) CGP 57148, a tyrosine kinase inhibitor, inhibits the growth of cells expressing BCR-ABL, TEL-ABL and TEL-PDGFR fusion proteins. Blood 90:4947–4952

Chan LC, Karhi KK, Rayter SI, Heisterkamp N, Eridani S, Powles R, Lawler SD, Groffen J, Foulkes JG, Greaves MF, et al (1987) A novel abl protein expressed in Philadelphia chromosome positive acute lymphoblastic leukaemia. Nature 325:635–7

Clark SS, McLaughlin J, Timmons M, Pendergast AM, Ben-Neriah Y, Dow LW, Crist W, Rovera G, Smith SD, Witte ON (1988) Expression of a distinctive BCR-ABL oncogene in Ph1-positive acute lymphocytic leukemia (ALL). Science 239:775–777

Cools J, DeAngelo DJ, Gotlib J, Stover EH, Legare RD, Cortes J, Kutok J, Clark J, Galinsky I, Griffin JD, Cross NC, Tefferi A, Malone J, Alam R, Schrier SL, Schmid J, Rose M, Vandenberghe P, Verhoef G, Boogaerts M, Wlodarska I, Kantarjian H, Marynen P, Coutre SE, Stone R, Gilliland DG (2003) A tyrosine kinase created by fusion of the PDGFRA and FIP1L1 genes as a therapeutic target of imatinib in idiopathic hypereosinophilic syndrome. N Engl J Med 348:1201–14

Corbin AS, Buchdunger E, Pascal F, Druker BJ (2002) Analysis of the structural basis of specificity of inhibition of the Abl kinase by STI571. J Biol Chem 277:32214–32219

Corless CL, McGreevey L, Haley A, Town A, Heinrich MC (2002) KIT mutations are common in incidental gastrointestinal stromal tumors one centimeter or less in size. Am J Pathol 160:1567–72

Daley GQ, Van Etten RA, Baltimore D (1990) Induction of chronic myelogenous leukemia in mice by the P210bcr/abl gene of the Philadelphia chromosome. Science 247:824–830

de Klein A, van Kessel AG, Grosveld G, Bartram CR, Hagemeijer A, Bootsma D, Spurr NK, Heisterkamp N, Groffen J, Stephenson JR (1982) A cellular oncogene is translocated to the Philadelphia chromosome in chronic myelocytic leukemia. Nature 300:765–767

Deininger MW, Goldman JM, Lydon N, Melo JV (1997) The tyrosine kinase inhibitor CGP57148B selectively inhibits the growth of BCR-ABL-positive cells. Blood 90:3691–3698

Demetri GD, von Mehren M, Blanke CD, Van den Abbeele AD, Eisenberg B, Roberts PJ, Heinrich MC, Tuveson DA, Singer S, Janicek M, Fletcher JA, Silverman SG, Silberman SL, Capdeville R, Kiese B, Peng B, Dimitrijevic S, Druker BJ, Corless C, Fletcher CD, Joensuu H (2002) Efficacy and safety of imatinib mesylate in advanced gastrointestinal stromal tumors. N Engl J Med 347:472–480

Druker BJ, Tamura S, Buchdunger E, Ohno S, Segal GM, Fanning S, Zimmermann J, Lydon NB (1996) Effects of a selective inhibitor of the ABL tyrosine kinase on the growth of BCR-ABL positive cells. Nat Med 2:561–566

Druker BJ, Lydon NB (2000) Lessons learned from the development of an abl tyrosine kinase inhibitor for chronic myelogenous leukemia. J Clin Invest 105:3-7

Druker BJ, Sawyers CL, Kantarjian H, Resta DJ, Fernandes Reese S, Ford JM, Capdeville R, Talpaz M (2001a) Activity of a specific inhibitor of the Bcr-Abl tyrosine kinase in the blast crisis of chronic myeloid leukemia and acute lymphoblastic leukemia with the Philadelphia chromosome. N Engl J Med 344:1038–1042

Druker BJ, Talpaz M, Resta D, Peng B, Buchdunger E, Ford JM, Lydon NB, Kantarjian H, Capdeville R, Ohno-Jones S, Sawyers CL (2001b) Efficacy and safety of a specific inhibitor of the Bcr-Abl tyrosine kinase in chronic myeloid leukemia. N Engl J Med 344:1031–1037

Faderl S, Talpaz M, Estrov Z, Kantarjian HM (1999) Chronic myelogenous leukemia: biology and therapy. Ann Intern Med 131:207–219

Fletcher CD, Berman JJ, Corless C, Gorstein F, Lasota J, Longley BJ, Miettinen M, O'Leary TJ, Remotti H, Rubin BP, Shmookler B, Sobin LH, Weiss SW (2002) Diagnosis of gastrointestinal stromal tumors: a consensus approach. Hum Pathol 33:459–65

Golub TR, Barker GF, Lovett M, Gilliland DG (1994) Fusion of PDGF receptor beta to a novel ets-like gene, tel, in chronic myelomonocytic leukemia with t(5;12) chromosomal translocation. Cell 77:307–316

Gorre ME, Mohammed M, Ellwood K, Hsu N, Paquette R, Rao PN, Sawyers CL (2001) Clinical resistance to STI-571 cancer therapy caused by BCR-ABL gene mutation or amplification. Science 293:876–880

Gorre ME, Ellwood-Yen K, Chiosis G, Rosen N, Sawyers CL (2002) BCR-ABL point mutants isolated from patients with imatinib mesylate-resistant chronic myeloid leukemia remain sensitive to inhibitors of the BCR-ABL chaperone heat shock protein 90. Blood 100:3041–3044

Griffin JH, Leung J, Bruner RJ, Caligiuri MA, Briesewitz R (2003) Discovery of a fusion kinase in EOL-1 cells and idiopathic hypereosinophilic syndrome. Proc Natl Acad Sci U S A 100:7830–5

Heinrich MC, Griffith DJ, Druker BJ, Wait CL, Ott KA, Zigler AJ (2000) Inhibition of c-kit receptor tyrosine kinase activity by STI 571, a selective tyrosine kinase inhibitor. Blood 96:925–932

Heinrich MC, Blanke CD, Druker BJ, Corless CL (2002a) Inhibition of KIT tyrosine kinase activity: a novel molecular approach to the treatment of KIT-positive malignancies. J Clin Oncol 20:1692–703

Heinrich MC, Corless CL, Blanke CD, Demetri GD, Joensuu H, von Mehren M, McGreevey LS, Wait CL, Griffith D, Chen C-J, Haley A, Kiese B, Druker B, Roberts PJ, Eisenberg B, Singer S, Silberman S, Dimitrijevic S, Fletcher CDM, Fletcher JA (2002b) KIT mutational status predicts response to STI571 in patients with metastatic gastrointestinal stromal tumors (GISTs). Proc Am Soc Clin Onc 21:2a

Heinrich MC, Corless CL, Duensing A, McGreevey L, Chen CJ, Joseph N, Singer S, Griffith DJ, Haley A, Town A, Demetri GD, Fletcher CD, Fletcher JA (2003) PDGFRA activating mutations in gastrointestinal stromal tumors. Science 299:708–10

Heinrich MC, Rubin BP, Longley BJ, Fletcher JA (2002c) Biology and genetic aspects of gastrointestinal stromal tumors: KIT activation and cytogenetic alterations. Hum Pathol 33:484–95

Heisterkamp N, Jenster G, ten Hoeve J, Zovich D, Pattengale PK, Groffen J (1990) Acute leukaemia in bcr/abl transgenic mice. Nature 344:251–3

Hermans A, Heisterkamp N, von Lindern M, van Baal S, Meijer D, van der Plas D, Wiedemann LM, Groffen J, Bootsma D, Grosveld G (1987) Unique fusion of bcr and c-abl genes in Philadelphia chromosome positive acute lymphoblastic leukemia. Cell 51:33–40

Hirota S, Isozaki K, Moriyama Y, Hashimoto K, Nishida T, Ishiguro S, Kawano K, Hanada M, Kurata A, Takeda M, Muhammad Tunio G, Matsuzawa Y, Kanakura Y, Shinomura Y, Kitamura Y (1998) Gain-of-function mutations of c-kit in human gastrointestinal stromal tumors. Science 279:577–580

Hochhaus A, Kreil S, Corbin AS, La Rosée P, Müller MC, Lahaye T, Hanfstein B, Schoch C, Cross NCP, Berger U, Gschaidmeier H, Druker BJ, Hehlmann R (2002) Molecular and chromosomal mechanisms of resistance to imatinib (STI571) therapy. Leukemia 16:2190–2196

Hofmann WK, Jones LC, Lemp NA, de Vos S, Gschaidmeier H, Hoelzer D, Ottmann OG, Koeffler HP (2001) Ph(+) acute lymphoblastic leukemia resistant to the tyrosine kinase inhibitor STI571 has a unique BCR-ABL gene mutation. Blood 99:1860–1862

Hoover RR, Mahon FX, Melo JV, Daley GQ (2002) Overcoming STI571 resistance with the farnesyl transferase inhibitor SCH66336. Blood 100:1068–1071

Huettner CS, Zhang P, Van Etten RA, Tenen DG (2000) Reversibility of acute B-cell leukaemia induced by BCR-ABL1. Nat Genet 24:57–60

Hughes T, Kaeda J, Branford S, Rudzki Z, Hochhaus A, Capdeville R, Gathmann I, Bolton AE, Goldman JM, Radich J (2002) Molecular responses to imatinib (STI571) or interferon + Ara-C as initial therapy for CML: results in the IRIS study. Blood 100:93a

Joensuu H, Roberts PJ, Sarlomo-Rikala M, Andersson LC, Tervahartiala P, Tuveson D, Silberman S, Capdeville R, Dimitrijevic S, Druker B, Demetri GD (2001) Effect of the tyrosine kinase inhibitor STI571 in a patient with a metastatic gastrointestinal stromal tumor. N Engl J Med 344:1052–1056

Kantarjian H, Sawyers C, Hochhaus A, Guilhot F, Schiffer C, Gambacorti-Passerini C, Niederwieser D, Resta D, Capdeville R, Zoellner U, Talpaz M, Druker B (2002) Hematologic and cytogenetic responses to imatinib mesylate in chronic myelogenous leukemia. N Engl J Med 346:645–652

Kasper B, Fruehauf S, Schiedlmeier B, Buchdunger E, Ho AD, Zeller WJ (1999) Favorable therapeutic index of a p210(BCR-ABL)-specific tyrosine kinase inhibitor; activity on lineage-committed and primitive chronic myelogenous leukemia progenitors. Cancer Chemother Pharmacol 44:433–438

Kelliher MA, McLaughlin J, Witte ON, Rosenberg N (1990) Induction of a chronic myelogenous leukemia-like syndrome in mice with v-abl and BCR/ABL. Proc Natl Acad Sci USA 87:6649–6653

La Rosee P, Corbin AS, Stoffregen EP, Deininger MW, Druker BJ (2002a) Activity of the Bcr-Abl kinase inhibitor PD180970 against clinically relevant Bcr-Abl isoforms that cause resistance to imatinib mesylate (Gleevec, STI571). Cancer Res 62:7149–7153

La Rosee P, Johnson K, O'Dwyer ME, Druker BJ (2002b) In vitro studies of the combination of imatinib mesylate (Gleevec) and arsenic trioxide (Trisenox) in chronic myelogenous leukemia. Exp Hematol 30:729–737

Lugo TG, Pendergast AM, Muller AJ, Witte ON (1990) Tyrosine kinase activity and transformation potency of bcr-abl oncogene products. Science 247:1079–1082

Ma Y, Zeng S, Metcalfe DD, Akin C, Dimitrijevic S, Butterfield JH, McMahon G, Longley BJ (2002) The c-KIT mutation causing human mastocytosis is resistant to STI571 and other KIT kinase inhibitors; kinases with enzymatic site mutations show different inhibitor sensitivity profiles than wild-type kinases and those with regulatory-type mutations. Blood 99:1741–4

Magnusson MK, Meade KE, Nakamura R, Barrett J, Dunbar CE (2002) Activity of STI571 in chronic myelomonocytic leukemia with a platelet-derived growth factor beta receptor fusion oncogene. Blood 100:1088–91

Maki RG, Awan RA, Dixon RH, Jhanwar S, Antonescu CR (2002) Differential sensitivity to imatinib of 2 patients with metastatic sarcoma arising from dermatofibrosarcoma protuberans. Int J Cancer 100:623–626

Ng EH, Pollock RE, Munsell MF, Atkinson EN, Romsdahl MM (1992) Prognostic factors influencing survival in gastrointestinal leiomyosarcomas. Implications for surgical management and staging. Ann Surg 215:68–77

Nowell PC, Hungerford DA (1960) A minute chromosome in human chronic granulocytic leukemia. Science 132:1497–1501

O'Brien SG, Guilhot F, Larson RA, Gathmann I, Baccarani M, Cervantes C, Cornelissen J, Fischer T, Hochhaus A, Hughes T, Kantarjian H, Lechner K, Nielsen JL, Rousselot P, Reiffers J, Saglio G, Shepherd J, Simonsson S, Gratwohl A, Goldman JM, Taylor K, Verhoef G, Bolton AE, Capdeville R, Druker BJ (2003) Imatinib compared with interferon and low-dose cytarabine for newly diagnosed chronic-phase chronic myeloid leukemia. N Engl J Med 348:994–1004

Oda T, Heaney C, Hagopian J, Okuda K, Griffin JD, Druker BJ (1994) CRKL is the major tyrosine phosphorylated protein in neutrophils from patients with chronic myelogenous leukemia. J Biol Chem 269:22925–22928

Ottmann OG, Druker BJ, Sawyers CL, Goldman JM, Reiffers J, Silver RT, Tura S, Fischer T, Deininger MW, Schiffer CA, Baccarani M, Gratwohl A, Hochhaus A, Hoelzer D, Fernandes-Reese S, Gathmann I, Capdeville R, O'Brien SG (2002) A phase 2 study of imatinib in patients with relapsed or refractory Philadelphia chromosome-positive acute lymphoid leukemias. Blood 100:1965–1971

Peng B, Hayes M, Racine-Poon A, Druker BJ, Talpaz M, Sawyers CL, Resta D, Ford JM, Lloyd P, Capdeville R (2001) Clinical investigation of the pharmacokinetic/pharmacodynamic relationship for Glivec (STI571): a novel inhibitor of signal transduction. Proc Am Soc Clin Oncol 20:71a

Roche-Lestienne C, Soenen-Cornu V, Grardel-Duflos N, Lai JL, Philippe N, Facon T, Fenaux P, Preudhomme C (2002) Several types of mutations of the Abl gene can be found in chronic myeloid leukemia patients resistant to STI571, and they can pre-exist to the onset of treatment. Blood 100:1014–1018

Rowley JD (1973) A new consistent abnormality in chronic myelogenous leukaemia identified by quinacrine fluorescence and Giemsa staining. Nature 243:290–293

Rubin BP, Singer S, Tsao C, Duensing A, Lux ML, Ruiz R, Hibbard MK, Chen CJ, Xiao S, Tuveson DA, Demetri GD, Fletcher CDM, Fletcher JA (2001) KIT activation is a ubiquitous feature of gastrointestinal stromal tumors. Cancer Research 61:8118–8121

Rubin BP, Schuetze SM, Eary JF, Norwood TH, Mirza S, Conrad EU, Bruckner JD (2002) Molecular targeting of platelet-derived growth factor B by imatinib mesylate in a patient with metastatic dermatofibrosarcoma protuberans. J Clin Oncol 20:3586–91

Sawyers CL (1999) Chronic myeloid leukemia. N Engl J Med 340:1330–1340

Sawyers CL, Hochhaus A, Feldman E, Goldman JM, Miller CB, Ottmann OG, Schiffer CA, Talpaz M, Guilhot F, Deininger MWN, Fischer T, O'Brien SG, Stone RM, Gambacorti-Passerini CB, Russell NH, Reiffers JJ, Shea TC, Chapuis B, Coutre S, Tura S, Morra E, Larson RA, Saven A, Peschel C, Gratwohl A, Mandelli F, Ben-Am M, Gathmann I, Capdeville R, Paquette RL, Druker BJ (2002) Imatinib induces hematologic and cytogenetic responses in patients with chronic myeloid leukemia in myeloid blast crisis: results of a phase II study. Blood 99:3530–3539

Schwaller J, Anastasiadou E, Cain D, Kutok J, Wojiski S, Williams IR, LaStarza R, Crescenzi B, Sternberg DW, Andreasson P, Schiavo R, Siena S, Mecucci C, Gilliland DG (2001) H4(D10S170), a gene frequently rearranged in papillary thyroid carcinoma, is fused to the platelet-derived growth factor receptor beta gene in atypical chronic myeloid leukemia with t(5;10)(q33;q22). Blood 97:3910–8

Shah NP, Nicoll JM, Nagar B, Gorre ME, Paquette RL, Kuriyan J, Sawyers CL (2002) Multiple BCR-ABL kinase domain mutations confer polyclonal resistance to the tyrosine kinase inhibitor imatinib (STI571) in chronic phase and blast crisis chronic myeloid leukemia. Cancer Cell 2:117–125

Shtivelman E, Lifshitz B, Gale RP, Canaani E (1985) Fused transcript of abl and bcr genes in chronic myelogenous leukaemia. Nature 315:550–554

Simon MP, Pedeutour F, Sirvent N, Grosgeorge J, Minoletti F, Coindre JM, Terrier-Lacombe MJ, Mandahl N, Craver RD, Blin N, Sozzi G, Turc-Carel C, O'Brien KP, Kedra D, Fransson I, Guilbaud C, Dumanski JP (1997) Deregulation of the platelet-derived growth factor B-chain gene via fusion with collagen gene COL1A1 in dermatofibrosarcoma protuberans and giant-cell fibroblastoma. Nat Genet 15:95–98

Sjoblom T, Shimizu A, O'Brien KP, Pietras K, Dal Cin P, Buchdunger E, Dumanski JP, Ostman A, Heldin CH (2001) Growth inhibition of dermatofibrosarcoma protuberans tumors by the platelet-derived growth factor receptor antagonist STI571 through induction of apoptosis. Cancer Res 61:5778–5783

Talpaz M, Silver RT, Druker BJ, Goldman JM, Gambacorti-Passerini C, Guilhot F, Schiffer CA, Fischer T, Deininger MWN, Lennard AL, Hochhaus A, Ottmann OG, Gratwohl A, Baccarani M, Stone R, Tura S, Mahon F-X, Fernandes-Reese S, Gathmann I, Capdeville R, Kantarjian HM, Sawyers CL (2002) Imatinib induces durable hematologic and cytogenetic responses in patients with accelerated phase chronic myeloid leukemia: results of a phase 2 study. Blood 99:1928–1937

Topaly J, Zeller WJ, Fruehauf S (2001) Synergistic activity of the new ABL-specific tyrosine kinase inhibitor STI571 and chemotherapeutic drugs on BCR-ABL-positive chronic myelogenous leukemia cells. Leukemia 15:342–347

Tuveson DA, Willis NA, Jacks T, Griffin JD, Singer S, Fletcher CD, Fletcher JA, Demetri GD (2001) STI571 inactivation of the gastrointestinal stromal tumor c-KIT oncoprotein: biological and clinical implications. Oncogene 20:5054–8

van Oosterom AT, Judson I, Verweij J, Stroobants S, Donato di Paola E, Dimitrijevic S, Martens M, Webb A, Sciot R, Van Glabbeke M, Silberman S, Nielsen OS (2001) Safety and efficacy of imatinib (STI571) in metastatic gastrointestinal stromal tumours: a phase I study. Lancet 358:1421–1423

von Bubnoff N, Schneller F, Peschel C, Duyster J (2002) BCR-ABL gene mutations in relation to clinical resistance of Philadelphia-chromosome-positive leukaemia to STI571: a prospective study. Lancet 359:487–491

HEP (2005) 167:411–432

Isoquinolinesulfonamide: A Specific Inhibitor of Rho-Kinase and the Clinical Aspect of Anti-Rho-Kinase Therapy

H. Hidaka[1] (✉) · Y. Suzuki[2] · M. Shibuya[3] · Y. Sasaki[4]

[1] Western Therapeutics Institute, 100-32 Yagotohonmachi, Showa-ku, 466-0825 Nagoya, Japan
hhidaka@aqua.ocn.ne.jp
[2] Department of Neurosurgery, Nagoya Daini Red Cross Hospital, 2-9 Myoken, Showa-ku, 466-8650 Nagoya, Japan
[3] Chukyo Hospital, 1-1-10 Sanjo, Minami-ku, 457-8510 Nagoya, Japan
[4] Department of Pharmacology, Pharmaceutical Science, Kitasato University, 5-9-1 Shirokane, Minato-ku, 108-8641 Tokyo, Japan

Abstract The light of molecular pharmacology research has been focused on protein kinase inhibitor sulfonamide derivatives since 1978. Our studies on naphthalene and isoquinoline sulfonamide derivatives over the last 25 years have achieved a pronounced contribution toward elucidating the physiological function of various protein kinases and, moreover, toward developing a new type of medicine. This chapter relates to the discovery of new protein kinase inhibitors, their mechanisms of action, and their clinical application in Japan.

Keywords Calmodulin antagonist · W-7 · Naphthalenesulfonamide · Isoquinolinesulfonamide · H-7 · H-8 · H-9 · HA1077 · Rho kinase inhibitor · Vasodilator · Phosphorylation of MLC_{20} · Vasospasm · Cerebral ischemia · Subarachnoid hemorrhage · Cerebral infarction

1
Discovery of Isoquinolinesulfonamide as a Protein Kinase Inhibitor

1.1
History of Discovery

Chemical compounds incorporating a sulfonamide residue have been synthesized for therapeutic purposes for over 70 years. In the period 1930–1950, many compounds were patented. Prontosil was produced as an anti-bacterial agent, and several kinds of sulfonamide derivatives appeared as diuretic agents. Other sulfonylureas were synthesized for different indications and used clinically for diabetes mellitus. However, none of the patents on sulfonamides, as their use as medicines declined, was maintained any more in the period of 1950–1970.

In the latter half of the 1970s, Hidaka et al. brought a new and unexpected focus on certain sulfonamide derivatives (Fig. 1). In 1978, a newly synthesized compound, *N*-(6-aminohexyl)-5-chloro-1-naphthalene-sulfonamide (W-7) was reported to inhibit contractile response of vascular smooth muscle in concentrations ranging from 1 to 300 μM by affecting actomyosin ATPase activity (Hidaka et al. 1978a). The molecular mechanism of W-7 action was then more thoroughly investigated (Hidaka et al. 1978b; Hidaka et al. 1979). W-7 inhibited the superprecipitation of aorta smooth muscle actomyosin, and the addition of the modulator protein calmodulin (CaM) neutralized, in a dose-dependent fashion, the inhibition of actomyosin superprecipitation by W-7 in a dose-dependent fashion.

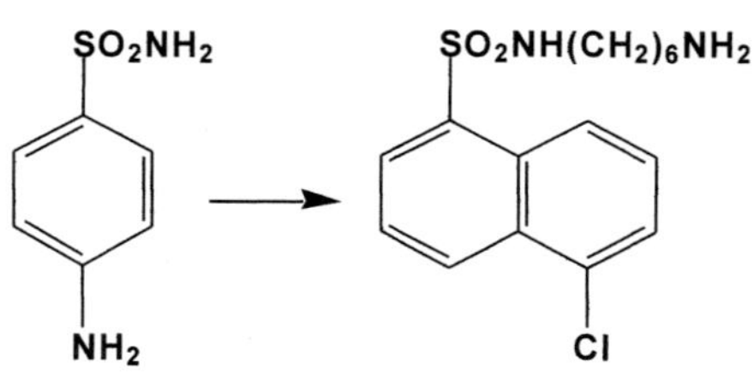

Prontsil **(Roughton et al., 1932)** **W-7** **(Hidaka et al., 1978)**

Fig. 1 Structure of sulfonamide derivatives Prontosil and W-7, anti-bacterial agent and calmodulin antagonist, respectively

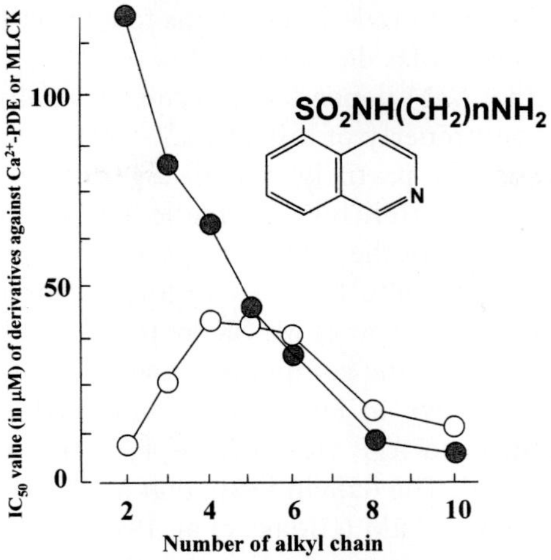

Fig. 2 Effect of naphthalenesulfonamides with various alkyl chains on calmodulin-dependent PDE and MLCK. The *closed* and *open circles* represent Ca^{2+}/calmodulin-dependent PDE and MLCK, respectively

In the process of elucidating the mechanism of action of W-7, we found W-7 to bind CaM only in the presence of calcium, indicating that it inhibited the activities of CaM-dependent enzymes by preventing the binding of CaM to these enzymes (Tanaka and Hidaka 1980a). The studies indicated that W-7 was a calmodulin antagonist (Hidaka and Tanaka 1983). This was the first time that the target molecule of a sulfonamide had been clarified.

As shown in Fig. 1, W-7 has six alkyl carbon chains. We have studied the effect of W-7 and its derivatives on Ca^{2+}/CaM-dependent enzymes such as Ca^{2+}/CaM-dependent cyclic nucleotide phosphodiesterase (Ca^{2+}-PDE) and myosin light chain kinase (MLCK) (Saito et al. 1987). We have synthesized several naphthalenesulfonamides with different alkyl chains, from 2–10, and examined their inhibitory effects on at least two different calcium-dependent enzymes (Fig. 2). The inhibitory activities on Ca^{2+}-PDE increased when the alkyl-carbon chain was elongated, while the inhibitory activities for MLCK did not always increase with a similar elongation of the alkyl-carbon chain. Contrasting results were clearly observed in the inhibitory activities of naphthalenesulfonamide derivatives with shorter alkyl-carbon chains (from 2–4) toward Ca^{2+}-PDE and MLCK. Inhibition of Ca^{2+}-PDE by ML-9, a naphthalenesulfonamide with a hexahydro-1,4-diazepine substituent corresponding to the length of two alkyl carbon chains between amino residues, was very weak, but the inhibition of MLCK by ML-9 was about ten times stronger (Saito et al. 1987). These different inhibitory potencies strongly suggested that the naphthalenesulfonamide ML-9 was a specific inhibitor of MLCK. The results also suggested that the inhibition of MLCK produced by ML-9 did not seem to be related to CaM but perhaps to a novel mechanism. Therefore, we performed the studies described below.

It is well-known that CaM-dependent enzymes partially digested by trypsin share the common property of loss of Ca^{2+}-CaM dependence (Tanaka et al. 1980b). In other words, partially trypsin-digested preparations of calcium-dependent enzymes exhibit full enzymatic activity even in the absence of Ca^{2+}-CaM. The removal of the inhibitory domain by proteolysis results in conversion of the enzymes into their active forms. Therefore, we prepared the Ca^{2+}/CaM-independent form of MLCK by partial proteolysis in order to evaluate the direct action of the compounds toward MLCK. We obtained results similar to those shown in Fig. 2. ML-9 inhibited Ca^{2+}/CaM-independent MLCK with respect to ATP with a K_i of 4.1 μM, but it inhibited CaM action with a K_i of 50 μM. The data indicate that ML-9 inhibits MLCK directly without interaction with CaM (Hidaka et al. 1991).

We therefore began studies to find and design new protein kinase inhibitors, considering that the compound with two alkyl chains between amino residues—which is more closely related to quinoline, isoquinoline, and quinazoline rather than naphthalene—inhibits Ca^{2+}/CaM-independent MLCK. Following these ideas, we have succeeded in finding the structure of new protein kinase inhibitors as shown in Fig. 3 (Hidaka et al. 1984). H-9 shown in Fig. 4 was a suitable ligand for affinity chromatography. By using an H-9 affinity column, we purified various protein kinases successfully from tissues (Inagaki et al. 1985). Our results also suggested that a number of different protein kinases could be isolated through this column chromatography approach. This is very important information not only for the purification of protein kinases, but also for estimation of the relative affinities of each of the protein kinases for isoquinolinesulfonamide. As shown in Fig. 4, cyclic AMP-dependent kinase (PKA), cyclic GMP-dependent kinase (PKG), and protein kinase C (PKC) were purified by H-9 affinity column chromatography (Inagaki et al. 1985).

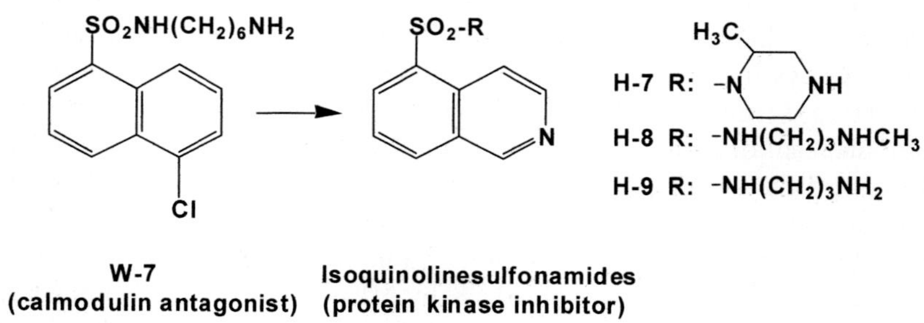

Fig. 3 The structure of isoquinolinesulfonamide derivatives that are protein kinase inhibitors

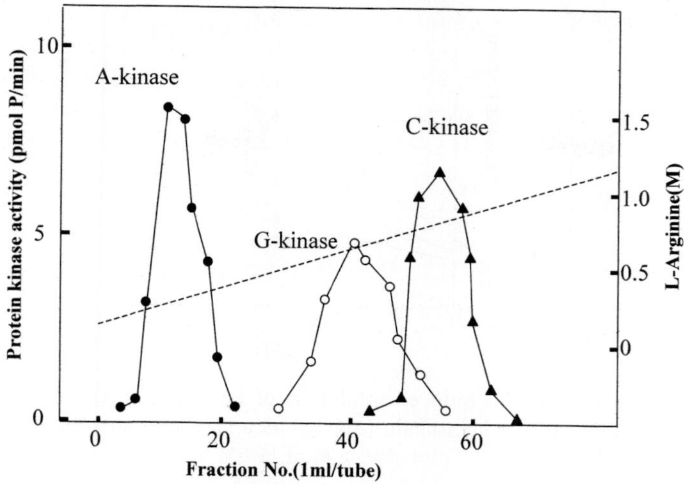

Fig. 4 H-9 affinity chromatography for purification of protein kinases. The mixed fraction, which contains PKC, PKA, and PKG partially purified from diethylaminoethyl (DEAE) column chromatography of 100,000×*g* supernatant of rat brain, was applied to H-9-immobilized Sepharose 4B column, and then the three protein kinases were separately eluted from the column by an l-arginine gradient

By application of this affinity column to a trial of purification of PKC, we found that we could purify PKC and we also uncovered the existence of the γ-isoform of PKC (Ohno et al. 1987). Among the inhibitor derivatives, H-7 was found to be relatively specific for protein kinase C.

1.2
Why Are Isoquinolinesulfonamides Specific for Protein Kinases?

As shown in Fig. 5, H-7 inhibited protein kinase C in competitive fashion with respect to ATP. It should be noticed that the same special arrangement of H-7 and ATP was revealed by co-crystallization of ATP or H-7 with PKA (Fig. 6) (Engh et al. 1996). This hypothesis is supported by our previous data that the isoquinolinesulfonamide H-8 inhibited all examined protein kinases competitively with respect to ATP, and the addition of H-8 protected the catalytic subunit of PKA from irreversible inactivation by the ATP analog *p*-fluorosulfonylbenzoyl-5′-adenosine (FSBA) in a dose-dependent manner. Our data (Hagiwara et al. 1987) also indicated that when the quantitative binding of H-8 to PKA was measured under conditions of thermodynamic equilibrium using a gel filtration method, the catalytic subunit bound approximately 1 mol of drug/mol of protein with apparent half-maximal binding at 1.0 μM drug. Differences in the inhibitory potencies of the isoquinolinesulfonamide derivatives tested against various protein kinases were dependent on the stereo structure of the isoquinolinesulfonamide substituent. For example, as

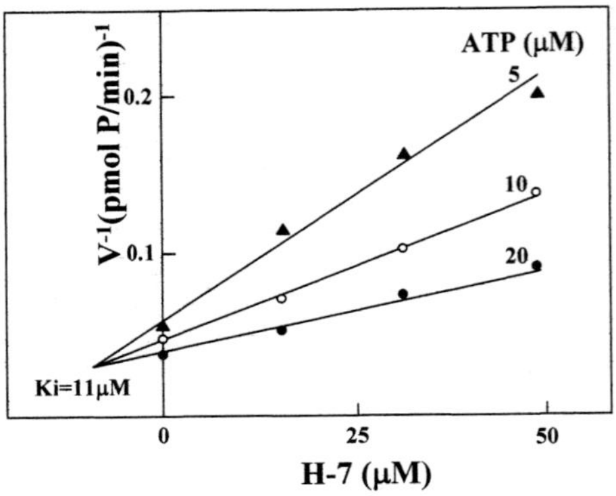

Fig. 5 Kinetic analysis of H-7-induced inhibition of PKC. The PKC reaction was performed with 20-kDa myosin light chain (MLC_{20}) as a substrate and PKC partially prepared from rabbit brain. A Dixon plot gives a K_i of 11 μM for H-7

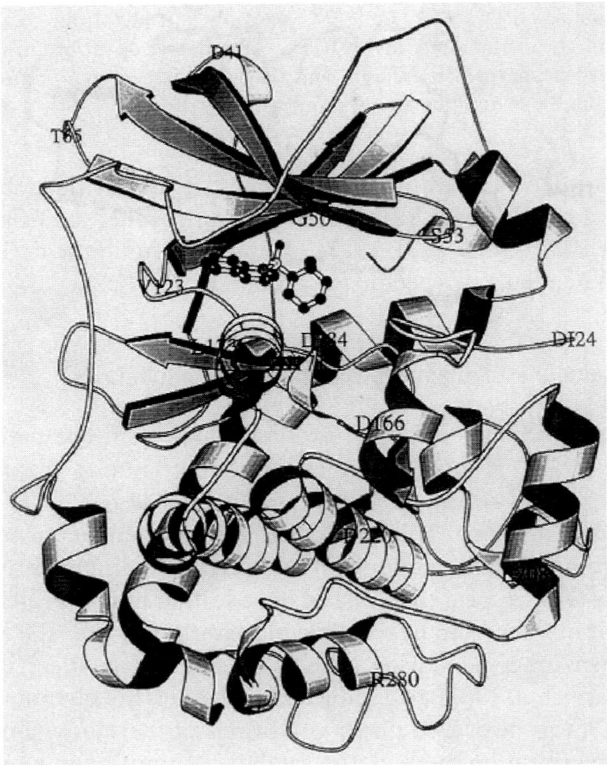

Fig. 6 Secondary structure of bovine PKA catalytic subunit in complex with H-7. The C-terminal region is displayed with DI24. (The figure was drawn by Bossemeyer and is cited with his permission)

Table 1 Protein kinase inhibitors: sulfonamide derivatives and others

	Compound	R	Mechanism	Pharmacological effect	
Sulfonamide derivatives	W-7	$-(CH_2)_6NH_2$	CaM antagonism	Vascular relaxation	<100
	ML-9	R1-*1	MLCK inhibition	Vascular relaxation	<10
	H-8	$-(CH_2)_2NHCH_3$	A-PK inhibition	Sperm motility ↓	<50
	H-89	$-(CH_2)_2NHCH_2$-CH=CH-C_6H_6-Cl	A-PK inhibition	Neurite growth ↓	<30
	H-7	R2-*2	PK-C inhibition	5HT release ↑	<50
	H-9	$-(CH_2)_2NH_2$	PK-C inhibition	PK-C purification	<50
	KN-62	*3	CaM KII inhibition	GABA release ↓	<30
	CKI-7	$-(CH_2)_2NH_2$	Casein kinase inhibition	?	<30
	HA1077	R2-*1	Rho-K inhibition	Vascular relaxation	<10
Others	Staurosporin		Multi kinase inhibition	Ornithine decarboxylase induction ↑	<1.0
	K252a		Multi kinase inhibition	5HT release ↓	<10
	Sphingolipids		PK-C inhibition	?	<100

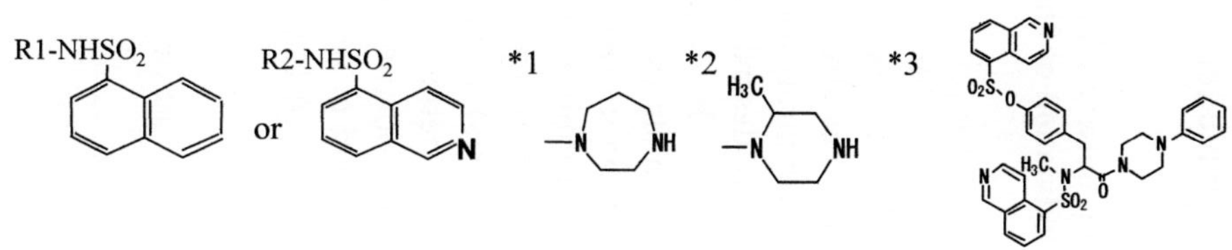

shown in Table 1, differing sensitivity toward protein kinases may be mainly dependent on the substituent structure. From the standpoint of protein kinases, our previous study (Hagiwara et al. 1987) suggested that the specificity of the PKA-specific inhibitor, H-8 (isoquinolinesulfonamide), for PKA was related closely to the β-subsite of ATP-binding site of PKA.

2
Rho-Kinase Inhibitor and Its Pharmacological Properties

2.1
Relationship Between Rho-Kinase Inhibition and the Modulation of Physiological Function

Among many isoquinolinesulfonamide derivatives, we selected HA1077 as a therapeutic agent for the treatment of cerebral vascular spasm (Takayasu et al. 1986). This compound (HA1077) was shown to be an excellent therapeutic agent and has already been utilized in 100,000 patients in Japan who suffered from cerebral vascular spasm (Shibuya et al. 1992). The clinical effects of HA1077 are described in another section.

HA1077 was shown to have a wide spectrum of action against various vasoconstriction states including vasospasm. The compound relaxed both the calcium ionophore (A23187)-induced and the receptor agonist-induced contractions of rabbit aorta to a similar extent; the ED_{50} (the concentration of the compound producing 50% inhibition of vasoconstriction induced by various agonists) values were micromolar in potency (Asano et al. 1987). Therefore, to better understand the mechanisms involved, we determined the inhibitory potential on various kinds of enzymes relevant to the contraction mechanism of smooth muscle (Table 2). Like other isoquinolinesulfonamide derivatives, HA1077 inhibited the activity of various protein kinases

Table 2 Inhibitory activity of Rho-kinase inhibitors against several kinds of serine/threonine protein kinase

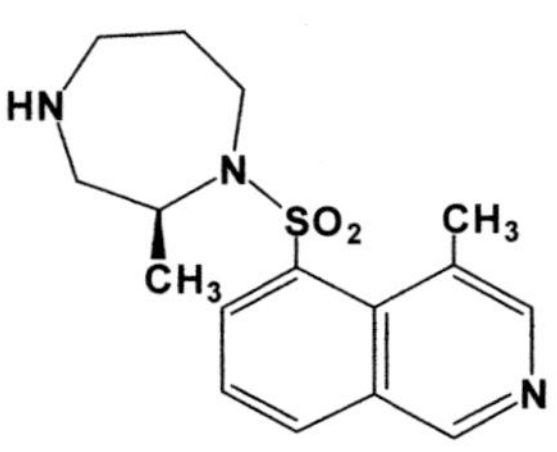

H1152

Protein kinases	K_i (μM) H7	HA1077	H1152	Y-276322
Rho-kinase	0.457	0.33	0.0016	0.14
PKA	5.7	1.0	0.63	25
PKC	7.7	9.3	9.27	26
MLCK	170	55	10.1	>250
PAK[a]	<100	<100	<100	<100

[a] p21-Activated kinase.

with various K_i values in ATP-competitive fashion with a range of K_i values. The K_i values for Rho kinase and PKC were comparatively low, 0.35 and 0.90 μM, respectively. In an isolated arterial strip stimulated with $PGF_{2\alpha}$, we determined that HA1077 inhibits the phosphorylation of the regulatory myosin light chain (MLC_{20}), in particular the diphosphorylation step was more sensitive than the monophosphorylation reaction (Seto et al. 1991).

HA1077 was an effective inhibitor of arterial contraction and MLC_{20} diphosphorylation at sub-micromolar concentrations, but the K_i for MLCK was 55 μM. This fact indicates that the inhibition of MLCK by HA1077 was not likely to be related to its pharmacological action. Subsequently, we and others have demonstrated that MLC diphosphorylation was associated with an inhibition of myosin-phosphatase through the phosphorylation of the myosin binding subunit (MBS 130 kDa) of protein phosphatase 1 by Rho kinase (Kimura et al. 1996; Nagumo et al. 2000). In fact, we demonstrated that HA1077 inhibits $PGF_{2\alpha}$-induced arterial contraction co-incident with inhibition of MBS-phosphatase (Ito et al. 2003). We believed it was likely that Rho kinase inhibition was likely to be responsible for the mechanism of action of HA1077 and that it could explain its pharmacological activities. Moreover, we discovered that HA1077 also inhibits the phosphorylation of calponin in a porcine coronary artery stimulated with $PGF_{2\alpha}$ (Nagumo et al. 1998). At present, calponin phosphorylation is recognized to be alternatively catalyzed by both PKC and Rho kinase (Kaneko et al. 2000). The regulation of myosin

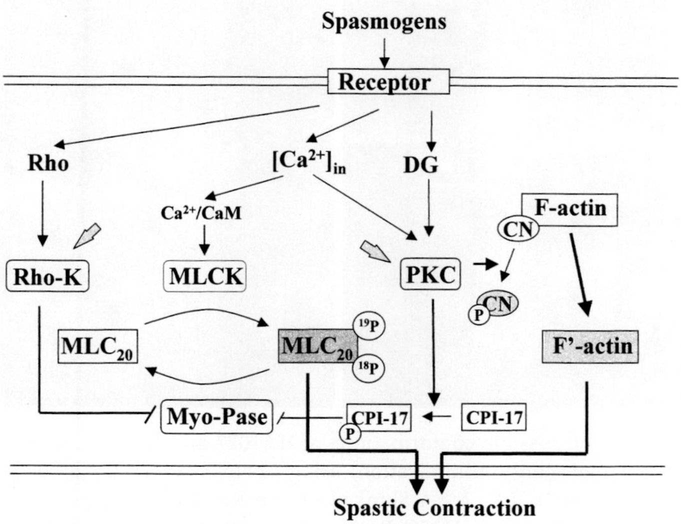

Fig. 7 Site of action of the Rho-kinase inhibitor HA1077 in arterial smooth muscle. *Arrowheads* show the target proteins, Rho-kinase and PKC. *Myo-Pase*, myosin phosphatase 1 with 130 kDa myosin binding subunit; *CN*, calponin; *CPI-17*, 17-kDa inhibitor protein of type 1 phosphatase; *DA*, diacylglycerol

phosphatase activity and calponin phosphorylation, which is dependent on Rho kinase or/and PKC, seems to control the calcium sensitivity of smooth muscle contraction. Taken together, HA1077 may have two sites of action in the mechanism of inhibition of smooth muscle contraction (Fig. 7).

2.2 A Novel Rho-Kinase Inhibitor and Its Perspective

We have made an effort to develop a highly potent and much more specific inhibitor of Rho kinase (Ikenoya et al. 2002). The characteristics of H1152 are summarized in Table 2. In in vitro systems, H1152 potently inhibited Rho kinase activity in a competitive fashion with respect to ATP. As the introduction of two methyl moieties into the HA1077 molecule drastically increases the inhibitory activity against Rho kinase, we analyzed and compared the conformations of H1152 and HA1077 using a computer molecular modeling program. Figure 8 shows that the introduction of the two methyl moieties produces steric hindrance between isoquinoline and homopiperazine moieties, thereby preventing some configurations of H1152 and suggesting that this inhibitor assumes a more rigid configuration than HA1077. In vivo, H1152 specifically inhibited the phosphorylation of myristoylated alanine-rich C-kinase substrate (MARCKS) in human neuronal (NT)-2 cells

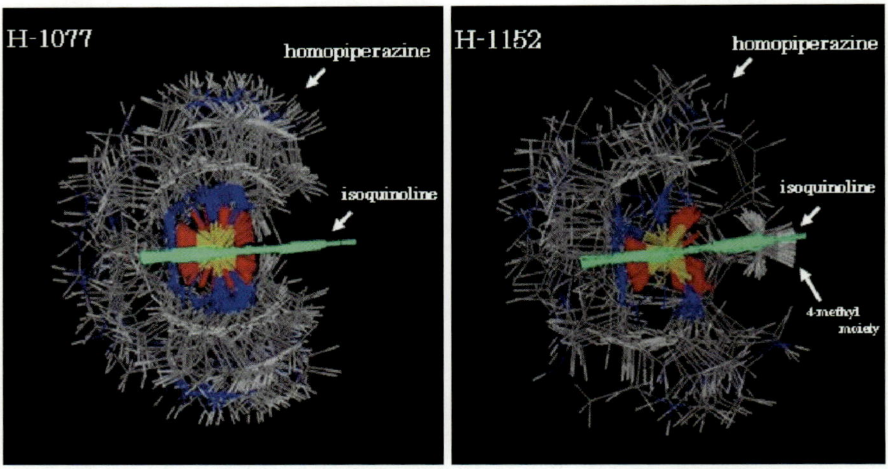

Fig. 8 Comparison of possible conformations of HA1077 and H1152. Systematic conformation analyses and energy minimization, using Chem-X molecular modeling package (version 2000.1; Accerlys K.K. 2-8-4 Shinkawa Chuo-Ku, Tokyo, Japan), assumed stable conformations of HA1077 and H1152. Bonds were rotated in steps of 30°. Energy minimizations were performed employing MM2 force field and default options. The pictures were drawn using MAESTRO software (Schrodinger, Portland OR, USA). (The figure was drawn by Dr. Masami Shiratsuchi and Dr. Hisashi Nakashima, Kowa, Japan, and is cited with permission)

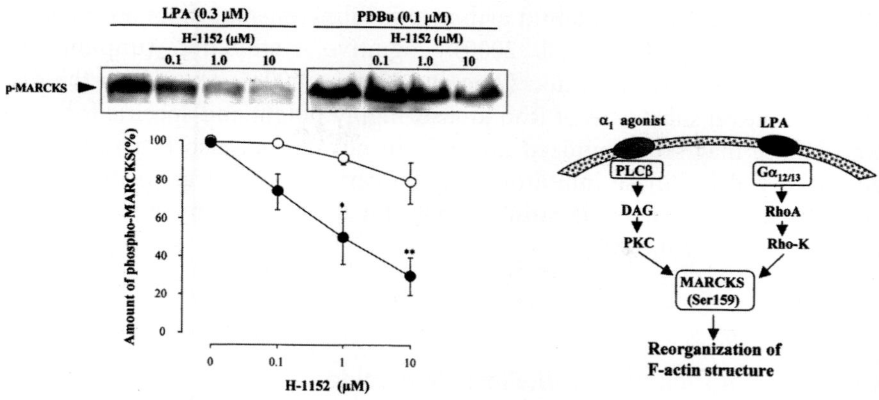

Fig. 9 Inhibition of MARCKS phosphorylation at Ser159 by H1152 in human neuronal (NT)-2 cells stimulated with 0.3 μM lysophosphatidic acid or 0.1 μM phorbol dibutyrate (*left panel*). Schematic outline of MARCKS phosphorylation pathways initiated by various stimuli (*right panel*)

stimulated with LPA, but not with phorbol ester (Fig. 9). Previously, we showed that the phosphorylation of MARCKS at Ser159 is catalyzed by Rho kinase as well as PKC (Nagumo et al. 2001). H1152 was used to probe a novel signal transduction pathway for the MARCKS phosphorylation by Rho kinase in LPS-stimulated neuronal cells. MARCKS is assumed to participate in neurotransmitter release through the reorganization or modulation of F-actin structure in neuronal terminals (Trifaro et al. 2002). It is plausible that the F-actin cross-linking activity of MARCKS participates in the dynamics of actin meshwork in a so-called active zone under the presynaptic membranes, and then the reorganization of actin meshwork facilitates the approach of synaptic vesicles to the active zone. Taken together, these data raise the important possibility and hypothesis that a Rho kinase inhibitor may modulate reorganization of the actin-meshwork, suppressing the trafficking of synaptic vesicles and subsequently inhibiting the release of neurotransmitter.

In neuronal cells and the CNS, Rho kinase is becoming recognized as a potent regulator of neurogenic events, such as the axon elongation and retraction cycle, axon guidance and synaptogenesis, and neurite extension in cultured cells (Kozma et al. 1997; Bito et al. 2000). These concepts seem to be based on the results of molecular and pharmacological experiments using cells expressing a Rho kinase mutant and/or treated with Rho kinase inhibitors. However, little is known about the target molecule of Rho kinase in neuronal cells and CNS.

These is a growing body of evidence that Rho kinase is involved in an increasing number of severe pathologies including angina pectoris (Katsumata et al. 1997), myocardial infarction (Yamamoto et al. 2000), bronchial asthma

(Chiba et al. 1999), rheumatoid arthritis, insulin-resistant diabetes mellitus, arteriosclerosis (Fukui et al. 2000), cognitive dysfunction (unpublished data), and astrocyte activation (Abe and Misawa 2003). Thus, with the discovery of novel substrates of Rho kinase, highly potent and specific forms of Rho kinase may be recognized not only in normal but also in pathological conditions. Rho kinase inhibitors may be very important as medicines for such diseases as well as diagnostic probes for Rho kinase-involved physiology (Moolenaar et al. 1997).

3 Clinical Application of Isoquinolinesulfonamide to Human Cerebral Vascular Diseases

Cerebral vasospasm is the leading cause of poor postoperative outcome of patients with subarachnoid hemorrhage due to ruptured aneurysms. Constriction of the arterial lumen begins about 4 days after the hemorrhage. Patients begin to show symptoms and signs of spasm at about the seventh day which last for 2–3 weeks. However, the spastic arteries begin to dilate by themselves after the fourth week if the patient can tolerate the ischemic insult. The primary cause of spasm is the degradation products of red blood cells in subarachnoid clot. However, further details of the mechanism have yet to be clarified. Both constriction of smooth muscle cells and inflammation seem to be involved. After the patient is secured from further bleeding by a successful neck clipping or intravascular treatment by GDC (Guglielmi detachable coil), 30% of the patients suffer from vasospasm in various forms, resulting in neurological deficits that range from mild cognitive dysfunction, sensorimotor paralysis, and aphasia, to death. Although, nimodipine, a calcium entry blocker, is widely used in the Western world, its effect has not always been satisfactory. HA1077 has been used in about 12,000 patients each year since it was approved in Japan in 1995. A recent comparative study in China between HA1077 and nimodipine on patients with subarachnoid hemorrhage (SAH) showed that HA1077 is equal to or better than nimodipine (unpublished data).

In this chapter, clinical effects as well as pharmacological analysis of HA1077 using model animals with experimental vasospasm or cerebral infarction will be further described.

3.1
Demonstration of the Therapeutic Effect of HA1077 on Cerebral Vasospasm and Infarction Using Model Animals

3.1.1
Effect on Subarachnoid Hemorrhage

Mongrel dogs of either sex weighing 7.5–13 kg or male beagle dogs weighing 7–10 kg were used as a two hemorrhage canine model of SAH. These model dogs reliably produce a chronic and intractable cerebral vasospasm similar to that seen in humans. A significant vasospasm was observed angiographically on day 7 after SAH in every dog. The diameter of the basilar artery diminished to 50%–60% of the control value obtained before SAH (on day 1). Chronic cerebral vasospasm in this model was not reversible by intravenous high doses of aminophylline, nifedipine, nimodipine, or papaverine (Varsos et al. 1983).

The intravenous administration of 0.5–10 mg/kg/30 min HA1077 caused a dilation of the basilar artery dose-dependently on day 7. HA1077 lowered the mean arterial blood pressure only at high doses of 3 and 10 mg/kg (Takayasu et al. 1986).

Prophylactic administration of HA1077 infused intravenously for 30 min twice daily from day 1 after SAH significantly prevented the development of chronic cerebral vasospasm, as demonstrated by angiography (Fig. 10). SAH produced a significant decrease in regional cerebral blood flow (rCBF), and blood velocity, with no remarkable change in blood volume. These results were supported by previous clinical investigations showing similar observations in patients with SAH (Grubb et al. 1977; Yamakami et al. 1983). This phenomenon is probably explained by the pathophysiology whereby the large, radiographically visible vessels contract without contraction of the arteriolar resistance vessels. A bolus intravenous injection of HA1077 dose-dependently increased the rCBF and blood velocity, without significantly changing the blood volume on day 7 after SAH.

It has been known that SAH induces marked pathological changes in cerebral arteries. In the light micrographs and transmission electron micrographs of the basilar arteries, severe constriction of the artery plus folding and corrugation of the elastic lamina were apparent. The endothelial cells were compressed between tight folds of the elastic lamina during a period of prolonged contraction, and these physiological mechanisms may provoke endothelial damage. Scanning electron micrographs of the endothelial surface of the basilar artery demonstrated endothelial disruption such as platelet aggregation, adhesion of red blood cells and leukocytes to the endothelial surface, and endothelial desquamation. Substances released from the platelets and leukocytes adhering to the luminal surface accelerate the constriction of spastic artery. The blood velocity may increase in a narrow segment

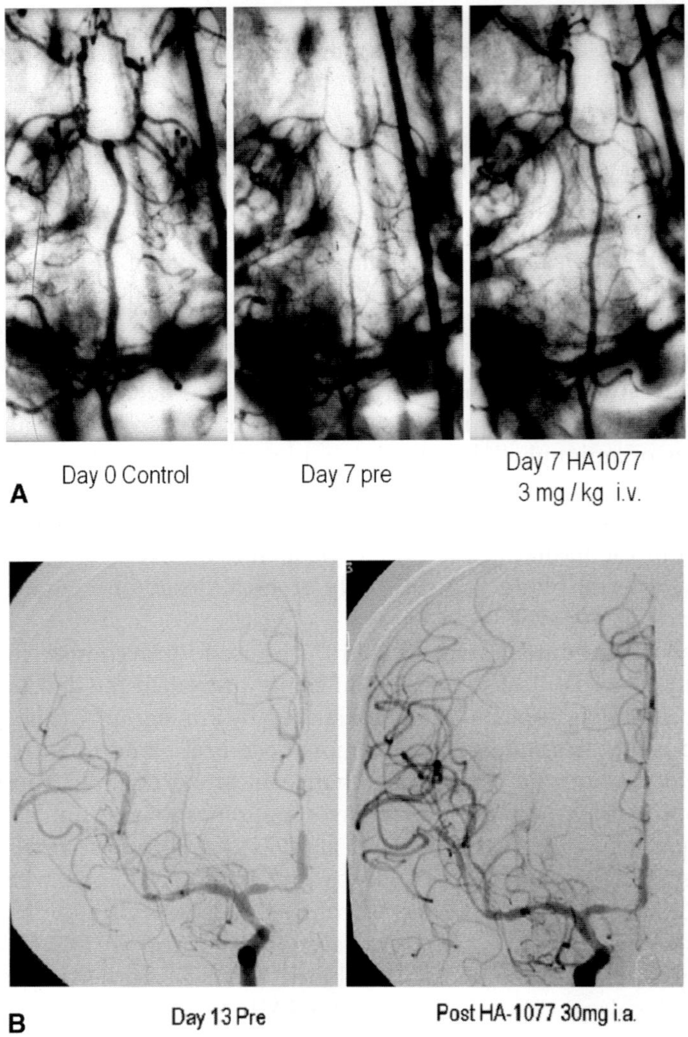

Fig. 10 A Effect of intravenous HA1077 on canine vasospasm. *Left*, control angiogram on day 0 before the subarachnoid blood injection. *Center*, day 7 before HA1077, shows a marked narrowing of the basilar artery. *Right*, 30 min after intravenous administration of 3 mg/kg HA1077, shows marked dilatation of the basilar artery. **B** Effect of intra-arterial administration of HA1077 in a patient with a ruptured fusiform aneurysm in the basilar artery. *Left*, right carotid angiogram on day 13 shows multiple segmental narrowing in the carotid, anterior, and middle cerebral arteries. *Right*, marked dilatation of the spastic arteries is seen after intra-arterial administration of 30 mg of HA1077. Patient's consciousness level improved after HA1077

of spastic vessels. This higher velocity of blood flow increases shear stress and damages the endothelial surface. However, pathological damage of cerebral arteries in HA1077-treated dogs was absent or minimal in contrast with the control dogs (Satoh et al. 1999a).

Activated neutrophils may play a major role in the pathogenesis of cerebral arterial vasospasm or cerebral injury. Such processes cause neutrophils to degranulate, aggregate, adhere to the endothelium, infiltrate, and release highly reactive compounds that promote inflammatory local responses. Oxygen radicals released from neutrophils are considered to be toxic to endothelial cells and to cause endothelial damage. Additionally, it is considered that free radicals from neutrophils induce cellular injury with inactivation of nitric oxide, a known vasodilator (Kajita et al 1994). We reported that inactivation of nitric oxide by superoxide anions contributes to the development of vasospasm (Suzuki et al. 1992). A later report (Arai et al. 1993) demonstrated that HA1077 can prevent the production of superoxide anions in neutrophils as well as the migration of neutrophils.

3.1.2 Effect on Cerebral Ischemia

The neuroprotective properties of HA1077 were evaluated in two animal models of cerebral ischemia: transient bilateral carotid artery occlusion in Mongolian gerbils and cerebromicroembolization in rats (Satoh et al. 1996). The common carotid arteries in male gerbils were clamped with microclips for 5 min. The brains were removed 7 days later and coronal sections through the hippocampus were prepared and stained with hematoxylin and eosin. The degree of neuronal damage was assessed in the CA1 region of the hippocampus by quantifying the number of pyramidal cell bodies per millimeter. The average of the neuronal cell density of the normal gerbil was 211±5 cells/mm, and the average in the ischemic control group of gerbils was 17.8±2.1 cells/mm. HA1077 significantly diminished the loss of CA1 neurons in hippocampus with the average of neuronal cell density of 101.0±22.0 cells/mm. Nimodipine, a calcium entry blocker and ozagrel, a thromboxane A_2 synthase inhibitor, did not significantly protect against the ischemia-induced neuronal loss.

Multiple infarctions were produced in the cerebral hemispheres of rats by the injection of the 50-μM microspheres into the left internal carotid artery, and neurological impairment was evaluated 24 h later. The assessment of neurological function following cerebral microembolization is a subjective test and would only give an indication as to alterations in function, but all rats in the control group showed typical symptoms of stroke such as truncal curvature, circling behavior, and rolling behavior. Although distribution of the infarction was unpredictable, the structures most frequently involved were the hippocampus, thalamus, and cortex, and the total size of infarctions was comparatively constant.

Neurological function and size of infarction was significantly improved in the HA1077-treated animals. HA1077 also suppressed the increased water content in ischemic brain tissues. Administration of HA1077 significantly improved the ischemia-induced impairment of neurological function, as well as impairment in the morphology.

It has been reported that the intravenous infusion of HA1077 increased rCBF and glucose utilization at various sites, including thalamus, cortex, and hippocampus (Sako et al. 1991; Tsuchiya et al. 1993). These sites were consistent with the infarct areas. The results suggest that HA1077 protects the brain from ischemic infarction by improving hemodynamic and metabolic function, at least in part.

Neutrophil accumulation in cerebral ischemic infarcts was observed in the ipsilateral hemisphere of ischemic brains, while there were few neutrophils in the normal brain area. Accumulation of leukocytes is known to be greater in the region of more severe ischemia and the central zone of the ischemia in acute embolic stroke in humans. Neutrophil infiltration into the ischemic area of the brain may be involved in the pathogenesis of ischemic injury and neurological impairment. As HA1077 can prevent the production of superoxide anions in neutrophils as well as the migration of neutrophils, this may be an important part of mechanism in neuroprotective effects of HA1077 (Satoh et al. 1999b). HA1077 had no significant effect on the magnitude of body temperature. This suggests that neuroprotective effect of HA1077 is not due to hypothermia.

3.2 Clinical Application of HA1077 to 100,000 Patients

3.2.1 Anti-vasospasmic Effect

HA1077 is unique in dilating spastic arteries not only by local (intra-arterial) application but also by systemic (intravenous, i.v.) administration with doses not causing significant hypotension (Takayasu et al. 1986). Usual calcium entry blockers such as nicardipine or diltiazem result in poor vasodilating effects even in doses that show significant hypotension. In order to select an appropriate dosage for use in a double-blind trial, various doses of HA1077 (20–180 mg/day) were given to separate groups of patients. Each dose of the drug was given in 100 ml of saline, infused for 30 min, two or three times a day for 14 days after clipping the aneurysm. Severe angiographic spasm decreased with increasing doses of HA1077. No severe vasospasm was seen in a group receiving 40–60 mg, three times a day. However, patients on high doses of HA1077 occasionally suffered mild hypotension,

Table 3 Summary: double-blind trial of fasudil (HA1077)

	Placebo	HA1077	*p* Value
1. Angiographic vasospasm (mod. or sev.)	61%	38%	$p<0.01$
2. Symptomatic vasospasm	50%	35%	$p<0.05$
3. Low-density area on CT scan (mod. or sev.)	38%	16%	$p<0.01$
4. Poor ADL (<vasospasm)	26%	12%	$p<0.05$
All causes	40%	34%	n.s.
5. Adverse reactions	6%	4%	n.s.

Mod., moderate; n.s., not significantly different; sev., severe.

especially dehydrated, small or older patients. No other side effects have been reported (Shibuya et al. 1990). Thus, three doses of 30 mg per day for 14 days was chosen for the double-blind trial. A placebo-controlled prospective double-blind trial was performed in 280 patients whose aneurysm was clipped within 3 days after the hemorrhage (Shibuya et al. 1992). The results of the double-blind trial (Table 3) showed that HA1077 significantly decreased symptomatic spasm from 50% to 35% ($p<0.05$), angiographic spasm from 61% to 38% ($p<0.01$, Fig. 11), and cerebral infarction which was seen as a low density area (LDA) on computed tomography (CT) from 38% to 16% ($p<0.01$). Poor outcome or ADL (active daily life) due to vasospasm was decreased from 26% to 12% ($p<0.05$). HA1077 is the only drug that showed significant effects by angiography and CT scan. Similar effects of

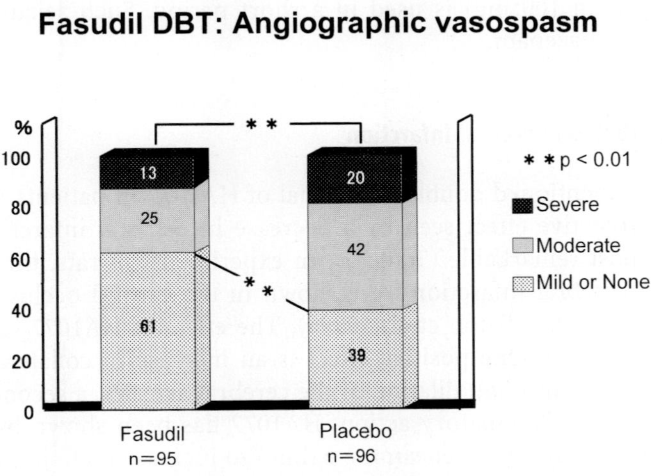

Fig. 11 Incidence of angiographically detected vasospasm. The patients in the fasudil (HA1077) group were administrated three times 30 mg HA1077 each day for 14 days, and the patients in placebo were given physiological saline. Values are percentages of the total within each group. Significant differences for moderate and severe spasm were found: $p=0.0023$

HA1077 have been shown in patients after it was commercialized. The currently approved dosage of HA1077 (30 mg, i.v., three times a day, for 14 days), HA1077 can ameliorate about half of the damage caused by vasospasm. This is an encouraging result and further improvement can be expected by increasing the dosage of HA1077. However, careful titration of the dosage of HA1077 must be undertaken to guard against hypotension. A close watch for fluid balance is also important, since HA1077 sometimes causes dehydration and hemoconcentration by increasing renal blood flow and urine volume, which may cause a further deterioration of ischemic injury in patients with vasospasm.

3.2.2
Intra-arterial Use of HA1077

Even when receiving intravenous treatment with HA1077, there are some patients who develop signs of vasospasm, usually at about 7–10 days after the hemorrhage. Intra-arterial use of HA1077 is effective in such cases. Thirty to 60 mg of HA1077 is given in divided doses through the arterial catheter during DSA (digital subtraction angiography). Intra-arterial HA1077 can dilate most of the spastic arteries. However, its clinical usefulness is limited to about 50% of the patients, because its effect may be only short acting or infarction had already been completed (Tachibana et al. 1999). The vasodilating effect of HA1077 is similar to that of papaverine, but HA1077 is superior to papaverine with fewer side effects. The only side effect reported with intra-arterial administration of HA1077 is seizure, especially when a large dose (more than 100 mg) is used in a short period. Such seizures can be treatable with diazepam.

3.2.3
Effect of HA1077 on Cerebral Infarction

In the above-mentioned double-blind trial of HA1077 in patients with SAH, the brain-protective effect seen by a decrease in cerebral infarction on CT scans was most remarkable (Table 3). In experiments in rats, the effects of HA1077 on cerebral infarction were shown in the carotid occlusion model (Tsuchiya et al. 1993; Satoh et al. 1999a). The effect of HA1077 on cerebral ischemia is twofold. One positive effect is an increase in collateral circulation in penumbra through dilation of the cerebral arteries, a second positive effect is an anti-inflammatory action. HA1077 has been shown by HMPAO (Tc-99m hexamethyl propyleneamine oxime) to increase rCBF in patients after SAH. Interestingly, it increased rCBF in the region of cerebral vasospasm without changing blood flow in normal regions. In other words, it increased rCBF more specifically in spastic regions, thus avoiding development of a so-called steal phenomenon. This is unique to HA1077. It is usual for calcium entry blockers to dilate normal arteries more than spastic arteries causing systemic hypotension, which is generally not desirable.

HA1077 had been shown to inhibit migration of white blood cells to the ischemic brain in rats (Satoh et al. 1999a,b). In addition, in in vitro system, HA1077 inhibits production of free radicals by NADPH oxidase in WBC through the inhibition of PKC (Arai et al. 1993). Decrease of free radical production by inhibition of PKC seems to be an important part of the effectiveness of HA1077. As HA1077 inhibits the phosphorylation of calponin in the intact artery, the effects of HA1077 on both cerebral vasospasm and infarction can be attributed to both vasodilatation and anti-inflammation. In a recent clinical study, a double-blind trial of HA1077 in patients with acute cerebral infarction due to thrombosis showed that HA1077 significantly decreased motor weakness and improved ADL (unpublished data). Effectiveness of HA1077 has experimentally been suggested in many other diseases where Rho kinase is believed to be involved, including angina pectoris (Katsumata et al. 1997), bronchial asthma (Chiba et al. 1999), rheumatoid arthritis, insulin-resistant diabetes mellitus, and arteriosclerosis (unpublished data).

In conclusion, HA1077 was found to be a novel compound inhibiting Rho kinase. This compound has been used clinically, especially for the therapy of cerebral vasospasm or cerebral infarction. Studies of model systems in animals with vasospasm or cerebral infarction have provided evidence to advance the study of HA1077 into the therapy of human vasospasm or cerebral infarction. Clinical trials of nearly 100,000 patients treated with HA1077 in Japan since 1995 have demonstrated that the Rho kinase inhibitor, HA1077 is quite a useful agent for the treatment with vasospasm.

Rho kinase has recently been considered one of the key enzymes involved in the development of vasospasm. The inhibition of Rho kinase by HA1077 has opened the door to an enhanced understanding of mechanisms involved not only in cerebral vasospasm and infarction but also many other diseases. The studies also have the potential to open an entirely new generation of therapeutic opportunities and important tools to study disease pathways and mechanisms.

Acknowledgements Critical reading of this manuscript was made by Dr. Barry Berkowitz, Director, Strong Pharmaceuticals, LLC, Massachusetts, USA.

References

Abe K, Misawa M (2003) Astrocyte stellation induced by Rho kinase inhibitors in culture. Brain Res Dev Brain Res 143:99–104

Arai M, Sasaki Y, Nozawa R (1993) Inhibition by the protein kinase inhibitor HA1077 on the activation of NADPH oxidase in human neutrophils. Biochem Pharmacol 46:1487–1490

Asano T, Ikegaki I, Satoh S, Suzuki Y, Shibuya M, Takayasu M, Hidaka H (1987) Mechanism of action of a novel antivasospasm drug, HA1077. J Pharmacol Exp Ther 241:1033–1040

Bito H, Furuyashiki T, Ishihara H, Shibasaki Y, Ohashi K, Mizuno K, Maekawa M, Ishizaki T, Narumiya S (2000) A critical role for a Rho-associated kinase, p160ROCK, in determining axon outgrowth in mammalian CNS neurons. Neuron 26:431–441

Chiba Y, Takada Y, Miyamoto S, Mitsui-Saito M, Karaki H, Misawa M (1999) Augmented acetylcholine-induced, Rho-mediated Ca^{2+} sensitization of bronchial smooth muscle contraction in antigen-induced airway hyperactive rats. Br J Pharmacol 127:597–600

Engh RA, Girod A, Kinzel V, Huber R, Bossmeyer D (1996) Crystal structures of catalytic subunit of cAMP-dependent protein kinase in complex with isoquinolinesulfonyl protein kinase inhibitors H7, H8 and H89. J Biol Chem 271:26157–26164

Fukui R, Amakawa M, Hoshiga M, Shibata N, Kohbayashi E, Seto M, Sasaki Y, Ueno T, Negoro N, Nakakoji T, II M, Nishiguchi F, Ishihara T, Ohsawa N (2000) Increased migration in late G_1 phase in cultured smooth muscle cells. Am J Physiol Cell Physiol 279:C999-C1007

Grubb RL Jr, Raichle ME, Eichling JO, Gado MH (1977) Effects of subarachnoid hemorrhage on cerebral blood volume, blood flow, and oxygen utilization in humans. J Neurosurg 46:446–453

Hagiwara M, Inagaki M, Hidaka H (1987) Specific binding of a novel compound, *N*-[2-(methylamino)ethyl]-5-isoquinolinesulfonamide (H-8) to the active site of cAMP-dependent protein kinase. Mol Pharmacol 31:523–528

Hidaka H, Tanaka T (1983) Naphthalenesulfonamides as calmodulin antagonists. Methods Enzymol 102:185–194

Hidaka H, Yamaki T, Asano M, Totsuka T (1978a) Involvement of calcium in cyclic nucleotide metabolism in human smooth muscle. Blood Vessels 15:55–64

Hidaka H, Asano M, Iwadare S, Matsumoto I, Totsuka T, Aoki N (1978b) A novel vascular relaxing agent, N-(6-aminohexyl)-5-chloro-1-naphthalenesulfonamide which affects vascular smooth muscle actomyosin. J Pharmacol Exp Ther 207:8–15

Hidaka H, Yamaki T, Totsuka T, Asano M (1979) Selective inhibitors of Ca^{2+}-binding modulator of phosphodiesterase produce vascular relaxation and inhibit actin-myosin interaction. Mol Pharmacol 15:49–59

Hidaka H, Inagaki M, Kawamoto S, Sasaki Y (1984) Isoquinolinesulfonamides, novel and potent inhibitors of cyclic nucleotide dependent protein kinase and protein kinase C. Biochemistry 23:5036–5041

Hidaka H, Watanabe M, Kobayashi R (1991) Properties and use of H-series compounds as protein kinase inhibitors. Methods Enzymol 201:328–339

Ikenoya M, Hidaka H, Hosoya T, Suzuki M, Yamamoto N, Sasaki Y (2002) Inhibition of rho-kinase induced myristoylated alanine-rich C kinase substrate (MARCKS) phosphorylation in human neuronal cells by H-1152, a novel and specific Rho-kinase inhibitor. J Neurochem 81:9–16

Inagaki M, Watanabe M, Hidaka H (1985) N-(2-aminoethyl)-5- isoquinolinesulfonamide, a newly synthesized protein kinase inhibitor, functions as a ligand affinity chromatography. J Biol Chem 260:2922–2925

Ito K, Shimomura E, Iwanaga T, Shiraishi M, Shindo K, Nakamura J, Nagumo H, Seto M, Sasaki Y, Takuwa Y (2003) Essential role of rho kinase in the Ca^{2+} sensitization of prostaglandin F(2alpha)-induced contraction of rabbit aortae. J Physiol 546:823–836

Kajita Y, Suzuki Y, Oyama H, Tanazawa T, Takayasu M, Shibuya M, Sugita K (1994) Combined effect of L-arginie and superoxide dismutase on the spastic basilar artery after subarachnoid hemorrhage in dogs. J Neurosurg 80:476–483

Kaneko T, Amano M, Maeda A, Goto H, Takahashi K, Ito M, Kaibuchi K (2000) Identification of calponin as a novel substrate of Rho-kinase. Biochem Biophys Res Commun 273:110–116

Katsumata N, Shimokawa H, Seto M, Kozai T, Yamawaki T, Kuwata K, Egashira K, Ikegaki I, Asano T, Sasaki Y, Takeshita A (1997) Enhanced myosin light chain phosphorylations as a central mechanism for coronary artery spasm in a swine model with interleukin-1 beta. Circulation 96:4357–4363

Kimura K, Ito M, Amano M, Chihara K, Fukuta Y, Nakafuku M, Yamamori B, Feng J, Nakano T, Okawa K, Iwamatsu A, Kaibuchi K (1996) Regulation of myosin phosphatase by Rho and Rho-associated kinase (Rho-kinase). Science 273:245–248

Kozma R, Sarner S, Ahmed S, Lim L (1997) Rho family GTPases and neuronal growth cone remodelling. Relationship between increased complexity induced Cdc42Hs, Rac1, and acetylcholine and collapse induced by RhoA and lysophosphatidic acid. Mol Cell Biol 17:1201–1211

Moolenaar WH, Kranenburg O, Postma FR, Zondag GC (1997) Lysophosphatidic acid: G-protein signalling and cellular responses. Curr Opin Cell Biol 9:168–173

Nagumo H, Seto M, Sakurada K, Walsh MP, Sasaki Y (1998) HA1077, a protein kinase inhibitor, inhibits calponin phosphorylation on Ser175 in porcine coronary artery. Eur J Pharmacol 360:257–264

Nagumo H, Sasaki Y, Ono Y, Okamoto H, Seto M, Takuwa Y (2000) Rho kinase inhibitor HA-1077 prevents Rho-mediated myosin phosphatase inhibition in smooth muscle cells. Am J Physiol Cell Physiol 278:C57–65

Nagumo H, Ikenoya M, Sakurada K, Furuya K, Ikuhara, T, Hiraoka H, Sasaki Y (2001) Rho-associated kinase phosphorylates MARCKS in human neuronal cells. Biochem Biophys Res Commun 280:605–609

Ohno, S, Kawasaki H, Imajoh S, Suzuki K, Inagaki M, Yokokura H, Sakoh T, Hidaka H (1987) Tissue-specific expression of three distinct types of rabbit protein kinase C. Nature 325:161–166

Saito M, Ishikawa T, Matsushima S, Naka M, Hidaka H (1987) Selective inhibition of catalytic activity of smooth muscle myosin light chain kinase. J Biol Chem 262:7796–7801

Sako K, Tsuchiya M, Yonemasu Y, Asano T (1991) HA1077, a novel calcium antagonistic antivasospasm drug, increases both cerebral blood flow and glucose metabolism in conscious rats. Eur J Pharmacol 209:39–43

Satoh S, Ikegaki I, Suzuki Y, Asano T, Shibuya M, Hidaka H (1996) Neuroprotective properties of a protein kinase inhibitor against ischemia-induced neuronal damage in rats and gerbils. Br J Pharmacol 118:1592–1598

Satoh S, Yamamoto Y, Toshima Y, Ikegaki I, Asano T, Suzuki Y, Shibuya M (1999a) Fasudil, a protein kinase inhibitor, prevents the development of endothelial injury and neutrophil infiltration in a two-haemorrhage canine subarachnoid model. J Clin Neurosci 6:394–399

Satoh S, Kobayashi T, Hitomi A, Ikegaki I, Suzuki Y, Shibuya M, Yoshida J, Asano T (1999b) Inhibition of neutrophil migration by a protein kinase inhibitor for the treatment of ischemic brain infarction. Jpn J Pharmacol 80:41–48

Seto M, Sasaki Y, Hidaka H, Sasaki Y (1991) Effects of HA1077, a protein kinase inhibitor, on myosin phosphorylation and tension in smooth muscle. Eur J Pharmacol 195:267–272

Shibuya M, Suzuki Y, Sugita K, Saito I, Sasaki T, Takakura K, Okamoto S, Kikuchi H, Takemae T, Hidaka H (1990) Dose escalation trial of a novel calcium antagonist

AT877, in patients with aneurysmal subarachnoid haemorrhage. Acta Neurochir (Wien) 107:11–15
Shibuya M, Suzuki Y, Sugita K, Saito I, Sasaki T, Takakura K, Nagata I, Kikuchi H, Takemae T, Hidaka H, Nakashima M (1992) Effect of AT877 on cerebral vasospasm after aneurysmal subarachnoid hemorrhage. J Neurosurg 76:571–577
Suzuki Y, Satoh S, Kimura M, Oyama H, Asano T, Shibuya M, Sugita K (1992) Effects of vasopressin and oxytocin on canine cerebral circulation in vivo. J Neurosurg 77:424–431
Tachibana E, Harada T, Shibuya M, Saito K, Takayasu M, Suzuki Y, Yoshida J (1999) Intra-arterial infusion of fasudil hydrochloride for treating vasospasm following subarachnoid haemorrhage. Acta Neurochir (Wien) 141:13–19
Takayasu M, Suzuki Y, Shibuya M, Asano T, Kanamori M, Okada T, Kageyama N, Hidaka H (1986) The effects of HA compound calcium antagonists on delayed cerebral vasospasm in dogs. J Neurosurg 65:80–85
Tanaka T, Hidaka H (1980a) Hydrophobic regions function in calmodulin-enzymes interactions. J Biol Chem 255:11078–11080
Tanaka T, Naka M, Hidaka H (1980b) Activation of myosin light chain kinase by trypsin. Biochem Biophys Res Commun 92:313–318
Trifaro JM, Lejen T, Rose SD, Pene TD, Barkar ND, Seward EP (2002) Pathways that control cortical F-actin dynamics during secretion. Neurochem Res 27:1371–1385
Tsuchiya M, Sako K, Yonemasu Y, Asano T (1993) The effects of HA1077, a novel protein kinase inhibitor, on reductions of cerebral blood flow and glucose metabolism following acute and/or chronic bilateral carotid artery ligation in Wistar rats. Exp Brain Res 97:233–238
Varsos VG, Liszczak TM, Han DH, Kistler JP, Vielma J, Black PM, Heros RC, Zervas NT (1983) Delayed cerebral vasospasm is not reversible by aminophylline, nifedipine, or papaverine in a "two-hemorrhage" canine model. J Neurosurg 58:11–17
Yamakami I, Isobe K, Yamaura A, Nakamura T, Makino H (1983) Vasospasm and regional cerebral blood flow (rCBF) in patients with ruptured intracranial aneurysms: Serial rCBF studies with the Xenon-133 inhalation method. Neurosurgery 13:394–401
Yamamoto Y, Ikegaki I, Sasaki Y, Uchida T (2000) The protein kinase inhibitor fasudil protects against ischemic myocardial injury induced by endothelin-1 in the rabbit. J Cardiovasc Pharmacol 35:203–211

HEP (2005) 167:433–450

Discovery and Development of Iressa: The First in a New Class of Drugs Targeted at the Epidermal Growth Factor Receptor Tyrosine Kinase

A. E. Wakeling

AstraZeneca Pharmaceuticals, Alderley Park, Macclesfield, Cheshire, SK10 4TG, UK
alan.wakeling@astrazeneca.com

Abstract The epidermal growth factor receptor (EGFR) is a promising target for anti-cancer therapy because of its role in tumour growth, metastasis and angiogenesis, and tumour resistance to chemotherapy and radiotherapy. This chapter describes a low-molecular-weight EGFR tyrosine kinase inhibitor (EGFR-TKI), Iressa (gefitinib, ZD1839). Iressa is a potent EGFR-TKI which blocks EGF-stimulated EGFR autophosphorylation in tumour cells and selectively inhibits EGF-stimulated tumour cell growth. In studies with mice bearing a range of human tumour-derived xenografts, Iressa given orally, once daily, inhibited tumour growth in a dose-dependent manner. Long-term (>3 months) Iressa treatment of xenograft-bearing mice was well tolerated, and Iressa completely inhibited the growth of xenografts derived from A431 cells which highly express EGFR, and induced regression of advanced A431-derived tumours. No Iressa-resistant tumours appeared during treatment, but some tumours regrew following drug withdrawal. The level of expression of EGFR did not determine xenograft tumour sensitivity to Iressa. These preclinical studies indicated the potential utility of Iressa in the treatment of a wide range of human tumours, and established that continuous once-daily oral dosing might be a suitable therapeutic regimen. The first clinical studies with Iressa confirmed that an oral, once-daily, regimen is generally well tolerated and shows activity in cancer patients. Phase II clinical trials, in patients with advanced non-small-cell lung cancer (NSCLC) who had been previously treated with chemotherapy, demonstrated that Iressa at a daily dose of 250 or 500 mg has a favourable safety profile and has activity. The lower (250 mg/day) dose was better tolerated and as effective as the 500 mg/day dose. In these phase II studies, the level of expression of EGFR did not predict response to Iressa treatment. In phase III clinical trials, addition of Iressa to standard two-drug chemotherapy regimens, in previously untreated NSCLC patients, failed to improve disease-free or overall survival. Studies are now underway to investigate how Iressa can be used as an alternative to or in sequence with chemotherapy in NSCLC, and to explore its efficacy in other tumours including head and neck, breast and colorectal.

Keywords Iressa · Gefitinib · ZD1839 · Epidermal growth factor receptor · EGFR tyrosine kinase inhibitor · NSCLC

1 Rationale

The application of molecular genetic techniques to cancer biology has elucidated multiple, interacting biochemical pathways involved in the malignant transformation and unrestricted growth of epithelial cells from which the majority of human solid tumours originate (Hunter 1997; Blume-Jensen and Hunter 2001). The first complete description of a biochemical pathway originating at the cell surface, propagating signals from the tumour cell environment and leading to changes in gene transcription and tumour cell proliferation, began with the recognition that the epidermal growth factor receptor (EGFR) is the normal cellular homologue (proto-oncogene) of the viral oncogene v-erbB, the oncogenic protein of the avian erythroblastosis virus (Downward et al. 1984). This description culminated in the recognition that the ras-raf-mitogen-activated protein kinase (MAPK) pathway transmits signals activated by binding of EGF or transforming growth factor alpha (TGF-α) to the EGFR (Schlessinger 1993). At the same time, the first reports that squamous cell carcinomas express high levels of EGFR at the cell surface (Gusterson et al. 1984), and that the presence of EGFR indicates a poor prognosis in breast cancer patients (Sainsbury et al. 1985), were published. Subsequently, it became clear that high levels of EGFR expression are a common manifestation of the malignant phenotype in many solid human tumours including those of the lung (Gullick 1991; Salomon et al. 1995; Nicholson et al. 2001).

The EGF receptor (also designated ErbB1/HER1) is the prototype of a large family of cell-surface receptor tyrosine kinases (RTKs) that possess intrinsic tyrosine kinase activity and transmit growth factors signals across the cell membrane. The ErbB family of RTKs has four members (EGFR/ErbB1/HER1, ErbB2/HER2/neu, ErbB3/HER3 and ErbB4/HER4), and at least ten ligands which include EGF, transforming growth factor (TGF)-α and the heregulins. These ligands preferentially induce different ErbB homo- and hetero-dimers conferring a high degree of signalling diversity (Yarden and Ulrich 1988; Olayioye et al. 2000; Yarden and Sliwkowski 2001). RTKs share a common structure encompassing an extracellular ligand-binding domain, a short transmembrane domain and an intracellular domain which has tyrosine kinase (TK) activity. Binding of EGF or TGF-α to EGFR stimulates receptor homo- or hetero-dimerisation, intramolecular autophosphorylation of specific tyrosine residues of EGFR (or other ErbBs in heterodimers) providing 'docking sites' for the assembly of signal transduction complexes, and direct phosphorylation of specific tyrosine residues in substrate proteins (Yarden and Ulrich 1988). Delineation of the molecular mode of action of the EGFR, together with the demonstration that mutation or overexpression of ErbB2, as well as EGFR, causes cellular transformation and is associated with poor prognosis in breast cancer (Slamon et al. 1987), provided a convincing case that these receptors represent a potential target for novel anti-tumour therapies. Proof of principle for this idea was first provided by the successful application of trastuzumab (Herceptin), a monoclonal anti-ErbB2 antibody, in the treatment of breast cancer patients whose tumours overexpress ErbB2 (Cobleigh et al. 1999). An alternative therapeutic approach is directed at inhibition of the EGFR tyrosine kinase (EGFR-TK) activity with small molecular weight enzyme inhibitors (Boschelli 1999; Woodburn 1999; Ciardiello and Tortora 2001; Grünwald and Hidalgo 2003).

Because the cytoplasmic tyrosine kinase domains of the receptor protein tyrosine kinase 'super family' are highly homologous, particularly within sub-families like the ErbB/HER family, an important issue at the beginning of the drug discovery program which led to Iressa, was whether or not it would be possible to find inhibitors selective for EGFR. An encouraging precedent for a synthetic chemistry-based approach to EGFR-TK inhibition was provided by the work of Yaish et al. (1988), who described small molecule inhibitors of EGFR-TK activity which did not inhibit the TK activity of the insulin receptor. Since RTKs are expressed in normal tissues as well as in tumours (Yano et al. 2003), selectivity for EGFR was deemed an important attribute for a drug candidate molecule in order to reduce as far as possible the likely undesirable sequelae of generic inhibition of receptor tyrosine kinase activity. The potential issue of toxicity associated with EGFR blockade in normal tissues was recognised; however, it was felt that the high level of activity of EGFR signalling in tumours implied by overexpression of the EGFR, compared with normal tissues, could provide an opportunity to define an acceptable therapeutic ratio between efficacy and toxicity. By analogy with previous experience of oestrogen receptor-targeted treatment of breast cancer with tamoxifen (Nolvadex) and fulvestrant (Faslodex), the aim was to develop a well-tolerated cytostatic agent suitable for long-term use in cancer patients. A drug discovery program was initiated in 1990 at ICI Pharmaceuticals (the predecessor company of Zeneca Pharmaceuticals, in turn a predecessor of AstraZeneca Pharmaceuticals), using a biochemical screen to test compounds representative of the chemical diversity in the company compound inventory, in a substrate tyrosine phosphorylation assay, with EGFR-TK prepared from a human tumour cell line (A431) that highly expresses EGFR. Lead identification was enhanced by the application of structure-based searching (Ward et al. 1994). The discovery of potent selective EGFR-TK inhibitors of the anilinoquinazoline class (Barker and Davies 1992; Fry et al. 1994; Wakeling et al. 1996) was the first step towards selecting a candidate drug molecule, ZD1839, with which to test the efficacy-versus-toxicity question (Barker et al. 2001). This chapter describes the properties of Iressa, (gefitinib, ZD1839), an orally active EGFR-TK inhibitor, and clinical experience to date in cancer therapy with Iressa.

2 Pharmacology

2.1 Enzyme Inhibition

Chemical compounds were tested as potential inhibitors of EGFR-TK activity in a substrate phosphorylation assay with a synthetic peptide substrate and a plasma membrane preparation derived from human A431 cells, which overexpress the EGFR. This assay first identified the anilinoquinazoline class of EGFR-TK inhibitors (Ward et al. 1994; Wakeling et al. 1996), and subsequently the candidate drug EGFR-TK inhibitor, ZD1839 (Gibson et al. 1997; Barker et al. 2001; Wakeling et al. 2002), designated Iressa. Iressa potency and kinase selectivity was demonstrated by comparing its activity against EGFR-TK with that against several other tyrosine and serine-threonine kinases (Wakeling et al. 2002). Enzyme kinetic methods described by Ward et al. (1994) showed that Iressa is competitive with ATP (K_i=2.1±0.2 nM) and non-competitive with substrate (K_i=15.0±1.0 nM). Thus, Iressa inhibits EGFR-TK activity by competing directly with ATP at the enzyme active site. EGF binding to EGFR stabilises a kinase active dimeric form of EGFR and stimulates intermolecular autophosphorylation of receptor homo- or hetero-(erbB)-dimers. Iressa inhibits EGF-stimulated EGFR autophosphorylation in several human tumour cell lines cells (Wakeling et al. 2002). Iressa blocked EGF-stimulated EGFR autophosphorylation in a dose-dependent and complete manner; complete inhibition was achieved at 0.16 μM in Du145 (prostate) and A549 (lung) cells, and at 0.8 μM Iressa in KB (oral squamous) and HT29 (colon) cells. Drug wash-out studies showed that this inhibition was sustained for at least 24 h following a 2-h drug treatment.

Investigation of TK inhibitory selectivity in cell lines expressing EGFR or ErbB2 showed that Iressa, at concentrations up to 5 μM, does not directly inhibit ErbB2 tyrosine phosphorylation (Christensen et al. 2001; Moulder et al. 2001; Normanno et al. 2002).

2.2
Inhibition of Tumour Cell Growth In Vitro

An important aspect of our drug discovery strategy required a test which would distinguish between specific EGFR-TKI-mediated effects on cell growth and non-target-specific cell growth inhibition or cytotoxicity. For this purpose we selected the human KB cell line derived from a vulval squamous tumour (Wakeling et al. 1997). KB cells grow well in basal conditions, that is in growth medium supplemented with 5% charcoal-treated calf serum (to deplete serum growth factors), and redouble their growth rate upon addition of EGF to the growth medium. Iressa inhibited EGF-stimulated growth much more potently than basal growth (IC_{50} 0.054 μM compared with 8.8 μM) demonstrating that Iressa specifically inhibits EGF-stimulated tumour cell growth (Wakeling et al. 2002).

Selectivity of cell growth inhibition by Iressa was also exemplified in studies with normal tissue-derived human cells (HUVEC, human umbilical vein endothelial cells) which are stimulated to grow by several different growth factors. Iressa inhibited EGF-stimulated HUVEC cell growth with a potency similar to that recorded for EGF-stimulated KB cells (<0.1 μM) whereas at least tenfold greater concentrations were needed to significantly affect FGF- or VEGF-stimulated HUVEC growth (Wakeling et al. 2002).

Numerous investigators have shown that Iressa inhibits the proliferation of many different tumour cell lines; this growth inhibition is accompanied by inhibition of EGFR phosphorylation and of downstream signalling through the ERK MAP kinase(s) and PKB/Akt pathways, but tumour cell sensitivity to Iressa was not determined by the level of EGFR expression (Ciardiello et al. 2000; Albanell et al. 2001; Anderson et al. 2001; Moasser et al. 2001; Barnes et al. 2003; Vicentini et al. 2003). Although Iressa does not directly inhibit ErbB2 phosphorylation, it effectively inhibits the growth of ErbB2-overexpressing tumour cells, and inhibitory efficacy did not depend on the relative levels of expression of ErbB2 and EGFR (Anderson et al. 2001; Moasser et al. 2001; Moulder et al. 2001). Inhibition of ErbB2 signalling by Iressa may be mediated by induction of inactive ligand-heteromeric receptor complexes containing ErbB2 and ErbB3 (Lichtner et al. 2001; Anido et al. 2003). Thus, Iressa may inhibit heregulin-mediated tumour cell growth as well as that mediated by EGFR ligands. As well as inhibiting tumour cell proliferation, Iressa treatment increases apoptosis (Ciardiello et al. 2000; Gilmore et al. 2002; Normanno et al. 2002), reduces motility and invasiveness (Fujimura et al. 2002; Barnes et al. 2003) and decreases angiogenesis in some tumour cells (Ciardiello et al. 2001; Hirata et al. 2002). Iressa is a particularly effective inhibitor of the growth of anti-oestrogen-resistant breast cancer cells (McLelland et al. 2001; Knowlden et al. 2003), of taxane-resistant, hormone-independent breast cancer cells (Ciardiello et al. 2002) and enhances the anti-tumour activity of cytotoxic drugs (Ciardiello et al.

2001, 2002; Magne et al. 2002) and of radiation treatment (Bianco el 2002; Huang et al. 2002; Williams et al. 2002) in vitro.

2.3
In Vivo Anti-tumour Activity

Testing of drug candidate TK inhibitors for in vivo anti-tumour activity was carried out with KB cell-derived human squamous tumour xenografts grown in nude mice. Structural chemistry necessary for in vivo anti-tumour activity, and the importance of sustaining concentrations of drug in the blood sufficient to inhibit EGFR-TK activity throughout each 24-h period following once-daily, oral dosing, were defined using this model. Iressa was chosen as a drug development candidate because it achieves high and sustained blood levels, in vivo, over a 24-h period (Barker et al. 2001). The potential spectrum of anti-tumour activity for Iressa in patients was assessed in xenografts of major solid human tumours representing a wide range of tissues of origin (Wakeling et al. 2002). The anti-tumour efficacy of Iressa varied widely between tumours. Dose-dependent growth inhibition was noted for A431 (human vulval squamous), A549 (lung), Du145 (prostate), HCT15, HT29 and LoVo (colon), and KB (oral squamous) tumours (dosing regimen 3–200 mg/kg, po, once daily). Maximum anti-tumour efficacy ranged from tumour regression of A431, through tumour stasis in A549 and Du145 tumours, to no effect on P246, (broncho-epithelial), MKN45, (gastric) and AR42 J, (pancreatic) tumours. No correlation was apparent between xenograft response to Iressa and expression levels of EGFR in the cognate tumour cell lines.

In long-term treatment studies, Iressa provided complete control of tumour growth; when drug treatment was withdrawn after 4 months, most but not all tumours resumed growth, demonstrating that Iressa has a cytostatic effect. When drug treatment was delayed until tumours were well-established, Iressa caused complete regression of all A431 tumours. Drug withdrawal again allowed tumour regrowth. No evidence for the development of drug resistance emerged during these studies with A431 tumours, since no tumour regrew during Iressa treatment (Wakeling et al. 2002). To assess the pharmacodynamic action of Iressa treatment, A431 tumours were excised 6 h after the last of four daily doses of 0, 12.5, 50 and 200 mg/kg Iressa, or at 2, 4, 6, 24, 30 and 36 h after a single 50 mg/kg dose. Total RNA was extracted from the tumours to quantify c-fos mRNA by RT-PCR. C-fos expression was inhibited in a dose-dependent manner; at the anti-tumour ED_{50} dose (50 mg/kg), c-fos mRNA was reduced by 94% and was completely blocked (>99%) at the 200-mg/kg dose. In mice treated with a single 50-mg/kg po dose of Iressa, c-fos expression reached a nadir (5% versus control) at 6 h and did not fully recover until 36 h later. These studies were consistent with a cytostatic effect on tumour cell growth, and suggested that continuous drug treatment is required to maintain control of tumour growth.

Xenograft studies have demonstrated Iressa's potential clinical efficacy alone (Anderson et al. 2001; Moasser et al. 2001; Fujimara et al. 2002; Sewell et al. 2002; Matsuo et al. 2003), in combination with single agent chemotherapy (Ciardiello et al. 2000; Sirotnak et al. 2000), radiotherapy (Bianco el 2002; Huang et al. 2002; Williams et al. 2002) or hormone therapy (Sirotnak et al. 2002; Schiff et al. 2004), and in combination with other targeted treatments (Moulder et al. 2001;Tortora et al. 2003). Animal model studies have also demonstrated that Iressa may have utility in early disease, for example, in the adjuvant or chemopreventative treatment of breast cancer. Iressa inhibited the proliferation of xenografts of normal breast and of ductal carcinoma in situ (Chan et al. 2001, 2002), and suppressed the development of mammary tumours in mouse mammary tumour virus (MMTV)-c-erbB2 transgenic mice (Lu et al. 2003). Since no correlation has been established between response and expression of EGFR in any of these studies, it is clear that receptor expression does not indicate the degree to which any individual tumour is *dependent* for growth on the EGFR signalling pathway. Biomarkers that might predict drug response or resistance have yet to be defined. Some studies have implicated persistent activation of the AKT/PKB pathway in resistance to EGFR-TK inhibition. For example, loss of PTEN (Bianco et al. 2003), high AKT activity (Janmaat et al. 2003) and increased insulin-like growth factor (IGF)-1R signalling (Chakravarti et al. 2002) all confer decreased sensitivity to anti-EGFR treatments. Comparison of gene expression profiles in Iressa-sensitive and -resistant tumour cell lines or xenografts could provide markers of activity for evaluation in biopsies from drug treated patients (Zembutsu et al. 2003).

3 Clinical Studies

3.1 Phase I Trials

Early investigations of the pharmacokinetics and oral bioavailability of Iressa were carried out in healthy male volunteers (Swaisland et al. 2001). These studies demonstrated that peak plasma drug concentration occurred 3–7 h after administration, the concentration–time curve was dose-proportional from 10- to 100-mg doses, and the terminal elimination half-life was 28 h. These studies indicated the potential for a convenient once-daily oral administration schedule. In preliminary studies to investigate the efficacy and tolerability of Iressa, patients with a variety of solid tumours were treated once daily with oral doses up to 1,000 mg of Iressa (Baselga et al. 2002;

Herbst et al. 2002; Ranson et al. 2002; LoRusso et al. 2003; Nakagawa et al. 2003). Iressa was generally well-tolerated; the most common side effects were mild to moderate diarrhoea and rash (grade 1/2), which was reversible. The incidence and severity of side effects increased with increasing dose, but there were none of the severe adverse events involving the haemopoietic, digestive and nervous systems commonly associated with cytotoxic chemotherapy. The maximum tolerated dose (MTD) was greater than or equal to 700 mg/day. Anti-tumour activity was observed in a number of tumour types, notably non-small-cell lung cancer (NSCLC; 10/100 patients with partial response), at doses exceeding or equal to 150 mg/day. Consistent with these clinical observations, biomarker studies in skin samples taken from Iressa-treated patients showed that Iressa inhibited EGFR action to a similar extent at all doses meeting or exceeding 150 mg/day (Albanell et al. 2002). Iressa inhibited EGFR and MAPK phosphorylation, reduced keratinocyte proliferation index and increased apoptosis and expression of the CDK inhibitor $p27^{KIP1}$ and of STAT3. Dose selection for further study was intended to identify a dose for optimum anti-tumour activity, combining maximum efficacy with minimum adverse events, and avoiding the classical MTD approach generally applied to the study of novel cancer chemotherapeutics. Thus, two doses below the MTD, 250 mg/day and 500 mg/day, were chosen for evaluation in phase II trials. Responses with minimum toxicity had been seen at the 250-mg/day dose, and the 500-mg/day dose was the highest well-tolerated dose during prolonged treatment.

3.2 Phase II Trials

Following-up the encouraging responses seen in NSCLC patients in the phase I studies, two phase II clinical trials of Iressa monotherapy were conducted in patients with locally advanced or metastatic NSCLC who had previously been treated with platinum-based chemotherapy (Fukuoka et al. 2003; Kris et al. 2003). Trials IDEAL 1 and 2 (Iressa Dose Evaluation in Advanced Lung Cancer) evaluated two different doses, 250 and 500 mg/day, which were given daily until disease progression or withdrawal due to intolerable toxicity. Patients in IDEAL 1 were recruited from Europe, Japan, Australia and South Africa and had received one or two prior chemotherapy regimens, at least one of which contained platinum. Patients in IDEAL 2 were recruited from the USA and had received at least two prior regimens including platinum and docetaxel given either concurrently or separately. Both doses of Iressa produced similar anti-tumour effects but side effects were fewer and less severe at the lower dose. For the 250-mg/day dose, response rates in IDEAL 1 and 2 were 18.4% and 11.8%, respectively. Since many NSCLC patients have frequent and severe symptoms, the impact of treatment with Iressa on symptoms was investigated. Symptom improvement was recorded in approximately 40% of patients (40.3% in IDEAL 1 and 43.1% in IDEAL 2), and such improvements occurred very rapidly with a median time to improvement of 8 and 10 days after beginning Iressa treatment (Douillard et al. 2002). Symptom improvement correlated with objective tumour response and was associated with increased overall survival; for example, in IDEAL 2, median overall survival in patients with symptom improvement was 13.6 months, compared with 3.7 months for patients without symptom improvement. The most frequent drug-related adverse events in the IDEAL trials were skin rash (47% and 43% in IDEAL 1 and 2, respectively) and diarrhoea (40% and 48%), which were generally mild in nature (grade 1/2).

Determination of tumour EGFR status was not an entry criterion for the IDEAL trials, but tumour biopsies taken during these trials have been analysed for EGFR expression. An immunohistochemical (IHC) assay estimated the intensity of EGFR membrane staining intensity using a four-point scale (0, 1+, 2+, 3+ for no, weak, moderate and strong staining, respectively) (Janas et al. 2003). The correlation of membrane staining intensity with the probability of objective tumour response or symptom improvement was investigated. The mean proportion of cells staining 2+ or 3+ in tumours from patients who responded was 31.3% compared with 37.5% in those who did not respond. In both trials there were patients who responded but in whom tumour EGFR expression was very low (Bailey et al. 2003). Therefore, this analysis failed to reveal a consistent association between EGFR expression and response to Iressa in NSCLC patients.

Phase II clinical trials in several other tumours are underway. A study of Iressa monotherapy (500 mg/day) in patients with recurrent or metastatic squamous cell carcinoma of the head and neck (SCCHN), showed promising anti-tumour activity. The response rate was 10.6%, the disease control rate was 53% and median overall survival was 8.1 months. Toxicity was modest; skin toxicities (Grade 1/2) were observed in 48% of patients, and diarrhoea (grade 3 in three patients) was observed in 50% of patients (Cohen et al. 2003). In colon cancer, a phase II study (n=32) investigating combination therapy of Iressa (500 mg/day) with FOLFOX-4, a triple-combination standard treatment regimen for patients with advanced colorectal cancer, showed response rates of 75% for previously untreated patients and 23% for patients who had relapsed after chemotherapy. This compares well with historical response rates of 30%–55% and 9%, from the phase III trial programme of FOLFOX in first and second-line therapy, respectively. This combination therapy was generally well tolerated with the most common grade 3/4 adverse event being diarrhoea (Cho et al. 2003). In breast cancer, two phase II studies investigated Iressa monotherapy (500 mg/day) in patients with advanced disease. In one study, 10 of 31 patients (32%) had stable disease for at least 3 months (Baselga et al. 2003). In a second study, one of nine patients with acquired tamoxifen-resistant, oestrogen-receptor positive breast had a partial response and five had stable disease. One of 18 patients with oestrogen-receptor-negative breast cancer had a partial response and one patient had stable disease (Robertson et al. 2003).

3.3 Phase III Trials

The standard first treatment for patients with advanced NSCLC is combination chemotherapy with a platinum-based, two-drug regimen (e.g. cisplatin or carboplatin combined with gemcitabine, docetaxel or paclitaxel). Based on preclinical studies which showed that Iressa enhanced the efficacy of individual cytotoxic agents against a range of human tumour cell lines and xenografts—independent of the level of EGFR expression (Ciardiello et al. 2000; Sirotnak et al. 2000)—two phase III studies (Iressa NSCLC Trials Assessing Combination Treatment, INTACT 1 and 2) investigated Iressa combination with chemotherapy in more than 2,000 previously untreated NSCLC patients. Patients in INTACT 1 received cisplatin and gemcitabine, while patients in INTACT 2 received carboplatin and paclitaxel, and in both trials the chemotherapy was combined with Iressa 250 mg/day, Iressa 500 mg/day, or placebo. In both studies, addition of Iressa to chemotherapy failed to improve response rate, disease-free survival, or overall survival compared with chemotherapy given alone (Giaccone et al. 2004; Herbst et al. 2004). However, these placebo-controlled studies confirmed the favourable safety profile of Iressa reported in the IDEAL trials. Except for addition of dose-dependent diarrhoea and skin rash, which was less frequent in the 250-mg/day group, the toxicity profile was similar to that in patients receiving chemotherapy alone. The failure to translate the added benefit of combining Iressa and chemotherapy, anticipated from animal model studies (Ciardiello et al. 2000; Sirotnak et al. 2000), into the clinical setting in the INTACT trials is disappointing but should not be interpreted to mean that such combinations will be inappropriate in all settings (other stages of disease/other tumours/other agents). No animal studies were performed examining concurrent treatment with two cytotoxic agents and Iressa.

4 Future Prospects

Clinical trials with Iressa and other EGFR-targeted drugs (e.g. erlotinib/Tarceva and cetuximab/Erbitux) have clearly demonstrated that this new approach to cancer therapy is of great benefit for some patients (Grunwald and Hidalgo 2003). However, it is equally clear that some patients in an unselected population with, for example, advanced NSCLC, do not derive significant benefits from treatment with this class of drugs. Unlike the case of breast cancer patients, where trastuzumab (Herceptin) treatment is determined by the presence or absence of overexpression of ErbB2, the very small number of clinical studies on linkage between tumour EGFR expression and response to EGFR-targeted therapies have so far failed to establish any correlation. Currently, the best indicator of response to gefitinib is symptom improvement, which typically occurs early during the course of treatment and is associated with tumour response, time to progression and overall survival (Cella et al. 2003). A huge challenge for the future is to identify either pathological or mechanism-based biomarkers which accurately predict the likelihood of therapeutic benefit from treatment with EGFR inhibitors. Formidable intellectual and technical barriers must be surmounted to achieve this objective. For example, to what extent would a complete knowledge of the expression or activity levels of all signal transducers, downstream of or linked to EGFR, help in patient stratification, and how might the best quantitative methods for putative biomarker measurement be defined and applied in the routine pathology laboratory setting? Measurement of EGFR expression by IHC presents major problems for routine application, since there is no consensus on methods for tumour sampling, storage, preparation and analysis. Many translational science laboratories are focussing their attention on the use of IHC methods to measure activated receptors [e.g. phosphorylated (p) EGFR and other ErbBs] and key downstream mediators like pMAPK and pAKT, as well as putative endpoints of drug action, like changes in cell cycle status (eg $p27^{KIP1}$), proliferative rate (eg Ki67/Mib1) and apoptosis (eg Tunel) in Iressa-treated patients (Albanell et al. 2001, 2002; Cappuzzo et al. 2003; Daneshmand et al. 2003; Mukohara et al. 2003; Rojo et al. 2003). Because of the inaccessibility to diagnostic biopsy sampling of many tumours, and the cost and complexity of biomarker analyses, the age of targeted drug treatment tailored to the (individual) tumour remains elusive. In immediate practical terms, the fact that Iressa is generally well tolerated means that there is no reason to exclude patients from treatment. Furthermore, as symptom improvement and tumour response generally occur soon after the start of treatment (IDEAL trials), the patients who do benefit from Iressa treatment will be rapidly identified.

In the longer term, the application of oncogenomic and/or proteomic analysis to tumour diagnostic samples may open a realistic prospect for individually targeted treatment. Important pilot studies in Iressa-treated xenograft models (Zembutsu et al. 2003) and patient samples have begun (Natale et al. 2003), and the increasing availability and use of frozen tumour tissue microarrays (Fejzo and Slamon 2001) hold great promise for the future.

References

Albanell J, Codony-Servat J, Rojo F, Del Campo JM, Sauleda S, Anido J, Raspall G, Giralt J, Rosello J, Nicholson RI, Mendelsohn J, Baselga J (2001) Activated extracellular signal-regulated kinases: association with epidermal growth factor receptor/transforming growth factor α expression in head and neck squamous carcinoma and inhibition by anti-epidermal growth factor receptor treatments. Cancer Res 61:6500–6510

Albanell J, Rojo F, Averbuch S, Feyereislova A, Mascaro JM, Herbst R, LoRusso P, Rischin D, Sauleda S, Gee J, Nicholson RI, Baselga J (2002) Pharmacodynamic studies of the epidermal growth factor receptor inhibitor ZD1839 in skin from cancer patients: histopathologic and molecular consequences of receptor inhibition. J Clin Oncol 20:110 - 124

Anderson NG, Ahmad T, Chan K, Dobson R, Bundred NJ (2001) ZD1839 (Iressa), a novel epidermal growth factor receptor (EGFR) tyrosine kinase inhibitor, potently inhibits the growth of EGFR-positive cancer cell lines with or without erbB2 overexpression. Int J Cancer 94:774–782

Anido J, Matar P, Albanell J, Guzman M, Rojo F, Arribas J, Averbuch S, Baselga J (2003) ZD1839, a specific epidermal growth factor receptor (EGFR) tyrosine kinase inhibitor, induces the formation of inactive EGFR/HER2 and EGFR/HER3 heterodimers and prevents heregulin signalling in HER2-overexpressing breast cancer cells. Clin Cancer Res 9:1274–1283

Bailey LR, Kris M, Wolf M, et al (2003) Tumor EGFR membrane staining is not clinically relevant for predicting response in patients receiving gefitinib ('Iressa', ZD1839) monotherapy for pretreated advanced non-small-cell lung cancer: IDEAL 1 and 2. Proc Am Assoc Cancer Res 44:abstr LB-170

Barker AJ, Davies DH (1992) Therapeutic preparations containing quinazoline derivatives. European Patent EP-520722-A

Barker AJ, Gibson KH, Grundy W, Godfrey AA, Barlow JJ, Healy MP, Woodburn JR, Ashton SE, Curry BJ, Scarlett L, Henthorn L, Richards L (2001) Studies leading to the identification of ZD1839 (Iressa): an orally active, selective epidermal growth factor receptor tyrosine kinase inhibitor targeted to the treatment of cancer. Bioorg Med Chem Lett 11:1911–1914

Barnes CJ, Bagheri-Yarmand R, Mandal M, Yang ZB, Clayman GL, Hong WK, Kumar R (2003) Suppression of epidermal growth factor receptor, mitogen-activated protein kinase, and Pak1 pathways and invasiveness of human cutaneous squamous cancer cells by the tyrosine kinase inhibitor ZD1839 (Iressa). Mol Cancer Ther 2:345–351

Baselga J, Rischin D, Ranson M, Calvert H, Raymond E, Kieback DG, Kaye SB, Gianni L, Harris A, Bjork T, Averbuch S, Feyereislova A, Swaisland H, Rojo F, Albanell J (2002) Phase I safety, pharmacokinetic, and pharmacodynamic trial of ZD1839, a selective oral epidermal growth factor receptor tyrosine kinase inhibitor, in patients with five selected solid tumor types. J Clin Oncol 20:4292–4302

Baselga J, Albanell J, Ruiz A, Lluch A, Gascon P, Guillen V, Gonzalez S, Sauleda S, Koehler M, Rojo F (2003) Phase II and tumor pharmacodynamic study of gefitinib ('Iressa', ZD1839) in patients with advanced breast cancer. (Oral presentation at ASCO)

Bianco C, Tortora G, Bianco R, Caputo R, Veneziani BM, Damiano V, Troiani T, Fontanini G, Raben D, Pepe S, Bianco AR, Ciardiello F (2002) Enhancement of antitumor activity of ionizing radiation by combined treatment with the selective epidermal growth factor receptor-tyrosine kinase inhibitor ZD1839 (Iressa). Clin Cancer Res 8:3250–3258

Bianco R, Shin I, Ritter CA, Yakes FM, Basso A, Rosen N, Tsurutani J, Dennis PA, Mills GB, Arteaga CL (2003) Loss of PTEN/MMAC1/TEP in EGF receptor-expressing tumor cells counteracts the antitumor action of EGFR tyrosine kinase inhibitors. Oncogene 22:2812–2822

Blume-Jensen P, Hunter T (2001) Oncogenic kinase signalling. Nature 411:355–365

Boschelli DH (1999) Small molecule inhibitors of receptor tyrosine kinases. Drugs of the Future 24:515–537

Cappuzzo F, Gregorc V, Rossi E, Cancellieri A, Magrini E, Paties CT, Ceresoli G, Lombardo L, Bartolini S, Calandri C, De Rosa M, Villa E, Crino L (2003) Gefitinib in pretreated non-small-cell lung cancer (NSCLC): Analysis of efficacy and correlation with HER2 and epidermal growth factor receptor expression in locally advanced or metastatic NSCLC. J Clin Oncol 21:2658–2663

Cella D, Natale RB, Lynch TJ, Lee C, Carbone D, Douillard J-Y, Kay A, Wolf M, Heyes A, Ward J (2003) Disease-related symptoms in advanced non-small-cell lung cancer as measured by the Lung Cancer Subscale of the FACT-L questionnaire: clinically meaningful improvement with gefitinib ('Iressa', ZD1839). Poster 2531 presented at the ASCO, Chicago, IL, USA, May 31-June 3, 2003

Chakravarti A, Loeffler JS, Dyson NJ (2002) Insulin-like growth factor receptor I mediates resistance to anti-epidermal growth factor receptor therapy in primary human glioblastoma cells through continued activation of phosphoinositide 3-kinase signalling. Cancer Res 62;200–207

Chan KC, Knox WF, Gandhi A, Slamon DJ, Potten CS, Bundred NJ (2001) Blockade of growth factor receptors in ductal carcinoma in situ inhibits epithelial proliferation. Br J Surg 88:412–418

Chan KC, Knox WF, Gee JM, Morris J, Nicholson RI, Potten CS, Bundred NJ (2002) Effect of epidermal growth factor receptor tyrosine kinase inhibition on epithelial proliferation in normal and premalignant breast. Cancer Res 62:122–128

Cho CD, Fisher GA, Halsey J, Jambalos CN, Advani RH, Wakelee H, Lum BL, Sikic BI (2003) A phase II study of gefitinib in combination with FOLFOX-4 (IFOX) in patients with unresectable or metastatic colorectal cancer. Program Proc Am Soc Clin Oncol 22:7

Christensen JG, Schreck RE, Chan E, Wang X, Yang C, Liu L, Cui J, Sun L, Wei J, Cherrington JM, Mendel DB (2001) High levels of HER-2 expression alter the ability of epidermal growth factor receptor (EGFR) family tyrosine kinase inhibitors to inhibit EGFR phosphorylation in vivo. Clin Cancer Res 7:4230–4238

Ciardiello F, Tortora G (2001) A novel approach in the treatment of cancer: targeting the epidermal growth factor receptor. Clin Cancer Res 7:2958–2970

Ciardiello F, Caputo R, Bianco R, Damiano V, Pomatico G, Placido S De, Bianco AR, Tortora G (2000) Antitumor effect and potentiation of cytotoxic drugs activity in human cancer cells by ZD-1839 (Iressa), an epidermal growth factor receptor-selective tyrosine kinase inhibitor. Clin Cancer Res 6:2053–2063

Ciardiello F, Caputo R, Bianco R, Damiano V, Fentanini G, Cuccato S, De Placido S, Bianco AR, Tortora G (2001) Inhibition of growth factor production and angiogenesis in human cancer cells by ZD1839 (Iressa), a selective epidermal growth factor receptor tyrosine kinase inhibitor. Clin Cancer Res 7:1459–1465

Ciardiello F, Caputo R, Borriello G, Del Bufalo D, Biroccio A, Zupi G, Bianco AR, Tortora G (2002) ZD1839 (Iressa), an EGFR-selective tyrosine kinase inhibitor, enhances taxane activity in bcl-2 overexpressing, multidrug-resistant MCF-7 ADR human breast cancer cells. Int J Cancer 98:463–469

Cobleigh MA, Vogel CL, Tripathy D, et al (1999) Multinational study of the efficacy and safety of humanized anti-HER2 monoclonal antibody in women who have HER2-overexpressing metastatic breast cancer that has progressed after chemotherapy for metastatic disease. J Clin Oncol 17:2639–2648

Cohen EW, Rosen F, Stadler WM, Recant W, Stenson K, Huo DZ, Vokes EE (2003) Phase II trial of ZD1839 in recurrent or metastatic squamous cell carcinoma of the head and neck. J Clin Oncol 21:1980–1987

Daneshmand M, Parolin D AE, Hirte HW, Major P, Goss G, Stewart D, Batist G, Miller WH Jr, Matthews S, Seymour L, Lorimer IAJ (2003) A pharmacodynamic study of the epidermal growth factor receptor tyrosine kinase inhibitor ZD1839 in metastatic colorectal cancer patients. Clin Cancer Res 9:2457–2464

Douillard JY, Giaccone G, Horai T, Noda K, Vansteenkiste JF, Takata I, Gatzemeier U, Fukuoka M, Macleod A, Feyereislova A, Averbuch S, Nogi Y, Heyes A, Baselga J (2002) Improvement in disease-related symptoms and quality of life in patients with advanced non-small-cell lung cancer (NSCLC) treated with ZD1839 ('Iressa') (IDEAL 1). Proc Am Soc Clin Oncol 21:299

Downward J, Yarden Y, Mayes E, Scrace G, Totty N, Stockwell P, Ullrich A, Schlessinger J, Waterfield MD (1984) Close similarity of epidermal growth factor and v-*erb-B* oncogene protein sequences. Nature 307:521–527

Fejzo MS, Slamon DJ (2001) Frozen tumor tissue microarray technology for analysis of tumor RNA, DNA, and proteins. Am J Pathol 159:1645–1650

Fry DW, Kraker AJ, McMichael A, Ambroso LA, Nelson JM, Leopold WR, Connors RW, Bridges AJ (1994) A specific inhibitor of the epidermal growth factor receptor tyrosine kinase. Science 265:1093–1095

Fujimura M, Hidaka T, Saito S (2002) Selective inhibition of the epidermal growth factor receptor by ZD1839 decreases the growth and invasion of ovarian clear cell adenocarcinoma cells. Clin Cancer Res 8:2448–2454

Fukuoka M, Yano S, Giaccone G, Tamura T, Nakagawa K, Douillard JY, Nishiwaki Y, Vansteenkiste J, Kudoh S, Rischin D, Eek R, Horai T, Noda K, Takata I, Smit E, Averbuch S, Macleod A, Feyereislova A, Dong RP, Baselga J (2003) Multi-institutional randomized phase II trial of gefitinib for previously treated patients with advanced non-small-cell lung cancer. J Clin Oncol 21:2237–2246

Giaccone G, Herbst RS, Manegold C, Scagliotti G, Rosell R, Miller V, Natale RB, Schiller JH, Von Pawel J, Pluzanska A, Gatzemeier U, Grous J, Ochs JS, Averbuch SD, Wolf MK, Rennie P, Fandi A, Johnson DH (2004) Gefitinib in combination with gemcitabine and cisplatin in advanced non-small-cell lung cancer: a phase III trial–INTACT 1. J Clin Oncol 22:777–784

Gibson KH, Grundy W, Godfrey AA, Woodburn JR, Ashton SE, Curry BJ, Scarlett L, Barker AJ, Brown DS (1997) Epidermal growth factor receptor tyrosine kinase—structure-activity relationships and antitumor activity of novel quinazolines. Bioorg Med Chem Lett 7:2723–2728

Gilmore AP, Valentijn AJ, Wang PB, Ranger AM, Bundred N, O'Hare MJ, Wakeling A, Korsmeyer SJ, Streuli CH (2002) Activation of BAD by therapeutic inhibition of epidermal growth factor receptor and transactivation by insulin-like growth factor receptor. J Biol Chem 277:27643–27650

Grünwald V, Hidalgo M (2003) Developing inhibitors of the epidermal growth factor receptor for cancer treatment. J Natl Cancer Inst 95:851–867

Gullick WJ (1991) Prevalence of aberrant expression of the epidermal growth factor receptor in human cancers. Br Med Bull 47:87–98

Gusterson B, Cowley G, Smith JA, Ozanne B (1984) Cellular localisation of human epidermal growth factor receptor. Cell Biol Int Rep 8:649–658

Herbst RS, Maddox A-M, Rothenberg ML, Small EJ, Rubin EH, Baselga J, Rojo F, Hong WK, Swaisland H, Averbuch A, Ochs J, LoRusso PM (2002) Selective oral epidermal growth factor receptor tyrosine kinase inhibitor ZD1839 is generally well-tolerated and has activity in non-small-cell lung cancer and other solid tumors: results of a phase I trial. J Clin Oncol 20:3815–3825

Herbst RS, Giaccone G, Schiller JH, Natale RB, Miller V, Manegold C, Scagliotti G, Rosell R, Oliff I, Reeves JA, Wolf MK, Krebs AD, Averbuch SD, Ochs JS, Grous J, Fandi A, Johnson DH (2004) Gefitinib in combination with paclitaxel and carboplatin in advanced non-small-cell lung cancer: a phase III trial–INTACT 2. J Clin Oncol 22:785–794

Hirata A, Ogawa S, Kometani T, Kuwano T, Naito S, Kuwano M, Ono M (2002) ZD1839 (Iressa) induces antiangiogenic effects through inhibition of epidermal growth factor receptor tyrosine kinase. Cancer Res 62:2554–2560

Huang SM, Li J, Armstrong EA, Harari PM (2002) Modulation of radiation response and tumor-induced angiogenesis after epidermal growth factor receptor inhibition by ZD1839 (Iressa). Cancer Res 62:4300–4306

Hunter T (1997) Oncoprotein networks. Cell 88:333–346

Janas MS, Franklin WA, Schmidt K, et al (2003) Interobserver reproducibility of visually interpreted EGFR immunohistochemical staining in non-small-cell lung cancer. Proc Am Assoc Cancer Res 44:abstrLB-213

Janmaat ML, Kruyt F AE, Rodriguez JA, Giaccone G (2003) Response to epidermal growth factor receptor inhibitors in non-small cell lung cancer cells: Limited antiproliferative effects and absence of apoptosis associated with persistent activity of extracellular signal-regulated kinase or Akt kinase pathways. Clin Cancer Res 9:2316–2326

Knowlden JM, Hutcheson IR, Jones HE, Madden T, Gee J MW, Harper ME, Barrow D, Wakeling AE, Nicholson RI (2003) Elevated levels of epidermal growth factor receptor/c-erbB2 heterodimers mediate an autocrine growth regulatory pathway in tamoxifen-resistant MCF-7 cells. Endocrinology 144:1032–1044

Kris MG, Natale RB, Herbst RS, Lynch TJ Jr, Prager D, Belani CP, Schiller JH, Kelly K, Spiridonidis H, Sandler A, Cella D, Wolf MK, Averbuch SD, Ochs JJ, Kay AC (2003) Efficacy of gefitinib (ZD1839, Iressa), an inhibitor of the epidermal growth factor receptor tyrosine kinase, in symptomatic patients with non-small cell lung cancer. JAMA 290:2149–2158

Lichtner RB, Menrad A, Sommer A, Klar U, Schneider MR (2001) Inactive-inactive epidermal growth factor receptor/ligand complexes in intact carcinoma cells by quinazoline tyrosine kinase inhibitors. Cancer Res 61;5790–5795

LoRusso PM, herbst RS, Rischin D, Ranson M, Calvert H, Raymond E, Kieback D, Kaye S, Gianni L, Harris A, Bjork T, Maddox A-M, Rothenberg ML, Small EJ, Rubin EH, Feyereislova A, Heyes A, Averbuch SD, Ochs J, Baselga J (2003) Improvements in quality of life and disease-related symptoms in phase I trials of the selective oral epidermal growth factor receptor tyrosine kinase inhibitor ZD1839 in non-small cell lung cancer and other solid tumors. Clin Cancer Res 9:2040–2048

Lu C, Speers C, Ahzung Y, Xu, X, Hill H, Steinbis E, Celestino J, Shen Q, Kim H, Hilsenbeck SG, Mohsin SK, Wakelin AE, Osborne C, Brown PH (2003) The EGFR inhibitor ZD1839 (Gefitinib; "Iressa") suppresses the development of estrogen receptor-negative mammary tumors in transgenic mice. J Natl Cancer Inst (in press)

Magne N, Fischel JL, Dubreuil A, Formento P, Marcie S, Lagrange JL, Milano G (2002) Sequence-dependent effects of ZD1839 ('Iressa') in combination with cytotoxic treatment in human head and neck cancer. Br J Cancer 86:819–827

Matsuo M, Sakurai H, Saiki I (2003) ZD1839, a selective epidermal growth factor receptor tyrosine kinase inhibitor, shows activity using a hepatocellular carcinoma model. Mol Cancer Ther 2:557–561

McClelland RA, Barrow D, Madden TA, Dutkowski CM, Pamment J, Knowlden JM, Gee J MW, Nicholson RI (2001) Enhanced epidermal growth factor receptor signalling in MCF7 breast cancer cells after long-term culture in the presence of the pure antiestrogen ICI 182,780 (Faslodex). Endocrinol 142:2776–2788

Moasser MM, Basso A, Averbuch SD, Rosen N (2001) The tyrosine kinase inhibitor ZD1839 ('Iressa') inhibits HER2-driven signalling and suppresses the growth of HER2-overexpressing tumor cells. Cancer Res 61:7184 - 7188

Moulder SL, Yakes FM, Muthuswamy SK, Bianco R, Simpson JF, Arteaga CL (2001) Epidermal growth factor receptor (HER1) tyrosine kinase inhibitor ZD1839 (Iressa) inhibits HER2/neu (erbB2)-overexpressing breast cancer cells in vitro and in vivo. Cancer Res 61:8887–8895

Mukohara T, Kudoh S, Yamauchi S, Kimura T, Yoshimura N, Kanazawa H, Hirata K, Wanibuchi H, Fukushima S, Inoue K, Yoshikawa J (2003) Expression of epidermal growth factor receptor (EGFR) and downstream-activated peptides in surgically excised non-small-cell lung cancer (NSCLC). Lung Cancer 41:123–130

Nakagawa K, Tamura T, Negoro S, Kudoh S, Yamamoto N, Yamamoto N, Takeda K, Swaisland H, Nakatani I, Hirose M, Dong RP, Fukuoka M (2003) Phase I pharmacokinetic trial of the selective oral epidermal growth factor receptor tyrosine kinase inhibitor gefitinib ('Iressa', ZD 1839) in Japanese patients with solid malignant tumors. Ann Oncol 14:922–930

Natale RB, Shak S, Aronson N, Averbuch S, Fox W, Luthringer D, Clark K, Baker J, Cronin M, Agus DB (2003) Quantitative gene expression in non-small cell lung cancer from paraffin-embedded tissue specimens: Predicting response to gefitinib, an EGFR kinase inhibitor. Program Proc Am Soc Clin Oncol 22:190

Nicholson RI, Gee JMW, Harper ME (2001) EGFR and cancer prognosis. Eur J Cancer 37:S9–S15

Normanno N, Campiglio M, De Luca A, Somenzi G, Maiello M, Ciardiello F, Gianni L, Salomon DS, Menard S (2002) Cooperative inhibitory effect of ZD1839 (Iressa) in combination with trastuzumab (Herceptin) on human breast cancer cell growth. Ann Oncol 13:65–72

Olayioye MA, Neve RM, Lane HA, Hynes NE (2000) The erbB signalling network: receptor heterodimerization in development and cancer. EMBO J 13:3159–3167

Ranson M, Hammond LA, Ferry D, Kris M, Tullo A, Murray PI, Miler V, Averbuch S, Ochs J, Morris C, Feyereislova A, Swaisland H, Rowinsky EK (2002) ZD1839, a selective oral epidermal growth factor receptor-tyrosine kinase inhibitor, is well tolerated and active in patients with solid, malignant tumors: results of a phase I trial. J Clin Oncol 20:2240 - 2250

Robertson J FR, Gutteridge E, Cheung KL, Owers R, Koehler M, Hamilton L, Gee J, Nicholson RI (2003) Gefitinib (ZD1839) is active in acquired tamoxifen (TAM)-resistant oestrogen receptor (ER)-positive and ER-negative breast cancer: Results from a phase II study. Program Proc Am Soc Clin Oncol 22:7

Rojo F, Tabernero J, Van Cutsem E, Ohtsu A, Albanell J, Koizumi W, Peeters M, Averbuch S, Gallagher N, Baselga J (2003) Pharmacodynamic studies of tumor biopsy specimens from patients with advanced gastric carcinoma undergoing treatment with gefitinib (ZD1839). Program Proc Am Soc Clin Oncol 22:191

Sainsbury JRC, Malcolm AJ, Appleton DR, Farndon JR, Harris AL (1985) Presence of epidermal growth factor receptor as an indicator of poor prognosis in patients with breast cancer. J Clin Pathol 38:1225–1228

Salomon DS, Brandt R, Ciardiello F, Normanno N (1995) Epidermal growth factor-related peptides and their receptors in human malignancies. Crit Rev Oncol Hematol 19:183–232

Shou J, massarweh S, Osborne CK, Wakeling AE, Ali S, Schiff R (2004) Tamoxifen resistance: increased estrogen receptor-HER-2/neu crosstalk converts tamoxifen into an estrogen agonist in breast cancer. J Natl Cancer Inst (in press)

Schlessinger Y (1993) How receptor tyrosine kinases activate Ras. Trends Biochem Sci 18:273–275

Sewell JM, Macleod KG, Ritchie A, Smyth JF, Langdon SP (2002) Targeting the EGF receptor in ovarian cancer with the tyrosine kinase inhibitor ZD 1839 ('Iressa'). Br J Cancer 86:456–462

Sirotnak FM, Zakowski MF, Miller VA, Scher HI, Kris MG (2000) Efficacy of cytotoxic agents against human tumour xenografts is markedly enhanced by co-administration of ZD1839 (Iressa), an inhibitor of EGFR tyrosine kinase. Clin Cancer Res 6:4885–4892

Sirotnak FM, She YH, Lee F, Chen J, Scher, HI (2002) Studies with CWR22 xenografts in nude mice suggest that ZD1839 may have a role in the treatment of both androgen-dependent and androgen-independent human prostate cancer. Clin Cancer Res 8:3870–3876

Slamon DJ, Clark GM, Wong SG, Levin WJ, Ullrich A, McGuire WL (1987) Human breast cancer: correlation of relapse and survival with amplification of the HER-2/*neu* oncogene. Science 235:177–182

Swaisland H, Laight A, Stafford L, Jones H, Morris C, Dane A,Yates, R (2001) Pharmacokinetics and tolerability of the orally active selective epidermal growth factor receptor tyrosine kinase inhibitor ZD1839 in healthy volunteers. Clin Pharmacokinet 40:297–306

Tortora G, Caputo R, Damiano V, Caputo R, Troiani T, Veneziani BM, De Placido S, Bianco AR, Zangemeister WittkeU, Ciardiello F (2003) Combined targeted inhibition of bcl-2, bcl-XL, epidermal growth factor receptor, and protein kinase A type I causes potent antitumor, apoptotic, and antiangiogenic activity. Clin Cancer Res 9:866–871

Vicentini C, Festuccia C, Gravina GL, Angelucci A, Marronaro A, Bologna M (2003) Prostate cancer cell proliferation is strongly reduced by the epidermal growth factor receptor tyrosine kinase inhibitor ZD1839 in vitro on human cell lines and primary cultures. J Cancer Res Clin Oncol 129:165–174

Wakeling AE, Barker AJ, Davies DH, Brown DS, Green LR, Cartlidge SA, Woodburn J (1996) Specific inhibition of epidermal growth factor receptor tyrosine kinase by 4-anilinoquinazolines. Breast Cancer Res Treat 38:67–73

Wakeling AE, Barker AJ, Davies DH, Brown DS, Green LR, Cartlidge SA, WoodburnJR (1997) New targets for therapeutic attack. Endocrine-related Cancer 4:1–5

Wakeling AE, Guy S, Woodburn JR, Ashton SE, Curry B, Barker AJ, Gibson K (2002) ZD1839 (Iressa): an orally active inhibitor of epidermal growth factor signalling with potential for cancer therapy. Cancer Res 62:5749–5754

Ward WHJ, Cook PN, Slater AM, Davies DH, Holdgate GA, Green LR (1994) Epidermal growth factor receptor tyrosine kinase. Investigation of catalytic mechanism, structure-based searching and discovery of a potent inhibitor. Biochem Pharmacol 48:659-666

Williams KJ, Telfer BA, Stratford IJ, Wedge SR (2002) ZD1839 ('Iressa'), a specific oral epidermal growth factor receptor-tyrosine kinase inhibitor, potentiates radiotherapy in a human colorectal cancer xenograft model. Br J Cancer 86:1157–1161

Woodburn JR (1999) The epidermal growth factor receptor and its inhibition in cancer therapy. Pharmacol Ther 82:241–250

Yaish P, Gazit A, Gilon C, Levitzki A (1988) Blocking of EGF-dependent cell proliferation by EGF receptor kinase inhibitors. Science 242:933–935

Yano S, Kondo K, Yamaguchi M, Richmond G, Hutchison M, Wakeling AE, Averbuch S, Wadsworth P (2003) Distribution and function of EGFR in human tissue and the effect of EGFR tyrosine kinase inhibition. Anticancer Res 23:3639–3650

Yarden Y, Ullrich A (1988) Growth factor receptor tyrosine kinases. Annu Rev Biochem 57:443–478

Yarden Y, Sliwkowski MX (2001) Untangling the ErbB signalling network. Nat Rev Mol Cell Biol 2:127–137

Zembutsu H, Ohnishi Y, Daigo Y, Katagiri T, Kikuchi T, Kakiuchi S, Nishime C, Hirata K, Nakamura Y (2003) Gene-expression profiles of human tumor xenografts in nude mice treated orally with the EGFR tyrosine kinase inhibitor ZD1839. Int J Oncol 23:29–39

Subject Index

Printing: Saladruck, Berlin
Binding: Stein+Lehmann, Berlin